Ann K. Suszek

15095 Long Lake Hwy.

Alpena, Mich.

Ph. 595-6029

Second Edition

ESSENTIALS OF NURSING

A Medical-Surgical Text for Practical Nurses

CLAIRE BRACKMAN KEANE, R.N., B.S.

Consultant in Nursing, Department of Sociology
and Anthropology, University of Georgia.
Formerly Director, Athens General Hospital School
of Practical Nursing, and Clinical Instructor, Athens
School of Practical Nursing, Athens, Georgia.
Formerly Director of Nursing Education and Instructor
in Medical-Surgical Nursing, Grady Memorial
Hospital School of Nursing, Atlanta, Georgia.

W. B. SAUNDERS COMPANY Philadelphia London Toronto

W. B. Saunders Company: West Washington Square
Philadelphia, Pa.   19105

12 Dyott Street
London, WC1A 1DB

833 Oxford Street
Toronto 18, Ontario

ESSENTIALS OF NURSING

ISBN 0-7216-5311-1

Print No.:   9   8   7   6   5

Love your patient, not for what you can help him to be, but for what he is. With mutual respect and trust you can both become something better.

PREFACE

The changes and additions included in this second edition of *Essentials of Nursing* are based on suggestions and comments from many instructors and students of practical nursing. Their sincere interest and intelligent critiques only serve to point up the fact that the teaching of practical nurses is indeed a challenging role and that practical nurse students and graduates have a very real thirst for knowledge. It would not be possible to include in one text the great wealth of material needed to quench that thirst. Our goal has been, instead, to greatly enlarge the basic information presented in this text and to guide the reader, through references and suggested reading lists, to other sources of information.

The vocabulary list at the beginning of each chapter and the outline at the end of each chapter are included at the request of instructors and students, who are also responsible for the glossary that is included in this revision.

Chapters on first aid and emergency nursing and communicable disease nursing have been written in an effort to meet the needs of today's practical nurse.

The revised text is based on the same principle as the first edition of *Essentials of Nursing*; that is, that one learns best by progressing from the known to the unknown, from the general to the specific, from the concrete to the abstract and from the simple to the complex. The reader is introduced to a broad concept of illness and the ways in which illness affects the individual patient, his family and his community.

Chapters 2, 3 and 4 help the student understand the body's usual response to illness and injury and the ways in which diseases are diagnosed. Chapter 5 gives the student a basic understanding of the surgical patient and the needs and special problems that may be brought about by anesthesia and surgery. Chapter 6 has been enlarged to discuss newer equipment, intensive care units, and other aspects of care of the critically ill in the modern hospital. Chapter 7 is about the care of the aged and chronically ill and the physical, emotional and financial problems characteristic of these patients. Chapter 8 is a completely new chapter on nursing care of the patient with an infectious disease. Chapter 9 deals with nursing care of the cancer patient.

Although curriculum plans for schools of practical nursing may vary widely, most schools continue to use the anatomical systems as a basis for organizing courses in medical-surgical nursing. It is for this reason that we have divided the chapters in the second half of the book according to body systems. The text may be used anywhere in the course of instruction. If it is introduced early in the course, anatomy and physiology, pharmacology, diet therapy, and nursing procedures may all be taught at the time at which they

v

apply to specific conditions of illness. For example, Chapter 13 discusses the respiratory system. The normal structure and functions of the organs of respiration are taught first. Then the student is ready for the general principles of nursing that apply to abnormal conditions of the respiratory system. Nursing procedures such as throat irrigations, steam inhalations and croup tents are demonstrated in the nursing laboratory as they apply to the treatment of specific illness. Diets used as part of the treatment also may be taught at this time. Drugs affecting the respiratory system and used in abnormalities of respiration also may be included in the course of instruction. In this way it is felt that the student can more easily grasp an integrated body of knowledge, rather than memorize isolated facts that she may or may not be able to apply to nursing situations in the clinical area.

Illustrations in the text have been almost doubled in number. The tables in the first edition have elicited favorable comment from readers and so they have been included and revised only as necessary for clarity. Clinical case problems presented at the end of each chapter have also been increased in number and it is hoped that they will stimulate critical thinking and serve as exercises in the application of the problem-solving technique in nursing situations.

The author is indebted to the many persons who have offered their help and suggestions for revision of this text. A special thanks must go to the instructors and students who took time to talk with me about the text or were interested enough to write their comments and criticisms.

CLAIRE B. KEANE

CONTENTS

Chapter 1

INTRODUCTION TO NURSING CONDITIONS OF ILLNESS

VOCABULARY

Anxiety
Depression
Disability
Facade

THE NURSE AND HER PATIENT

When a student practical nurse first goes into the clinical area and begins to put into practice the skills she has mastered in the classroom, she is prepared to do many things for her patients. How well she will be able to carry out the procedures she has been taught will depend on her concept of nursing care. If she has only a vague idea of *why* she must do the things she has learned *how* to do, and if she considers nursing as a mechanical type of service to be doled out to every patient in exactly the same way, her clinical experience will have little meaning and her patients will suffer the consequences.

First of all the nurse should understand that nursing care is simply *doing for the patient those things which he cannot do for himself to assure his physical and mental comfort.* Secondly, the kind of nursing care he will need depends on: (1) his particular condition of illness, (2) his ability to care for himself during the various stages of his illness, and (3) the manner in which he, as an individual, responds to his illness physically, mentally and emotionally.

In some illnesses a patient will not need skilled nursing care at all. He may visit his physician in a clinic or doctor's office, receive instructions in regard to medications and treatments necessary, and then return to his home and follow these instructions intelligently and accurately. In other types of illness the patient may be totally dependent on the nursing staff of the hospital for most of his physical needs, because his illness has rendered him completely helpless. An example of extreme helplessness would be the patient with respiratory failure who must have a tracheostomy performed and requires the help of an artificial respirator so that adequate respiration can be maintained.

These are the two extremes of need created by illness. No assistance from the nurse is needed in one case; total dependency on the nursing staff for maintenance of the most basic bodily functions is present in the other. Between these two extremes we will find varying degrees of dependency in patients. Their needs will require different levels of nursing skills and will demand certain kinds of scientific knowledge. And each patient will have needs that are unique to him. The function of the

1

nurse has been described as one in which she is to "assist the individual, sick or well, in the performance of those activities contributing to health or its recovery (or to peaceful death) that he would perform unaided if he had the necessary strength, will or knowledge. And to do this in such a way as to help him gain independence as rapidly as possible."[6]

In order for the nurse to know the needs of a patient she must first know *him* as a person and she must try to see his problems as he sees them. Virginia Henderson, a noted leader and educator in nursing, puts it this way: "She [the nurse] must, in a sense, get 'inside the skin' of each of her patients. She is temporarily the consciousness of the unconscious, the love of life for the suicidal, the leg of the amputee, the eyes of the newly blind, a means of locomotion for the infant, knowledge and confidence for the young mother, the 'mouthpiece' for those too weak or withdrawn to speak."

The practical nurse, as a recognized member of the nursing team, will be expected to meet many of the needs of the person who is ill. The level of nursing care she may give is determined by the nursing skills she is able to perform and the scientific knowledge she has acquired as a student practical nurse. Because of the limitations of her education in nursing, the practical nurse will not be able to solve all the nursing problems brought about by conditions of illness and she cannot meet all the needs of her patient. She jeopardizes her own peace of mind and the welfare of her patient when she attempts to function above her level of nursing. However, if the practical nurse is to function efficiently and intelligently, she must have a basic knowledge of the various effects of illness on an individual and she must use this knowledge in the care of her patients. It is not enough that she knows what to do in certain situations; she must also know what NOT to do when the patient's condition demands care beyond the level she is prepared to give.

EFFECTS OF ILLNESS ON THE PATIENT

Physical Effects of Illness. Most persons are quite familiar with the physical effects of illness on an individual. They realize that a person who is ill is unable to function as he normally would because of certain physical changes which have taken place in his body. But we cannot limit the definition of illness to physical factors alone. We do not nurse a broken leg, a peptic ulcer, or an inflamed gallbladder. We nurse the whole patient. Total nursing care means attention to every detail that concerns the individual patient.

Mr. Thomas in Room 306 is not a peptic ulcer. He is a human being who has a wife and children, works in the community in which he lives, and has certain likes and dislikes, emotions, and thoughts. He has his own unique way of reacting to his illness and to the persons with whom he comes in contact, whether he is ill or well. The manner in which he reacts to his illness will depend on his age, personality, place in the family and community, past experience with illness, and emotional stability. All the things which go together to make him the person he is must be included in the over-all picture of Mr. Thomas and his illness.

Figure 1-1 shows these various factors which influence an individual's reaction to illness and will help the practical nurse realize the importance of considering each of her patients as a unique person, who is in many ways different from any other patient she has ever known.

Emotional Aspects of Illness. Emotions are actually emergency reactions to stimuli. When something disturbs a person he reacts by physically moving about, expressing his displeasure vocally or in some way showing his physical

Personal Factors		Environmental Factors
Age		Cultural background
Personality		Past experience with illness in others
Emotional stability		Knowledge of modern medicine and
Role in the family group	⟶ Patient ⟵	methods of treatment
Religious and spiritual attitudes		Community in which he lives
Standing in the community		Available sources of help
General state of health prior to present illness		

Figure 1-1. Factors influencing the patient's reaction to illness.

response to the situation that has upset him. He also reacts emotionally with fear, worry, dread, anxiety, resentment or depression. Emotions are inseparably woven into an individual's make-up and they greatly affect his outlook on life and his ability to cope with the problems of life.

In nursing we must realize that illness and injury serve as stimuli to the patient's emotions and produce certain reactions within the individual. We cannot always predict the manner in which a patient will respond to his illness emotionally, but we do know that such reactions are inevitable.

It is not always possible to determine immediately the way a patient feels about his illness and the resultant helplessness and dependency. Many persons hide their true emotions under a facade of apparent calm and acceptance. It is not the responsibility of the nurse to delve deep into the recesses of the patient's mind and probe for evidence of emotional unrest. We are not suggesting that she practice a kind of pseudo-psychotherapy on each of her patients, because this may produce some very harmful results, and may serve to alienate her patient rather than gain his trust and confidence. It is important, however, that the nurse understand the patient's need for expressing himself freely without fear of reprimand for his childishness. Nothing can be more exasperating than a pat on the head and the admonition to stop worrying when one truly has a problem to cause worry and anxiety. The nurse

must also consider her own actions and the effect these have on her patient.

Imagine a formerly healthy and active individual's reaction to being placed in a situation in which everyone is busily working, using words and initials he doesn't understand, and showing precious little interest in him beyond their dedication to administering medications and treatments. He is stripped of his usual attire and given a hospital gown to wear. Someone walks in immediately after supper, removes his water pitcher and glass, and places a sign over his bed. The sign reads *N.P.O.*, and when he asks the meaning of the letters he is told, "You're having a G.I. series in the morning." Now, few of us would settle comfortably in our beds and have a good night's sleep after this experience. We surely would not feel secure in the knowledge that we were in the hands of people sincerely interested in us as human beings with our own personal hopes and fears.

One cannot always judge an individual's true feelings by his behavior. The patient who is frightened may cover up his fear by being loud and demanding, giving little thanks to anyone for services rendered, and appearing to be completely unsatisfied with whatever is done for him. The wise nurse realizes that this patient is afraid and that he is covering up his fear by exhibiting a demanding attitude toward those responsible for his care. She will not attempt to dominate this patient or "teach him a lesson" for his childish behavior by ignoring his requests for more attention. She will realize that the patient who acts this way really needs *more* attention, and *more* of her time for listening to his complaints and re-assuring him that everything possible is being done to help him recover from his illness.

Another patient may react to his illness by becoming quiet and with-drawn. He apparently asks for nothing more than to be left alone to cope with his problems himself. It may not be possible for the nurse to help this pa-tient, but she should never miss an opportunity to let this patient talk when he shows an inclination to do so. It is only by being a good listener and allow-ing the patient to express himself that she can ever find out what is troubling him.

Many emotional problems of the pa-tient in the hospital can be avoided if the nurse will realize the true meaning and purpose of nursing. She is taking care of the patient because he needs her and because she has chosen service to others as her way of life. In rendering that service to her patients the nurse is aware that the emotions of fear, anxiety, depression, or resentment are natural responses to a physical disability that inflicts some degree of helplessness on the patient. These emotions are an integral part of the patient and his ill-ness, and must receive attention the same as his physical symptoms.

Spiritual Aspects of Illness. Nurses, doctors, and other members of the health team who are daily concerned with prolonging life and maintaining health in the human body are some-times in danger of losing sight of the immortal soul encased in that body. All of us would do well to remember that the average human being can expect to live on this earth approximately 70 or 80 years, whereas most religions teach that the soul will exist forever. Cer-tainly then, we should not overlook the spiritual welfare of our patients when taking care of their physical needs.

Religion is a private affair with most people and it is usually with some apprehension that the subject is brought up and discussed, even among friends. The nurse must realize this, and while she should respect the patient's feelings and beliefs in the matter of religion and show concern for his spiritual well-being, she certainly is not expected to pry into the spiritual life of her patient.

It is important too that she realize the relationship between spiritual strength and physical strength. Illness often brings a person face to face with the true meaning of life and death for the first time in his life. Some patients find comfort in meditation and contempla-tion of the realities of life and the mean-ing of illness and death. They feel closer to God when they are physically inactive (and perhaps somewhat help-less), and they are spiritually strength-ened rather than weakened by their illness. Others will worry and fret about the pain and suffering imposed upon them, unable to see any reason for such afflictions, and resentful that such a thing has had to happen to them. They may also fear death and refuse to dis-cuss the matter with anyone.

Obviously, the best person to satisfy the spiritual needs of a patient is one who has received special training and education in ministering to the spiritual life of others. Hospitals vary in the religious and spiritual services offered to patients. In some hospitals a chaplain makes regular visits to all patients; in others there are no chaplains and the nurse may need to call the patient's minister if he should make such a request. She should make the call promptly, with respect for her patient's beliefs whether she happens to agree with them or not. A minister should not be called unless the patient or his family requests it, and no attempt should be made to impose the nurse's religion on her patient or his family. Her attitude should be one of respect and sincerity, alert to the slightest indi-cation that her patient wishes spiritual guidance from a priest, minister, or rabbi.

The nurse must remember, too, that her attitude and actions in the presence of the patient and his family can serve as a source of inspiration to them. At times, a patient may not want a minister called, but will ask the nurse to "pray with" him. There is no need for embarrassment in this situation. She might simply ask the patient if he has any particular prayer he wishes read, and if not, the Lord's Prayer is one that is familiar and comforting.

EFFECTS OF ILLNESS ON THE FAMILY

No normal, emotionally stable person wants to be ill. It is a great inconvenience to him and also affects those who know and love him. The family, friends and other social groups can, in turn, have a deep and lasting effect on the success of medical treatment and the restoration of the patient to his former status, or at least to an acceptable way of life.

The inconveniences and hardships imposed on the family by an illness will depend to some extent on the patient's place in the household. If it is the father and wage-earner for the family who is ill, or the mother on whom the family depends for making the house into a home, everyone in the family group will be greatly inconvenienced. The person who is ill may worry and become upset because he or she can no longer assume responsibilities for the family and arrangements must be made for someone else to take over his former duties. This may be a temporary or a permanent arrangement, depending on the type of illness and whether or not the patient will be able to resume his former activities. Whatever the case, definite and practical plans must be made to keep the family together. Juvenile delinquency, overdependence on welfare agencies, and other socioeconomic problems can grow out of a disturbance in the family life.

Illness within the family will usually make the ties stronger or weaker. A family that is closely knit will most likely draw still closer together and work together for the good of all. A family group that has always been at odds with one another and unable to work together will probably drift even farther apart under the pressures of misfortune. There are exceptions, of course, but the general rule is that additional problems most often aggravate a situation rather than minimize the problems already existing.

Sometimes, as in the case of the aged or chronically ill for whom there is no hope of recovery, the family will breathe a sigh of relief as they admit a troublesome relative to the hospital or nursing home. They apparently feel that they have done all they can for the person and now someone else can bear the burden. As time goes on, visits from the family become less and less frequent until it is only on holidays and special occasions that the patient sees those he had thought loved him.

The practical nurse must realize that she cannot be a substitute for the patient's family, nor can she take sides for or against their attitude of indifference toward the patient. She can give these neglected patients her love and affection as a nurse, and show that she is interested in their welfare and anxious to help them lead useful lives, but she must be aware of her position as an outsider to the family. She should also realize that there is danger in becoming too emotionally involved with these patients and that sentimentality can hinder her performance as a nurse. The nurse's only recourse is to encourage closer family ties, letting those who do come to visit the patient know how much their thoughtfulness means to the patient and how important their interest is to his general well-being.

The oversolicitous and indulgent family can sometimes do as much harm as the indifferent one. They need help in understanding the treatments necessary, especially rest and diet. Too many visitors, too many flowers, and too much rich food are the usual excesses the nurse must guard against.

EFFECTS OF ILLNESS ON THE COMMUNITY

The family is the basic unit of society. The community, as a larger and more complex group of society, is composed of individuals and their families living within a certain area. Whenever one or more of these individuals within the group becomes ill and can no longer function in the community, the whole group is affected. Illness is costly to the community in terms of money and in the loss of essential services.

First let us consider the loss in regard to the number of dollars spent. Take as an example two members of a community; one is the only doctor in a small town. He becomes ill and is unable to continue practicing medicine for several weeks. His patients will need to pay for transportation to another area where they can receive medical care, and they will incur additional expenses because their doctor is ill. Now let us suppose that the town drunk and part-time painter collapses in the street with a stroke and is rushed off to the hospital. Few of his neighbors will consider that his illness is going to cost them money, yet this man will require expensive care in a tax-paid institution, and if he has provided money for his family, they will have to seek other sources of income now that he can no longer work. They will probably turn to a tax-paid and community-supported agency for help. These are just a few examples of the cost of illness to the community.

We cannot measure the loss to the community in terms of money only. There is a loss of service, because in our type of society today we are all dependent on one another for services of some kind. Every person who earns a living or maintains a home serves his fellow man. Doctor, lawyer, nurse, housewife, mechanic, grocer, farmer, airline pilot, or whatever, it is difficult to find an adult who does not serve others. The illness of any one person in the group will inconvenience the others in some way. Long-term illnesses place the heaviest burden on all concerned, but even a short-term, acute illness will take its toll.

INDIVIDUALS AND AGENCIES SERVING THE NEEDS OF THE PATIENT

When a person becomes ill he is often faced with many problems he cannot solve without assistance from others. We are fortunate in this country in having many agencies, both governmental and voluntary, which are interested in the health of our citizens and dedicated to the task of helping those in need. These agencies serve a very useful purpose in our society and contribute much to the health and welfare of our citizens. They are also necessary, for even though each individual and his family should assume responsibility for their own welfare, illness may present problems too overwhelming for them to handle. Figure 1-2 shows the general categories of the patient's needs that must be met and the individuals, groups, and agencies which best serve those needs.

The practical nurse is encouraged to familiarize herself with all resources of assistance for her patient so that she might know the ways in which her patient can receive help in meeting his needs, which go beyond those of simple nursing care.

The Role of the Licensed Practical Nurse. The position of the practical nurse in the field of nursing is not as clearly defined as some would like it to be, but we must realize that there have been many changes in nursing in the past few decades, and practical nursing as we know it today is comparatively new. Gone are the days of unskilled helpers who donned white uniforms, called themselves practical nurses, and

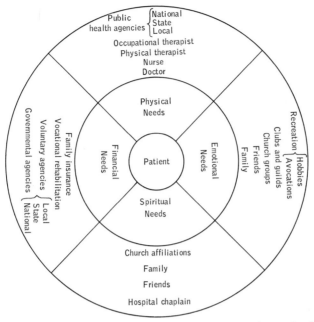

Figure 1-2. Some of the many individuals and agencies serving the needs of the patient.

functioned only as "sitters" or attendants in the home and hospital. Today's licensed practical nurse is prepared by education and experience to fulfill her role as a recognized member of the nursing team. In the Statement of Functions of the Licensed Practical Nurse issued in 1964 by the American Nurses' Association the role of the licensed practical/vocational nurse is described as follows:

"The work of the LPN is an integral part of nursing. The licensed practical nurse gives nursing care under the supervision of the registered professional nurse or physician to patients in simple nursing situations. In more complex situations the licensed practical nurse functions as an assistant to the registered professional nurse. A simple nursing situation is one that is relatively free of scientific complexity. In a simple nursing situation the clinical state of the patient is relatively stable and the measures of care offered by the physician require abilities based on a comparatively fixed and limited body of scientific facts and can be performed by following a defined procedure step by step. In a more complex

situation, the licensed practical nurse facilitates patient care by meeting specific nursing requirements of patients as directed, such as preparing equipment, supplies and facilities for patient care, helping the professional nurse to perform nursing measures, and communicating significant observations to the registered professional nurse."

The shortage of nurses in hospitals, institutions for the aged and infirm, and doctors' offices has sometimes given rise to the practice of pushing the practical nurse beyond her level of nursing care. Some registered nurses, fearful that practical nurses will replace them in the various areas of nursing, have complained bitterly about the situation and resent the fact that in some instances no limitations seem to be placed on the practical nurse. Hospital administrators and others who are responsible for staffing various medical institutions answer that they must allow practical nurses full responsibility for nursing care because there is no one else to do the work. In the midst of all this furor stands the practical nurse wondering what she is to do. On the one hand she is pressured into going beyond her limits in the practice of nursing and on the other hand she is resented when she accepts too much responsibility for patient care.

We can see, then, that it is not easy to define clearly the role of the practical nurse, but this does not excuse us from our responsibility in establishing some guiding principles. No one organization or institution can control the functions of all the practical nurses in this country and no one can predict the exact situations in which a practical nurse might find herself. Much of the responsibility for determining the limitations of the practical nurse must rest with the practical nurse herself. She must use her common sense and exercise good judgment in deciding the situations she can handle and those which are best left to others better qualified to meet the needs of the patient. She must keep abreast of the legal restrictions set up for the practice of nursing at different levels and she must know the policies of the institution in which she works. In many instances her conscience must be her guide. If the practical nurse has a sound knowledge of the fundamentals of nursing in conditions of illness and is capable of recognizing varying degrees of helplessness and dependency in a patient, she should be able to recognize nursing problems which require the services of a registered nurse or physician.

In analyzing the phrase, "limitations of the practical nurse," we should not overlook the real meaning of the word "practical." A practical plan is a plan that is sensible and useful, and can be applied to a situation with a minimum of speculation and detail. In a literal sense, a practical nurse is one who can apply her knowledge to some useful end. Her role is that of the person who manifests her knowledge in practice and in action.

It is unfortunate that we must use the word "limitations" when we speak of the functions of the practical nurse because this seems to imply a deficiency of intelligence or native ability. Such is not the case, of course. The limitations are determined by the amount of education required and the length of time spent in preparation for the practice of nursing. The fact that a practical nurse spends only one year in school (as compared to three or more years for the professional nurse) necessarily limits the amount of scientific information and nursing skills she can acquire. If the practical nurse wishes to function more efficiently on her level, she may acquire more education through postgraduate courses for the practical nurse, and by reading literature on nursing practices and learning through experience, but she cannot function above the level of practical nursing without acquiring the *formal* education necessary.

CLINICAL CASE PROBLEMS

1. Miss Thomas is a practical nurse student who is assigned to the care of three patients from 7:00 A.M. to 11:00 A.M. She has been a student for three months and works under the direct supervision of her clinical instructor. When she receives her morning report at 7:00 A.M. Miss Thomas learns the following about her patients:

Mr. Allman, age 35, sustained multiple and deep lacerations of the arms, received when he fell through a pane of glass while working at a construction site. He has been in the hospital for three days and is very despondent because he cannot use his arms to care for himself and has been told that he will need extensive physical therapy before he regains full use of them.

Mrs. Smith, age 50, is scheduled for surgery at 8:00 A.M. She has been prepared for surgery and has received all of the preoperative medications.

Mrs. Johnson, age 26, has undergone appendectomy, is in her third postoperative day, and is to be dismissed from the hospital today.

How should the student nurse go about organizing her work and carrying out her assignments?

What problems might she expect Mr. Allman to present?

How can she use the information she has in solving these problems?

REFERENCES

1. American Journal of Nursing: "Statement of Functions of the Licensed Practical Nurse." March, 1964, p. 93.
2. Bush, C. H.: *Personal and Vocational Relationships for Practical Nurses.* Philadelphia, W. B. Saunders Co., 1961.
3. Cooley, C. H.: *Social Aspects of Illness.* Philadelphia, W. B. Saunders Co., 1951.
4. Dennis, R. J.: "Ways of Caring." Am. Journ. Nurs., Feb., 1964, p. 107.
5. Gazaway, R.: *Human Relationships in Nursing,* 2nd edition. Philadelphia, W. B. Saunders Co., 1959.
6. Henderson, V.: "The Nature of Nursing." Am. Journ. Nurs., Aug., 1964, p. 62.
7. Ross, C. F.: *Personal and Vocational Relationships in Practical Nursing.* Philadelphia, J. B. Lippincott Co., 1961.
8. Sorenson, G. S.: "Dependency—A Factor in Nursing Care." Am. Journ. Nurs., Aug., 1966, p. 1761.
9. Turner, C. E.: *Personal and Community Health,* 11th edition. St. Louis, C. V. Mosby Co., 1959.

SUGGESTED STUDENT READING

1. Babcock, C. H.: "Stress and Illness." Practical Nursing, May, 1962, p. 16, and June, 1962, p. 18.
2. Boulette, T. R.: "Anxiety and the Nurse." Journ. Pract. Nurs., Aug., 1967, p. 28.
3. Dennis, R. J.: "Ways of Caring." Am. Journ. Nurs., Feb., 1964, p. 107.
4. Drummond, E. E.: "Impact of a Father's Illness." Am. Journ. Nurs., Aug., 1964, p. 89.
5. Ellerbrock, M. C., Sr.: "This I Believe." Nurs. Outlook, March, 1967, p. 38.
6. Groton, J.: "Mental Health Roles in Practical Nursing." Journ. Pract. Nurs., Oct., 1965, p. 37.
7. McTernan, E. J.: "The LPN on the Patient–Care Team." Journ. Pract. Nurs., 1966, p. 44.

OUTLINE FOR CHAPTER 1

I. The Nurse and Her Patient

A. Nursing care is doing for the patient those things which he cannot do for himself to assure his physical and mental comfort.

B. Nursing care needed will depend on: (1) particular condition of illness, (2) patient's ability to care for himself, and (3) manner in which patient responds to his illness.

C. Practical nurse will need a basic knowledge of the various effects of illness on an individual.

II. Effects of Illness on the Patient

A. Physical effects.

B. Emotional effects.

C. Spiritual aspects of illness.

III. Effects of Illness on the Family

A. Inconvenience and hardships may be financial, emotional, and physical.

B. The nurse cannot be a substitute for the family. She must consider their needs and their importance to the patient.

IV. Effects of Illness on the Community

A. Illness is costly in terms of money and loss of essential services.

V. Individuals and Agencies Serving the Needs of the Patient

A. Physicians, nurses, and members of the health team.

B. Agencies may be governmental or voluntary.

VI. Role of the Practical Nurse

A. An important member of the nursing team.

B. Works under the supervision of a registered professional nurse or physician.

Chapter 2

CAUSES OF DISEASE
AND THE BODY'S
RESPONSE TO ILLNESS

INTRODUCTION

Because we cannot fully understand the abnormal until we know what is normal, we must know something about the normal structure and functions of the human body before we can understand disease. Anyone exposed to the essentials of anatomy and physiology cannot fail to appreciate the importance of cells and tissues within the body because of the vital functions these millions of cells perform. They usually do their jobs so well we take them for granted and tend to forget their importance, but we must remember that these minute organisms are essential to our existence and unless they continue to function properly we cannot stay healthy.

Medical science was hampered in its study of disease until the microscope, x-ray and other laboratory equipment were developed to study the cell. Prior to these developments, internal changes in cell structure and function were generally assumed to be present but they could not be clearly defined and classified. The modern branch of medicine concerned with the study of changes in cell structure and function as a result of disease is called pathology. The physician practicing medicine must rely heavily on the pathologist for accurate diagnosis and the treatment of disease.

Generally the changes brought about by disease can be divided into the following categories: (1) changes in the structure of cells and tissues, as for example hardening of the arteries (arteriosclerosis); (2) changes in function, such as in decreased absorption and excretion of urine by a diseased kidney; and (3) chemical changes, as an increase in the blood sugar when diabetes is present.[7]

Though the practical nurse cannot be expected to know and understand the many pathological changes which occur

10

as a result of disease, she must be aware that these changes are taking place, be alert to external symptoms indicating internal changes, and be familiar with the nursing care required by the patient exhibiting these symptoms.

CAUSES OF DISEASE

The human body is composed of a complex variety of parts, each component part being dependent in some manner on the other. Because of this interdependence the determination of the exact cause of disease is extremely difficult. In some areas where the cause has been unquestionably proven, as in many infectious diseases, the mortality and incidence rate have greatly declined. This is especially true of diphtheria, meningitis, and pneumonia, all three of which were leading causes of death in the United States in 1900. Today these diseases have been replaced on the list by arteriosclerosis, diabetes, and cancer. This does not necessarily mean that the degenerative diseases are more prevalent now than they once were. It does mean, however, that we have eliminated acute infectious diseases as leading causes of death in young people. We now consider most infectious diseases preventable, and it is important that we continue to seek to know the cause of disease, for it is in knowing and understanding the cause that we take the first step toward prevention.

Causes of disease usually fall under one of two general headings: (1) predisposing causes and (2) specific or immediate causes. A weak and malnourished person, for example, will more readily succumb to pneumonia than one who is healthy and able to resist an invasion of bacteria. In this case the poor state of health was a predisposing cause, the bacteria the immediate cause.

Specific Causes of Disease

CONGENITAL DEFECTS. A congenital defect is one which results from an abnormal development during fetal life and is apparent at birth or immediately after. Those obvious from external signs include clubfoot, cleft palate and harelip, and spina bifida. Others that involve internal organs may not make

Table 1. *Predisposing Causes of Disease*

CAUSE	EXAMPLE
Extremes of temperature	Chilling predisposes one to respiratory infections
Extreme humidity	Fungi, such as the one causing "athlete's foot," thrive in a moist environment
Excessive dryness	Mucous membranes of respiratory tract lose ability to rid the tract of bacteria
Age	Mumps, measles, etc., more common in children; arteriosclerosis most likely to occur after 45 years of age
Heredity	Hemophilia
Sex	Leukemia more common in males
Race	Sickle-cell anemia occurs exclusively in Negro race

themselves known until several hours or days after birth. Obstructions within the alimentary canal, for example, will not become evident until the baby has started to take nourishment.

GENETIC DISORDERS. These are physical and mental defects that are transmitted through the genes. Genes are units of heredity; they transmit the physical, biochemical, and physiological traits that children inherit from their parents. Genetic disorders may or may not be apparent at the time of birth and they need not be present in the parents of the child who has inherited the disorder.

Diseases included under genetic disorders are *sickle cell anemia, thalassemia* and other blood dyscrasias resulting from abnormalities in hemoglobin.

Some genetic disorders are inborn errors of metabolism in which there may be faulty or incomplete metabolism of carbohydrates, proteins or fats. We know that metabolism is the sum of all the physical and chemical processes taking place in the body and there are many individual steps involved in these processes. The absence of a necessary enzyme can lead to a metabolic "block" which then results in the accumulation of products formed part of the way through the metabolic process; or there may be a deficiency of a product that is normally found in the series of metabolic reactions. *Galactosemia* and *phenylketonuria* (PKU) are examples of inborn errors of metabolism. In galactosemia there is a lack of the enzyme necessary for proper metabolism of galactose (a sugar). This enzyme normally would change galactose, which cannot be utilized by the body, into glucose, which can be used. Since the galactose cannot be utilized, it accumulates in the blood. In PKU there is a disturbance in the metabolism of an amino acid (phenylalanine). This results in a lack of a substance necessary for the production of the hormones adrenalin and thyroxin. A deficiency of these hormones leads to severe mental retardation un-

less the condition is detected early in the infant's life and corrected.

In some genetic disorders there is an imbalance of genetic material; for example there are too many or too few chromosomes. Such imbalances can lead to severe mental and physical defects. *Down's syndrome* (Mongolism) is an example of this type of genetic disorder. The infant with Down's syndrome has 47 chromosomes instead of the normal 46.

Research into genetic disorders and an increasing awareness of the importance of early diagnosis and treatment have greatly improved the prognosis and reduced the danger of permanent disability from such defects.

INJURY TO TISSUES. These injuries may be physical or chemical. Physical injury as a result of physical violence is known as *trauma*. Accidents are, of course, responsible for most injuries of this kind. Excessive exposure to heat or radiation can also be considered under physical injuries to tissues. Chemical injuries result from caustics, poisons, and toxins, all of which are detrimental to the body's cells and tissues.

PARASITES. A parasite is an organism which lives in or on another animal, depending on the host for his supply of nourishment. These unwanted guests are usually found in the intestinal tract, but they may also be found in other parts of the body, such as muscle tissue, blood stream, and liver. Tapeworms, roundworms, and pinworms are examples of parasites.

OBSTRUCTIONS. Many organs of the body are constructed as hollow tubes to allow for the passage of vital liquids and solids through them. Nourishment is carried to the various tissues through these organs and waste products excreted. Whenever there is a narrowing or complete closure of these hollow organs with a resulting obstruction to the flow of liquids or solids through them, there follows damage to the organ and the adjacent tissues it has served. A kidney which cannot be properly drained of urine because of kinking of the ureter will become filled with urine and its tissues will be damaged.

DEFICIENCY DISEASES. These are a result of an inadequate intake or the body's improper utilization of essential nutrients. The most common deficiency diseases are vitamin deficiencies.

DEGENERATIVE DISEASES. *Necrosis*, or death of tissues, results from practically every severe disease process; thus, any disease which continues unchecked will eventually bring about death of the cells of the affected part.

Sclerosis is a hardening of the tissues or organs resulting in impaired function. The diseases in which this type of degenerative process is found are arterial diseases such as hardening of the arteries (arteriosclerosis).

NEOPLASMS. A neoplasm is literally a *new growth*. Frequently the word "tumor" is used to describe a neoplasm even though this is not a true description. Tumor simply means a swelling and does not necessarily mean the development of new cells. The new cells in a neoplasm do not behave as normal cells do; they serve no purpose and become troublesome when they interfere with the functions of normal tissues. A neoplasm may be benign or malignant. *Benign neoplasms*, as their name implies, do not wreak as much havoc as malignant ones, but they should never be thought of as completely harmless. They may develop into malignant growths or grow so large as to cause damage to nearby tissues and organs.

Malignant growths are referred to as *cancerous*. The cells of a malignant growth interfere with and sometimes destroy the cells of normal tissue; they use up essential nutrients intended for the normal cells and usually multiply and spread rapidly. This spreading of the malignant cells to other parts of the body from their original site is called *metastasis*.

Neoplasms also may be classified according to their origin. Those which include new growth of bone, fat, blood vessels or lymphatic tissue are of *mesenchymal* origin. Malignant tumors of this type are called *sarcomas*. Epithelial neoplasms arise from the coverings of the internal and external surfaces of the body, such as the skin and mucous membranes. The term *carcinoma* refers to malignant tumors of this type. Neoplasms that contain more than one type of tissue are called *teratomas*. These are mixed tumors that represent all three germ layers of the body tissues and they often show attempts at organ formation.

INFECTIONS. When we say that a part of the body is "infected" we mean that disease-causing bacteria, fungi, or viruses are present. Inflammation is a characteristic of infection but not all inflammations are a result of an infection. For this reason the two words should not be used synonymously. Inflammation is actually the body's response to some irritating agent, its attempt to defend itself. A sunburn is an example of an inflammation in which there are no bacteria and no infection present. If the burn is very deep, however, and the wound is not kept sterile, bacteria will invade the tissues and an infection will result.

Types of Bacteria. Organisms capable of producing disease in humans are called *pathogenic*. Not all bacteria, yeasts, and molds are pathogenic, however, and many serve useful functions in the body as aids to digestion and absorption of food. Those which usually are not harmful to cells and tissues are called *nonpathogenic*.

Bacteria belong to the plant family, as do viruses, yeasts and molds, and they are classified according to their characteristics. There is no need for the practical nurse to learn and know all the many varieties under these classifications. Since bacteria are the most common causative agents in infections, however, and because the practical nurse will hear the terms "strep throat" and "staphylococcal infection," she may wish to understand something about these terms and what they mean.

Generally, bacteria are divided into three main groups according to their shapes (see Fig. 2-1): (1) cocci (round), (2) bacilli (rod-shaped), and (3) spirochetes (spiral or corkscrew).

Since bacteria in their natural state are seen through the microscope as tiny, colorless organisms, they must be stained with a dye. This dye is usually methylene blue and the procedure is called the Gram stain after the scientist who first used this method of classifying bacteria. Those bacteria which "take" the dye are called *gram-positive*. Those which will not retain the color are called *gram-negative*. All streptococci and all staphylococci are gram-positive. The bacillus which causes tuberculosis is gram-negative.

Bacteria may be grown in the laboratory in a specially prepared broth or jelly. They become visible to the naked eye as a large group or colony of specific types, all members of the colony having grown from one microscopic cell. The manner in which these bacteria arrange themselves as a group is also a means of classifying them. Some grow in pairs (diplococci), some in chains (streptococci), and some in clusters (staphylococci).

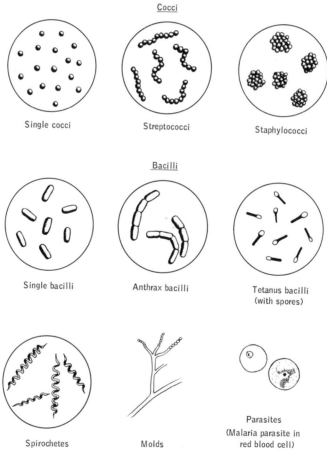

Cocci

Single cocci   Streptococci   Staphylococci

Bacilli

Single bacilli   Anthrax bacilli   Tetanus bacilli (with spores)

Spirochetes   Molds   Parasites (Malaria parasite in red blood cell)

Figure 2-1. Drawings of various pathogenic microorganisms as they appear under the microscope. Their shape and groupings determine their classification.

Thus we see that "strep throat" (short for streptococcal infection of the throat) is an infection caused by round organisms which grow in chains. A "staph" infection is an abbreviated way of saying that there is an infection present caused by round organisms which grow in clusters.

Viruses. Viruses are extremely small living pathogenic organisms that are increasingly causing disease and death. They are known to be responsible for at least 50 diseases in humans, among them the common cold, poliomyelitis, most childhood diseases, and a variety of respiratory disorders. Investigations are underway to determine whether viruses are a contributing factor in the development of cancer.

The study of viruses is difficult because they are so small; they cannot be seen without an electron microscope. The process of growing colonies of viruses similar to cultures of bacteria is difficult because viruses propagate only within living cells. Another difficulty in research on viruses as a cause of disease in man is the problem of growing human viruses in experimental animals. Before their effects on animals can be determined the viruses often change their characteristics and in effect evolve into different viruses. This characteristic of adaptability in the virus means that scientists who start out working with the same virus in different laboratories may, after some time, find themselves working with different viruses. Because of this adaptability and changing of characteristics the diagnosis and treatment of viral diseases can be very difficult. In addition, establishing immunity against certain viruses may be almost impossible, primarily because immunity is specific and immunity against one virus will not guarantee immunity against another type. This does not mean that there is no immunity for any viral disease. We already have an immune vaccine for smallpox, measles and mumps, all of which are viral diseases.

Biologists and biochemists are interested in viruses because they are excellent subjects for the study of the fundamental processes of cell growth and multiplication.

Classification of viruses can be based on a variety of characteristics including size, nucleic acid composition and affinity for certain types of tissues in the human body.

Fungi. A fungus is any member of a class of vegetable organisms of a low order of development, including molds and yeasts (see Fig. 2-2). They thrive

Table 2. *Classification of Viruses**

NUCLEIC ACID	VIRUS GROUP	SIZE, Mμ	TYPES PATHOGENIC TO MAN
RNA	Picorna	17-30	Poliovirus; Coxsackie viruses A and B; echovirus; rhinovirus (common cold)
	Reovirus	74	Types 1, 2, 3
	Arbovirus	20-100	Encephalitis (many varieties)
	Myxovirus	80-200	Influenza; mumps; parainfluenza; measles; respiratory syncytial
DNA	Papovavirus	40-55	Papilloma (wart)
	Adenovirus	68-85	Common cold (28 types)
	Herpesvirus	120-180	Herpes simplex; herpes zoster; cytomegalovirus
	Poxvirus	150-300	Variola (smallpox) Varicella (chickenpox)

*From French: Nurses' Guide to Diagnostic Procedures. 2nd edition. Copyright McGraw Hill, Inc., 1967. Used by permission of McGraw-Hill Book Company.

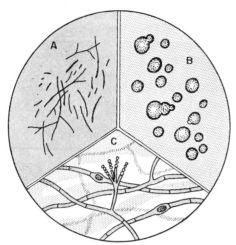

Figure 2-2.   Fungal types. *A*, Actinomycete. *B*, Yeast. *C*, Mold. (From Brooks: *Basic Facts of Medical Microbiology*, W. B. Saunders Co., Philadelphia.)

in warm, moist places and are easily spread. A fungal infection of the skin, hair, and nails is called a *dermatomycosis*. Examples of this type of fungal infection include athlete's foot and ringworm. Systemic fungal infections *(systemic mycoses)* are usually acquired by inhalation of the spores of the fungus, and the primary site of infection is the lung. From there the infection may spread throughout the body by the lymph vessels or blood stream. Histoplasmosis, blastomycosis, and actinomycosis are examples of systemic mycoses. The recent discovery of specific antifungal drugs, such as griseofulvin and amphotericin B, has greatly changed the prognosis for fungal infections with the result that long-standing cases that have resisted other forms of treatment now can be completely cured.

Nursing Implications. We must realize that bacteria, viruses, and fungi are always present in our environment. They are likely to be present in much greater numbers in a hospital where infections of all kinds are constantly being treated, and a proportionately large number of people within the hospital walls are quite likely to serve as carriers and sources of infectious agents.

From the beginning of her experiences as a practical nurse, the student is admonished to wash her hands before and after every nursing procedure. Though this may seem a simple and sometimes annoying task, its importance can never be overstated. The principles of cleanliness and good personal hygiene that are taught at the beginning of and throughout the course of practical nursing are of vital importance in the prevention of cross-infection and self contamination. In all nursing procedures we are taught to clean and dry equipment after it is used, and we must never underestimate the importance of plain soap, water and "elbow grease." In Chapter 8 of this text are presented the special procedures necessary for isolation and care of patients with specific infectious diseases, but the underlying principles of cleanliness are the same in all nursing procedures. Unfortunately we cannot see infectious agents without special microscopes, but we must be aware that they are always with us. By applying your knowledge of infectious agents to all aspects of nursing care you will do much to protect your patients, yourself, and your family from needless sickness and misery.

THE BODY'S RESPONSE TO ILLNESS AND INJURY

Introduction. The human body responds to an attack by pathogenic organisms or other foreign substances in the same general manner that a normal individual will respond to anything that endangers his welfare. He will take measures to defend himself against the attack and then engage in active battle if necessary to preserve his life.

The body's lines of defense consist of the skin and mucous membranes, which serve as a protective covering, and the inflammatory process, which serves as a type of internal defense. As long as the skin and mucous membranes remain intact without breaks in their surfaces the body is comparatively safe against the multitude of pathogenic micro-organisms in its environment. Should this line of defense fail, however, the body responds by setting into motion a process known as inflammation.

The body is able to resist many infections and toxic conditions because of the functions of the reticuloendothelial system and the leukocytes of the blood. The reticuloendothelial system is composed of cells and tissues which are capable of forming immune bodies against foreign substances. This process is called the *antigen-antibody reaction* and it is discussed in more detail later in this chapter. The most important function of the leukocytes is *phagocytosis*, which means that these white cells engulf and ingest the foreign particles.

The Process of Inflammation. In every inflammatory process there are two opposing forces at work: the aggressors and the defenders. The aggressors may be bacteria or viruses, or the toxins produced by these organisms. In some instances the inflammatory process may be initiated by chemical, mechanical, or other local injury and damage to the tissue. The outcome of the battle between the aggressors and the defenders depends, as in any battle of this kind, on the preparedness, strength, and resources of the defenders and their ability to resist and overpower the aggressors.

In the human body there are three possibilities:

1. The inflammation may be localized (the enemy cornered, so to speak) and eventually the battle against the aggressors is won. This is referred to as *localization and resolution*, which means that there is a resolving of the battle with victory going to the defenders and no permanent damage done to the tissues. A boil is an example of this type of inflammation.

2. There may be a localization of the inflammation, but because of repeated injury, inflammatory reactions and attempts at repair, the tissues involved are destroyed and can no longer function. An example of this is nephrosclerosis or death of the kidney cells with a loss of the kidney's ability to excrete urine, as a result of chronic nephritis.

3. The last possibility is one in which attempts at localization fail and a widespread inflammation results. Unless the body is able to overcome this overwhelming infection the result will be death of the individual. Fortunately the body is usually able to localize the infection and, with the aid of our modern antibiotic drugs, there is less likelihood of fatal infections.

What happens internally when the body is successful in restricting the infection to one area? We know from external signs such as *redness, heat, swelling*, and *pain* in that area that an inflammation is present. Internally several changes are also taking place:

1. Vascular changes. As soon as tissue injury occurs, whether by bacteria, heat, chemicals or physical trauma, a substance called *necrosin* is liberated by the damaged cells. It enters the surrounding fluids and affects the adjacent capillaries so that there is an increased flow of fluid and protein to the area. The blood flow slows down and becomes sluggish; thus very few bacteria are transported to other parts of the body. If the inflammation is due to factors other than infection, the reduced blood flow to and from the inflamed area delays the spread of toxic substances produced by the breakdown and death of the damaged cells.

2. Leukocytosis. The inflamed tissues liberate a substance known as *leukocytosis promoting factor*. As the name implies this substance causes increased production and release of leukocytes from the bone marrow. The leukocytes gather in large numbers at the site of the inflammation. There a group of leukocytes called *phagocytes* engulf and ingest bacterial cells and dispose of

them. Other white cells *(lymphocytes)* carry enzymes which dissolve or digest bacteria.

3. Exudation. The third activity going on during the inflammatory process is called *exudation.* This is the formation of a thick substance known as pus. This exudate is composed of fluid from the blood (plasma) and debris from the scene of the battle. It helps to wash away dead bacteria, tissue cells, and blood cells. It also brings immune bodies to the area as well as necessary enzymes, all of which are helpful in removing the debris. It is necessary that this exudate have an outlet so that the body might begin repair of the damage done. That is why the surgical procedure called "incision and drainage" is sometimes needed for abscesses, etc., when drainage cannot be achieved in any other way. In some cases a strip of rubber or tubing is placed in the wound by the surgeon to facilitate drainage.

4. Repair. The process of repairing the damage done by the inflammation begins almost immediately after inflammation starts. Fluid begins to flow into the area and immature cells of connective tissue and endothelial tissue begin to fill the space left by the "clean-up crew." These young cells grow and form a network of tissue called *granulation tissue.* If the inflammatory process is in the skin the granulation tissue is gradually replaced by new endothelial cells. Sometimes the granulation process is overstimulated by a prolonged infection or by repeated wet dressings. When this happens, overenthusiastic production of granulation tissue results in the formation of what is known as *proud flesh.*

5. Scar formation. This is a natural result of the repairing process. There is a general shrinkage of the capillaries and connective tissue cells, causing them to have the glossy and taut appearance of scar tissue with which we are all familiar. Internally the formation of scar tissue may form adhesions which are sometimes troublesome, in that these tough fibrous tissues may interfere with the normal functions of the internal organs around which they are formed.

Antigen-Antibody Reaction. Usually the invading agent causing the body to utilize its internal defenses is some type of protein. Bacteria and viruses are mainly protein, as are the toxins produced by bacteria. Fortunately, the body processes are especially geared for the formation of substances which act against such foreign protein substances. The battle between the invaders and the defenders is called the antigen-antibody reaction. The *antigens* are the invading substances; they may be bacteria, viruses, or a protein to which an individual is especially sensitive. Antigens stimulate the formation of specific proteins which act against them in defense of the body. These specific proteins are called *antibodies.* They are almost all formed in the lymph nodes, spleen, bone marrow and lymphoid tissue of the gastrointestinal tract. As soon as an antigen enters the body the plasma cells of these tissues begin to multiply very rapidly, thus increasing the production of antibodies.

How do the antibodies go about destroying their enemies the antigens? Remember that the antibodies are specific agents; that is, the plasma cells produce only the type of antibody needed to destroy the particular type of antigen present in the body. Thus, when the antigen is a *toxin,* or poisonous substance, the antibody produced is an *antitoxin* capable of neutralizing the toxin. Other antibodies combine with a specific type of antigen causing its precipitation and rendering it ineffective. These antibodies are called *precipitins.*

Some antibodies (called *agglutinins*) attach themselves to the surface of the antigens, causing them to clump together (agglutinate) and assume a heavy, nonaggressive aggregate form, thereby rendering them harmless. We know that red blood cells will agglubacilli, and most recently the polio vaccine, are all examples of agents used to produce an active immunity in humans.

This method of stimulating the production of immunizing substances in the body is quite successful in situations in which there is time to wait for the person to build up his own defenses. But what can be done if a person has no immunity and contracts the disease? Obviously there is no point in adding insult to injury by injecting more antigens into his body. Thus we come to the third type of immunity: *passive immunity.*

Passive Immunity. As the name implies, passive immunity is acquired through the efforts of someone else. Usually the "someone else" is a horse or a rabbit. The serum from the blood of one of these animals contains ready-made antibodies and antitoxins. This is done in the laboratory by giving increasingly stronger injections of specific antigens to the animals over a period of time so that they build up the necessary antibodies and antitoxins. The most common diseases in which passive immunity is an effective means of treatment to bolster the patient's defenses are diphtheria and tetanus. Immune serum is also useful in treating victims of bites from venomous snakes. It must be remembered, however, that these injections giving passive immunity should be given in the earliest stages of the disease, as they can only help prevent damage to tissues; they cannot repair damage already done.

Sometimes passive immunity is established before the disease is contracted. In instances of contact with a disease such as measles, when the exposed person is considered too weak to withstand the rigors of a full-blown disease, gamma globulin is given to prepare the body in advance and lessen the severity of the disease should the person exposed contract the disease.

The fetus in the uterus can *passively* receive some natural immunity from its mother. Most antibodies in the mother's blood stream can pass through the placenta and become mixed with the blood of the fetus, so that they are present in the infant's blood at birth. Thus an expectant mother who has a high level of immunity to diphtheria, tetanus, and whooping cough can be assured that her newborn baby will have some immunity to these diseases. This is only a *temporary* arrangement, however, and the child must be immunized again when it has reached the age of two or three months.

Actually, all passive immunity is useful only as a temporary safety measure and cannot be expected to guarantee a permanent safeguard against attacks from specific disease. In fact, for such diseases the antibody content may drop to a very low level over a period of years, even with active immunity. It is then necessary that the body be reminded of the need to produce more antibodies. To achieve this, single doses of antigens are given. These are so-called "booster doses."

Allergies. Basically, all allergic reactions result from antigen-antibody reactions that occur in contact with cells. When the reaction occurs, for reasons not yet fully understood, the cells begin to swell, and some of them rupture, releasing substances such as histamine, heparin and choline into the body fluids. Some of these substances are toxic. Histamine, or a histamine-like substance, is believed to be responsible for many of the serious reactions in allergy. Drugs called antihistamines are frequently used to relieve the symptoms of an allergic reaction.

The allergic reaction may be immediate or delayed. It also may be very mild and present only minor symptoms such as a rash or watery eyes, or it may be severe and produce *anaphylaxis,* which is characterized by circulatory collapse and can be fatal.

Factors influencing the types of response are: (1) the kind of antigen, (2) concentrations of antigens and antibodies, (3) the kind of antibody, and (4) the location and kind of tissue cells involved.

Since allergic reactions are antigen-antibody reactions, an allergy will not develop until an individual has become "sensitized." This means that on first contact with an *allergen* (antigen that causes allergic reactions) there will be no specific antibodies present in his body; therefore no antigen-antibody reactions can occur. Upon the second exposure to the antigen, however, the antibodies are available and the reaction takes place. Many allergens are proteins, and they include animal proteins such as those present in milk, eggs, meat and fish, and plant proteins such as those present in pollen.

Treatment of Allergy. It is thought that allergies occur only when a person is mildly immunized against an allergen. For example, an infant may be temporarily allergic to a substance such as egg albumin or meat extracts, but as he becomes more exposed to the allergen he develops more immunity and eventually the allergy disappears. The *desensitization* of patients suffering from an allergy is based on this principle. Under the supervision of an allergist the allergen is given to the patient in small but progressively larger doses over a period of time until he builds up sufficient antibodies to have an immunity.

Antihistamine drugs work as blocking agents to the histamine released during an antigen-antibody reaction. They are especially useful in preventing the effects of histamine in hay fever, urticaria (hives), and anaphylaxis.

Epinephrine acts as a neutralizing agent and is used to counteract the effects of histamine in an allergic reaction. It causes constriction of the blood vessels, which is the reverse of the histamine effect. It also produces dilatation of the bronchi, which is helpful in the relief of asthma or other respiratory difficulties due to an allergy.

Cortisone and hydrocortisone, which are hormones of the adrenal cortex, are sometimes used in the treatment of allergy. These hormones are anti-inflammatory agents that reduce the effects of the reaction. In large doses they also act to depress the formation of antibodies.

Nursing care of a patient with an allergy will depend on the way in which the allergy is manifested. Skin disorders resulting from an allergic reaction are discussed in Chapter 10; respiratory disorders are discussed in Chapter 13. Whatever the type of allergic disorder, it is well to remember that the emotional state of the patient will greatly affect the progress of the disease and the effectiveness of the treatment. His environment should be as quiet and non-stimulating as possible. Situations that produce anxiety, fear or anger should be avoided, and the nurse must do whatever she can to help the patient achieve serenity and peace of mind.

Prevention of Serious Allergic Reactions. Everyone concerned with the administration of medications should be aware of the dangers of giving drugs to patients who are highly sensitive. One should always ask the patient about specific allergies before administering any antibiotic or immunizing agent. The sera from animals, when injected into humans for the purpose of immunization, may produce serious or even fatal results in hypersensitive individuals. Others may be allergic to the substance (for example egg white or chick embryo) used for growth and nourishment of the cultured organism. Although the nurse cannot always foresee the development of a serious allergic reaction, she must be prepared for such an eventuality. Epinephrine (Adrenalin) should always be readily at hand when allergy-producing drugs are administered. The symptoms of an allergic reaction should be familiar to the nurse and if they appear she should notify the physician at once. These symptoms include apprehension, generalized rash or hives, choking sensation, wheezing, cough, incontinence, shock, fever, loss of consciousness and convulsions. In anaphylaxis death may occur in five to ten minutes.

CLINICAL CASE PROBLEMS

1. A neighbor of yours asks why the doctor has told her to apply hot compresses to a small abscess on her arm. She states that cool compresses relieve the pain and throbbing and she would rather use these than the hot compresses.

> How would you explain the need for her to continue the hot compresses as ordered by her doctor?
> Suppose that a few days later the same neighbor told you that her doctor had incised the abscess and inserted a drain. How would you explain the purpose of the drain?

2. A 19-year-old girl is brought to the emergency clinic with injuries received while riding horseback. Her past record of immunizations is not known but the girl states that she often has hay fever. The doctor orders tetanus antitoxin given.

> What precautions should be taken in the administration of this immunizing agent?
> What is the emergency treatment for a serious allergic reaction?

3. A child who has been exposed to measles is given an injection of gamma globulin. A month later he still has shown no sign of having contracted measles and so he is given the measles vaccine.

> What type of immunity is established by injections of gamma globulin?
> Of what benefit is gamma globulin to a person who has been exposed to an infectious disease?
> What type of immunity is established by administration of measles vaccine?

REFERENCES

1. Beland, I. L.: *Clinical Nursing: Pathophysiological and Psychosocial Approaches.* New York, The Macmillan Co., 1965.
2. Brunner, L. S., et al.: *Textbook of Medical-Surgical Nursing.* Philadelphia, J. B. Lippincott Co., 1964.
3. Frobisher, M., Jr., Sommermeyer, L., and Goodale, R. H.: *Microbiology and Pathology for Nurses,* 5th edition. Philadelphia, W. B. Saunders Co., 1960.
4. Johnson, K. J.: "Allergic Infections." Am. Journ. Nurs., July, 1965, p. 212.
5. Salsbury, C. R.: *Introduction to Pathology,* 2nd edition. New York, The Macmillan Co., 1946.
6. Shafer, J., and Sweet, L.: "Allergic Reactions to Drugs." Am. Journ. Nurs., Oct., 1965, p. 100.
7. Sinclair, C. G.: *Microbiology and Pathology,* 6th edition. Philadelphia, F. A. Davis Co.
8. Utz, J. P., and Benson, M. E.: "Systemic Mycoses." Amer. Journ. Nurs., Sept., 1965, p. 103.

SUGGESTED STUDENT READING

1. "Allergy." Practical Nursing Oct., 1960, p. 18.
2. McLean, J. A.: "Hay Fever." Am. Journ. Nurs., July, 1961, p. 85.
3. Mueller, H. L.: "Serious Allergic Reaction to Insect Stings," Am. Journ. Nurs., Aug., 1960, p. 1110.

OUTLINE FOR CHAPTER 2

I. Introduction

A. Pathology—the study of changes in cell structure, chemistry or function to determine the cause of disease.

II. Causes of Disease

A. Predisposing causes of illness—those which "pave the way" for disease.

B. Specific causes—the immediate, known causes.

1. Congenital defects—result from abnormal fetal development.
2. Genetic disorders—defects transmitted through genes.
3. Injury—physical or chemical trauma.
4. Parasites—organisms living in or on other animals.
5. Obstructions—narrowing or closure of hollow organs.
6. Deficiency diseases—caused by inadequate intake or poor absorption.

7. Degenerative diseases — a breakdown of tissues and impairment of function.
8. Neoplasms — new growths, benign or malignant.
9. Infection — invasion by a disease-producing organism.
   a. Bacteria — belong to the plant family and are classified according to their characteristics such as shape, grouping and ability to take a dye.
   b. Viruses — minute organisms seen only with an electron microscope. Viral infections are difficult to diagnose, to treat and to provide immunity against.
   c. Fungi — a member of a class of vegetable organisms which thrive in warm, moist places.
   d. Nursing functions in prevention of infection are based on principles of cleanliness and good personal hygiene. Importance of handwashing should never be underestimated in prevention of infection.

III. Body's Response to Illness and Injury

A. Defenses: (1) skin and mucous membranes, (2) inflammatory process, and (3) antigen-antibody reaction.
1. Process of inflammation.
   a. Initiated by invading organisms, foreign substances, or chemical or mechanical injury.
   b. Three possible outcomes — localization, local destruction of tissue, or widespread inflammation.
   c. External symptoms — heat, swelling and pain.
   d. Internal changes — vascular changes, leukocytosis, exudation and scar formation.
2. Antigen-antibody reaction — antigens (bacteria, viruses, etc.) stimulate formation of specific proteins (antibodies) which act against the antigens. Types of antibodies include antitoxins, precipitins, agglutinins, lysins, and opsonins.
3. Immunity — a security against a particular disease or toxin.
   a. Types of immunity: (1) natural — an innate resistance to disease, (2) active — obtained by having an attack of the disease or being given antigens which cause the body to produce antibodies, and (3) passive — obtained by receiving "ready-made" antibodies in immune serum or gamma globulin.
4. Allergies — also a result of antigen-antibody reaction and accompanied by the release of histamine, which is believed to be responsible for symptoms of serious allergic reactions.
   a. Severity of allergic reactions varies with the individual. The more sensitive person may suffer serious illness or death.
   b. "Desensitization" is based on gradual increase of immunity to specific allergens by administering small doses of the specific antigen and stimulating production of antibodies.
   c. Antihistamines, epinephrine and cortisone are drugs most commonly used in control of allergy.
   d. Prevention of serious allergic reactions important in the administration of certain drugs and immunizing agents.

Chapter 3

SYMPTOMS OF ILLNESS

Vocabulary

Aspiration	Enzyme
Capillary	Flatus
Catalyst	Hallucination
Contraction	Reaction
Delusion	Toxic
Dilatation	Vascular
Disoriented	Vital

INTRODUCTION

The diagnosis of disease from the symptoms presented by the patient and the prescription of treatment for illness lie within the realm of the physician. But when continued treatment and personal care are required, it is the nurse who spends the longest periods of time with the patient. During his absence from the bedside the physician must rely on the nursing staff for intelligent observation and accurate reporting of the patient's progress and the symptoms his illness produces. Of all the duties involved in nursing care, observation is probably the most vital. Florence Nightingale, in describing the role of the nurse, said, "Without the habit of ready and correct observation, we [nurses] shall be useless for all our devotion."[5]

This talent for "ready and correct observation" is not easily achieved, and can only be developed with experience and a full understanding of what intelligent observation really means. It is much more than merely watching. First, there must be a sincere interest in the patient, a willingness to listen to his complaints, and an understanding of his individual personality and personal reactions to his illness. Secondly, the observer must have a sound knowledge of the usual course of the patient's particular condition or illness so that she can recognize deviations from that course. Third, the observer must make a critical judgment between the usual and the unusual, and finally, she must make a decision of action based on her observations.

An example of this is a situation in which the practical nurse observes a patient having slight respiratory distress. She changes his position to facilitate breathing but the dyspnea does not improve and the patient becomes restless. The nurse knows that this patient has had gastric surgery and she realizes that dyspnea is not usually associated with this condition. She recognizes this as an unusual occurrence and decides to report the patient's dyspnea to the nurse in charge. This practical nurse has made an intelligent observation and chosen a wise course of action on the basis of her observations.

25

The nurse can learn much about her patient by observing his general appearance. With experience she will understand that facial expressions, posture in bed, bodily movements, and ability to cooperate are all significant clues to the physical and mental condition of a patient.

There are also specific signs which nurses must learn to look for while caring for patients. These signs of the presence of illness, or a change in the progress of an illness, are called *symptoms*. They are the warning signals that something is amiss. These symptoms may be *subjective* or *objective*. Subjective symptoms are those the patient must tell us about; for example, itching, pain, nausea, and fatigue are subjective symptoms. Objective symptoms are those which can be determined with instruments and laboratory tests, or those which we can see for ourselves. Pallor, high blood pressure, increased blood sugar, or skin rash are examples of objective symptoms.

Since the practical nurse is not called upon to diagnose an illness she is not expected to understand all of the symptoms of specific diseases. She should, however, be aware of the more common symptoms of illness and what these symptoms mean to the patient in terms of discomfort and danger. Later in this text, symptoms of specific diseases will be discussed, but there are many symptoms which are common to a variety of diseases. These symptoms are presented in the following discussion.

COMMON SYMPTOMS

An understanding of the *cardinal symptoms*, sometimes referred to as the vital signs, is basic to any type of skilled nursing care. These cardinal symptoms include (1) temperature, (2) pulse, (3) respiration, and (4) blood pressure.

Temperature. An elevation of the body temperature so that it is one or more degrees above normal is called a *fever*. This elevation is determined by taking the patient's temperature with a clinical thermometer. There are other indications that a fever is present. These include flushed face, hot dry skin, a facial expression of anxiety, and rapid, shallow breathing.

The main cause of fever is the presence of an infection or inflammation somewhere in the body. Tissue necrosis, dehydration, toxic substances and nervous disorders may also cause a rise in the body temperature.

Because fever is a defense reaction of the body during an acute infection, and thus may be considered advantageous, no nursing measures to reduce the body temperature should be taken without a doctor's specific order to do so. There are some comfort measures which the nurse may take, such as frequent bathing of the face and hands, rubbing the back with alcohol, and providing for sufficient intake of fluids. In prolonged fever the patient is usually placed on bed rest with bathroom privileges. His room should be kept quiet and darkened to decrease irritability. The mucous membranes of the nose and mouth will require special attention to prevent their becoming excessively dry and cracked. The diet should be high in calories during a fever.

When the fever becomes excessively high there is some danger of damage to tissue cells, and the physician will then order specific measures to reduce the body temperature. These methods will vary, but usually include sponging the patient with a solution of alcohol and water to cool the surface of the body by evaporation. Ice bags applied to the head, axillae and groin, a cool-water enema, and antipyretic drugs such as aspirin will also reduce the body temperature. Caution should be taken that the body temperature is not lowered too suddenly. The nurse should check the temperature of a feverish patient 30 minutes after temperature measures have been taken and at least every two hours thereafter unless otherwise ordered.

Chills, with violent shivering, often accompany or immediately precede high temperatures. These uncontrollable muscular activities are the body's attempt to raise the temperature (as a defense against infection) by increased muscular activity. The patient suffering from a chill will need extra warmth in the form of blankets and hot water bottles. When the chill subsides, the patient's linens may be wet with perspiration and extreme care should be taken that he is not exposed to drafts. The linen should be changed with as little fanning of the covers as possible. It should also be remembered that with profuse perspiration there has been a loss of body fluids which must be replaced by fluids orally or intravenously.

Pulse. Irregularities in the rhythm of the pulse beat are called *arrhythmias*. There may be a difference between the length of time between beats, or a difference in the force of the beats. In either case these should be reported when observed. They may occur in apparently normal persons or they may indicate a serious disease.

An increase in the rate of the pulse to over 130 beats per minute is considered to be an indication that the heart contractions are not behaving normally. This increase in the rate of the heart beat is called *tachycardia*, and is usually an indication of an increase in the basal metabolism resulting from a need for a greater supply of blood somewhere in the body. It may be present in persons who are merely excited, of course, and this is a normal reaction, but a fast pulse also frequently accompanies fever, hyperthyroidism, congestive heart failure, and hemorrhage.

A slowing of the heart rate to below 60 per minute is called *bradycardia*. This is considered normal for some persons (for example, young male adults and athletes), but it may also be an indication of a disease. Wherever there is a possibility of brain damage from head injury, the slowing of the pulse is a very alarming sign and should be reported

at once. Bradycardia in some cardiac patients might also be considered dangerous. Some drugs, such as digitalis, slow the heart beat and should not be given if the pulse rate is below 60 per minute.

Respiration. The rate of the rhythmic inhalation and exhalation of air is controlled by three factors: (1) the respiratory center in the brain, (2) nerve impulses of the autonomic nervous system, and (3) the chemical composition of the blood. A disturbance of any of these three can cause a change in the rate of respiration.

Dyspnea is a term used for difficult breathing and is a symptom common to many diseases of the respiratory tract, heart, or brain. It is usually accompanied by *cyanosis*, a bluish tint to the skin most noticeable around the lips and fingertips. The patient with dyspnea has a characteristic expression of anxiety; the eyes become prominent and the nostrils dilated. The patient appears to struggle for air and he may use the phrase "short of breath" to describe his condition. Usually the administration of oxygen will relieve these symptoms unless there is some severe obstruction in the respiratory tract. The nurse should be aware of a patient's fear and do all that she can to allay his anxieties. Unless contraindicated, the patient breathes best sitting upright with the chin raised well off the chest, as this will straighten the thoracic cavity and air passages, allowing for the intake of a full breath of air.

If it is necessary for the patient to maintain this position of *orthopnea* for a period of time, he may sleep more comfortably if an overbed table is placed over his bed, raised to the height of his chest and covered with pillows. The patient's arms are then placed across the pillow and his head allowed to rest between his arms (Fig. 3-1). Since dyspnea is aggravated by a full stomach, patients presenting this symptom fare better on small, frequent feedings.

Cheyne-Stokes respiration is the term

Figure 3-1. Orthopneic position, used when the patient has difficulty breathing and is more comfortable in a sitting position. Pillows are used to support back. Other pillows are placed on overbed table to support weight of arms, shoulders, and head. (From Montag and Swenson: *The Fundamentals of Nursing Care*, 3rd edition. W. B. Saunders Co., Philadelphia.)

used to describe a type of respiration characterized by periods of dyspnea followed by periods of *apnea* (absence of breathing). These periods alternate with regularity. During the period of apnea there is comparative rest, while during the phase of dyspnea the patient may become restless. Cheyne-Stokes respiration is a serious symptom and in acute illness it often signals approaching death.

Blood Pressure. The degree of pressure of blood volume against the arterial walls, commonly called blood pressure, varies with individuals. A disease in any part of the circulatory system can change this pressure to very high or very low readings.

Hypertension (high blood pressure) becomes dangerous when it places such a strain on the arterial walls that they may rupture, resulting in damage to the surrounding tissues. The most likely place for this to occur is within the cranial cavity where there is less room for expansion of the blood vessels. This is what sometimes happens at the time

of a cerebrovascular accident or "stroke."

There are various theories as to the exact cause of hypertension, but we do know that it often accompanies circulatory diseases, such as arteriosclerosis, and kidney diseases. Generally, the treatment for high blood pressure consists of rest and quiet, a dietary regimen aimed at preventing obesity, and administration of drugs which dilate the blood vessels. Hypertension and hypertensive heart disease are discussed in more detail in Chapter 12 of this text.

Hypotension is in itself not dangerous unless it becomes extreme, as in shock and hemorrhage. (See Chapter 5, Preoperative and Postoperative Care.) Anemia sometimes is accompanied by hypotension but, as one authority has said, "Therapeutically the patient with low blood pressure may be congratulated." It is the marked deviation from what is normal for the patient that is cause for alarm. The blood pressure must be checked carefully in patients with head injuries and any marked change in the readings reported immediately, as it may indicate changes in the pressure within the cranial cavity and resultant brain damage.

FLUID AND ELECTROLYTE BALANCE

Introduction. More than half of the body is composed of water which contains dissolved organic and mineral nutrients and waste products. The taking in of nutrients and the excretion of waste products is a continuous life-long process internally, within the cells and tissues, just as it is with the total individual man. When something happens to disturb this internal process of intake and output, the balance is upset, and unless the situation is relieved, death of the tissues and eventual death of the individual will result.

Even though the body fluids are continuously in motion, passing through cell membranes and the walls of the blood and lymph vessels, physiologists consider these fluids to be compartmentalized. This means that the fluid in the cells, for example, is distinguished from the fluid in the tissue spaces between the cells. The fluid within the vascular system is called *plasma water*, the fluid in the tissue spaces between the cells is called *interstitial fluid* or *tissue fluid*, and the fluid within the cells is called *intracellular fluid*.

Dissolved in the various body fluids are substances which play an essential role in maintaining the normal fluid balance and in promoting normal function of the cells. These compounds are called *electrolytes*. As their name implies, once they are dissolved in water they are capable of conducting an electric current. The fluids within the various compartments contain different compositions of electrolytes. This difference causes an electrical charge to develop across the membrane of each cell, and it is this electrical charge which allows nerves to transmit impulses, muscles to contract and glandular cells

to secrete. We can see that the body fluids and the electrolytes dissolved in them are essential to normal functioning of the cells and consequently to the well-being of the entire body.

The principal electrolytes are potassium, calcium, magnesium, sodium and chloride. Potassium is important in growth of the cells, repair of tissue, transmission of impulses in nerves and muscles, and in many different aspects of metabolism. Calcium plays an integral part in the formation of a blood clot and is essential to normal functioning of the muscles. Sodium, magnesium and chloride are essential to chemical changes necessary for normal body function. Sodium is especially important in the maintenance of a normal fluid balance in the body.

A normal balance of body fluids depends on a balance between water added to the body, as in beverages, food, infusions and tube feeding, and water lost from the body through the skin, urine, stool and expired air. An elevated body temperature and sweating increase the loss of water. Too much water in the body is called *overhydration* or *edema*; a deficiency of water in the body is called *dehydration*.

Edema. When there is an excessive amount of fluid within the interstitial compartment (tissue fluid), the affected area becomes swollen and the condition is referred to as *edema*. The tissue in which this swelling is apparent is called *edematous* tissue. Edema is frequently a symptom of poor circulation, as in cardiovascular diseases, or of poor elimination of water from the kidneys, as in chronic kidney disease.

Pitting edema is a condition in which a small depression or pit occurs when one places his finger on the skin over an edematous area. This is caused by a shifting of the tissue fluid from the area beneath the pressure point to another nearby tissue area. In *non-pitting edema* the tissue fluid coagulates and cannot be moved to other areas by pressure. This type is also called *brawny edema. Dependent edema* most often affects the lower extremities and can be relieved by elevating the affected part. It is frequently a sign of decreased circulation of blood or lymph. *Pulmonary edema* results from a collection of fluid within the tissue spaces of the lungs.

The physician often requests daily weighing of the patient who has severe edema. This is done for the purpose of determining the amount of body fluids lost or gained over a period of time.

When daily weight is ordered, the practical nurse must be careful to obtain as accurate a reading as possible. Ideally, the patient should be weighed before breakfast and at the exact same time each day. The same scales should be used each time the patient is weighed and he should be wearing exactly the same type of clothing. The loss or gain of one or two pounds of body fluids can be quite significant in the course of the patient's illness.

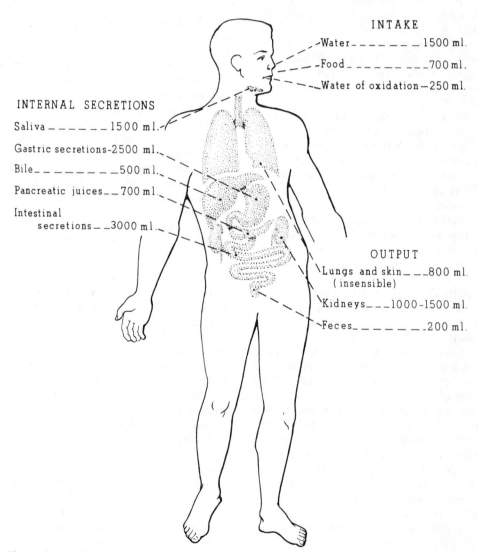

INTAKE
Water _ _ _ _ _ _ _ 1500 ml.
Food _ _ _ _ _ _ _ _ 700 ml.
Water of oxidation — 250 ml.

INTERNAL SECRETIONS
Saliva _ _ _ _ _ _ 1500 ml.
Gastric secretions - 2500 ml.
Bile _ _ _ _ _ _ _ 500 ml.
Pancreatic juices _ _ 700 ml.
Intestinal
    secretions _ _ 3000 ml.

OUTPUT
Lungs and skin _ _ _ 800 ml.
    (insensible)
Kidneys _ _ _ 1000 - 1500 ml.
Feces _ _ _ _ _ _ _ 200 ml.

Figure 3-2.   Balance between intake and output. (From Jacob & Francone: *Structure and Function in Man.* W. B. Saunders Co., Philadelphia.)

When nursing a patient with edema we must remember that the tissues and capillaries are not functioning normally and the skin is stretched beyond its normal limits. Care must be taken, then, to preserve the skin surface as much as possible, by keeping the linens dry and smooth and relieving the pressure of body weight by frequently turning the patient. It is also helpful in the relief of edema in the extremities to elevate the swollen limb above the level of the heart so as to facilitate drainage of the fluid out of the tissues. Since sodium holds water in the tissues, the patient with edema is usually placed on a low sodium diet.

Dehydration. The term *dehydration* refers to the removal or loss of water. The patient who is dehydrated has a deficiency of body fluids. Since these fluids are necessary for the transport of the substances dissolved in them, a depletion of fluids also means a disturbance in normal electrolyte concentrations in the body fluids.

The dehydrated patient will have skin that is very dry and wrinkled and has lost its elasticity. The eyes are sunken and the mucous membranes lose their moisture. The patient appears very weak and lethargic and may go into severe shock if the dehydration is extreme.

Treatment of dehydration is primarily concerned with replacement of lost fluids, either orally or intravenously. There also must be a replacement of the vital electrolytes lost with the body fluids. The physician determines the exact amount of water and the specific electrolytes needed. Often the fluid is given intravenously at a specific rate ordered by the physician. The nurse must be sure that the solution flows into the patient's vein at the exact number of drops per minute that the physician has ordered. Sodium chloride, potassium and calcium are frequently used in the intravenous fluids to quickly restore the electrolytes lost.

DISORDERS OF ELIMINATION

Introduction. All of the body's metabolic processes eventually produce waste products which must be eliminated from the body. If these substances are not eliminated properly they can become toxic, causing serious illness. Their accumulation also can lead to disturbances in the water and electrolyte balance and in the acid-base balance. It is also possible for loss of fluids, electrolytes, and stomach acids through severe vomiting to cause similar disturbances in the body's chemical balance.

Nausea and Vomiting. Nausea is a feeling of discomfort in the stomach region with an urge to vomit. Extreme nausea is usually accompanied by vomiting, which is defined as the expulsion of the contents of the stomach. The causes of nausea and vomiting are many and varied, including gastrointestinal disorders, radiation sickness, various drugs and chemicals swallowed or absorbed through the skin, anesthetics and pregnancy.

Relief of nausea and vomiting is usually best achieved by the administration of the antiemetic drugs now available. These drugs depress the vomiting reflex and also have a tranquilizing effect. They must be used with caution since they can cause oversedation and lower blood pressure.

Nursing measures during a vomiting episode include having the patient lie down and holding his head so that it is turned to one side to prevent aspiration of the vomitus into the respiratory tract. An emesis basin should be held close to the side of the face. A cool, damp washcloth should be used to wipe the patient's face, and a glass of ice water or mouthwash should be offered to the patient after vomiting so that the mouth can be rinsed. The vomitus is observed for odor, color, contents and approximate amount. It is best that the patient not take anything by mouth during severe nausea as it will only trigger further attacks of vomiting. When oral nourishment is allowed it should begin with small amounts of liquids and gradually progress to solid foods. If the nausea and vomiting persist over a prolonged period of time, intravenous feedings are necessary to replace the lost fluids.

Diarrhea. Diarrhea refers to the passing of frequent, watery stools. The number of stools per day varies and might range from three or four to as many as 15 or 20. The consistency of the stools, rather than the number per day, is the determining factor as to whether diarrhea is present. It is usually accompanied by cramplike pains in the abdomen, a result of hyperactive peristalsis and increased flatus.

Diarrhea may be a symptom of gastrointestinal diseases, such as an infectious inflammatory process, or obstruction of the intestinal tract due to fecal impaction or neoplasms.

The strength of the patient with diarrhea is rapidly spent. Nursing measures should be aimed at rest and eventual replacement of fluids. In acute diarrhea the stomach is kept empty for at least 24 hours to rest it. A soda water enema is sometimes given to remove irritating substances from the lower intestinal tract. Oral feeding, once it is allowed, consists of liquids at first, progressing gradually to more solid foods.

The practical nurse is responsible for noting and recording on the patient's chart the number of stools per day and the characteristics of the feces; that is, the color, consistency, and odor of the stool each time the patient has a bowel movement. If the stools are frequent and extremely watery, the patient can become dehydrated very rapidly. If symptoms of dehydration appear they should be reported to the nurse in charge or to the patient's physician.

Chronic diarrhea is usually accompanied by anemia because there is often loss of blood with the frequent stools. Food passing through the intestinal tract too rapidly cannot be properly digested and absorbed, and so malnutrition may also be present. The treatment in these cases consists of a bland diet, with vitamins and minerals added to help maintain good nutrition. Diarrheic patients are frequently nervous and embarrassed by their condition. The practical nurse can help these patients by maintaining a calm and dignified manner, providing a restful environment with privacy, and encouraging them to relax.

Constipation. When defining constipation we must remember that frequency of bowel movements is not the only criterion. For some individuals a daily bowel movement is normal; for others with different eating habits, body build or variance in physical activity, a bowel movement every three days may be normal. If the stools are extremely hard and dry or difficult to pass from the rectum, then the term constipation can be applied. Other symptoms include nausea, headache and feeling of fullness in the lower abdominal and rectal area.

Treatment of constipation depends on its cause. Good eating habits, establishment of a routine for evacuation and adequate exercise are all important in the prevention of constipation. Mild laxatives or enemas may be used to relieve occasional constipation, but a chronic condition in which there is incomplete or inadequate evacuation of the bowels requires medical attention to determine the cause. Obstructions in the intestines producing constipation can be caused by hernias, malignant or benign tumors and strictures. Decreased peristalsis due to disorders of the colon also can cause constipation.

Urinary Retention. In this condition urine is retained in the urinary bladder instead of being voided periodically. It is not to be confused with urinary suppression in which the kidneys fail to produce urine. A variety of conditions can cause urinary retention, such as emotional upsets, infections, inflammations, and stricture or compression of the urethra.

Under normal circumstances urination should take place several times a day with a total of 1000 to 1500 ml. of urine being voided during a 24-hour period. When the bladder cannot be emptied it becomes distended and the patient experiences extreme discomfort.

Nursing measures to induce voiding include placing the patient's hands in water, pouring warm water over the perineal area, and helping the patient to relax. It is also necessary that the patient is assured of privacy while he is attempting to void. For the male patient it is helpful to have him stand by the side of the bed to use the urinal when he cannot walk to the bathroom. Catheterization is a last resort to be used only when other measures fail to help the patient who has difficulty in voiding. No matter how carefully the procedure may be carried out, there is always the danger of introducing bacteria into the urinary tract when a catheter is inserted.

ACID-BASE BALANCE

Normally the body maintains a very delicate balance between acids and bases (alkalies) in the body fluids. This is done through complex chemical reactions that involve three major buffer systems. These buffers help regulate hydrogen ion concentrations, and in so doing, control the acid-base balance. Even slight changes in the chemical reactions in the cells can cause some reactions to speed up and others to slow down. These chemical reactions are vital to the life of the cell and occur in all organs of the body. When the chemical processes of the cells of an organ are accelerated or depressed the functions of the organs are similarly affected.

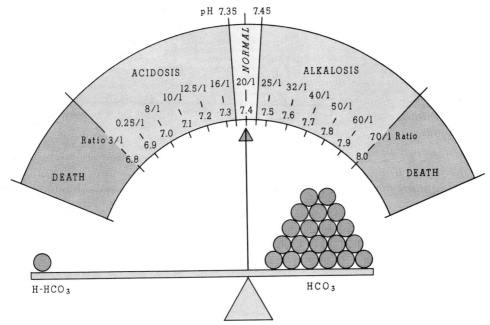

Carbonic acid in a ratio of 1:20 with bicarbonate salt
maintains a normal body pH

Figure 3-3. Acidosis and alkalosis showing ratio between carbonic acid and bicarbonate ion. (From Jacob and Francone: *Structure and Function in Man.* W. B. Saunders Co., Philadelphia.)

A shift in acid-base balance can present a variety of symptoms, ranging from mild to severe or even fatal reactions. In general, it is found that the patient with uncontrolled *acidosis* will die in coma, and the patient with uncontrolled *alkalosis* will die of tetany or convulsions.

Acidosis. A shift of the body fluids toward acidity produces the condition known as *acidosis.* Such a condition can occur in uncontrolled diabetes mellitus and starvation *(metabolic acidosis)*, or in respiratory disorders which interfere with adequate release of carbon dioxide from the lungs and thereby cause an accumulation of carbonic acid in the blood *(respiratory acidosis).*

Symptoms of acidosis include dyspnea with deep, periodic breathing, a sweet-smelling odor of fruit on the breath, disorientation, coma and eventually death if the condition is not treated. Symptoms are relieved by the administration of sodium bicarbonate or sodium lactate orally or intravenously. Treatment is aimed at controlling the condition causing the acidosis.

Alkalosis. The opposite of acidosis is *alkalosis* in which there are excess alkaline substances in the body fluids. Alkalosis can be caused by excessive vomiting or improper use of a gastric suction apparatus and by hyperventilation, when an individual breathes too rapidly. Symptoms include shallow respiration, a tingling sensation in the fingers, toes and lips, muscular cramps, tetany and convulsion. Respiratory alkalosis is relieved by administering carbon dioxide by mask, breathing into a paper bag, or holding one's breath. Severe alkalosis requires removal of its underlying cause.

CONVULSIONS

A convulsion or seizure is an attack of uncontrollable muscular contractions. Generally, there are three types of convulsion: (1) *tonic*, in which there is continued contraction of all muscles; (2) *clonic*, in which there is alternate contraction and relaxation of the muscles, giving the body a jerking motion; and (3) *jacksonian seizures*, in which the muscular twitching begins in one area and spreads to other parts of the body.

These attacks of uncontrollable muscular contractions may appear in many diseases. The most common ones are epilepsy, infectious diseases in which there are extremely high temperatures, tetanus, uremia, and brain injuries.

It is very important that the practical nurse be aware of the possibility that the patient may hurt himself during a convulsion. She must remain with the patient during the convulsion in order to observe him and to help protect him from injury. The bed should be fitted with side rails and the head of the bed well padded with a pillow or folded bath blanket. A tongue depressor padded with gauze should be at the bedside. This is placed between the patient's teeth to prevent biting the tongue or the inside of the mouth when the strong jaw muscles contract. No effort should be made to pry open the mouth, as this may loosen the patient's teeth. If the patient having the convulsion was not in his bed, but was up and had fallen to the floor during the seizure, no attempts should be made to move him during the seizure. The only choice then is to protect the patient from injury as much as possible, making sure that his head is placed on a pillow or blanket so that he does not injure the skull during the convulsion. No restraint should be used.

The following observations should be made during the convulsion and reported in detail on the patient's chart or directly to the nurse or doctor in charge.

1. When convulsion began and length of time it lasted.
2. Type of convulsion, whether tonic, clonic, or jacksonian.
3. Area of the body in which the con-

vulsion began and whether it was restricted to one particular part or was generalized over the entire body.

4. If the patient lost consciousness or was incontinent of urine or feces.

5. Effect of convulsion on the pulse and respiration of the patient.

6. Changes in skin color and whether or not there was profuse perspiration.

7. Any complaints the patient may have had before or after the convulsion.

DELIRIUM

The delirious patient is confused and disoriented as to place and time. Because of disturbances in the nerve cells of the brain he may suffer from delusions and hallucination, and he cannot act rationally until the delirium subsides. Fortunately, delirium is usually only temporary and can be relieved when the underlying cause is eliminated. Conditions that can produce delirium include infectious diseases which are accompanied by high fevers, alcoholism (*delirium tremens*) and drug addiction.

The nursing care of the delirious patient is primarily concerned with protecting the patient from harm and avoiding circumstances in his environment which may stimulate the brain and excite him. While delirium is present someone should remain with the patient to prevent him from injuring himself. Restraints should be used only when absolutely necessary as they may disturb the patient and increase his restlessness. One must be careful about windows and doors which the patient may try to use as a means of escape during his confusion.

Bright lights, noises and sudden movements of persons around the patient can serve as stimuli which aggravate the delirium and give rise to delusions. Conversation in the patient's presence should be kept at a minimum because of the possibility of his mis-interpreting what he hears, but the nurse should always explain in a calm voice what she is going to do for the patient and why it is being done. One must avoid arguing with a delirious person. It is often helpful to remind him where he is and who is caring for him, thus assisting him in orienting himself. Finally, an attitude of sympathy and understanding on the part of the nurse can help relieve the patient's anxiety. He cannot control his behavior and no amount of reprimanding or so-called disciplinary measures will relieve his unhappy situation. In fact, such practices will only further confuse and upset him.

INCONTINENCE

The patient who is unable to control his functions of elimination presents many physical and emotional problems for himself as well as for those who must care for him. We do not mean to imply that improvement of the situation is impossible, though at times it may appear so. If there is to be any progress made, it is necessary that the nurse begin with a positive attitude and discourage feelings of hopelessness on the part of the patient and his family. Once the nurse has convinced herself and the patient that something can be done she has already begun to do something about the problem. Since there are many different causes of incontinence, the next step is to try to determine why the patient cannot control the passage of feces and/or urine. If the incontinence is a result of trauma to the nerve pathways or muscular deficiencies in which there is no possibility of removing the cause or remedying the original condition, some type of permanent appliance or receptacle should be used. The use of these in specific diseases and surgical procedures will be discussed more fully later in the text.

All nursing measures will be aimed

at keeping the patient clean, odorless, and dry. A bit of imagination and use of waterproof materials available can help in improving ways of protecting the patient's clothing and bed linens. A regularity in routine of eating and elimination can also prevent episodes of embarrassment to the patient. It is rare that the first thing tried will work well and those easily discouraged will soon sink into despair. If, however, the nurse can imagine herself in the patient's place and try to appreciate how the family must feel, she will persist until her patient is at least more comfortable and socially acceptable.

JAUNDICE

Jaundice is a symptom, *not* a disease, and is the result of increased accumulation of bile pigments in the blood. To say that a patient has jaundice is similar to saying that he has nausea or dyspnea. Jaundice may be due to an obstruction of the flow of bile from the liver through the ducts to the gallbladder and intestines, to inability of the liver to clear normal amounts of bilirubin from the blood, or to increased destruction of red blood cells with the degradation of hemoglobin and release of bile pigments.

The patient who is jaundiced has a yellowish cast to his skin and the whites of his eyes. He may experience severe itching over his entire body as a result of deposits of crystals on his skin. He may suffer from mental confusion and extreme irritability. Because the liver is concerned with the production of vitamin K, many patients with jaundice have a pronounced tendency to bleed readily because of impaired formation of blood clots. In obstructive types of jaundice the urine will be dark from bile pigments excreted by the kidney, and the stools light or clay-colored because of decreased amounts or absence of bile pigments normally in feces.

Nursing care includes skin care to relieve itching. This means frequent sponge baths with a starch or vinegar solution, followed by application of calamine lotion. The patient is watched closely for signs of bleeding internally or externally and any changes in his condition should be reported immediately so that hemorrhage can be averted. The patient's environment should be nonstimulating with avoidance of bright lights, noises or other stimuli which can aggravate his irritability.

PAIN

Pain is such a universal symptom, common to so many diseases, that it is difficult to be specific in regard to the physical illnesses it accompanies. Individuals vary in their response to pain and what might be simply annoying to one person will be unbearable to another. Emotions also affect the degree of tolerance to pain. The patient who is mentally at ease will suffer less from discomfort than one who is emotionally disturbed and fearful. The practical nurse must guard against an air of indifference to pain in others and she should make no judgment as to its severity. Pain is a warning signal of distress within the body; the decision of whether it is real or not real rests with the physician.

In a sense, pain can be advantageous; in fact, we would have fewer people remaining ignorant of the early stages of disease if pain were always present at the beginning of an illness. Cancer rarely causes pain in its first stages of development and this is, of course, unfortunate, because by the time pain has entered into the clinical picture there is usually very little that can be done to cure the patient of cancer.

The extent and type of pain are sometimes difficult to evaluate. The physician depends on the nurse for intelligent, objective reporting of the patient's complaints. The exact words used by the patient in describing his discomfort will be most helpful to the doctor without added opinions and interpretations by the nurse. If the patient describes his pain as a "sharp, stabbing pain that doesn't go away," this is all that should be reported. It is not necessary that the practical nurse add her observations that the patient doesn't really appear to have as much pain as he says he has, *unless* the physician specifically asks for her opinion. This might be done in cases of potential addiction, or control of pain with gradually diminishing doses of a drug.

The problem of addiction in patients is one which the physician must constantly guard against. The nurse can assist the physician in the prevention of addiction by doing all she can to make her patient comfortable with simple nursing measures, and by reassuring her patient and providing him with moral support during his illness.

CLINICAL CASE PROBLEMS

1. A 3-month-old infant is admitted to the pediatric ward with fever and dehydration. The doctor has ordered temperature measures for a fever of 102°F. or over. Before admission the infant had convulsions as a result of the extremely high body temperature.

What specific nursing measures would you use to lower the infant's temperature?
If the infant convulses while you are caring for him what should you do?
How could vomiting and diarrhea cause this infant's severe dehydration?

2. A 68-year-old woman is admitted to the hospital with a diagnosis of uremia. She has edema of the extremities and is apparently semiconscious. She is also incontinent and though she has a very scanty output, the urine is extremely foul-smelling.

What special care must this patient be given to prevent decubitus ulcers?
What can you do about the incontinence to keep the patient clean and dry?
What special observations should you make if you have been told the patient is likely to have convulsions?

REFERENCES

1. Beland, I. L.: *Clinical Nursing: Pathophysical and Psychosocial Approaches.* New York, The Macmillan Co., 1965.
2. Brunner, L. S., et al.: *Textbook of Medical-Surgical Nursing.* Philadelphia, J. B. Lippincott Co., 1964.
3. Fuerst, C. V., and Wolff, L. V.: *Fundamentals of Nursing.* Philadelphia, J. B. Lippincott Co., 1956.
4. Guyton, A. C.: *Textbook of Medical Physiology.* Philadelphia, W. B. Saunders Co., 1966.
5. Harmer, B., and Henderson, V.: *Textbook of the Principles and Practice of Nursing,* 5th edition. New York, The Macmillan Co., 1960.
6. Healy, E. A., and McGurk, W.: "Effectiveness and Acceptance of Nurses' Notes." Nurs. Outlook, March, 1966, p. 32.
7. Jacob, S. W., and Francone, C. A.: *Structure and Function in Man.* Philadelphia, W. B. Saunders Co., 1966.
8. Montag, M. L., and Swenson, R. S.: *Fundamentals in Nursing Care,* 3rd edition. Philadelphia, W. B. Saunders Co., 1959.
9. Phelps, E. T.: "Fever, Its Causes and Effects." Am. Journ. Nurs., March, 1956, p. 319.
10. "Pointers on Measuring Blood Pressure." RN, May, 1962, p. 75.
11. Shafer, K. N., et al.: *Medical-Surgical Nursing,* 4th edition. St. Louis, Mo., C. V. Mosby Co., 1966.
12. Smith, D. W., and Gips, C. D.: *Care of the Adult Patient.* Philadelphia, J. B. Lippincott Co., 1966.

SUGGESTED STUDENT READING

1. Cunningham, L. S.: "What Are You Noting?" Journ. Pract. Nurs., Oct., 1964, p. 28
2. "Pointers on Measuring Blood Pressure." RN, May, 1962, p. 75.
3. Seide, D.: "Answering Your Questions about Hypertension." RN, July, 1960, p. 50.

OUTLINE FOR CHAPTER 3

I. Introduction

A. Nurse must develop good habits of observation, sound knowledge of usual course of various illnesses and good judgment in reporting of observations.

B. Symptoms are signs of an illness or a

change in the progress of disease.
1. Subjective symptoms—patient must tell about these.
2. Objective symptoms—those that can be determined by examination and observation.

II. Common Symptoms: Those Likely to Be Present in a Variety of Illnesses

A. Temperature—disorders include fever and chills.

B. Pulse—disorders include tachycardia, or increased heart beat, and bradycardia, or decreased heart beat. Other abnormalities may be those of volume.

C. Respiration—controlled by the respiratory center in the brain, nerve impulses and chemical composition of the blood. Disorders include dyspnea and Cheynes-Stokes respiration.

D. Blood pressure—the degree of pressure of blood volume against the arterial walls. Disorders include hypertension (high blood pressure) and hypotension (low blood pressure).

III. Fluid and Electrolyte Balance

A. Body fluids.
1. Plasma water—within the vascular system.
2. Interstitial fluid or tissue fluid—in the tissue spaces between cells.
3. Intracellular fluid—within the cells.

B. Electrolytes—substances dissolved in the body fluids. They are capable of conducting electric current and are vital to normal functioning of body cells.

C. Disturbances in fluid balance—overhydration or edema, and dehydration or deficiency of fluid.

IV. Disorders of Elimination

A. Faulty elimination can lead to accumulation of toxic substances in the body.

B. Nausea and vomiting may produce dehydration and electrolyte loss.

C. Diarrhea prevents adequate absorption of nutrients and water from the digestive tract; produces deficiency of water and nutrients.

D. Constipation—treatment depends on cause.

E. Urinary retention leads to bladder distention and discomfort.

V. Acid-Base Balance

A. Actually a regulation of hydrogen ion concentration in body fluids. A shift in the balance produces changes in the functions of cells and organs.

B. Acidosis—a shift toward acidity often seen in uncontrolled diabetes mellitus and lung disorders.

C. Alkalosis—an excess of alkaline substances in the blood caused by excessive vomiting or hyperventilation.

VI. Convulsions

A. Are seizures of uncontrollable muscular contractions. Types include tonic, clonic and jacksonian.

B. Nursing care includes intelligent observation and protection of the patient from injury.

C. Frequently associated with epilepsy and with high fevers in children.

VII. Delirium (Mental Confusion and Disorientation)

A. Protection of patient and providing a non-stimulating environment are important factors in nursing care.

B. Often accompanies high fevers, alcoholism and drug addiction.

VIII. Incontinence (Inability to Control Functions of Elimination)

A. Nurse must approach problem with a positive attitude.

B. Keep patient clean, odorless and dry.

IX. Pain (Extreme Discomfort)

A. Nurse evaluates patient's pain on the basis of what he tells her.

B. Those in pain need sympathetic understanding.

X. Jaundice

A. It is a symptom rather than a disease; the result of increased bile pigments in the blood.

B. May be due to (1) obstruction of the flow of bile from liver to intestines, (2) inability of liver cells to clear bilirubin from blood, or (3) increased destruction of red blood cells with degradation of hemoglobin.

C. Symptoms include yellowing of the skin and white of the eyes. In obstructive type the stools are clay-colored and the urine is dark.

D. Nursing care includes skin care to relieve itching (use starch baths or calamine lotion), observation for bleeding and provision of a quiet environment.

Chapter 4

DIAGNOSIS OF ILLNESS

VOCABULARY

Antibiotic	Meninges
Atom	Oxidation
Cauterize	Radiopaque
Element	Virulent
Fulguration	

INTRODUCTION

The diagnosing of illness has always presented a challenge to the physician. It is the very cornerstone of medical practice, for once the diagnosis has been made, the course of treatment will be comparatively clear. The word "diagnosis" is derived from two Greek words: *dia* — through, and *gnosis* — knowing or recognition. Thus the word implies an ability to see through and detect facts not easily determined. In primitive times man resorted to witchcraft and superstitious practices in an effort to explain the symptoms of illness. When the modern physician diagnoses an illness, he is still seeking the "demons of illness," but he has the advantages of many instruments and laboratory tests to aid him in his search. In the past few decades the use of laboratory tests as aids to diagnosis has become increasingly important and it is expected that in future years the medical team will become more dependent on the chemist, physicist, and radiologist in the battle against disease and illness.

PURPOSES OF SPECIAL DIAGNOSTIC TESTS

The physician uses information from laboratory tests in several ways: (1) As a method of determining the patient's general physical condition. Most patients will receive a complete blood count and urinalysis as a part of the initial examination in the physician's office or hospital because abnormal findings in the blood and urine are common to many diseases. (2) As a means of determining the cause of disease, e.g., cultures grown in the laboratory to isolate the causative organism. (3) As a verification of the diagnosis the physician may have already suspected from other findings. An example would be the glucose tolerance test, which, if positive, would indicate the presence of diabetes. (4) As a guide to the physician in his method of treating a certain disease. Anticoagulant drugs such as Dicumarol, for example, are given only after the prothrombin time of the patient has been determined. This is done daily

39

before each dose is ordered so that the physician can adjust his treatment according to the progress of the patient.

It is sometimes confusing to the practical nurse when she finds an order for collection of a specimen from one system of the body as a diagnostic test for quite a different organ or system. A tubeless gastric analysis, for instance, requires that specimens of urine be gathered at intervals even though this test measures the presence of free hydrochloric acid in the stomach. Urine samples may also be taken for tests done to obtain information about liver function. This is not too surprising, however, when we remember that all organs of the body are interdependent and interrelated and the physician interprets the various findings in relation to the *total* physical condition of his patient.

RESPONSIBILITIES OF THE NURSE

Although the diagnosis of illness is the responsibility of the physician, the nurse is expected to assist him in his search for reasons for the patient's symptoms.

The general physical examination is a routine preliminary to diagnosis and treatment. The practical nurse learns to assist the physician with the physical examination early in her training because it is a basic procedure in nursing. She learns the proper draping, positioning, and reassurance of the patient during the physical examination and the instruments the physician generally uses.

Special diagnostic tests are an equally important part of diagnosis and the practical nurse should understand her responsibilities in this area. Generally she is expected to: (1) prepare the patient and bring the necessary equipment to the bedside; (2) label the specimens accurately and be sure they are sent to the proper laboratory promptly, with accompanying information sheet as required by the laboratory; and (3)

collect specimens as required by the test.

Of all the nursing duties and responsibilities, none can be more exacting or more demanding than the proper preparation of a patient for diagnostic tests and the conscientious follow-through of the procedure to its completion. A spinal tap for diagnostic laboratory work cannot be considered finished until the specimen of spinal fluid has been placed safely in the laboratory technician's hands; a glucose tolerance test is not completed until the last specimen of urine has been collected, labeled, and taken to the laboratory. When there are several departments of the hospital involved in a procedure there is sometimes a tendency to let someone else worry about the details. This is inexcusable, however, and the practical nurse assisting with any diagnostic procedures must understand her responsibilities and accept them as she should.

BACTERIOLOGICAL STUDIES

In some instances it is necessary for the physician to know exactly what particular organism is causing a disease. In order to do this, fluid from the infected area of the body must be collected and taken to the laboratory. There the technician encourages the growth of the organism by placing it in circumstances favorable to its growth. This carefully controlled nourishing and growing of the organism is called "culturing." Since the organisms must be alive and able to reproduce when they reach the laboratory extreme care must be taken that the specimen collected for a culture is promptly sent to the laboratory. Care must also be taken that the organisms from sources other than the specimen do not get into the container used for collecting the specimen. The following rules must be strictly adhered to in the collection of body excretions intended for culture in the laboratory:

1. Use containers which are sterile and not cracked or broken.

2. Use standard tubes from the laboratory and collect the specimen directly into the tube when possible.

3. Keep inside of tube and stopper of tube free from contamination.

4. Do not use cotton plugs unless absolutely necessary. Cork stoppers are best. If cotton plugs are used they must not be allowed to become wet, either from the contents of the tube or from outside liquids.

5. Place plugs firmly in place, rotating them in a clockwise manner, after the specimen has been collected.

6. Be careful that the material is not spilled outside the container. If such material is spilled, report this immediately and determine from the laboratory technician what antiseptic should be used to destroy the organisms. Warn others of the spilled material and clean the area thoroughly as soon as possible.

7. Containers should not be filled more than halfway.

8. Containers must be kept in an upright position after specimen is collected and should be taken to the laboratory at once. Avoid shaking the container.[2]

URINALYSIS

The term "routine urinalysis" usually means the examination of a single specimen of urine collected after one voiding and under conditions of cleanliness. The amount of urine needed is usually 60 to 100 ml. (cc.), and the specimen should be fresh when examined. The doctor usually prefers that urine specimens be collected in the morning after a night's sleep. This is particularly true if the patient is an out-patient. In this case the practical nurse should inform the patient of the doctor's wishes in regard to the time the specimen is to be collected and the time it should be brought to the office or clinic.

The composition of normal urine may vary from time to time; this is an indication of good kidney function and is no cause for alarm. However, abnormal substances in the urine are an indication of disease. These ab-

Table 3. *Abnormal Constituents of Urine*

SUBSTANCE PRESENT	CONDITIONS INDICATED
1. Blood	Damage to tissues somewhere along the urinary tract.
2. Pus cells	Infection in the urinary system
3. Bacteria or other infectious organisms	Local infection of bladder or urinary tract
4. Proteins, mainly albumin	Kidney disease involving the glomeruli, hypertension, severe heart failure, toxic conditions or abnormal proteins in the blood
5. Acetone	Diabetes mellitus, ketosis accompanying starvation
6. Sugar	Diabetes mellitus or some other metabolic disorder
7. Bile	Obstruction of bile ducts from liver or gallbladder, or liver disease which interferes with normal bile removal

normal constituents include: (1) numerous red cells, (2) pus cells, (3) bacteria, (4) albumin, (5) sugar, (6) acetone, and (7) bile (see Table 3).

ANALYSIS OF BLOOD

The progress of medical science in its search for causes and effects of disease would be seriously hampered without the help of blood tests. We sometimes think of these tests as part of a dull routine but they must be considered among the greatest achievements of medical research. It is believed that in future years we will be able to examine the body fluids and detect diseases long before any other symptoms become apparent. Imagine what this would mean in terms of disease prevention and treatment of conditions such as cancer in the earliest stages!

The most common test done on the blood is the *cell count*. The red cells and white cells are counted in a sampling of blood and recorded in numbers per cubic millimeter (1/1000 of a cubic centimeter). A *differential* white count determines the number of various kinds of white cells present in the sampling of blood (see Fig. 4-1).

HEMOGLOBIN. Hemoglobin is a chemical compound of protein and iron. It is responsible for carrying oxygen in the blood and is the substance which gives red blood cells their color. A determination of the amount of hemoglobin in the red cells is important in the diagnosis of certain anemias. The normal range for hemoglobin is 14 gm. per 100 ml. of blood for women and 16 gm. for men. If, however, hemoglobin is recorded in percentage, the normal is considered to be from 80 to 100 per cent.

PLATELETS. Platelets are cells necessary for the clotting of blood. They are minute particles suspended in the blood and are much smaller than red blood cells. Information about the quantity of platelets in the blood is important in the treatment of diseases affecting, or affected by, the clotting of blood.

HEMATOCRIT. Hematocrit is a test done to measure the volume of cells

Figure 4-1. Various types of leukocytes that are counted and recorded in a *differential white cell count*. *A*, Lymphocyte. *B*, Monocyte. *C*, *D*, and *E*, Granulocytes. *C*, Neutrophile. *D*, Eosinophile. *E*, Basophile. (From Manner: *Elements of Anatomy and Physiology*, W. B. Saunders Co., Philadelphia.)

in relation to the volume of plasma. When there has been a loss of body fluids but no cell loss (as in dehydration) the cell volume is high in proportion to the amount of liquid (plasma). On the other hand, when either hemorrhage or anemia has depleted the supply of cells, the blood is "thinned" and the hematocrit or cell volume is low.

CLOTTING TIME (COAGULATION TIME). Clotting time is a test to measure the ability of the blood to form a clot (coagulate) in a given period of time. Naturally a prolonged clotting time indicates a danger of hemorrhage. There are some diseases in which there is a deficiency of one or more of the essential factors in clotting. In these diseases a knowledge of the patient's clotting time can be of great importance. The normal range for clotting time depends on the method used for testing. Ten to 25 minutes is a normal range for one test, whereas one to five minutes is normal in another test.

PROTHROMBIN TIME. In the formation of a clot, prothrombin is converted to thrombin. If the prothrombin level is very low the clot will form much more slowly than normal. The diseases most commonly associated with a low level of prothrombin are liver diseases and vitamin K deficiency. There are times, however, when the physician wishes to slow down the clotting process of the blood and he uses an anticoagulant drug such as Dicumarol to achieve this. Hampering clotting is sometimes done in the treatment of diseases in which there is a pathological formation of clots and one or more have lodged in the openings of vital blood vessels. In these patients the physician usually orders a daily prothrombin time before he orders an anticoagulant drug to be given. He will observe closely the level of prothrombin and attempt to keep the prothrombin level at 20 to 30 per cent of normal. The normal is considered to be 100 per cent.

BILIRUBIN. This substance is always present in the blood in small amounts because it is an end product of the breakdown of red cells. Our bodies are continuously manufacturing new red cells and breaking down and excreting the worn-out cells. We can expect, then, that there will always be some bilirubin in the blood stream as long as our bodies are performing this function. In fact, the yellow color of bile is chiefly due to the presence of the pigment bilirubin, which has been removed from the blood by the liver and excreted in the bile.

If, however, there is an excessive destruction of red cells, or if the liver becomes so diseased that it cannot handle a normal amount of bilirubin, this yellow pigment reaches a high level in the blood stream. When this happens the skin and mucous membranes of the body take on a yellowish cast and the patient is said to have *jaundice.* The purpose of doing a laboratory test is to determine the level of bilirubin in the blood stream before it gets high enough to produce jaundice.

UREA NITROGEN. This is another substance normally present in the blood in small amounts. The end product of protein metabolism is urea and the body rids itself of this waste product by way of the kidneys. We can conclude then that if an excessive amount of urea is present in the blood it is an indication that the kidneys are not functioning as they should. It is also a warning that certain tissues of the body are being exposed to damaging toxic substances. For example, urea affects the brain and nervous system in such a way that the nurse might expect a patient with a high blood urea nitrogen level to be extremely irritable, confused, and subject to convulsions. She will then be prepared for these symptoms and plan her nursing care accordingly.

BROMSULPHALEIN TEST. Another blood test used to determine the function of a specific organ is the *Brom-*

Table 4. *Blood Tests*

TEST	NORMAL RANGE	INCREASED IN	DECREASED IN
Red cell count	4,000,000 to 5,000,000 per cu. mm.	Severe dehydration, polycythemia	Anemia, hemorrhage
White cell count	5000 to 9000 per cu. mm.	Infections	Blood dyscrasias, drug poisoning
Hemoglobin	12 to 16 gm. per 100 cc. of blood 80 to 100% of normal	Same as increased R.B.C.	Anemias
Platelet count	200,000 to 500,000 per cu. mm.	Polycythemia, fractures	Thrombocytopenic purpura, aplastic anemias
Hematocrit	35 to 50 mm./100 cc. of blood	Dehydration, polycythemia	Anemias, after hemorrhage
Clotting time	Depends on type of test used, usually 3 to 7 min.	Longer in hemophilia	
Prothrombin time	70 to 100% of control		Liver disease and vitamin K deficiency, anticoagulant therapy
Bilirubin	0.1 to 1.0 mg./100 cc. of serum	Excessive destruction of red blood cells, liver disease	
Urea nitrogen (B.U.N.)	9 to 17 mg./100 cc. of whole blood	Certain kidney diseases	
Bromsulphalein	Less than 0.4 mg. of B.S.P. per 100 cc. of serum	Liver disease	
Sedimentation rate	Up to 20 mm. per hour	Infections, cell destruction	
Glucose	80 to 120 mg. per 100 cc. of blood	Diabetes, chronic liver disease, some metabolic diseases	
Chlorides	350 to 390 mg. per 100 cc. of serum	Some kidney disorders	Excessive vomiting and diarrhea.
Potassium	16 to 22 mg. per 100 cc. of serum	Cell damage and destruction	Severe diarrhea and diuresis, some kidney disorders
Sodium	315 to 355 mg. per 100 cc. of serum	Inadequate water intake	Diarrhea, heat exhaustion, Addison's disease

sulphalein (B.S.P.) *retention test.* Brom-sulphalein is a dye which under normal conditions is removed from the blood by the liver. If, after injection of the dye, there remains a large amount of the dye in the blood, it is assumed that the liver is not functioning properly. Some hypersensitive individuals may have a serious reaction to the dye; therefore an ampule of Adrenalin and a syringe for its administration should be readily available when the B.S.P. test is done.

SEDIMENTATION RATE. This is a test which measures the length of time it takes the red cells in a sample of whole blood to separate from the plasma and settle to the bottom of a glass test tube. The blood cells of a person suffering from infectious diseases and some other diseases, such as rheumatic fever and arthritis, will settle more rapidly than those of a normal person. This test is used frequently in determining the progress or regression of a disease and is used as an index to the success of treatment rather than specifically for diagnosis.

Chemical Substances in the Blood

Glucose is a sugar normally found in varying amounts in the blood. A marked increase is indicative of a serious metabolic disorder, most commonly diabetes mellitus.

Chloride, potassium, and sodium are essential salts dissolved in blood. They are concerned with maintaining the proper acid-base balance and water balance within the body tissues and fluids. A serious depletion of these essential substances can result in death. Decreases frequently follow excessive vomiting and diarrhea, certain chronic kidney diseases, and heat exhaustion. Increases may be found in conditions of severe cell damage and destruction, and inadequate water intake.

GASTROINTESTINAL CONTENTS

Disturbances of the gastrointestinal system are so common, and symptomatic of such a wide range of diseases, that examination of the stomach contents is one of the most widely used tests. Usually the stomach contents are examined for the amount of free hydrochloric acid present in the morning, before food is taken. If there is a marked increase in acid content, peptic ulcer may be suspected. In advanced carcinoma, pernicious anemia, gastritis, and gallbladder disease there is either a deficiency or total absence of hydrochloric acid. There are times when the physician may wish to rule out or verify his suspicion of bleeding in the intestinal tract even though there have been no vomiting of blood or obvious signs of blood in the stools. Then he will order the collection and laboratory examination of a specimen for *occult* (hidden) *blood*. The stomach contents are sometimes examined for microorganisms such as the tubercle bacillus. The contents of the stomach are aspirated by means of a tube and sent to the laboratory. If a stool specimen is ordered and the patient is unable to defecate, the physician may order a small tap water enema for the purpose of obtaining the specimen.

Parasites or their eggs (ova) are sometimes the object of the search in laboratory examinations of stool specimens. In most cases a "warm" stool specimen, kept at body temperature, is required for successful laboratory tests. Unless otherwise indicated, then, the practical nurse can assume that a stool specimen should be kept warm until delivered to the laboratory. In any case, the specimen should be fresh and brought to the laboratory immediately after collection.

CEREBROSPINAL FLUID

The cerebrospinal fluid circulates over the brain in the ventricles of the brain and through the spinal canal. It

Figure 4-2. *A*, The nurse positions the patient for a lumbar puncture and assists the physician by holding the patient in this position. *B*, The physician measures the pressure of the spinal fluid by attaching a manometer to the needle inserted into the spinal cavity. *C*, The nurse holds one culture tube while the physician collects sample of spinal fluid in another tube. (From Slosberg: Journal of Practical Nursing, October, 1965.)

surrounds the meninges and aids in protecting these structures by cushioning them against shocks. Normally the spinal fluid is clear and colorless. Its pressure of 5 to 7 mm. of mercury maintains optimal pressure within the cranial cavity.

Samples of cerebrospinal fluid are obtained through a lumbar or cisternal puncture (see Fig. 4-2). (See Chapter 18 for more information about these procedures.) Examinations of the fluid samples, especially cell counts and bacterial studies, must be done as quickly as possible, so there should be no delay in getting them to the laboratory after they are collected. All specimens obtained must be handled with extreme care to avoid contamination of the fluid and also to avoid self-contamination, since many infectious diseases involving the spinal fluid are caused by a highly virulent organism.

An increase in cerebrospinal fluid pressure may indicate brain tumor, hemorrhage or infection within the cranial cavity. In cases of obstruction of the flow of spinal fluid in the spinal canal, the pressure remains normal or decreases below the point of obstruction and increases above that point. Examples of disorders that can produce such an obstruction include tumors, blood clots and severance of the spinal cord.

ANALYSIS OF SPUTUM

Sputum refers to the liquid material brought up from the lungs by coughing.

Table 5. *Typical Spinal Fluid Findings**

CONDITION	WBC	RBC	TOTAL PROTEIN	GLUCOSE	COLLOIDAL-GOLD TEST	SEROLOGY
Normal	0-5	0	20-40 mg. 100 ml.	60-80% of blood glucose	0000000000-0	Neg.
Bacterial infection	200 or more (polys)	0	Elevated	Lowered	Not done	Not done
Viral infection	100 or more (lymphs)	0	Normal to slightly elevated	Normal	Not done	Not done
Tuberculous infection	50-100 (lymphs)	0	Elevated	Lowered	Not done	Not done
CNS syphilis	10-60 (lymphs)	0	Normal to slightly elevated	Normal	Luetic: 0123100000-0 Paretic: 5555542100-0	Pos.
Multiple sclerosis	0-5	0	Normal to slightly elevated	Normal	5555542100-0	Neg.
Tumor	Normal	0	Elevated	Normal	Not done	Not done
Hemorrhage	Influenced by mixture with blood		Markedly elevated, owing to presence of blood	Not accurate, owing to presence of blood	Not done	Not done

*From French: Nurses' Guide to Diagnostic Procedures, 2nd edition. Copyright McGraw-Hill, Inc., 1967. Used by permission of Dr. Charles Poser.

Table 6. *Some Common Laboratory Tests*

NAME OF TEST	SPECIMEN USED	PREPARATION OF PATIENT	NORMAL RANGE	REMARKS
Carbon dioxide (CO_2) combining power	Blood	No special preparation necessary	52-58 vol/100 ml. serum (22-30 mEq./liter)	Elevated in alkalosis, decreased in acidosis
Cephalin flocculation (Hanger's test)	Serum	Patient must be fasting	Negative to 2 plus	A rough measure of serum proteins; gives an estimate of liver cell function
Colloidal gold	Cerebrospinal fluid	No special prep	No change in color; negative curve	Useful in diagnosis of multiple sclerosis
Coombs' test: indirect	Blood, especially cord blood	No special prep	Negative for antibodies	Used in studies of acquired hemolytic anemias and in testing for anticipated erythroblastosis
direct	Blood serum	No special prep	Negative for antibodies	Used in transfusion crossmatching and in testing maternal serum for anti-Rh antibodies
Fishberg's concentration	Urine to be collected at 10:00 and 11:00 a.m.	Patient must have no food or water from the evening meal at 6:00 p.m. until after the test the following morning	Specific gravity of 1.020 or greater	In the absence of diabetes mellitus a specific gravity of less than 1.020 indicates impairment of kidney function

Table 6. *Some Common Laboratory Tests* (Continued)

NAME OF TEST	SPECIMEN USED	PREPARATION OF PATIENT	NORMAL RANGE	REMARKS
Glucose tolerance	Blood and urine specimens are obtained 30 minutes before ingestion of glucose, and every hour from 4 to 5 hours	Patient must be fasting. Water is allowed during the test but no food may be taken. No smoking is allowed during the test. Exercise is limited	Urine should be negative for sugar; blood sugar should be approx. 80 mg. per 100 ml. at the end of the test	Useful in ruling out diabetes and in diagnosing hyperinsulinism
Nonprotein nitrogen (NPN)	Blood	No special prep	15-30 mg./100 ml. of blood	Elevated levels are present in kidney disease, urinary retention or suppression
Protein-bound iodine (PHI)	Blood	Iodine is restricted from the diet for 3 days prior to the test. This includes restriction of the intake of iodized salt	5-8 mg./100 ml. of serum	Serves as a source of information about thyroid function since iodine is essential to the synthesis of thyroxin. Increased levels indicate impaired thyroid function.
Phenolsulphonphthalein (PSP)	Urine specimens collected 15 minutes, 1 and 2 hours after injection of dye	Patient may have light breakfast and one glass of water, but no coffee or tea	40 to 60% excretion 1st hour; and an additional 20 to 25% 2nd hour	Poor excretion indicates kidney damage.
Van den Bergh's (bilirubin)	Blood	Patient must be fasting	Direct, 0.0 to 0.1 mg./100 ml. serum; indirect, 0.2 to 0.4 mg./100 ml. of serum.	Used as a measure of liver function, since the liver removes bilirubin from the blood; also used in evaluating hemolytic anemias
VDRL	Blood	No special prep	Negative to precipitation due to antigen-antibody reaction.	Used as a screening test to determine the presence of syphilis. If positive, further tests are necessary .

It is *not* the saliva or secretion from the nose and throat and the nurse should explain this fully to her patient when she prepares him for the procedure of collecting a sputum specimen. Unless the doctor orders a 24-hour specimen collected for the purpose of determining the amount as well as the contents of the sputum, the best time to secure a specimen is in the morning before breakfast. Secretions which may have collected in the lungs and bronchi during the night will give the laboratory technician more information. The sputum may be examined for the presence of certain organisms or blood and pus cells.

X-RAY STUDIES

Normal sight depends on the response of the eye to light rays. In order for us to see an object it is necessary for rays of light to be present. We know that ordinary light cannot penetrate some objects of certain density and for this reason we are not able to see beyond or into these objects. When there is a complete absence of light rays we are in total darkness and cannot see "our hands before our faces."

In the year 1895, a German physicist by the name of Roentgen discovered some unusually penetrating rays, which he produced by directing a stream of electrically charged particles onto a metal surface. He did not know nor fully understand how these radiations or rays worked so he called them x-rays ("x" being the symbol for the unknown quantity). As Dr. Roentgen experimented with these rays he found that he could direct them through certain materials and their outline would be left on films placed in back of them.

X-ray films are *negatives*. They are not pictures in the true sense of the word. When the x-rays pass through structures such as skin and fat they do so readily and leave a dark area on the film. If, however, the rays strike a denser structure such as bone, they are slowed down in their progress and will make a much lighter mark on the film. Thus objects of greater density appear lighter on the x-ray film and objects of lesser density appear darker on the film. It is important that this be understood before one can fully realize the importance of removing flatus etc. from the intestinal tract during x-rays of the abdominal area. If flatus or fecal material are present they will cast dark and confusing shadows on the film, making the interpretation of the film difficult for the radiologist.

Hollow tubes and organs such as those in the intestinal tract and urinary system can be filled with barium or very dense radiopaque dyes containing iodine. Following the instillation of the opaque substance, x-ray films are taken. Obstruction from tumors, twisting or kinking, and other abnormalities of the organ can then be readily diagnosed. The normal hollow organ will fill readily and can be outlined on the film, whereas obstruction of a tube or organ will prevent filling beyond that point and the exact location of the difficulty can be pinpointed. This is generally what occurs when a GI series, barium enema, gallbladder series, or pyelogram is done. These specific diagnostic tests are discussed more fully under diseases of their respective systems later in this text.

Fluoroscopy is a method of x-ray in which there are no "still pictures" taken. Fluoroscopy might be compared to a motion picture, whereas x-ray is comparable to a photograph, although neither is a picture in a true sense of the word. During a fluoroscopy the physician can watch a particular organ at work, for example the action of the heart or the flow of barium through the stomach and small intestine (see Fig. 4-3).

Preparation of the Patient for Diagnostic X-ray Films. The nursing procedures necessary for preparing the patient for x-ray will depend on the area being filmed and the purpose of

Although preparation of the patient for a B.M.R. varies slightly in different institutions, it is generally true that the hospitalized patient is to be left undisturbed the morning of the test, and is taken to the laboratory on a stretcher if the apparatus is not to be brought to the bedside. A careful explanation of the need for restriction of food and water intake and limited physical activity during the evening and night before the test should be given to the patient so as to gain his full cooperation. If the patient is not in the hospital, but must travel from his home to the laboratory for the test, he is usually asked to come several hours before the test is given so that he might rest.

In measuring the metabolic rate there is a comparison made between the individual's heat production and the predicted heat production for a person of his age, sex, and body build. The rate is expressed in terms of plus or minus; thus a person with −20 reading has a heat production and oxygen intake 20 per cent lower than would be considered normal for him.

ELECTROCARDIOGRAM (E.K.G.)

An *electrocardiogram* is a means of studying the heart muscle activity by observing the effects of the electric current flowing from the heart. Electric current means the rate of movement of electrical charges through a conductor just as water current refers to the rate of flow of water molecules through a pipe or other conductor.

Activity of the heart muscle generates negative charges of electricity. For an electrocardiogram, electrodes are placed on various parts of the body. These electrodes pick up the electric impulses which are then magnified 3000 times or more and conducted through wires (leads) to a very sensitive needle attached to a graph (see Fig. 4-5). As the impulses cause the needle to vibrate, a recording of the movement is made on a moving paper at the front of the electrocardiograph machine. The tracing made on the paper is called an electrocardiogram. Information obtained by the electrocardiographic tracings includes rhythm of the heart beat, site of the pacemaker of the heart, size of the ventricles, and abnormal currents passing through the heart muscle.

The electrocardiogram is used to diagnose heart disorders that interfere with proper contraction and relaxation of the heart muscle. It cannot always detect potential heart disease or other disorders of the cardiovascular system.

Preparation of the patient ·for an

Figure 4-5. *A*, Standard leads in electrocardiography. *B*, Normal electrocardiogram shows pattern of P, Q, R, S, and T waves in rhythmic cardiac cycle. (From Meltzer: American Journal of Nursing, December, 1965.)

electrocardiogram should include some brief explanation of the way in which the machine works. It is natural for the patient to have some fear of a machine that obviously is concerned with electricity. If he understands that the machine transmits electricity *from* his body and in no way conducts electricity toward him, he will be less apprehensive and more cooperative.

ELECTROENCEPHALOGRAM (E.E.G.)

An *electroencephalogram* is a tracing of the electric impulses from the brain. These impulses, generated by activity of brain tissue, are picked up by electrodes placed on the scalp. A vacuum tube radio amplifier magnifies the electric impulses more than a million times, causing them to move an electromagnetic pen that records the brain waves on the electrograph paper.

The electroencephalogram aids in the diagnosis and treatment of epilepsy, brain tumor, and other diseases of and injury to the brain.

RADIOISOTOPES

In order to understand the use of radioisotopes in diagnosis we must first have some knowledge of the terms used in this relatively new field. The word radioisotope is made up of the words *radioactive* and *isotope*. A radioisotope is an isotope that is radioactive; that is, it gives off "rays" or streams of particles that can be detected by special equipment. Isotopes are different forms of the same element. For example, an isotope of iodine has the same ordinary chemical and physical properties as an atom of iodine, but it differs in the number of neutrons in its nucleus (mass number); it is not exactly the same as an atom of iodine.

Most chemical elements are not radioactive. They possess a balanced ratio of protons to neutrons in their nuclei and do not give off any form of radiation. Those elements (such as radium) which do not have this balanced ratio are said to be unstable. All unstable elements try to achieve stability by altering the ratio of protons to neutrons. They do this by releasing with great energy particles from the nucleus. These particles form the rays which constitute radiation. Elements which are naturally stable and therefore not radioactive can be made unstable by bombarding them with large numbers of free neutrons in a nuclear reactor. Cobalt-59 is a stable, nonradioactive element. When atoms of cobalt-59 are placed in a nuclear reactor some of the atoms will absorb an extra neutron in their nuclei. This upsets the atom's balanced ratio of protons to neutrons, and each atom so altered becomes cobalt-60, a radioactive isotope of cobalt-59.

A radioisotope behaves in the body in the same way as its nonradioactive counterpart. This means it follows the same metabolic pathways and is concentrated in the same organs and tissues. Because the radioisotope gives off some form of radiation, it can be followed and located by an externally placed detector. This then gives the diagnostician information about the function of an organ or tissue, or it can locate and give the type and degree of abnormality that may be present in the organ or tissue.

Radioactive iodine, for example, can be used in the diagnosis of thyroid disorders because the thyroid gland takes up and utilizes iodine in the synthesis of its hormone thyroxin. Some diagnostic procedures use radioisotopes for the sampling and radioactive counting of blood, urine, and other body fluids and tissues. Counting gives an indication of the concentration or density of such substances.

The term *scanning* is used to describe a procedure whereby a detector moves slowly over a body area and produces a "picture" composed of a series or grouping of dots. The dots are produced by the rays or emanations from the radioisotope concentrated in the area.

Most diagnostic tests utilizing radioisotopes are done in an out-patient clinic. Some explanation should be given the patient as to what specific test is to be done and its purpose. Scanning requires that the patient remain almost motionless during the procedure so that a clear, well-defined picture can be obtained. This may be difficult for the patient unless he is positioned comfortably before the scanning is begun. In some cases sedation may be necessary. Although all radioactive materials require special handling and precautions, radioisotopes in the dosage used for most diagnostic tests do not require any special precautions once the test is completed. This also should be explained to the patient before he is dismissed from the clinic.

CLINICAL CASE PROBLEMS

1. Mr. Gordon, age 42, is admitted to the hospital for diagnostic tests. He has had indigestion, upper abdominal pain, and gastric distress for several months. Recently he started vomiting small amounts of blood and his physician suspects a gastric ulcer or carcinoma of the stomach. Mr. Gordon is a very tense individual who worries about the things that will be done to him during the diagnostic tests.

How can you help this patient and prevent some of his anxiety?
What preparation will be necessary for a gastrointestinal series of x-rays?
What is a tubeless gastric analysis?

2. Mrs. Franklin is a patient, age 77, admitted to the hospital with a heart condition. She has never been in a hospital before and is very apprehensive about all the treatments and tests being done. When an E.K.G. is ordered for the patient and the technician begins the procedure Mrs. Franklin becomes very upset about the electrical apparatus.

How can you help prepare this patient for the procedure?
Why do you think this person is so frightened?

3. You have been assigned to the care of Mrs. Long who is to be prepared for a barium enema in the morning.

How will you explain to this patient the treatment necessary in preparation for a barium enema?
What steps will you take in preparing her?

4. You are asked to assist with a spinal puncture that is being done for the purpose of obtaining a specimen of cerebrospinal fluid for culture.

What equipment should be assembled for this procedure?
Do you know your responsibilities in assisting the physician who is doing a spinal puncture?
What precautions must be taken with a specimen that is to be used for a culture?
What other kinds of laboratory tests are commonly done on cerebrospinal fluid?

5. Mr. English, age 49, is admitted to the hospital with symptoms of chronic cough and weight loss. His physician has ordered a sputum analysis.

How would you instruct Mr. English in regard to the sputum specimen?
What is the ideal time for obtaining a specimen?

REFERENCES

1. French, R. M.: *Nurse's Guide to Diagnostic Procedures*, 2nd edition. New York, McGraw-Hill Book Co., 1967.
2. Garb, S.: *Laboratory Tests in Common Use*, 2nd edition. New York, Springer Publishing Co., 1960.
3. Goostray, S., and Schwenck, R.: *A Textbook of Chemistry*, 8th edition. New York, The Macmillan Co., 1961.
4. Harmer, B., and Henderson, V.: *Textbook of the Principles and Practice of Nursing*. 5th edition. New York, The Macmillan Co., 1960.
5. *Nursing Clinics of North America*, vol. 2. no. 1.

Philadelphia, W. B. Saunders Co., March, 1967.
6. Price, A.: *The Art, Science, and Spirit of Nursing,* 2nd edition. Philadelphia, W. B. Saunders Co., 1959.
7. Sackheim, G.: *Practical Physics for Nurses,* 2nd edition. Philadelphia, W. B. Saunders Co., 1962.
8. Shafer, K. N., et al.: *Medical-Surgical Nursing,* 2nd edition. St. Louis, Mo., C. V. Mosby Co., 1961.
9. Sister Mary Louise: *The Operating Room Technician.* St. Louis, Mo., C. V. Mosby Co., 1965.

SUGGESTED STUDENT READING

1. Eisenberg, S. W., Napoli, R. P., and Radding, B.: "Proctosigmoidoscopy." Am. Journ. Nurs., Jan., 1965, p. 113.
2. Hammer, L. G., Sawyer, J. G., et al.: "The Three-Maneuver Enema." Am. Journ. Nurs., Aug., 1962, p. 72.
3. Miller, R. E., and Gerard, S.: "The Nurse on the Radiological Team." Am. Journ. Nurs., July, 1964, p. 128.
4. Mohammed, M. F. B.: "Urinalysis." Am. Journ. Nurs., June, 1964, p. 87.

OUTLINE FOR CHAPTER 4

I. Introduction

A. The chemist, radiologist and pathologist aid the physician in diagnosis of an illness.

II. Purposes of Special Diagnostic Tests

A. To determine the patient's general physical condition.
B. To find the cause of illness.
C. As a verification of diagnosis.
D. As a guide for treatment.

III. Responsibilities of the Nurse

A. Assist with physical examination.
B. Prepare patient and explain procedure to him; assemble equipment.
C. Collect and label specimens as directed.

IV. Bacteriological Studies (Study of Bacteria)

A. Use proper procedure for collection of specimens for culturing of organisms.
B. Avoid contamination of specimens as well as of environment.

V. Urinalysis (Examination of Urine)

A. Abnormal constituents include red cells, pus cells, bacteria, albumin sugar, acetone and bile.

VI. Analysis of Blood

A. Cell count most common test.
B. Hemoglobin—important in diagnosing certain anemias.
C. Platelets—used in diagnosing disorders in blood clotting.
D. Hematocrit—measures volume of cells in relation to volume of plasma.
E. Clotting time—measures ability of blood to coagulate and form clot.
F. Prothrombin time—used to diagnose conditions in which there is difficulty in clot formation. Also used to determine clotting status of patient receiving anticoagulant drug.
G. Bilirubin—a bile pigment normally present in the blood in small amounts. A high level of bilirubin produces jaundice.

VII. Gastrointestinal Contents

A. Stomach contents tested for free acid, occult blood and microorganisms such as the tubercle bacillus.
B. Stools examined for parasites and occult blood.

VIII. Cerebrospinal Fluid (Obtained from Spinal Cavity by Spinal Puncture)

A. Specimen examined for cell counts, bacterial studies and protein content.
B. Pressure of spinal fluid may be tested at time specimen is withdrawn.

IX. Analysis of Sputum (Examination of Liquid Material Brought up from Lungs)

A. Analyzed for certain organisms, blood or pus cells.

X. X-ray Studies (Use of Roentgen Rays which Are Capable of Penetrating Soft Tissues of the Body)

A. Proper preparation of patient necessary for adequate studies of hollow organs. Radiopaque dye used to visualize those structures.
B. Fluoroscopy—filming organs by x-ray while they are in motion.

XI. *Endoscopic Examinations*

A. Utilization of a special instrument that is inserted into hollow organs.

B. Bronchoscope, cystoscope and gastroscope are examples of instruments used.

XII. *Basal Metabolic Rate (B.M.R.)*

A. Measurement of the lowest possible rate of metabolism.

B. Patient must be at rest physically and mentally.

C. Measures oxygen intake.

XIII. *Electrocardiogram (E.K.G. or E.C.G.) (Study of Heart Muscle Activity)*

A. Used to diagnose cardiac disorders that affect muscular contraction of heart.

XIV. *Electroencephalogram (E.E.G.) (Tracings of Electric Impulses from the Brain)*

XV. *Radioisotopes (Radioactive Isotopes)*

A. Useful in diagnosis because they give off radiations that can be detected by special equipment.

B. Used in diagnosis of thyroid disorders to "count" blood, urine and body fluid concentrations, and to help locate abnormal growths in certain organs.

Chapter 5

THE SURGICAL PATIENT

INTRODUCTION

The nursing care of the surgical patient is generally divided into three phases: (1) the preoperative period, (2) the operative and immediate postoperative period, and (3) the period of convalescence and rehabilitation. The length of time each of these periods involves varies according to the type of surgery and the general physical condition of the patient.

The preoperative period includes physical, mental, and emotional preparation for the surgical procedure. The operative period includes the time the patient is under anesthesia and recovering from the anesthesia. In most hospitals the patient is kept in a special area usually called the recovery room until this phase of surgery and anesthesia is completed. The postoperative period of convalescence and rehabilitation demands the attention of many members of the medical team and may include the occupational therapist, physical therapist, and social worker. The practical nurse must understand the various aspects of surgery so that she might be better prepared to render total nursing care to her patient.

PREOPERATIVE PERIOD

Emotional and Psychological Preparation. Preparation of the patient for surgery actually begins when the surgeon first decides that an operation is necessary and explains to his patient the need for surgery and the kind of operation which will be done. It is usually something of a shock to the individual and his family to learn that surgical treatment is necessary and this change in the routine of their everyday lives will place some personal and financial burdens on them. For some patients the surgery will alter their lives permanently, leaving them handicapped in some way, and requiring an adjustment in their lives and the lives of their families. Others may expect to be greatly helped by the surgical procedure, but even they will have some fears and misgivings about the prospect of having anesthesia and surgery.

All of us fear the unknown. The surgical patient who has never had surgery before or is not familiar with hospital routine will have many questions about what is in store for him now that he realizes surgery is necessary. It is to the advantage of all concerned that these

58

questions be satisfactorily answered and that the patient have a general idea of what he might expect before and after surgery.

We know that there should always be an effective means of communication between hospital personnel and the patient. What do we mean by good communication? Our first thought is usually communication by the spoken word. But the patient may not feel free to ask questions or to voice his apprehension about surgery and anesthesia. The first step then, is to instill a feeling of confidence and trust in our ability, and to demonstrate by our attitudes and actions that we are sincerely interested in the patient as an individual. When questions are asked of us we must exercise extreme care in the answers we give. We are often as much misunderstood by what we *don't* say as by what we *do* say. It is far better, then, if the patient asks a practical nurse a question she is not qualified to answer, for her to say simply that she doesn't know but that the nurse in charge or the physician can tell him what he wishes to know. An example of this is a question such as, "Will the doctor remove my whole stomach or just the part where the ulcer is?" Obviously she is not qualified to explain the intentions of the surgeon. A general question, however, such as "Will I wake up in my own room after surgery?" can be answered quite easily.

The patient should be encouraged to ask questions about certain aspects of his care that he does not understand and he should be given answers promptly and accurately. It is extremely frustrating and a bit frightening for him when his questions are evaded or answered in a vague manner at a time when everything happening to him seems so important. And indeed it is important to him and to his recovery. The relaxed and confident patient is under less strain physically as well as mentally and will recover more rapidly than one who is confused, angry, or fearful.

We must not forget the patient's family in the emotional preparation for surgery. They should be informed of the usual routines, including the premedication the evening and morning of surgery, which will make the patient somewhat groggy and incoherent just before he goes to the operating room. It is also helpful if the family realizes that the length of time the patient is away from his room does not necessarily represent the length of the operation. There are sometimes slight delays in getting the procedure started in the operating room. And then, after surgery, most hospitals have a recovery unit where the patient is kept under close observation until he is considered out of immediate danger and awake from anesthesia. This simple explanation of what they can expect and how long they may have to wait to see the patient after the operation helps to prevent much unnecessary worry and anguish about their loved one.

It is also reassuring to the patient and his family if they have some idea of the treatments which may be necessary postoperatively. So many people associate the administration of oxygen, blood transfusions, or IV fluids, and the presence of a Levin tube or other drainage apparatus with a critical situation. If they understand that many of these treatments are commonplace in surgical procedures they will realize these do not indicate the patient has "taken a turn for the worse."

Spiritual Preparation. Since most of us have a justifiable fear of anesthesia and surgery it is comforting to have some moral and spiritual support before surgery. The patient or his family may ask that a spiritual advisor be called in. This is a very important aspect of preoperative care and must not be overlooked in the many activities of physical preparation. The practical nurse who displays a sincere interest in every aspect of her patient's care will do all that she can to help him gain peace of mind.

Physical Preparation of the Patient for Surgery

Preoperative Examination. Before he undertakes surgery the physician will try to have his patient in the best possible condition. In emergencies, of course, he cannot always manage this, but in planned surgery he may postpone the operation for days or weeks until the patient is physically able to withstand the rigors of anesthesia and major surgery.

On admission to the hospital the surgical patient will have a hemoglobin and blood count ordered. If the laboratory reports indicate any abnormalities, measures will be taken to improve the general health of the patient before surgery is scheduled.

A urinalysis is also done to eliminate the possibility of an infection or other disease of the urinary system. Surgery puts an additional strain on the circulatory, urinary, and respiratory systems. Thus the heart and lungs will be carefully examined for pathological conditions. These are all the responsibilities of the physician but the practical nurse may need to explain to the patient the need for these tests before surgery. Once the patient is confident that everything is being done to assure him of a safe and successful operation, he will become more relaxed and cooperative.

Preparation of the Skin. The skin and hair are both harborers of many microorganisms. It is not possible to make the skin completely sterile, but most of the organisms may be removed by shaving and scrubbing the area with green soap or hexachlorophene. The exact procedure for cleansing the operative area varies according to the wishes of the surgeon and the accepted procedure of the hospital. In some types of bone surgery sterile towels or dressings are applied after the area is cleansed. However, some surgeons believe that dressings tend to increase perspiration, bringing deep-seated bacteria to the surface of the skin. When the practical nurse has no definite orders as to how the surgeon wishes the area to be prepared she should ask for specific instructions from the nurse in charge. These instructions should designate the total area to be shaved and scrubbed as well as the method to be used.

Restriction of Oral Intake. The surgeon will leave written orders regarding restriction of food and drink before surgery. It may be necessary for the practical nurse to explain to the patient that he is not allowed anything by mouth because of the danger of vomiting with subsequent aspiration of the vomitus into the air passages during or immediately after surgery. In some cases a gastric tube may be inserted into the stomach by way of a nostril and gastric suction started the evening or morning before surgery. This tube is to be clamped off and left in place just before the patient is taken to the operating room. It may reassure the patient if he understands that gastric suction eliminates much unnecessary distention, nausea and vomiting postoperatively, all of which place strain on the sutures and are exhausting and unpleasant for him.

Elimination. Surgery involving the abdominal cavity, rectum, or perineum usually requires a cleansing of the lower intestinal tract by catharsis and/or enemas. This preparation will reduce the possibility of contamination of the operative area during anesthesia when the sphincter muscles are relaxed and will also help to eliminate distention following surgery. Patients having rectal surgery or other operative procedures in which the surgeon does not wish the patient to have a bowel movement for several days after surgery often have "enemas until clear" ordered preoperatively. These are very exhausting and should be given slowly and with care, allowing the patient to rest between enemas.

Rest and Sedation. The body needs all of its strength and physical resources when coping with surgical procedures.

Fear of unknown

Lack of confidence in surgeons and nurses

Worry over family

Unable to communicate with nurses

Fear of anesthesia

Fear of invalidism

Confidence in surgeon

Informed about events to come

Good rapport with nurses

Family safe and comfortable

Rehabilitation planned

Nurse's Preoperative Care

Explains nursing procedures
Explains hospital routine
Answers questions
Listens to patient and family
Shows interest in family
Obtains spiritual advisor when requested
Cooperates with other members of medical team

Surgeon's Preoperative Care

Explains surgical procedure
Assists patient in planning rehabilitation
Explains anesthesia--type to be used
     and how it will affect patient

Figure 5-1. Preparation of the patient for surgery.

Thus the patient should have a restful night with adequate sleep the night before surgery. A barbiturate is usually ordered but this does not always guarantee that the patient will sleep well. The nurse should check frequently during the night to make sure the patient is sleeping. If he is awake and seems restless and fearful she should stay with him for a while, answer his questions and try to allay his fears. It may be necessary to secure an order to repeat the sedation given at bedtime. If the patient is sleeping well he should not be disturbed for routine procedures during the night and morning of surgery.

The Operative Permit. Before the surgeon can perform an operation he must have written permission, signed by the patient or his guardian. This written permit protects the surgeon against "claims of unauthorized operations and protects the patient against unsanctioned surgery."[3] In most hospitals this permit is a printed form which will have the patient sign before surgery. This permit is then attached to the patient's chart and sent to the operating room with the chart (see Fig. 5-2).

Immediate Preoperative Care. The patient must wear a hospital gown to the operating room. The hair should be covered with a towel or cap and in some hospitals surgical boots are put on the patient. Women with very long hair should have it combed and plaited

AUTHORITY TO OPERATE

a.m.

Date........................... 19...... Time...............p.m.

I hereby authorize the physician or physicians in charge of the care of

_____

(Name of Patient)

to administer any treatment; or to administer such anesthetics; and perform such operations as may be deemed necessary or advisable in the diagnosis and treatment of this patient.

Witness _____   Signed _____

(Patient or Nearest Relative)

Witness _____   _____

(Relationship)

Authorization must be signed by the patient, or by the nearest relative in the case of a minor, or when patient is physically or mentally incompetent.

Figure 5-2. Sample operative permit. These are used when surgical procedures are performed and must be completely filled out and properly signed before the operation is begun.

into braids and all hairpins must be removed from the hair. If the patient wishes to wear a wedding ring this should be secured in place with a loop of gauze or tape slipped through the ring and tied to the wrist. Watches and other valuables must be removed from the bedside table and placed under lock and key according to the hospital policy. Dentures are usually removed, placed in a denture cup and kept in a designated place according to hospital policy. Sometimes the anesthesiologist will request that the dentures be left in place because they help to maintain the contour of the face and facilitate the administration of inhalation anesthesia.

An identification bracelet or tag is attached to the patient's wrist to avoid any error or mix-up of patients in the operating room.

Unless there is a urinary catheter in place, preoperative patients are offered the bedpan or urinal just before going to surgery. As stated before, the sphincter muscles may become completely relaxed during anesthesia and the patient might be incontinent and contaminate the operative field.

In the evaluation of the vital signs postoperatively it is helpful to know the patient's blood pressure, pulse and respiration rate before he is sent to the operating room.

The preoperative medication must be administered at exactly the time ordered by the surgeon or anesthesiologist. This is essential because the amount of anesthesia and time of induction have been calculated according to the hour the premedication was expected to be given. A delay in the preoperative medication may cause difficulties for the patient and a great inconvenience to the person administering the anesthesia. All preliminary preparations should be done before the medication is given so that it will have maximum effect.

Preoperative medications are given to (1) promote rest and relaxation, (2) decrease secretion of mucus and other body fluids, and (3) enhance the effects of the anesthetic. The sedatives that are usually used are the barbiturates such as phenobarbital or Seconal. The dry-

ing agents may include atropine or scopolamine. Narcotics such as morphine or Demerol are given to supplement the anesthetic.

Many hospitals have a check list to be filled out by the nurse in charge before the patient is taken to the operating room. This eliminates the danger of omitting any part of the preoperative preparation (see Fig. 5-3).

ANESTHESIA

Anesthesia (the loss of sensory perception) came into use as an accepted part of surgical procedure in the 1840's. With the advent of drugs which safely

CLEARANCE RECORD FOR SURGICAL OPERATIONS

NAME _____ HOSP. NO. _____ DATE _____

	YES	NO	REMARKS
1. Written permission for surgery	✓		
2. Blood count and hemoglobin	✓		
3. Urinalysis	✓		
4. History and physical	✓		
5. Valuables a. Removed and placed in cabinet b. Tied to patient's wrist	✓		none
6. Dentures removed			
7. Identification bracelet on patient	✓		
8. Vital signs 30 min. preoperatively a. BP /32/84 b. Pulse 90 c. Resp 18			
9. Preoperative medication given			at 7:45 a.m.
10. Bleeding and clotting time (for T & As)			
11. Consultation sheet for sterilization for first Cesarean section			

Figure 5-3. Clearance record for surgical operations.

produced anesthesia, the performance of surgical operations became a more widely accepted and successful means of treating disease and injury. Few of us would accept surgery without the advantage of being insensible to pain during the operation, and the modern surgical procedures requiring several hours would be impossible without adequate anesthesia.

The first anesthetics used were ether and nitrous oxide. It is interesting to note that these drugs were used as a source of entertainment and amusement before anyone considered using them in medical practice. Nitrous oxide, commonly called "laughing gas," was sometimes administered to a volunteer from the audience of a side show for the purpose of watching the antics of the victim as he was transported into a state of euphoria and became hysterical with laughter. During the 1800's, ether "frolics" were also a source of entertainment (crude and dangerous as it may seem to us) in which medical students and other persons with access to the drug inhaled a small amount of ether and subsequently enjoyed a feeling of lighthearted gaiety. Today, both of these drugs are in common use in surgery and considered to be among the safest and most effective anesthetics for major surgery.

There are three main objectives in the administration of an anesthetic: (1) to prevent pain, (2) to achieve adequate muscle relaxation, and (3) to calm fear, allay anxiety, and give forgetfulness.[1]

Types of Anesthesia. In order to achieve the objectives mentioned above there are a variety of anesthetics available. The choice of anesthesia rests with the anesthesiologist and depends on the type of surgery to be performed, age and physical condition of the patient, and his ability to tolerate the anesthetic. The types of anesthesia may be classified according to the method of administration. They include inhalants, intravenous anesthetics, local anesthetics, spinal anesthetics, and refrigeration anesthesia.

INHALANTS. These include ether, nitrous oxide, trilene, and cyclopropane. Most of these gases and liquids are highly inflammable and demand extreme caution to guard against electric sparks in their presence. Ether causes an irritation of the mucous membranes, resulting in large amounts of mucus in the respiratory tract. Patients receiving ether will, therefore, need frequent suctioning while unconscious, and must be encouraged to take deep breaths and cough up the bronchial secretions once they have awakened. They will frequently have nausea and vomiting of the mucus which has collected in the stomach and esophagus.

INTRAVENOUS ANESTHETICS. The drug must commonly used for this type of anesthesia is Pentothal, a fast-acting barbiturate, which produces immediate unconsciousness when it is administered. A patient who has received this anesthetic must be watched closely during the immediate postoperative period for cyanosis, restlessness, and dyspnea, which are signs of laryngeal spasm, a condition sometimes associated with the administration of Pentothal.

LOCAL OR REGIONAL ANESTHESIA. In this type of anesthesia, only the area of the surgical incision and adjacent tissues are deadened to the pain involved and the patient remains awake. This method is used most frequently for minor surgery, diagnostic tests, and examinations. Drugs most commonly used are procaine, tetracaine and dibucaine. Some hypersensitive individuals may suffer a severe reaction to the drugs used in local anesthesia, and circulatory failure and death may occur. The practical nurse assisting with procedures in which a local anesthetic is used should be alert to signs of hypersensitivity in the patient and be prepared for the administration of oxygen and an emergency drug such as Adrenalin in the event that a reaction develops. Usually, if there is any possibility of an idiosyncrasy to the anesthetizing drug, the physician will do a skin test before injecting a local anesthetic.

Topical Anesthesia. This is a form of local anesthesia in which the drug is applied directly on the surface of the area to be treated. It is used frequently in examinations or treatments of the eye, nose, and throat.

SPINAL ANESTHESIA. The spinal cord serves as a pathway for nerve impulses passing to and from the brain. By injecting a drug into the spinal cavity around the spinal cord these impulses are blocked and there is complete loss of feeling in all areas of the body below the site of injection. This is what is done when a spinal anesthesia is given. Obviously this type of anesthesia can only be used for surgery below the diaphragm but it is very effective and produces complete muscular relaxation even though the patient remains awake during the operation.

The postoperative care of the patient receiving spinal anesthesia is basically the same as for a general anesthesia, although there are usually fewer gastrointestinal and respiratory complications to be guarded against following spinal anesthesia. On the other hand, the nurse must realize that respiratory difficulties and cardiovascular complications can develop when spinal anesthesia is given. If the anesthesia ascends beyond the point of injection, innervation of the respiratory muscles and blood vessels is effected. This produces depression of respiration and a lowering of the blood pressure. In case respiratory embarrassment occurs artificial respiration by machine or the mouth-to-mouth method must be employed. Hypotension is treated by the administration of drugs such as ephedrine or methoxyl unless the lowered blood pressure is caused by blood loss. The patient may not be placed in shock position with the head lowered until at least 20 minutes after injection of the anesthetic.

As the anesthesia wears off, the patient may complain that he cannot move his legs and that they feel numb and heavy. This is to be expected at first and will gradually subside. The patient is kept flat in bed for a minimum of 8 hours, and longer if he experiences headache or dizziness. Some confusion and dizziness may be due to the preoperative drugs given; in this event side rails are applied and the patient is watched carefully until he is no longer dizzy and confused. He may be turned from side to side unless there are specific orders to the contrary. The first few times the patient is allowed out of bed there must be someone in attendance to protect him from falls and injury because he may experience some difficulty in maintaining his balance.

REFRIGERATION ANESTHESIA. This type of anesthesia is produced by lowering the temperature of a part (usually a lower limb) until the extreme cold retards the conduction of nerve impulses. It sometimes is supplemented by the administration of another anesthetic. Advantages of refrigeration anesthesia include minimal bleeding during and after surgery, less possibility of physical shock, and elimination of the hazards of inhalation anesthesia for patients who are weak and debilitated.

This type of anesthesia is especially useful for amputations in the treatment of arteriosclerotic gangrene. The area to be anesthetized is packed in ice or wrapped in a special electric refrigeration unit. Tourniquets are applied to prevent chilling of the rest of the body. The length of time necessary for anesthetizing the area ranges from 1 to 3 hours, depending on the size of the area to be anesthetized and the type of equipment used. Duration of the anesthesia is about one hour.

HYPOTHERMIA

The term *hypothermia* refers to a reduction of body temperature. Its purpose in surgery is to lower metabolism and thereby decrease the need for oxygen. In many types of surgery involving the heart, blood vessels or brain, it is necessary to interrupt the flow of blood through the body. By lowering the body temperature to between 32° C. (89.6° F.) and 26° C. (78.8° F.), the metabolic needs of the vital organs are reduced and they are less likely to be damaged by a decreased supply of blood and oxygen. Hypothermia also may be used in the treatment of diseases accompanied by a high fever.

There are several ways in which hypothermia can be achieved. In *external hypothermia* the patient's body is wrapped in a cooling blanket, packed in ice or submerged in a tub of ice water. This is done after the patient has been anesthetized and immediately before the surgical procedure is performed.

In *extracorporeal* cooling the patient's blood is cooled outside the body. It is removed from a major vessel, circulated through a refrigerant unit for cooling, and then returned to the body by way of another large blood vessel. This is the quickest way to achieve hypothermia and is usually the method used for patients undergoing surgery.

The reduction of body temperature by drugs which affect the heat regulating center in the brain is called *internal hypothermia*. The drug most often used is chlorpromazine hydrochloride (Thorazine) and it is given in combination with sedatives such as Demerol and Phenergan. Internal hypothermia usually reduces the body temperature by no more than three or four degrees.

During the rewarming process the patient's temperature is raised gradually. Care must be taken to avoid burns if warm baths or diathermy are used. The rewarming procedure is discontinued when the body temperature is within one or two degrees of normal. Observations during the rewarming include checking the pulse, blood pressure and respiration as well as the temperature. Any sudden change must be reported immediately.

POSTOPERATIVE PERIOD

Immediate Postoperative Care. This is a critical period for the patient, one which demands close and constant observation by persons well trained and equipped to handle any emergency which may arise. The ideal situation is, as mentioned before, placing the patient in a special section of the hospital such as a recovery unit, where trained personnel may give him individual and constant attention until he is considered safely past immediate danger.

The following statement will give the practical nurse some idea of the kind of attention necessary during the immediate postoperative period.

Figure 5-4. Position for immediate postoperative patient which permits drainage of mucus from the mouth and general relaxation. (From Winters: *Protective Body Mechanics in Daily Life and in Nursing.* W. B. Saunders Co., Philadelphia.)

Table 7.   *Postoperative Care*

I. Control of pain	Nursing measures to provide maximum comfort and reassurance of the patient Analgesic drugs
II. Maintenance of drainage	Urinary catheters Gastric suction Thoracic drainage Bile drainage Drainage from surgical wounds
III. Maintenance of fluid and electrolyte balance	Intravenous fluids and minerals Oral intake Observation and recording of output
IV. Relief of abdominal distention, nausea and vomiting	Rectal tube Gastric suction Ice collar Antiemetic drugs
V. Prevention of complications:	
A. Shock B. Hemorrhage	Close observation for signs of shock and hemorrhage
C. Blood clots in vascular system	Frequent turning Early ambulation
D. Hypostatic pneumonia	Encourage coughing and deep breathing and turn frequently
E. Decubiti	Frequent turning Skin care
F. Contractures	Proper positioning Exercise
G. Wound infection	Adherence to the basic principles of cleanliness and asepsis

Whether a patient is conscious or unconscious at the conclusion of the operation, his protection reflexes may be depressed. Careful observation is necessary to determine that (1) the airway remains patent [open], (2) respiration remains adequate and of normal character, (3) color and turgor of the skin remain good and that the skin remains dry, (4) pulse remains adequate in quality, rate, and rhythm, (5) blood pressure remains within normal limits, and (6) vomitus or secretions are not aspirated.[1]

During the time that the patient is beginning to recover from the effects of anesthesia the nurse must also give some attention to simple nursing measures which can relieve some of his discomfort. Because the patient has had nothing by mouth for 8 hours or more he may experience severe thirst. If there are no contraindications the nurse may offer him small sips of water, otherwise his lips can be moistened with a gauze square dipped in ice water. If he is receiving intravenous fluids it is wise to restrain the arm loosely so that in his state of semiconsciousness he will not fling his arm about and dislodge the needle. Plastic armboards shaped to fit the arm are more comfortable than the straight armboards made of wood, but in either case the bony prominences of the arm should be well padded and the hand supported so that it is not hanging off the edge of the board.

Many surgical procedures extend over a period of hours, which means that the patient has been lying motionless, in a fixed position, on a hard table for that length of time. No wonder, then, that the patient often complains of backache when he first wakes up. Turning the patient on his side and administering a gentle back rub will help. If he cannot be turned, the lumbar region may be supported with a small pillow or folded bath towel.

Nausea and vomiting following anesthesia are not uncommon. Supportive measures such as holding the patient's head or turning it to the side to prevent aspiration of the vomitus if he is not fully awake are most helpful and reassuring to the patient. He will also appreciate a few sips of water to rinse his mouth after the siege of vomiting is over.

While the patient is apparently still under anesthesia the nursing staff and other persons within his hearing should be careful in their conversations. Many times the patient misinterprets the bits of conversation he hears and becomes unduly alarmed and disturbed. It is best to avoid talking except when absolutely necessary and then the voice should be kept low unless the patient is being addressed. Whispering is inexcusable.

Other measures must include turning the patient every hour and encouraging deep breathing and coughing. This is necessary to improve circulation of the blood and expansion and aeration of the lungs. If the blood flow is allowed to become sluggish there is danger that clots may form and give rise to a thrombus. The lungs must be expanded and secretions coughed up so that hypostatic pneumonia will not occur. In turning the patient the nurse must guard against handling the patient too roughly or turning him too quickly. A sudden overstimulation might result in a drop in blood pressure.

Complications During the Postoperative Period. The two most common and serious complications of surgery are shock and hemorrhage. These two terms represent separate and distinct complications, although hemorrhage, if unchecked, will rapidly lead to a state of shock.

SHOCK. The word "shock" actually represents a group of symptoms resulting from a failure of the blood vessels near the surface of the body to function properly. This collapse of the peripheral vessels leads to a serious decrease in the supply of circulating fluids to the vital organs. The pathological changes which occur internally lead to the following signs and symptoms: the skin is pale and clammy and cold, the temperature is subnormal, the pulse rapid and weak, and the respiration rapid and shallow. The blood pressure during shock may drop to 90 mm. systolic pressure. If the pressure continues to drop and remains below 50 mm. for very long there is permanent damage to the vital centers of the body.

Treatment and Nursing Care. The simplest form of shock is fainting. The more serious types of shock (for example after severe trauma) may become extreme and result in death if the process is not quickly reversed by treatment. Because a surgical incision and major surgical procedure are unavoidably traumatic to the body, the postoperative patient must be watched very closely for symptoms of shock. The blood pressure, pulse and respiration must be taken at frequent intervals. Observation of the color and general condition of the skin are equally important, as is the patient's state of consciousness, because the patient may lose consciousness if shock is severe or prolonged.

Elevation of the foot of the bed by adjustment of the Gatch bed to Trendelenburg position or placing "shock blocks" under the foot of the bed will help increase the flow of blood to vital organs. Application of heat in the form of blankets or hot water bottles is no longer advocated because it is believed to bring the flow of blood to the peripheral vessels and thus further deprive the vital organs of their blood supply. It is sufficient merely to keep the body warm enough to protect the patient from excessive heat loss through the skin. Intravenous fluids, plasma or whole blood may be ordered by the physician to increase the blood volume. Other medications and treatments ordered for the patient in shock must be carried out with dispatch, as the loss of time due to inefficiency or apathy may lead to the loss of a life.

HEMORRHAGE. Hemorrhage (hemo— blood, rrhage—excessive flow) is the flow of blood from the body in amounts sufficient to endanger health and life. Postoperatively, hemorrhage might occur when a ligature slips off a vessel tied during surgery or when a drainage tube causes erosion in the wall of a blood vessel. The patient suffering from hemorrhage, whatever the cause, must receive immediate treatment or death will eventually be the outcome.

Hemorrhage may occur internally or externally. External hemorrhage is, of course, much more obvious and easily determined, but in both types the patient's vital signs are of extreme importance in evaluating his condition. Generally hemorrhage is accompanied by a drop in blood pressure and an increase in pulse and respiration. The patient may become restless and complain of thirst and feeling cold. The skin will be pale and moist and the extremities mottled and cold to the touch. If the hemorrhage continues unchecked the lips and conjunctiva will become extremely pale and the patient will complain of weakness, fatigue, and spots before his eyes.

The treatment of hemorrhage is to stop the flow of blood and to replace by transfusion that which has been lost. In emergencies, the blood loss may be diminished by pressure dressings over the area, manual restriction of the blood flow to the area with tourniquets, or pressure on the so-called "pressure points" of the body. If the hemorrhage is postoperative, the patient may be taken back to the operating room and the bleeding vessel retied.

During the postoperative period, then, we can see the importance of checking the blood pressure, pulse and respiration at frequent and regular intervals to determine whether the patient is bleeding internally or going into shock. During this time and for several days or more postoperatively the dressing must be carefully observed for signs of fresh bleeding. It is also important that all body excretions be closely observed for evidence of internal bleeding. This is also true for drainage from tubes or surgical drains.

If a patient does show signs of hemorrhage the nursing staff must move quickly but with a minimum of excitement. The patient is usually frightened and partially aware of what is going on and any unnecessary anxiety on his part will only aggravate the bleeding. Conversations among the nursing personnel must be kept at a minimum in his presence, and evidence of the hemorrhage, such as blood-soaked dressings or soiled linen and gown, should be quickly removed from sight. It will be necessary to reassure the patient frequently and demonstrate by a calm, efficient bearing that everything is under control and will turn out well.

WOUND INFECTION. With the advent of antibiotics (the so-called "miracle drugs") the word infection has become less frightening and we have become more complacent about the need for precautions against wound infection following surgery. We must not use antibiotics as an excuse for careless nursing. In the first place, there are many microorganisms that have developed a resistance to the antibiotic drugs. This is particularly true of many strains of staphylococci which are capable of causing painful and stubborn infections. Secondly, even though the infection eventually may be overcome, the patient has been unnecessarily subjected to discomfort, inconvenience and added expense.

Prevention of wound infection begins before surgery and continues until the surgical wound is healed. It includes careful attention to rules of surgical asepsis and also entails the less glamorous cleaning chores that must continue from day to day. It is expected that table tops and other visible surfaces in the patient's room will be kept free of dust, but what about the lower rungs and wheels of beds, stretchers, chairs, etc.? Are we constantly aware of the fantastic rate of reproduction that is characteristic of pathogenic microorganisms, and do we realize that many are resistant to all but the strongest of disinfectants? And what about handwashing? Each time the nurse begins any procedure involving direct contact with a postoperative patient she should wash her hands for at least one full minute under running water.

One must never let familiarity with "routine" nursing procedures give her a feeling of complacency or security. Wound infection is a very real hazard which has become increasingly more prevalent in recent years, and it is all the more tragic because it can be prevented. That fact should make us more aware than ever of the need for applying the basic principles of cleanliness and sanitation.

Convalescence and Rehabilitation. The period of convalescence from surgery has been greatly shortened by modern surgical techniques. Surgical procedures are less traumatic than formerly because of the development of improved surgical instruments and equipment. The practice of encouraging early ambulation and rapid return to physical activities has given the patients (and the nurses) a more optimistic view of surgical procedures and have helped the patient in his recovery and return to his former life.

Rehabilitation is the restoring of the patient to as near his former state of health and activity as possible. For the surgical patient rehabilitation may include readjustment to a completely new and better way of life, as is necessary when the surgery is restorative and the patient is able to be more active physically than he formerly might have been. Other types of surgery will render the patient more handicapped and helpless to some degree. Surgical procedures which require the use of a prosthesis or special appliances (such as a permanent colostomy) demand much time and specially trained personnel to help the patient learn to live with his handicap. In rehabilitation, probably more than any other phase of nursing, we can see the advantages of a well-coordinated medical team. It is in this phase of care that the physiotherapist, occupational therapist, social worker, and public health nurse can make their greatest contribution toward the care of the patient and his restoration to a life more productive and thus more bearable.

For further information on rehabilitation the reader is referred to Chapter 7 of this text.

CLINICAL CASE PROBLEMS

1. Mrs. Smith, age 43, is admitted to the surgical unit of the hospital with a diagnosis of acute cholecystitis and obesity. She is the mother of five children and her husband has been dead for four years. Mrs. Smith works in a sewing plant to support her family. Her oldest son, age 19, also works to provide an income for the family.

This patient has never been hospitalized before except for the birth of her last three children. She is extremely apprehensive about her illness and is worried about her children and the financial status of the family now that she cannot work.

Several days after her admission to the hospital the acute inflammation responds to treatment sufficiently to permit surgical removal of the gallbladder. The patient gives her consent to the surgery, but she is very frightened and seems to feel that she will never be well again.

> What problems can you see in this situation?
> How can you help reassure Mrs. Smith before surgery?

In what ways might you help Mrs. Smith with her problem of obesity?

2. You are assigned to the care of a 20-year-old woman who has just returned from surgery for removal of a small tumor of the breast. You overheard the head nurse tell another staff nurse that the tumor was benign. In spite of the minor nature of the surgery, the patient has shown signs of shock in the recovery room and requires careful attention when she is returned to her room. When she recovers from the anesthesia the patient is very nauseated and uncomfortable.

What special observations should you make while caring for this patient?
How can you help relieve the nausea and vomiting?
If the patient asked you whether the tumor was benign or malignant, and you were not really sure because nothing had yet been recorded on her chart, what would your answer be?

3. This is your first day on duty on a surgical ward.
What specific policies and procedures are required by your hospital when a patient undergoes surgery?
Is there a clearance record or check list to be completed?

REFERENCES

1. Breckinridge, F. J., and Bruno, P.: "Nursing Care of the Anesthetized Patient." Am. Journ. Nurs., July, 1962, p. 74.
2. Brunner, L. S., et al.: *Textbook of Medical-Surgical Nursing.* Philadelphia, J. B. Lippincott Co., 1964.
3. Harmer, B., and Henderson, V.: *Textbook of the Principles and Practice of Nursing,* 5th edition. New York, The Macmillan Co., 1960.
4. LeMaitre, C., and Finnegan, J.: *The Patient in Surgery.* Philadelphia, W. B. Saunders Co., 1966.
5. Price, A. L.: *The Art, Science, and Spirit of Nursing,* 3rd edition. Philadelphia, W. B. Saunders Co., 1966.
6. Shafer, K. N., Sawyer, J. R., et al.: *Medical-Surgical Nursing,* 4th edition. St. Louis, Mo., C. V. Mosby Co., 1966.
7. Smith, D. W., and Gips, C. D.: *Care of the Adult Patient.* Philadelphia, J. B. Lippincott Co., 1966.

SUGGESTED STUDENT READING

1. Breckinridge, F. J., and Bruno, P.: "Nursing Care of the Anesthetized Patient." Am. Journ. Nurs., July, 1962, p. 74.
2. Carneval, D.: "Preop Anxiety." Am. Journ. Nurs., July, 1966, p. 1536.
3. Clark, R. B.: "The Case for Spinal Anesthesia." Am. Journ. Nurs., Feb., 1967, p. 294.
4. Elder, F.: "Effective Support for the Preoperative Patient." RN, May, 1962, p. 47.
5. Healy, K. M.: "Does Preoperative Instruction Make a Difference?" Am. Journ. Nurs., Jan., 1968, p. 63.
6. Hickey, M. C.: "Hypothermia." Am. Journ. Nurs., Jan., 1965, p. 116.
7. Landis, E. M.: "Some Pointers on Postoperative Care." RN, July, 1962, p. 54.

OUTLINE FOR CHAPTER 5

I. Introduction

A. Nursing care divided into three phases: preoperative, operative and immediate postoperative, and convalescence and rehabilitation.
B. Length of each period varies with individual patient.

II. Preoperative Period

A. Emotional and psychological preparation:
   1. Listen to patient and answer his questions to the best of your ability.
   2. Prepare patient and family so that they will know what to expect during postoperative period.
B. Spiritual preparation for peace of mind.
C. Physical preparation:
   1. Preoperative examination to determine patient's physical status.
   2. Preparation of skin to reduce chance of postoperative infection.
   3. Restriction of oral intake to avoid complications of nausea, vomiting and distention after surgery.
   4. Cleansing of intestinal tract if ordered to avoid contamination of operative site.
   5. Rest and sedation to conserve strength and energy of patient.
   6. Operative permit must be signed to avoid legal difficulties.
   7. Immediate preoperative care is done according to hospital's policies and procedures and directions of the

patient's physician. Medications must be given on time.

III. Anesthesia — Loss of Sensory Perception

A. Given to prevent pain, achieve muscular relaxation, and allay anxiety.
B. Types include:
1. Inhalants.
2. Intravenous anesthetics.
3. Local or regional anesthetics.
4. Spinal anesthesia (drug is injected into spinal cavity, anesthesia achieved below point of injection).
5. Refrigeration anesthesia (temperature of a part is lowered so that conduction of nerve impulses is retarded).

IV. Postoperative Period

A. Immediate postoperative period is a critical time demanding close and constant observation to determine if:
1. Airway is open.
2. Respiration is adequate.
3. Color and turgor of skin are normal.
4. Pulse is adequate.
5. Blood pressure is within normal limits.
B. Prevent aspiration during vomiting episodes.

C. Avoid noise and conversation within patient's hearing.
D. Turn patient frequently to avoid circulatory stasis and respiratory failure.
E. Handle gently.
F. Complications to be watched for include shock, hemorrhage and wound infection.

V. Hypothermia — Reduction of Body Temperature

A. Used in some types of surgery to lower metabolism and decrease the need for oxygen.
B. Methods:
1. External hypothermia: using ice packs or other forms of external cold.
2. Extracorporeal hypothermia: rerouting the blood outside the body, through a cooling unit, and back into the body.
3. Administration of drugs.
D. During rewarming period patient's vital signs are noted at frequent intervals.

VI. Convalescence and Rehabilitation

A. Length of time will vary depending on type of surgery and patient's reaction.
B. Ultimate goal is return of the patient to as near his former state of health and activity as possible.

Chapter 6

THE CRITICALLY ILL PATIENT

VOCABULARY

Aerosols
Anaerobic
Asphyxiation
Bronchioles

Expectorate
Reflex
Stasis

INTRODUCTION

The patient who is critically ill is in a crucial situation: he is at the crossroads of life and death. He usually will require assistance in one or more vital functions such as breathing, maintaining adequate circulation, and control of elimination. He often has sudden changes in his condition that require skilled and competent nursing care.

The duties of the practical nurse caring for the critically ill patient encompass many roles. She must be a skilled bedside nurse, intelligent observer, accurate reporter, friend and confidante and student. The practical nurse working in the intensive care unit or caring for an acutely ill patient in any other area of the hospital must give the best she has to offer in bedside nursing. She must follow all the principles of nursing care that she has been taught, she must discipline herself to watch her patient closely without being distracted, and she must perform each of her many tasks with complete accuracy. There is no room for compromise in nursing a patient whose very life may depend on intelligent observation, good judgment and quick action.

Since critically ill patients do not always recover from their illness, death is a relatively frequent occurrence in the intensive care unit. The practical nurse must, therefore, be emotionally mature, with a firm philosophy of life that will sustain her in trying times.

There often is a profusion of complicated equipment surrounding the critically ill patient. This equipment can be frightening to the patient and he may feel that he is losing his individuality and identity as a human being in such an environment. The nurse must guard against giving the impression that she is more concerned with care of the equipment than with care of the patient. Most intensive care units have a ratio of at least one nurse per patient; usually there are more nurses than patients on these units. This means that the practical nurse can, and should, get to know her patient intimately; she should use her time to establish a good relationship with him. By treating her patient as an individual she can gain his respect and cooperation.

Finally, and perhaps most important, the role of the practical nurse caring for the critically ill patient is that of a student. She must always be eager to

73

learn and willing to study, and must actively participate in the in-service education programs provided by the hospital. The truly educated person knows how much he doesn't know. The rapid development of new techniques and new equipment used in patient care demands continuous study from those who wish to keep pace.

INTENSIVE CARE UNITS

Within the past few years there have developed special units within the hospital where patients can receive around-the-clock nursing care of the most detailed kind. These intensive care units (I.C.U.'s) are designed so that patients who require maximum nursing

Figure 6-1. *A,* Under the watchful eye of the head nurse, LPN Edna Feamster operates oxygen equipment for ICU patient. *B,* Two LPN's in the Neurology ICU turn patient on Stryker frame. Patient is almost totally paralyzed following an automobile accident. *C,* LPN Rosa Blocker assists Dr. John Harris as he operates the cardiac monitor machine which notes any irregularities or changes in pattern of heart beats. The monitor is used on patients who have just had heart attacks. The LPN must let the doctor know of any changes in the patient's condition. (From Bradford: Journal of Practical Nursing, November, 1966.)

care and constant observation can be located in one specific area where special equipment, drugs and personnel will be readily available. They are usually planned so that all beds are visible from the nurses' station. The visitors' room usually is separate from the unit so that the family and friends may be near the patient but will not disturb him or interfere with his care.

Special equipment in the intensive care unit usually includes the following: (This may vary, however, according to the type of patient admitted to a specific unit.)

1. Cardiac monitor for the heart patient. The monitoring equipment is attached to the patient for the purpose of relaying continuous electrocardiographic information on an oscilloscope. In this way the heart rhythm is continuously observed.

2. An artificial pacemaker that stimulates the heart by a series of electric shocks.

3. Respiratory resuscitative equipment that is used to reinstate breathing and maintain adequate exchange of gases in the lungs.

4. Reverse isolation set-up which protects the patient from contamination. It is used frequently for patients with extensive burns or for those who have lowered resistance to infection.

5. Oxygen apparatus, usually a wall unit.

6. Suction machine, also usually a wall unit.

7. Hypothermia blanket for control of body temperature.

8. Circolectric bed, Stryker frame or other equipment for patients who cannot be turned easily.

9. Special drugs that are used in acute illnesses, for example, heart stimulants, diuretics, vasodilators, and vasodepressors.

GENERAL PRINCIPLES OF NURSING CARE OF THE CRITICALLY ILL

The basic principles underlying the nursing care of the critically ill will remain the same even though diagnoses and special treatments will vary with individual patients. Usually it can be assumed that diseases resulting from involvement of the brain and central nervous system, severe trauma, toxemias from drugs, serious infections, failure of the kidneys or liver, or profound shock will all produce a very serious and critical illness. These conditions will require additional care beyond the usual treatments necessary for the primary disease. This special nursing care must embrace each of the following considerations:

1. Determination of the patient's state of consciousness and the presence or absence of the body's normal protective reflexes, as for example, the gag reflex which normally protects the body from aspiration of fluids or solids into the respiratory tract.

2. Maintenance of respiration with

Figure 6-2. This patient who is confined to a Circolectric bed has had a tumor in the back of his neck removed and has been in traction for a month. LPN Marie Amey turns him every two hours so that he can be in the most comfortable position. The Circolectric bed elevates the patient for any treatment or feeding. (From Bradford: Journal of Practical Nursing, November, 1966.)

Figure 6-3. *A*, The Life Island isolator. The master console is at the foot of the bed with two ultraviolet lighted pass-through locks, a control panel, and air filtering system. All items enter and leave the isolator through the pass-through locks. *B*, All items (except oral medications) entering the isolator are sterile. Aseptic pass-through technique is used by the nurse. (From Seidler: *Nursing Clinics of North America*, December, 1966.)

adequate intake and circulation of oxygen to the tissues, and the release and elimination of carbon dioxide.

3. Regulation of the intake of fluids and essential nutritious elements, minerals, and vitamins.

4. Maintenance of the correct body temperature.

5. Proper excretion of wastes from the body.

6. Maintenance of adequate peripheral circulation.

STATE OF CONSCIOUSNESS

The word "unconscious" is actually a relative term because there are varyings levels of consciousness. To be fully conscious is to be aware of one's surroundings and to respond to various stimuli in a normal manner. If one is totally *unconscious* or *comatose* there will be a total absence of any response to stimuli and even the involuntary reflexes will not be present. The *semicomatose* or semiconscious patient will respond to painful stimuli, but he is usually unaware of his environment most of the time, and will only briefly show signs of wakefulness before sinking back into a deep sleep.

A suggested outline for the nurse who is assessing a patient's state of consciousness is presented below. The author does not present it as an exhaustive listing of the assessment process, but comments that it can be modified by individual patients. It is not presented in order of priority.

Patient's Response to Auditory-Visual Stimuli*

1. Is the patient easily aroused when called by name? How easily?

2. How readily does he respond to the spoken word? In what manner?

*Reprinted from American Journal of Nursing: "Responsiveness as a Measure of Consciousness," M. A. Gardner, May, 1968, page 1034.

3. Does he acknowledge the assessor's presence by verbal, nonverbal (moving eyes, head) response? Is he quiet or restless?

4. Is he unusually distracted by usual environment stimuli during the assessment? How shown?

5. Does he return to the pretesting state when stimulus is withdrawn?

6. What is the nature of his verbal response? (Groans, muttering, yes, no, etc.)

7. Does he respond to loud auditory stimuli? To bright lights? How? Is he withdrawn or combative?

8. Is he able to follow simple, first-level commands such as "Raise your right hand"? Are his responses correct or distorted? Is he able to respond to second-level and third-level commands in proper sequence? (For example, "raise your right hand," "pick up the pencil on your bedside table," "put that pencil in your left hand.")

Patient's Response to Tacticle-Painful Stimuli

1. Does he react to gentle shaking? Does he move away from the source of movement? Are movements accompanied by a facial grimace or audible response?

2. Are his movements purposeful? For example, does he move voluntarily in bed to change position automatically? Does he respond when the blood pressure cuff is applied? Is it a helpful gesture or a withdrawal? Does he attempt to protect himself from repeated stimuli?

3. Does he withdraw when painful stimuli are introduced, for example, pinching the biceps or Achilles tendons or stimulation of the sole of the foot? Is the withdrawal prompt and purposeful? Is the response selective to the area or is there general body withdrawal? Is the withdrawal accompanied or followed by abnormal movements or rigidity? Is there a pattern to his

withdrawal? Is the response equal on both sides of his body?

Persons who are comatose, or apparently are unconscious and unable to respond, must have continued observation of their vital signs and accurate reporting of any change in these signs as long as they are unable to respond normally. There is one important point in the care of the unconscious patient which cannot be stressed too often, and which must be clearly understood by those who care for him. *His ability to hear and fully understand what is being said in his presence cannot be determined by outward appearance of his state of consciousness.* It is best to assume that the patient can always hear you, whether he gives any indication of hearing you or not. The nurse must explain all procedures and treatments to the patient at all times, just as though he were mentally and physically able to respond.

Whispering is always in bad taste and is especially annoying to the person who is the subject of the whispered conversation. If it is necessary to speak with the patient's family or other members of the nursing staff, it is best to talk with them in a low voice outside the patient's room. Caution must also be used in the conversations held within the patient's hearing. It is a fact that some patients who have been thought to be totally unconscious, and therefore unable to hear, have later repeated to the attendants or family the conversations they heard during their illness. This should be warning enough to use care in the things we say when caring for the supposedly unconscious patient.

MAINTENANCE OF RESPIRATION

"Normal respiration depends on (1) a supply of oxygen in the air; (2) an open airway; (3) sufficient and healthy lung tissue; (4) nervous and chemical control; (5) an intact rib cage and diaphragm; (6) sufficient hemoglobin in an ample volume of blood; and (7) a healthy heart to pump blood through an intact circulation."[12]

We can see then that many factors can and do affect the process of respiration beyond the simple act of breathing. Most of these factors are the responsibility of the physician; however, *maintenance of an airway* and *providing a sufficient supply of oxygen in the air* must also be the concern of the practical nurse assisting in the care of the patient. If the supply of oxygen in the atmosphere of the patient's room is not sufficient for his needs the physician will increase the level of oxygen by ordering oxygen therapy for the patient. The nurse then has the responsibility of maintaining the oxygen concentration of the air the patient breathes at the level designated by the physician.

It is obvious that oxygen therapy is all but useless if the respiratory tract is obstructed and there is little or no air flowing into the patient's lungs. Many times, however, the value of simple nursing measures is overlooked in a frenzied concern over the proper functioning of complicated machinery and bedside equipment. The first concern of the practical nurse then, is the correct positioning of the patient so that each part of the body concerned with the intake and outflow of air is in a position of maximum function.

Proper Positioning of the Patient

We know the advantages of proper posture while walking, standing, and sitting; these principles of good posture are equally important to the patient lying in bed. The average person pictures an unconscious individual lying on his back, pillow under the head, chin resting on the chest, and one or both arms lying across the abdomen or chest. This is sometimes referred to as the "coffin" position, and indeed it is an accurate description. It is a posture more appropriate to death than to life.

The reasons for avoiding this position in an unconscious person become quite clear when we consider the ways such a position hampers respiration. First, the tracheal opening is narrowed considerably when the head is bent forward. Secondly, a person in the supine position, even without a pillow under his head, is in danger of aspirating vomitus and mouth secretions. In addition, the tongue may fall to the back of the throat, thereby obstructing the flow of air. Thirdly, the weight of one or both arms on the chest interferes with complete expansion of the thoracic cavity.

The best position to insure optimum breathing is on the side, (slightly more than 90 degrees) with the neck extended and the head and chin supported with a small pillow. The uppermost leg is flexed and the uppermost arm is also bent and brought in front of the patient and supported by a pillow. Sometimes the patient's particular condition of illness may prevent positioning the patient in this manner. In this case the practical nurse should consult with the nurse in charge or the physician and determine the proper positioning of the patient.

Maintenance of an Open Airway

Once she is assured that her patient is in the proper position for optimal breathing, the nurse must help him rid the bronchial tree of secretions. If the patient is completely unresponsive and cannot cough up and expectorate the secretions, a throat suction machine is used. The following rules should be observed when using this machine:

1. The bottle used for collecting wastes suctioned from the throat is never filled above the line designated on the bottle.

2. The catheter is pinched off until it has been inserted into the throat. This prevents damage to the mucous membranes. After the catheter is in the throat it is released and then moved gently up and down the throat so as to clear all areas of mucus.

3. During the suctioning procedure the catheter may become plugged with thick mucus. It must then be removed from the throat and placed in a glass of water or saline to rinse the catheter and remove the plug of mucus.

4. The catheter and tubing must always be rinsed clean after each suctioning by placing the catheter in a glass of water while the motor is still on.

There are times when the physician may place a tube or "airway" made of metal, rubber, or plastic into the throat of an unconscious patient to facilitate suctioning and also to prevent the tongue from falling back and obstructing the trachea. When an airway is in place the catheter is inserted through the opening of the airway and mucus is removed from the throat.

5. When the nasal passages require suctioning, it is recommended that two catheters be used, one for the nose and the other for the throat or tracheostomy opening. This will help minimize infection of the throat and the surgical incision.

Tracheostomy. DEFINITION. *Tracheostomy* is surgical incision into the trachea for the purpose of inserting a tube through which the patient breathes (see Fig. 6-4). It is done when there is complete obstruction of the trachea above the point of the incision and may be an emergency measure, or it may be done in anticipation of obstruction from edema or a growing malignancy.

The tracheostomy set consists of three parts: (1) the outer cannula which is hollow and must never be removed by the practical nurse; (2) the inner cannula which is also hollow and fits inside the outer cannula (this inner tube may be removed for cleaning); and (3) the obturator, a cone-tipped object which is used during the insertion of the tubes and is shaped to fit into the tubes. The obturator may be inserted to obstruct the inner cannula when the patient is learning to breathe normally again.

Figure 6-4. *A*, Tracheostomy tube in place. Note dressing around tubing and tapes that tie around neck and hold tubes in place. *B*, Inset shows tracheostomy tube and obturator that is inserted and used as a guide when the tube is first put into the trachea. The obturator may also be used later to help the patient adjust to normal breathing before the tracheostomy tube is removed. *C*, Position of tracheostomy tube and nasogastric feeding tube. (A and B, from Ferguson & Sholtes: *Eliason's Surgical Nursing*, 11th Ed., J. B. Lippincott Co., Philadelphia. C, from Totman and Lehman: American Journal of Nursing, March, 1964.)

NURSING CARE OF THE PATIENT WITH
A TRACHEOSTOMY. The nurse must
always remember that the patient with
a tracheostomy cannot speak or make
any vocal sounds as long as the tracheostomy is open because the air he
inhales and exhales does not pass
through the vocal cords. If he is conscious and able to move he should be
given a call bell whenever it is necessary
to leave him alone so that he will have
a way to summon help quickly. If he is
able to write he should be provided with
a pad of paper and pencil or a magic
slate so that he can communicate his
needs to the nurse. If he is not able to
move he must not be left alone for any
reason as there is danger of a mucus
plug obstructing the tracheostomy tube
and causing asphyxiation and possible
death.

The cleaning and care of the tracheostomy tube and special nursing care
of the patient demand constant attention. The practical nurse who is not
familiar with this special care should
gain experience through observation
and assisting with the care of the tracheostomy before she attempts to accept

such a responsibility. In some institutions she may be allowed to take on
more responsibility than the information given here will prepare her for. In
this case it is recommended that the
practical nurse request additional information and instruction from the
physician or nurse in charge. It must
be remembered that *the patient with a
new tracheostomy incision is always in danger of asphyxiation.*

The special considerations in the
nursing care of a tracheostomy patient
are as follows:

1. The outer tube is held in place by
a woven cotton tape which encircles
the neck and ties at the back. This tape
must never be cut or untied by the practical nurse because of the possibility that
the patient may cough the outer cannula
out of the incision.

2. An extra tracheostomy set should
be kept in the patient's room at all times.

3. All equipment for cleaning and
care of the tracheostomy should be kept
at the bedside.

4. When we inhale under normal
conditions the air is warmed and moistened as it passes through the nose and

Figure 6-5. Atraumatic, aseptic tracheal suctioning is important throughout the patient's illness.
(From Nett and Petty: American Journal of Nursing, September, 1967.)

throat. The patient with a tracheostomy does not breathe normally; thus the air he breathes must be warmed and moistened artificially. A small vaporizer at the bedside will usually accomplish this.

5. Secretions must be removed as soon as they appear at the opening of the tracheostomy tube to prevent their aspiration back into the tube. Great care must be used in wiping or suctioning these secretions so as to avoid trauma to the surgical wound (see Fig. 6-5).

6. Gauze dressings around the tracheostomy opening must be bound with tape so that loose strings will not be aspirated into the tube. Many hospitals have special dressings to be used around a tracheostomy to avoid this hazard.

7. The inner and outer cannulae are often made of very soft metal and may easily be bent by careless handling or improper cleaning methods. The inner cannula should be removed and cleaned on the inside with a pipe cleaner.

8. Until he becomes accustomed to breathing through the tube, and because he cannot speak, the patient may be very apprehensive and easily upset by fits of coughing. He will need continued reassurance and competent, well-informed nurses in attendance.

THE CUFFED TRACHEOSTOMY TUBE. This is a specially designed tracheostomy tube that is used when a patient in acute respiratory failure must receive assisted ventilation with a positive pressure respirator. (Respirators are discussed below.) The tracheal end of the tracheostomy tube is encircled by a small balloon. When this balloon is inflated it fills the space between the tracheostomy tube and the trachea, thereby providing a seal and preventing the escape of air around the tube. When positive pressure is administered, the air passes through the tracheostomy tube *only*, thus providing sufficient pressure to inflate the lungs. The cuffed tracheostomy tube also reduces the chance of aspiration of mucus and fluids in those patients whose protective reflexes in the larynx and trachea are impaired.

Since the lumen of the tube is the only source of air for the patient he must be watched closely for signs of obstruction of the tube. If the lumen is not suctioned frequently and kept open, the patient will suffocate. To avoid depression of the surface blood vessels in the tracheal wall and resultant necrosis, the cuff must be inflated just enough to seal the trachea without causing extreme pressure against the tracheal wall. A complaint from the patient that he has a sensation of tightness or choking must be reported immediately as this may indicate overinflation of the cuff.

Oxygen Therapy

Purposes of Oxygen Therapy. The air we breathe contains about 20 per cent oxygen. Under normal circumstances this percentage is quite adequate; but, when there is an obstruction of the intake of air or impaired circulation of the oxygen to the body tissues by way of the blood stream, the percentage of oxygen intake must be increased. The condition brought about by insufficient amounts of oxygen in the body is called *hypoxia*. The symptoms accompanying hypoxia are a result of damage to cells due to a lack of the oxygen so vital to their existence.

Tissues vary in their oxygen requirements. The cerebral cells, for example, receive 20 per cent of the body's oxygen supply and can live for only a few minutes if their supply of oxygen is cut off. Other cells, such as those of the myocardium, can survive as long as 30 to 40 minutes without a fresh supply of oxygen. We can see why it has been said that hypoxia not only stops the machine, but also wrecks the machinery.

The patient who is suffering from anoxia will complain of headaches and slight visual disturbances, his pulse will become rapid, and his respirations will increase. Restlessness is also present and cyanosis soon develops if the condition is not relieved. In order to pro-

Comparison of Methods of Applying Oxygen Therapy

	Efficiency	Comfort	Cost	Causes of Failure	Dangers
Tent	Satisfactory if well applied and regularly tested	Excellent	Very high	Improper application and leaks insufficient care and testing	Rare fire danger from sparks
Box	Satisfactory if well applied and regularly tested	Good	Moderate (¼ cost of tent)	Improper application and leaks	Almost no danger
Catheter	Excellent with reasonable attention to details	Fair usually acceptable sometimes poorly tolerated	Low	Leakage especially from water bottle attachments	Gastric distension or rarely rupture (if used without a stop on catheter)
Cannula	Poor	Good	Low	Inefficiency of method especially in restless patients	Practically none
Plastic Face Mask	Poor	Good	Low	Inefficiency of method especially in restless patients	Practically none

Figure 6-6. Note that administration of oxygen by nasal catheter provides greatest efficiency and low cost but may be poorly tolerated by some patients. Oxygen tent and box are satisfactory methods but attention must be paid to proper care and prevention of leaks. (From Burgess: American Journal of Nursing, December, 1965.)

vide the body cells with an adequate supply of oxygen it may be necessary to administer oxygen by tent, nasal catheter, or mask. The efficiency, cost and dangers of each method are presented in Figure 6-6.

OXYGEN BY TENT. Oxygen is heavier than air. It is possible for a considerable amount to be lost by seepage through the mattress when oxygen is administered by tent, unless a rubber sheet is placed over the mattress un-

der the tent area. To make the tent airtight, the sides of the tent are tucked well under the mattress and the front of the tent is folded inside an extra top sheet or bath blanket across the bed. The ends of the sheet are then tucked in at the sides of the bed (see Figs. 6-7 and 6-8).

All holes and tears in the tent must be repaired. When it is necessary to open the side zippers, the nurse should work as quickly as possible and do as

Figure 6-7. The top bedding has been brought up over the patient's chest. An additional sheet is placed across the bed and the tent edge placed over it. (From Brown: *Medical Nursing*, 3rd Ed., W. B. Saunders Co., Philadelphia.)

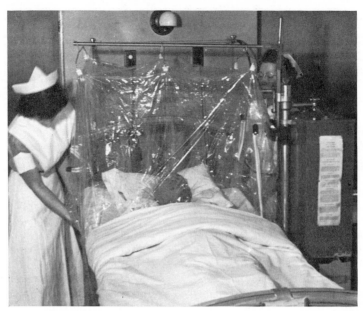

Figure 6-8. The sheet is then folded over the edge of the tent and each end is tucked securely under the mattress, thus preventing a loss of oxygen from the tent. (From Brown: *Medical Nursing*, 3rd Ed., W. B. Saunders Co., Philadelphia.)

much for the patient at one time as is practical so that there is a minimal loss of oxygen. Though speed is important, the patient should not be given the impression that he is being rushed through a procedure. Some persons suffer from claustrophobia when they are confined inside a tent. They become frightened and worry about the possibility of something going wrong with the apparatus and the supply of oxygen being cut off. These patients will need constant reassurance that the nurse is nearby and observing the apparatus very closely.

OXYGEN BY MASK. (See Fig. 6-9.) If oxygen is administered by mask, care must be taken that the mask fits snugly and follows the contour of the face. It is comforting to the patient to have the mask removed periodically so that the face can be gently cleansed and powdered to prevent irritation of the skin. Obviously this must be done quickly so that the patient does not suffer from a lack of oxygen while the mask has been removed.

OXYGEN BY NASAL CATHETER. (See Fig. 6-10A.) There are several types of nasal catheters available for the administration of oxygen. They are inserted in the nostril and held in place by adhesive tape or a small disk designed to prevent aspiration of the catheter into the bronchial tree. These catheters will need periodic changing, and special attention must be given to the nasal mucosa which may become somewhat irritated by the tube. Another hazard of the nasal catheter is the possibility of rupturing the stomach by passing the catheter into the esophagus. This can be avoided by placing a stop on the catheter (see Fig. 6-10A).

Precautions to Be Taken When Oxygen Is Used. Oxygen is NOT EXPLOSIVE. IT DOES SUPPORT COMBUSTION, which means that any spark or flame can cause a major fire in a very short period of time. The precautions necessary for the prevention of such a catastrophe are usually very clearly stated in every

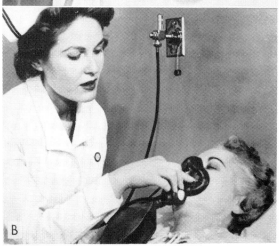

Figure 6-9. *A,* An oronasal meter type mask, which covers both the nose and mouth. Band around the head holds mask in place. *B,* Partial rebreathing mask. It is also held in place by head band (not shown). Note wall outlet for oxygen. (From Linde Company, Division Union Carbide Corp., New York.)

hospital policy book or procedure manual. These precautions include:

1. No smoking signs posted in the area where oxygen is being administered.

2. Use of cotton blankets rather than wool blankets on the patient's bed.

3. Substituting a hand bell for the electric call bell.

4. Discontinuing the flow of oxygen while any electric equipment such as an E.K.G. machine or suction machine is being used at the bedside.

Other precautions include attention to factors that can interfere with the flow of oxygen from the tank to the patient. These may include kinks in the tubing, loose connections and faulty humidifying apparatus. If there is some question as to whether oxygen is flowing properly, listen for the hissing sound of air passing into the catheter, mask or tent. To determine whether tubing is open and oxygen is passing through it hold your finger over the end of the tube momentarily and then release it. You should hear a "pfft" sound as the oxygen escapes through the end of the tube. Remember that it is not unusual to find that a patient who is supposedly

Figure 6-10. *A*, A stop placed 12.5 cm. from the catheter tip insures safe insertion in the oropharynx of any adult patient and prevents the catheter from extending into the patient's esophagus. *B*, Face mask is better for short-term therapy than for prolonged oxygen therapy. *C*, Double nasal cannula is best when only a slight increase in oxygen is needed. (From Burgess: American Journal of Nursing, December, 1965.)

receiving oxygen therapy is actually getting less oxygen than he would under normal circumstances. The physician decides when the patient is to receive oxygen and by what method and in what concentration, but it is the nurse who must see to it that the patient receives that which is ordered.

Hazards of Oxygen Therapy. Paradoxically, the very oxygen that is needed to sustain life can be toxic. In very high concentrations and given over a period of time, oxygen can actually depress respiration and cause the patient to become cyanotic and comatose. After about 48 hours of administering oxygen in high concentrations and under positive pressure, the lungs fail to expand properly. This is especially true when pure oxygen is being given via a cuffed tracheostomy tube.

The nurse is responsible for seeing to it that oxygen is administered in the concentration ordered by the physician. She also must encourage her patient to take deep breaths periodically if he is able to do so. If the patient complains of discomfort under the sternum, or has a cough or very shallow respiration, these symptoms should be reported to the physician in charge as they may indicate oxygen toxication.

Hyperbaric Oxygenation

The normal atmospheric pressure is approximately 14.9 pounds per square inch. Man is adapted to live in this atmospheric pressure and is rarely subjected to fluctuations in pressure unless he ascends to high altitudes or descends to certain depths beneath the sea. The term *hyperbaric pressure* refers to an increase in atmospheric pressure. Such an increase will bring about an increase in the amount of dissolved gases in the blood and body fluids. When a patient is placed in a hyperbaric oxygenation chamber the amount of oxygen available to the body tissues becomes greatly increased.

Hyperbaric oxygenation is not a new concept. Pressure chambers were used as early as the 1800's for treatment of a variety of ills. Today the chambers are considered most helpful in treating patients with anaerobic infections, carbon monoxide poisoning and acute obstruction to the blood supply of an extremity. Some chambers are fairly small; others are large enough to accommodate an entire surgical team and surgical equipment as well as the patient, and are used during corrective surgery for congenital heart diseases in which there is severe cyanosis of the patient (see Fig. 6-11).

The use of hyperbaric oxygenation is not without its hazards and those who work on the hyperbaric team must be specially trained and skilled in the care of the patient in such situations.

Respirators

Introduction. In the past the patient in acute respiratory failure was usually placed in an iron lung and his condition was most often neurogenic, as in bulbar

Figure 6-11. An operating room team at work in the hyperbaric oxygen chamber at Mount Sinai Hospital. (From Venger: *Nursing Clinics of North America,* March, 1966.)

A

B

Figure 6-12 A & B

Figure 6-12. *A*, Operation of the Bird respirator. Check oxygen inlet (6) and oxygen supply to the respirator. Establish the prescribed pressure by rotating the cross bar of the pressure limit (1). Later, when the respirator is attached to the patient, the needle on the pressure gauge (7) which has been resting at zero will move into the green area of the pressure gauge indicating the development of positive pressure in the patient's lungs. Pull the knob of the air mix (2) out all the way. This diverts oxygen into a mixing chamber with atmospheric air to give a 40% concentration. For automatic cycling, turn the dial of the expiratory timer (3) counterclockwise to the desired cycling rate. This determines the length of time between inspirations. It is important to allow sufficient time between cycles to permit gas exchange in the lungs. For spontaneous cycling, turn the dial clockwise to inactivate the timer. The manual control (8) tests the machine's action when spontaneous cycling does not exist and automatic cycling is not being used. Push the rod in until gas flow begins, then release it. The rod will return to its resting position. This action must be repeated for every cycle. The sensitivity indicator (4) restrains the flow of gas to the patient between inhalations. The control can be adjusted to allow the respirator to respond if the patient makes the slightest effort to breathe. When the patient is unable to start the inspiratory cycle on his own, turn the indicator counterclockwise to a lower number to increase the sensitivity. Care should be taken not to set this control for greater sensitivity than is necessary as the cycle will not allow for a postexpiratory phase. The flow rate (5) controls the inspiratory time and turns the respirator from OFF to ON. Use one hand to grasp the breathing head assembly with the palm over the breathing outlet (9), totally obstructing the flow. With the other hand, slowly open the flow rate in counterclockwise fashion until the respirator switches off. Check the nebulizer (10) by removing it from the tee (11). Hold it in a horizontal

88

Figure 6-12 C

position with the inlet stem pointing toward the floor. Connect the pressure line (12). Move the manual control in and out several times and look for nebulized particles from the nebulizer. Reinsert the nebulizer in the tee, checking the proper breathing position. Apply the respirator to the patient. When the patient has become adjusted to the respirator, the flow rate should be readjusted to increase inspiratory pressure as long as the respirator switches off at the end of each inspiration.

If negative pressure is to be incorporated in the Mark 8, it is initiated only on orders from the physician and after the positive phase has been established. Hold the rod of the manual control out temporarily to restrain the positive phase. Turn the knob of the negative pressure generator (13) counterclockwise until the prescribed pressure registers on the pressure gauge. Caution should be used, since higher negative values may lead to bronchiolar collapse. Rotate the sensitivity indicator into the negative scale on the sensitivity ring to match the pressure recorded on the pressure gauge. Release the manual control. If the respirator cycles prematurely after releasing the manual control, advance the sensitivity indicator into the negative scale until the unwanted cycles cease. *B*, Operation of Engstrom respirator. Make sure the respirator is plugged in and preferably grounded. Turn on machine by pushing button (A) on front. Adjust water lock level (knob on right side of machine) to maximum desired inspiratory pressure. Check water level (B) in humidifier. There should be no more than 3 inches depth in the bottom of the humidifier. Set speed control (C) to desired respiratory rate. Be sure not to set this until the machine is running. Select either spirometer or venturi (D). Choose venturi if negative pressure assisted expiration is desired. Set pressure control selector (E) to venturi. Set dosing valve (F) to required minute ventilation. Set dosing valve calibrator (G) so right compressor gauge (H) swings to the red mark. Set inspiratory flow rate (1) so that the rubber bag (J) is fully collapsed at the end of the inspiratory phase. Attach the patient through the tracheostomy or endotracheal tube to the long tubing with the Y-piece (K) at the end. Make sure that the glass bulb in the expiratory line (L) is level to catch condensation. Reset inspiratory flow rate with the patient on the respirator so that the bag is fully deflated at the end of the inspiratory phase, but so that no "bubbling over" occurs in the water lock. *C*, The Bennett respirator. (A and B, from McCallum: *Nursing Clinics of North America*, December, 1966. C, from McArdle: *Nursing Clinics of North America*, March, 1966.)

89

poliomyelitis. The iron lung has largely been replaced by more compact, efficient machines that improve ventilation of the lungs. These machines, called respirators, help the patient breathe more deeply, or breathe for him if he is in complete respiratory failure.

Types and Uses. There are two main types of respirators: those that provide controlled ventilation and those that give assisted ventilation. They may be used to: (1) provide patient-controlled pressure-breathing assistance for patients who are conscious and able to breathe spontaneously, (2) provide respiratory control for patients who cannot breathe, (3) relieve or overcome insufficient respiration, (4) deliver deep into the bronchial tree medications such as antibiotic and bronchodilator aerosols, or liquefying agents that make the mucus less tenacious and easier to cough up, and (5) provide a form of deep breathing exercise that "stretches" the respiratory muscles and improves their elastic tone and the circulation of the lungs. In both types of respirators there usually are controls for the administration of oxygen.

There are at least 50 models and designs of respirators in existence but the three most commonly used are the Bird, the Bennett and the Engstrom respirators. These are pictured in Figure 6-12.

Nursing Responsibilities. Those concerned with the care of patients having controlled or assisted ventilation must have a thorough understanding of the physiology of respiration and the use of respirators. Although the respirators may vary in design and purpose, there are some principles of nursing care applicable to all patients using respirators.

1. The patient who breathes spontaneously usually will breathe through a mouthpiece when assisted ventilation is used. He should be told to purse his lips around the mouthpiece but not to clench his teeth or obstruct the tube with his tongue. He must not breathe through his nose and if this is difficult at first he may use a nose clip.

2. He should be given a brief, simple explanation of the purpose of the ventilation and what he can expect from it. The pressure from the respirator helps him inflate his lungs as he inhales. His breathing triggers the machine and so he can control to some extent the amount of air flowing into his lungs. He should be told to pause after each exhalation.

3. If a mask is used it should be well fitted so there is no leakage of air.

4. Provide the patient with a quiet, relaxing atmosphere.

5. Check the dials frequently for accidental changes in the readings.

6. Watch for a drop in blood pressure or symptoms of respiratory alkalosis in patients having prolonged controlled ventilation.

7. Pay attention to the skin, state of nutrition and need for suctioning in patients who are paralyzed or comatose.

REGULATION OF FLUID INTAKE

Intravenous Therapy. The importance of an adequate intake of fluids for the maintenance of life has been discussed in Chapter 3. During a critical illness the patient will most likely be unable to take these essential fluids by mouth. The most common substitute for oral feedings is the administration of fluids by vein (intravenous therapy) or into the tissues by hypodermoclysis (see Fig. 6-13).

Intravenous therapy requires frequent checking of the apparatus for the proper rate of flow as ordered by the physician and for the assurance that the needle or catheter is still in the vein. If the needle is dislodged, the solution will infiltrate into surrounding tissues, causing pain and damage to the tissues. When the practical nurse observes a raised area around the tip of the needle, or an interruption in the

A

B

Figure 6-13. *A,* Intravenous administration of fluids. Note tape holding needle in vein and use of gauze square to serve as "bridge" so that needle is kept at proper angle in vein. Arm is held immobile by using arm board. *B,* Hypodermoclysis. Fluids are given directly into tissues. Tubing is looped and held with tape to prevent tension on needles. Thighs are site most frequently used for hypodermoclysis. (From Montag and Swenson: *Fundamentals in Nursing Care,* 3rd Ed., W. B. Saunders Co., Philadelphia.)

flow of solution, she should notify the nurse in charge immediately. It is extremely unwise to tamper with intravenous tubing or the needle during an infusion, as there is the possibility of allowing air to enter the tube, thus giving rise to an air embolus in the vein which could very easily be fatal to the patient.

All equipment from an infusion must be handled very carefully once it has been removed from the patient's vein. There is always the possibility that infectious hepatitis may be spread by way of contaminated equipment.

Sometimes when intravenous feedings are necessary for an extended length of time, or peripheral circulation is poor and there is collapse of the blood vessels, the physician must make an incision into the vein for the purpose of inserting a needle or plastic tubing. The site of this "cut down" into the vein must be treated with care during and after the infusion therapy. The incision is kept free from contamination until completely healed so as to avoid infection and thrombophlebitis.

Patients who are receiving continuous infusions require special mouth care since there is no food or drink being taken by mouth to stimulate the flow of saliva. If the patient is semiconscious or totally unconscious, he will probably breathe through his mouth most of the time, thus causing a drying of the mucous membranes.

When there is any doubt as to whether or not the patient is able to swallow, a few drops of water on a spoon may be placed on the back of the tongue and the patient instructed to swallow. If he cannot do so it is assumed that he cannot take anything by mouth without the danger of aspirating it into his lungs. A critically ill patient in this condition frequently suffers terribly from thirst even though he cannot express his discomfort. A sponge soaked with water will help to relieve his thirst. In addition, the mouth must be cleansed inside every two hours with either glycerine and lemon juice (to stimulate salivation) or a mouthwash. The application of a lubricant such as mineral oil or petroleum jelly to the lips will prevent drying and cracking. It is not wise to use an excess of either of these oils as they may be aspirated into the lungs and cause a lipoid pneumonia.

It may be well at this point to mention the eyes of the critically ill patient. Often these patients will not completely close their eyes even though they may be unconscious. In this instance warm boric acid solution or normal saline should be used to rinse the eyes several times a day. A drop of mineral oil in each eye after the rinsing will stimulate lacrimation and protect the eye from lint and dirt. Without this care it is possible for the cornea to become excessively dry, which can eventually lead to blindness.

Transfusion. The word "transfusion" refers to the transfer of whole blood from one person to another. In earlier times the only method used was by direct transfer. Today, blood is usually taken from the donor and stored in 500 ml. bottles in the blood bank until needed. With this modern method of transfusion, and the use of blood banks for proper storage and typing of blood, there is much less danger of reaction to blood transfusions than formerly. It is still a potentially dangerous procedure and the patient must be observed very carefully for a reaction during and after a transfusion.

Nurses must never become complacent about transfusions no matter how many times they may see them safely administered without incident. Any symptoms observed or any complaint

Table 8. *Parenteral Fluids*

TYPE	PURPOSE AND SPECIAL PRECAUTIONS
Amino acids	Used as supplemental protein feedings. Administer slowly to avoid nausea and vomiting
Dextrose or invert sugar (half dextrose, half levulose)	Provide carbohydrates. May cause vein damage if given in high concentrations. Invert sugar usually given at a rate of 1 gm. of dissolved sugar per kg. of body weight per hour. Dextrose administered 0.5 grains/kg. body weight/hour
Saline solution (sodium chloride)	Provides essential electrolytes. Too much may cause edema
Darrow's solution (potassium chloride)	Provides potassium, an essential electrolyte
Ethyl alcohol	A substitute for dextrose as a concentrated source of calories. Acts as a sedative and has a diuretic effect. Given slowly at first and then the rate of flow is increased

from the patient should be reported without delay. The word "reaction," when used in reference to the transfusion of blood or infusion of fluids, means a sensitivity to the substances being given by vein. These may include the blood itself or the minerals added to the blood or fluids to preserve them. The symptoms of a reaction may be so mild as to go completely unnoticed, or so severe that death is the outcome. In milder cases the patient develops a rash and complains of itching, or he may have chills and fever. In more severe cases the patient may experience dyspnea, coughing, flushed face, restlessness, and eventually there will occur collapse, coma, and death. When the symptoms of a reaction first appear the transfusion is stopped immediately and epinephrine may be given.

MAINTENANCE OF NORMAL BODY TEMPERATURE

Reduction of Elevated Temperatures. Extremes in body temperature frequently accompany critical illnesses and demand special attention from the nursing staff. Any patient on the critical list or in an intensive care unit must have his temperature checked at least every 4 hours. A very high temperature may be present in an infection or in disturbances of the heat-regulating center of the body. A tepid sponge bath, ice bags, and other measures for lowering the body temperature may be ordered by the physician when the patient's temperature becomes dangerously high.

Subnormal Temperatures. Patients with poor peripheral circulation will usually have a decrease in the body temperature. Others suffering from shock or in coma may also require extra warmth supplied by heating pads or hot water bottles. Since their skin is cold and damp, they should be kept out of drafts and as dry as possible, to

avoid pneumonia or an upper respiratory infection.

In applying additional warmth to any patient it must be remembered that *only enough heat to maintain normal body temperature is necessary.* Too much heat may cause excessive perspiration or loss of body fluids. It is generally agreed that patients suffering from hemorrhage should NOT have extra warmth applied. Should the practical nurse have some question in her mind as to the advisability of applying additional warmth, she must consult the nurse in charge.

EXCRETION OF WASTES

During a critical illness many of the usual functions of the body become seriously impaired and may cease altogether. The involvement of any vital organ concerned with the elimination of wastes, such as the kidneys or lungs, will soon lead to an accumulation of poisonous substances within the body tissues. Relief of this situation by artificial means offers some hope for acutely ill individuals in a critical situation. An example of this removal of wastes from the body is the artificial kidney, which is discussed in more detail in Chapter 15.

Other more general and less complicated methods of assisting the body to eliminate wastes include: (1) continued maintenance of proper respiration, (2) provision for adequate circulation of the blood and lymphatics by frequent turning of the patient and exercises when possible, (3) adequate bowel elimination through the use of enemas and/or mild laxatives, (4) drainage of urine from the bladder or kidney by catheter, and (5) proper cleansing and care of the skin.

EMERGENCY SITUATIONS

A sudden and serious change in the patient's status is not unusual in a critically ill patient. Those who care for such patients must be prepared for emergencies such as cardiac arrest or cessation of breathing. These and other emergency situations are discussed in Chapter 20.

MAINTENANCE OF CIRCULATION

Motion of muscular tissues within the body aids the flow of blood through the peripheral vessels and facilitates the return of venous flow to the heart. Critically ill patients who are unconscious or unable to move because of paralysis are likely to have a sluggish circulation of blood through the blood vessels. This predisposes the body to the formation of blood clots and the development of inflammation within the veins. Circulatory stasis will also lead to deterioration of the skin, particularly in areas where pressure of the body's weight decreases the flow of blood to the surface. In a critically ill patient, breaks in the skin which lead to decubitus ulcers may develop very quickly if measures are not taken to maintain good circulation. Changing the position of the patient who cannot turn himself

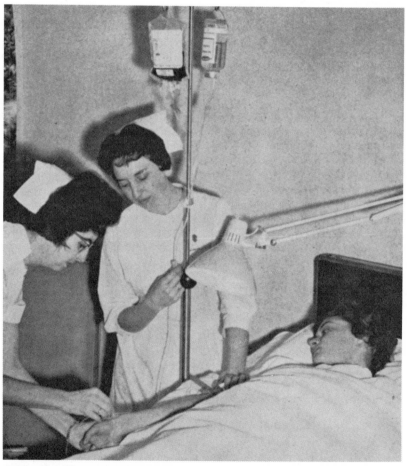

Figure 6-14. Careful cross-matching between the blood type of the patient and that of the prospective blood donor is mandatory before any blood transfusion can be administered. (From Buchanan: American Journal of Nursing, July, 1965.)

and passive exercises of the extremities are important in the maintenance of adequate circulation.

EMOTIONAL ASPECTS OF NURSING THE CRITICALLY ILL

Nurses devote their lives to preserving life and restoring to health those who are sick and injured. It sometimes happens, then, that when a nurse is faced with the death of a patient she has tried so hard to save, she is overcome with a sense of failure. If she has performed her duties faithfully and well, there is actually no justification for such an attitude. Each of us must face grief and death; it is a part of every life and our only recourse is to provide ourselves with a mature philosophy which will give some meaning to the unhappinesses which life brings.

When a patient is critically ill he is close to death. He may overcome his illness or he may succumb and die, but in either case he and his family need and deserve as much moral support as it is humanly possible to give them. The practical nurse, by the very nature of her role in nursing, is often very close to the patient and his family. She often spends more time at the bedside than other members of the nursing team and the patient and his family may find it easier to confide in her than in others with more authority. When grief and fear overcome the patient or his family it is often the nurse to whom they turn for moral support and spiritual strength. When this happens the nurse has an obligation to provide whatever comfort she is able to give, even though it may be easier to leave them alone and become as little involved with their problems as possible.

There are no pat answers to these problems of grief and despair. The nurse's ability to conduct herself with composure and tact must come from deep within herself. She must be a mature individual emotionally and spiritually, and she must be dedicated to the task of fulfilling her obligations to those she has pledged to serve in *all their needs.*

CLINICAL CASE PROBLEMS

1. Mr. Tower, age 30, has been admitted to the hospital's intensive care unit following injuries received in an automobile accident. He has a severe head injury and is semiconscious. A tracheostomy was performed in the emergency room to relieve obstruction of the trachea.

The third day after his admission Mr. Tower's condition remains critical because of his head injury and failure to respond to most stimuli in a normal manner. You are assigned to assist in the care of this patient.

> What special observations should be made while caring for this patient?
> What equipment should you be familiar with and able to operate while caring for this patient?
> If you learned that Mr. Tower is the father and sole support of four small children, what problems can you see in this situation?

2. Mrs. Thomas, age 53, is brought to the intensive care unit because of hemorrhage from a bleeding peptic ulcer. She is vomiting blood in large amounts and is receiving a blood transfusion which was started in the emergency room before admission to the intensive care unit. Mrs. Thomas is extremely weak and appears to be semiconscious.

> How should this patient be positioned to prevent aspiration of vomitus?
> What special observations must be made while caring for her?
> How can you handle the vomitus so that the patient and family are not unduly alarmed by the loss of blood?

3. Mrs. Long, age 73, is critically ill with a diagnosis of congestive heart failure. She has generalized edema, pulmonary congestion, and dyspnea with cyanosis. She apparently is comatose and does not respond when spoken to.

Her children are very concerned about the critical condition of their mother and realize that she is near death.

How should this patient be positioned in bed?

What special skin care will be necessary? Why?

What nursing measures may be used to help relieve the edema and dyspnea?

If the patient's son entered her room at the time you were caring for her and asked you if his mother was dying, what would you do?

REFERENCES

1. Adams, J. G.: "Hyperbaric Oxygen Therapy." Am. Journ. Nurs., June, 1964, p. 76.
2. Adriani, J.: "Venipuncture." Am. Journ. Nurs., March, 1963, p. 66.
3. Beland, I. L.: *Clinical Nursing—Pathophysical and Psychosocial Approaches.* New York, The Macmillan Co., 1965.
4. Brunner, L. S., et al.: *Textbook of Medical-Surgical Nursing.* Philadelphia, J. B. Lippincott Co., 1964.
5. Buchanan-Davidson, D. J.: "A Drop of Blood." Am. Journ. Nurs., July, 1965.
6. Burgess, A. M.: "A Comparison of Common Methods of Oxygen Therapy for Bed Patients." Am. Journ. Nurs., Dec., 1965, p. 96.
7. Burgess, R. E.: "Fluids and Electrolytes." Am. Journ, Nurs., Oct., 1965, p. 90.
8. Chow, R.: "Innovations in I.V. Equipment." Am. Journ. Nurs., March, 1962, p. 80.
9. Fielo, S. B.: "Teaching Fluid and Electrolyte Balance." Nurs. Outlook, March, 1965, p. 43.
10. Flatter, P. A.: "Hazards of Oxygen Therapy." Am. Journ. Nurs., Jan., 1968, p. 80.
11. Foster, M. A.: "Teaching Blood Groups and Reactions." Nurs. Outlook, Feb., 1966, p. 49.
12. Hadley, F., and Bordicks, K. J.: "Respiratory Difficulty." Am. Journ. Nurs., Oct., 1962, p. 64.
13. Harmer, B., and Henderson, V.: *Textbook of the Principles and Practice of Nursing,* 5th edition. New York, The Macmillan Co., 1960.
14. McCallum, H. P.: "The Nurse and the Respirator." *Nursing Clinics of North America,* vol. 1, no. 4. Philadelphia, W. B. Saunders Co., 1966.
15. Montag, M. L., and Swenson, R. S.: *Fundamentals in Nursing Care,* 3rd edition. Philadelphia, W. B. Saunders Co., 1958.
16. Neelon, V. J.: "Hyperbaric Oxygenation—Benefits and Hazards." Am. Journ. Nurs., Oct., 1964, p. 73.
17. Nett, L. M., and Petty, T. L.: "Acute Respiratory Failure." Am. Journ. Nurs., Sept., 1967, p. 1847.
18. Quint, J. C.: "Obstacles to Helping the Dying." Am. Journ. Nurs., July, 1966, p. 1568.
19. Shafer, K. N., Sawyer, J. R., et al.: *Medical-Surgical Nursing,* 4th edition. St. Louis, Mo., C. V. Mosby Co., 1967.
20. Smith, D. W., and Gips, C. D.: *Care of the Adult Patient,* 2nd edition. Philadelphia, J. B. Lippincott Co., 1966.
21. Sovie, M. D., and Israel, J. B.: "Use of the Cuffed Tracheostomy Tube." Am. Journ. Nurs., Sept., 1967, p. 1854.
22. Totman, L. E., and Lehman, R. H.: "Tracheostomy Care." Am. Journ. Nurs., March, 1964, p. 96.
23. Van den Bergh, R., and Davidson, R.: "Let's Talk About Death." Am. Journ. Nurs., Jan., 1966, p. 71.

SUGGESTED STUDENT READING

1. Bradford, C. M.: "The Intensive Care Unit and the LPN." Journ. Pract. Nurs., Nov., 1966, p. 35.
2. Brouillard, M. J.: "Nursing in the Intensive Care Unit." Practical Nursing, July-August, 1962, p. 14.
3. DeMeyer, J.: "Emphysema: Effective Positive-Pressure Breathing Therapy." RN, Jan., 1968, p. 42.
4. Dudley, M.: "Donor Blood and Its Major Uses:" RN, April, 1962, p. 47.
5. Engel, G. L.: "Grief and Grieving." Amer. Journ. Nurs., Sept., 1964, p. 93.
6. Hammes, J. J.: "Reflections on Intensive Care." Am. Journ. Nurs. Feb., 1968, p. 339.
7. Morris W. E.: "Parenteral Fluid Therapy." Journ. Pract. Nurs., Sept., 1966, p. 32.
8. Northington, J. M.: "Comfort for Your Dying Patient." RN, Oct., 1962, p. 63.
9. Perez, R.: "Tracheostomy." Practical Nursing. Nov., 1962, p. 14.

OUTLINE FOR CHAPTER 6

I. Introduction

A. Critically ill patients often require assistance with one or more vital functions; e.g., breathing.

II. Intensive Care Units

A. Specially designed units for patients requiring constant nursing care of the most detailed kind.

B. Contain special monitoring equipment, artificial pacemaker for the heart, respiratory resuscitative apparatus, oxygen supply, etc.

III. General Principles of Nursing Care

A. Determination of the patient's state of consciousness and presence or absence of protective reflexes.
B. Maintenance of respiration.
C. Adequate nutrition and elimination.
D. Adequate circulation.

IV. State of Consciousness

A. Unconscious or comatose patient gives no response to stimuli.
B. Semiconscious patient responds to painful stimuli but shows only brief periods of wakefulness.

V. Maintenance of Respiration

A. Factors influencing normal respiration include (1) supply of oxygen, (2) condition of lungs, (3) nervous and chemical control, (4) intact rib cage and diaphragm, (5) sufficient hemoglobin in an ample volume of blood, and (6) healthy heart.
B. Nurse's responsibility lies in maintaining an open airway and providing sufficient oxygen supply.
   1. Proper positioning necessary.
   2. Suctioning done as needed to maintain open airway.
   3. Tracheostomy done to relieve symptoms of obstruction of trachea and provide an open airway (cuffed tracheostomy tube allows for administration of positive pressure by respirator).
C. Oxygen therapy—used to relieve hypoxia.
   1. Methods include tent, nasal catheter prongs, and mask.
   2. Oxygen toxication can occur when patient is given pure oxygen over prolonged period of time.
D. Hyperbaric oxygenation—providing an increase in atmospheric pressure of patient's environment so that there is an increased amount of oxygen available to the body tissues.
E. Respirators—machines that do the work of breathing for the patient.
   1. Controlled ventilation: provides automatic inspiration and expiration for the patient who cannot breathe spontaneously. Assisted ventilation: provides help in deep breathing for the patient who has respiratory problems.
   2. Aerosols can be administered deep into bronchial tree by respirator.

   3. Nursing care includes adequate instruction to the patient and general hygienic care.

VI. Regulation of Fluid Intake

A. Parenteral therapy—administration of fluids, food or medications directly into the blood stream or tissues. Includes intravenous infusion and hypodermoclysis.
   1. Nursing responsibilities include (a) careful handling of equipment and frequent checking to be sure flow of fluid is not interrupted, and (b) mouth care to prevent drying and cracking of lips.
B. Blood transfusion—the transfer of whole blood from one person to another.
   1. "Transfusion reaction"—result of sensitivity to the blood or to minerals added as preservatives. Symptoms may vary from mild rash to fatal anaphylaxis.
   2. When reaction occurs the transfusion is stopped immediately and measures are taken to control sensitivity reaction.
   3. Nurse should always check blood type on label of bottle with patient's blood type recorded on chart before attaching any bottle of blood to transfusion apparatus.

VII. Maintenance of Normal Body Temperature

A. Measures to reduce elevated temperature are done on physician's order.
B. Subnormal body temperature may be due to poor circulation, shock or coma. Apply only enough heat to maintain normal body temperature.

VIII. Excretion of Wastes

A. By artificial means as in hemodialysis.
B. By continued maintenance of adequate respiration, provision for adequate circulation of blood and lymph, adequate bowel and bladder elimination and proper cleansing of skin.

IX. Maintenance of Circulation

A. Frequent changing of position and active and passive exercises.

X. Emotional Aspects

A. Patient and family will demand emotional maturity and spiritual depth on the part of the nurse.

Chapter 7

NURSING CARE OF THE AGED AND CHRONICALLY ILL

VOCABULARY

Altruistic
Disability
Interdependent
Poultice
Supine

Part I — THE AGED

INTRODUCTION

Before considering the care of the aged the practical nurse should have a clear understanding of some terms commonly used in connection with this type of care. First she might ask herself, "What is 'aging' and who are the 'aged'?" The process of aging actually begins at the moment of conception. Barring fatal illness or accident each of us will, as the days of our lives rush by, reach that stage in life referred to as old age. Yet we know that the number of years one lives isn't the only factor involved in deciding whether he is aged. A person's attitude toward life, his variety of interests and zest for living, his acceptance of new ideas, his opinion of himself and tolerance for the shortcomings of others all affect the speed with which he reaches a point of total dependence on others.

In this chapter, for the sake of clarity, we will consider the aged as those persons 65 years or older. This is the gen-erally accepted length of time a person must have lived before he is eligible for social security benefits or retirement from a wage earning job.

"Geriatrics" is a term taken from two Greek words: *Geras*, meaning old age, and *iatrikos*, meaning the care of. It is commonly understood to mean care of and service to the elderly. When the prefix *geras* is followed by the suffix *ology* it becomes the term "gerontology." This means study of the elderly, the aging process and the problems brought about by the process of aging. We often hear the word *senile*, which, used correctly, pertains to aging or growing old, but through improper usage and a misunderstanding of the term it has taken on a connotation of mental deterioration and is not a desirable term to use in referring to elderly people. Old people are senile, but the term should be used with caution and consideration of its implications.

Today the problems of care for the aged have become more evident as

98

medical science has found ways to conquer disease and prolong life.

There are more "senior citizens" in our midst than ever before in the history of our society. And within the past decade, to the everlasting credit of many altruistic groups, a number of volunteer and government agencies have sprung into existence for the purpose of actively helping to meet the problems of the aged.

Nursing, as a humanitarian occupation dedicated to the service of mankind, must take its share of the responsibility for the care of these older persons, because a large percentage of those over 65 have at least one chronic illness and older persons spend more time in general hospitals than the young. Practical nurses, in particular, will frequently find themselves assigned to the care of the elderly, often in hospitals, and sometimes in the home or in institutions operated for the purpose of offering shelter and housing for the aged.

For literature and current information on geriatrics there are several groups to which the practical nurse might apply. One such volunteer group is the Committee on Aging of the National Social Welfare Assembly, whose headquarters are at 345 East Forty-sixth Street, New York. The local public health department and geriatric section of the county medical society are also good sources of information and help in meeting the needs of the elderly.

MEDICARE*

On July 1, 1966 there became effective a governmental health insurance program designed to meet the health needs of the elderly. This program, called Medicare, encompasses two areas: a hospital insurance program to pay for part of the expenses of hospital and posthospital care, and a volun-

tary medical insurance program to help pay for a physician's services and other health services required by persons 65 or older. The benefits from each of the programs are as follows:

1. Hospital Insurance Program:
   a. Payment will be provided for 90 days of inpatient hospital services in an illness. The patient will have to pay a deductible of $40, but the government will pay the rest of the costs for the first 60 days. For the additional 30 days, the patient will pay $10 a day.
   b. In an extended care facility, the government will pay in full for 20 days of services in a spell of illness. After that, 80 more days of care will be partially paid for, with the patient sharing the cost by paying $5 a day.
   c. Outpatient hospital diagnostic services will be paid for, but the patient will pay the first $20 for each 20-day period of diagnostic services and 20 percent of the rest.
   d. Payments will be made for up to 100 visits by a home health agency for care at home in the year after discharge from a hospital or extended care facility. The patient does not share any of the cost.
2. Medical Insurance Program:
   a. Payment will be provided for physician's services, whether given in his office, a hospital, or in the patient's home.
   b. Payment will be provided for certain other medical and health services, such as diagnostic services, medical supplies and equipment, and prosthetic devices.
   c. Payment will be made for up to 100 visits by a home health agency during a calendar year without any requirement of prior hospitalization.
   d. The patient must pay the first $50 of these expenses in each calendar year. The program pays 80 percent of the rest.

Nurses are involved in implementation of the Medicare program in many ways. Patients who could not afford even the most basic of health needs now have an opportunity to share in the many advantages offered by modern

*Quoted from an article written by Arthur Hess, director of the Bureau of Health Insurance, Social Security Administration. Reprinted by permission of American Journal of Nursing. June, 1966 issue, p. 1295.

medical science. By stimulating the expansion of such facilities as outpatient services, extended care in nursing and convalescent homes, and home health programs, Medicare has provided a wider variety of job situations and greater challenges to practical nurses in all parts of the country. It has also increased the need for all types of personnel in the health field and granted recognition to the licensed practical nurse as an important member of the health team. By their education and experience licensed practical nurses are highly qualified to meet the nursing needs of older persons effectively.[12]

The far-reaching effects of Medicare can be appreciated by the following facts compiled after 18 months of operation of the plan:

1. Between July 1, 1966 and June 30, 1967, 5,000,000 Medicare patients had been admitted and two and one-half billion dollars had been paid to hospitals.

2. Between January 1, 1967 and January 1, 1968 some 200,000 persons were admitted to extended care facilities.

3. Home health agencies have provided for some 230,000 older citizens.

4. Under the voluntary medical insurance program 26 million bills have been submitted for medical services and $700 million have been paid out, 90 per cent of it for physicians' services.[19]

We can measure the number of persons helped and the amount of money spent in carrying out such a program, but it is difficult indeed to estimate its true value to the lonely and the desperate who have learned that there is a way in which they can be cared for and their health needs can be met. The nurse's task is to show that she not only cares *for* these persons, but that she truly cares *about* them.

UNDERSTANDING THE AGED

A nurse's feelings, possible prejudices, or biases toward a group of persons have a direct bearing on the caliber of care she will give individuals of that group. Thus the practical nurse must evaluate her feelings toward old age. She should think of it in relation to herself and her future years when she too will be over 65. Does she dread this time of her life and put off thinking about it? Has she neglected to prepare for it by failing to develop hobbies and a variety of interests outside nursing? Nurses have been accused of being narrow individuals with few interests outside the scope of medicine. The accusation is not entirely unjustified.

And what of the practical nurse's attitude toward old people while she is still comparatively young? Many persons have mixed feelings about elderly people. They may be amused at first by the little idiosyncrasies and strange quirks of the aged, but with constant close association, the amusement is short-lived and the "cute" mannerism becomes a "disgusting habit." Actually old people are neither amusing nor disgusting—at least not any more so than people of any other age. They are individual human beings and they long to be treated as such.

Perhaps the practical nurse has not been around the elderly enough to have any definite preconceived ideas and opinions about them. Our culture and the society in which we live have not prepared many of us for proper relations with the elderly. We have in America a definite social pattern of idolizing youth. Millions of dollars are spent each year by Americans trying to preserve their "youth," while in Nationalist China and other Eastern cultures it is a compliment to a person if he is mistakenly judged to be older than his years. Old age signifies wisdom and is treated with reverence. There are reasons for these differences: Ours is a comparatively young country, half our population is under 30, and everything is geared to a fast pace. We have had plenty of room for growing and going, without much thought, until recently, of what to do after we get there. Another influence has been the trend of population from rural living, in family homes sheltering several generations, to city life in rented apartments or small houses. The family unit no longer seems to include grandparents, and industry isn't interested in hiring anyone past 55. So there seems to be no place for them in the scheme of things. Many older people realize this and retire to the background, often to the point of losing their individuality and incentive for living. If they are ill the problem is even more serious.

Whatever the nurse's feelings toward and relations with the aged she should frequently try to take an objective view of the elderly and reevaluate her attitudes toward growing old. As she grows older she will realize that no one who is aging feels that he is getting old; the others are just getting younger.

The basic needs of the aged have been very simply defined as "the need for somewhere to live, something to do, someone to care."[2] When they are ill these needs, and more, must be met. The practical nurse, with her training and education centered on bedside nursing, is in an excellent position to give service and comfort to the aged. There is a rich and rewarding experience in store for those who dedicate themselves to this type of care. All the human qualities of warmth, love, and understanding are required of the geriatric nurse, plus an extra measure of each for those individuals who have lived much but still have much to give.

Perhaps it is because of lending credence to the expression "second childhood" that younger persons tend to treat the elderly as children. Nothing can be more destructive to human dignity and self-esteem than being treated as an infant or spoken to as if one were either deaf or stupid. Dr. Verwoerdt has written: "It is not uncommon practice to call aged patients by their first name, to speak loudly to them as if to shake them up, to talk about them in their presence, to smile or laugh at their oddities, and even to scold them for undesirable acts. On the other hand, it is not so difficult to combine *sincere respect* for the patient (in spite of his oddities) with *considerate helpfulness* (without infantalizing him)."[19]

In the very elderly and incapacitated patient it is extremely difficult sometimes to find ways of maintaining hope and purpose in the patient's life. But without such hope and purpose one only *exists*, he does not truly *live*. In our efforts to help such patients we must avoid the extremes of doing too much and of doing too little. A variety of interests and projects that occupy the hands or the mind can be offered, but the nurse's activities should be aimed at *motivating* the patient toward appropriate activity and self-care.

PHYSICAL CHANGES IN THE AGING

As stated above, aging is a normal process. It is a gradual "wearing out" of the organs. This does not mean that a disease exists in the organ, but should a disease develop it is *complicated* by the degeneration which has taken place in the organ. This breaking down of tissue, or degeneration, occurs in every organ of the body. Sometimes the body of the older person cannot repair this damage, and even when it does, the repair is not complete and the new cells are inferior in structure and function to those they have replaced[7] (see Fig. 7-1).

It is important that the practical nurse understand these pathological changes and adjust her nursing care accordingly. The object of her care will be to help restore her patient to a condition normal *for his age*; he cannot ever again have the health and strength of a 20-year-old if he is 70, but he can possibly be restored to a healthy 70-year-old.

NURSING CARE

Care of the Skin. Most nurses have been so thoroughly indoctrinated with

Figure 7-1. According to statistics from 1958, heart disease, cancer, and stroke take the heaviest toll of life among the older segments of the population. Many of the deaths that occur in middle life or later are not preventable in view of our limited knowledge about some degenerative diseases. (From *Health and Economic Conditions of the American Aged—A Chart Book,* U.S. Government Printing Office, Washington, D.C.)

the creed of the "daily bath" they are shocked at the thought of not performing this essential part of morning care. So when 80-year-old Mrs. Thomas, with a fractured femur, refuses her bath on the grounds that "I had a bath yesterday, I haven't stirred from this bed since then, therefore I am not dirty and do not need a bath," the nurse shakes her head at the strange ways of old ladies and then busily prepares the bath water anyway.

But Mrs. Thomas was right! Her sweat and oil glands are no longer as active, she perspires little and the daily bath can actually do her thin and dry skin more harm than good. A condition, well named "bath itch," occurs frequently in the elderly. It invariably begins as small raw areas over the shins and spreads over the body. It is best prevented by limiting the complete bath to one or two weekly, using mild soaps or natural detergent solutions. Bathing in between times should be arranged so as to insure good personal cleanliness, especially in the incontinent patient. After the bath, and perhaps as a substitute on the days a bath is not given, the skin may be gently massaged with lanolin or some oil-base lotions. Because the skin is so sensitive to trauma from burns and friction, great care should be used in the application of hot water bottles and in the method of massage.

Prevention of decubiti in the elderly begins with good nutrition and handling the skin as though it might break down any minute. In turning a patient the nurse must be sure to avoid pulling the undersheet roughly against the skin. This can best be done by turning the patient far enough to be able to pull the undersheet and tuck it without rubbing it across the patient's side or back.

"Pressure sores" is a name frequently

used to designate decubiti. It is a good name, for pressure on any one area of the skin, with resulting collection of heat and moisture and accompanying deprivation of an adequate blood supply, will eventually lead to an ulcer. For relief of this pressure frequent turning and proper positioning of the patient are necessary. This applies to patients of any age but particularly to the aged.

Older persons are particularly susceptible to respiratory infections and more sensitive to cold. Drafts, electric fans and extremes in room temperature should be avoided. Most prefer a room temperature above 70 degrees.

Care of the Nails and Hair. The nails, especially the toenails, undergo changes which make them so brittle and thick they should not be cut without first softening them by applying a warm castor oil poultice for a period of time. In the more difficult cases the poultices may need to be applied at intervals for several days. If the feet are kept dry and powdered well between the toes, fungus infections can be avoided. Fingernails must be kept clean and cut short, but as the cuticle is very susceptible to infection it should be softened with oil and pushed back rather than cut or trimmed with scissors.

It has been proved in mental institutions that even the most seriously deranged person will respond to an improvement in his physical appearance. Cosmetics and attractive clothing help the patient return more quickly to reality. An elderly person will react the same way and his physical appearance will greatly affect his attitude toward himself and others. Male patients who are shaved and neatly manicured with well-groomed hair are more likely to welcome visitors and show some interest in getting up and out into a more normal environment.

Dermatologists agree that most bases for powder and lipstick are not harmful to the skin of an elderly person. Thus the nurse may safely encourage her elderly female patients to "primp"

a little and give them the assistance they need in making themselves more attractive. Regardless of her age a normal woman should show interest in how she looks.

In cleansing the hair and scalp, excessive scrubbing should be avoided. A shampoo labeled as recommended for dry hair is the best and safest to use on elderly persons.

NUTRITION AND DIET

Likes and dislikes of the elderly in relation to food often become a point of irritation to the practical nurse striving so diligently to provide an adequate diet for her patient. However it is futile for her to try to change lifelong habits abruptly. Her only choice is to exercise great ingenuity in getting the patient to eat what he must have for maintenance of reasonable health. (Special diets as treatment for diseases are discussed elsewhere in this book.)

In spite of claims to the contrary, there is no special diet which will guarantee long life or continued health in old age. The needs of the aged are basically the same as those for any other age group except that the aged may need fewer calories as they become less active, and some modifications of the food may be necessary because of chewing and digestive difficulties. Such things as habit, ignorance of what constitutes a well-balanced diet, economic and emotional insecurity, and poorly fitting dentures or absence of teeth all contribute to the malnutrition present in most persons over the age of 60.

There is also poor absorption of calcium into the tissues of the older person; hence, ways of increasing the calcium intake must be found. Unfortunately most old people do not like milk. Substitutes such as cheese, ice cream, or foods cooked with milk will help make up for the lack of calcium in the diet of those who refuse to drink milk. Sometimes it is necessary to increase foods but there may be a strong objection from older persons to increasing the amount of solid foods they should eat. If so, nutritious liquid feedings may be planned and given. It is usually better to give frequent small feedings than to adhere strictly to the routine of three large meals a day.

Older persons also usually suffer from *achlorhydria*, a condition in which free hydrochloric acid is no longer present in the stomach. This absence of hydrochloric acid hinders digestion and interferes with the absorption of iron. For this reason anemia is often present in these people. In addition to the above, muscular actions of the digestive tract slow down with age and the intestinal mucosa is easily irritated by excessive bulk and rough residue from food.

An understanding of these changes which directly affect the appetite and digestion should make the practical nurse more patient and forbearing in handling feeding problems of the elderly.

Whenever possible the patient should feed himself. If he has great difficulty with liquids and hard-to-manage foods, the nurse can thoughtfully offer assistance without making him feel helpless. No mention should be made of the mess he might make in attempting to feed himself. The important point is to make sure he has an adequate intake of food. Some patients, however, are completely unable to feed themselves. When feeding an elderly person it is best to elevate his head and shoulders slightly and to have his spine straight with the shoulders back. This will aid digestion and prevent difficulties in swallowing. The gag reflex in the elderly usually does not function too well, creating danger of aspiration during eating and drinking. Therefore we must allow them ample time to chew their food thoroughly and swallow it completely, remembering that eating should be a pleasurable and leisurely experience.

Above all, the nurse must show she cares. Offering food and sharing our daily bread are expressions of love and demonstrations of our belief in the brotherhood of man. Frequently, then, one of the first signs of withdrawal from society is a refusal to eat. The principles of serving food attractively, providing appetizers and an atmosphere conducive to eating, and selecting foods with as much consideration for preference and taste as practical are no less important for the aged.

OTHER CONSIDERATIONS

Hearing. The hearing of the aged may not be as acute as that of other patients, and if for no other reason than common courtesy, the nurse should speak clearly in the presence of her patient. Older persons resent being treated as children, not being included in the general conversation of others, or being talked about in muffled tones as though they did not have the ability to understand what is being said.

It should be understood, however, that not all old people have difficulty in hearing and that the admonition to speak clearly is not a license to shout at the elderly; many people acquire the mistaken assumption that all old people are stone-deaf.

Sight. Usually dimness of vision or loss of sight is one of the first conditions which come to mind when thinking of old age and its infirmities. There is a condition especially common in older persons called "tunnel vision," in which the person sees only what is directly in front of him, as if he were in a tunnel or wearing side blinds. (Other diseases of the eyes and total loss of vision will be taken up in Chapter 19.) The practical nurse should do all she can to conserve the eyesight of her elderly patients and to report early symptoms of eye disease to the physician in charge.

The Bones. Poor vision, combined with duller reflexes and unstable balance, all take their toll in accidents among the aged. Fractured ribs and fractured femurs occur most often in persons over 60 for the reasons stated above, aggravated by a condition called *osteoporosis*. A large percentage of the aged suffer from this disease in which the bone cells are decalcified and the bones become porous. Osteoporosis is thought to be the indirect result of confinement to bed, in which case the bones are not used for support and weight-bearing and also are no longer subjected to the normal stresses of exercise.

Accidents. We can see, then, that prevention of accidents and fractures in the elderly should not be based on keeping them inactive and safely in bed, but rather on providing a safe environment for their much-needed activities. Good lighting, removal of obstacles such as footstools and other low objects which they might stumble over, sturdy handrails on stairs and all the other safety rules dictated by common sense must be used in the care of the elderly. In no instance, however, should the nurse appear oversolicitous and anxious about their welfare. Old people like to feel independent and to be given credit for having good sense.

Sleep and Recreation. Many younger persons do not realize that a man 75 years old may feel several different ages in the course of one day. Mr. Thompson awakens at 7:00 A.M. feeling every day of his 75 years. His joints are stiff and aching, his eyes dull and his hearing fuzzy, his disposition nasty. He growls at those around him and refuses most of his breakfast with the excuse that he is just not hungry. By 10:00 A.M. however, he asks for something to eat with the remark, "That breakfast wouldn't have filled a starving bird," and decides he wants to be up and doing. He works diligently in his garden for a while, acting as though he were 45 again, then he suddenly sits down in his favorite chair and is asleep in minutes. This may continue for the rest of the day—periods of activity and

periods of dozing and lethargy. This is a normal pattern for the aged and, as they very strongly resist change, it is best for the nurse to schedule her care around their moods as much as possible.

She must use imagination in choosing recreation for those who have nothing to do when they are in the mood for activity, remembering that the elderly need "something to do." When they show signs of tiring, the conscientous nurse will provide an atmosphere of rest, interrupting their naps only when necessary for medications or treatments, since older people usually require more sleep, at shorter intervals.

Elimination. Constipation in the elderly is generally a result of changes in the digestive tract aided by inactivity and poor eating habits. Because it is irritating to the intestinal mucosa, extremely rough bulk cannot be used as a means of eliminating this difficulty. The diet should include such vegetables as carrots and potatoes, which do not require much chewing, and some whole-grain cereals. Both of these food groups contain "soft" bulk.

Laxatives should be avoided; when they are necessary for temporary relief of constipation, mild ones are advisable for the elderly. Stool softeners that make defecation less difficult are preferred to laxatives and enemas. Since diarrhea is frequently a symptom of fecal impaction, its occurrence should be reported to the doctor or nurse in charge so that the impacted feces can be broken up manually and an oil retention enema given.

Benign hypertrophy of the prostate gland, so common in elderly men, is discussed elsewhere in this text. This is by no means, however, the only genitourinary problem to be considered in the elderly. Urinary incontinence, for one reason or another, frequently occurs, particularly after an injury or acute illness. Following either of these events the aged person becomes confused and fearful. He doesn't feel comfortable using a bedpan or urinal and isn't quite sure they won't leak or run over. A simple, tactful explanation with assurance of privacy may be all that is necessary to gain cooperation. Sometimes the "incontinent" patient isn't incontinent at all. He may just not get the impulse to void in time to notify someone of his need for a bedpan or urinal. All muscles of the aged lose some of their tone; this includes the sphincter muscles of the urinary and rectal outlets. For this reason the nurse may find she can prevent embarrassment to her elderly patients and unnecessary work for herself by offering them a bedpan or urinal at frequent and regular intervals. The practice of getting a patient out of bed regularly also has surprising results in the control of incontinence.

In spite of these techniques, urinary and fecal incontinence will continue in some patients. There are several appliances available for the collection or control of the flow of urine in the incontinent male patient. The problem is more difficult in the female. The practical nurse, after trying all recommended nursing measures, should seek assistance from the physician or nurse in charge.

MENTAL CHANGES

It would be a rash individual indeed who would state that the mental faculties of all humans decline at a steady rate after a given age, and thus conclude that all old people are stupid and forgetful. Medical science does not yet know all that is involved in the processes of learning and remembering. We do not know why some regress in their mental ability more rapidly than others in their old age. However, it is agreed that factors contributing toward "staying young" mentally include a *variety of interests in life, physical fitness, feeling needed,* and *companionship of others* (See Fig. 7-2). Old people need friends and contact with persons of all ages to keep themselves alert and mentally and emotionally healthy. The average person prefers people to things; thus the practical nurse cannot expect to satisfy her elderly patients completely simply by giving them something to do with their hands. She must learn to talk with and know her patients as individual human beings who need her warmth and understanding. She can learn much through conversations with the aged, though some may often tell her the same thing over and over again.

Old people enjoy recalling their youth. (No one likes to look back over his life and remember it as dull.) We can sometimes get them away from the oft-told tales by asking them about some detail in the story. If, for instance, Mr. Thompson, for the tenth time, launches into his favorite account of the day half his home town burned down, one might ask him how fire alarms were spread in his day, or what methods were used to extinguish the blaze. This will show genuine interest and give Mr. Thompson something else to talk about.

The important point is to let the older person set the pace in the conversation or activity in which *he* is interested. The nurse then respectfully injects new ideas and thoughts as her patient shows a willingness to accept them, even though she may meet with some resistance at first.

Many elderly persons with a chronic illness or disability manage fairly well in their home environment, but when they must be hospitalized they become confused and disoriented. In the new environment, away from familiar surroundings and persons whom he knows, the patient may be less able to think clearly and he may show signs of forgetfulness, wandering about his ward or room or becoming belligerent and uncooperative. He also may show signs of extreme tension, anxiety or anger that produce insomnia and further aggravate his confusion.

It is important to bear in mind that this mental confusion is most often only temporary and will subside when

Figure 7-2. Retirement at age 65 does not necessarily mean retirement from life. Many people take advantage of their retirement years to do some of the things they did not have time to do while they were employed full time. Each of us should prepare for the day when forced retirement leaves us with "nothing to do." *A*, J. C., a retired tobacco farmer, tired of loafing, bought into a small cafe, where he has fun meeting people. *B*, T. C., former heavy equipment contractor, started a second career as proprietor of a bait and tackle shop. *C*, J. P., former athletic director, took a job as a yacht club manager. (Photos by Dick Harmon in Today's Health, February, 1963.)

the patient returns to his home. One should also avoid labeling a patient as confused or uncooperative when he may have only short periods of confusion during his hospital stay. Never assume that the patient who shows confusion at times is always going to behave irrationally or that he cannot be reached through simple, direct conversation. For example, when he makes a statement that is obviously wrong, such as "It's time for my lunch," when it is actually bed time, correct him and point out the fact that it is dark outside and give him the correct time of day. Be quite sure, however, that you do not try to correct his statements when he may be right. He may continue a conversation he was having with a visitor after the visitor has gone. If this happens, simply point out that the visitor is no longer there and show a willingness to listen to what he is saying. Arguing with the confused patient may only add to his confusion; your goal is to help him think clearly as to time and place.

The elderly patient who is isolated

from others, removed from all time-orienting equipment such as a clock, radio or television, and deprived of the normal communications with persons outside his hospital room is much more likely to become confused and difficult to handle. If he must be restricted to his room, he should be visited frequently by a member of the nursing staff, if only for very brief periods of time. Ideally, he should be placed in a solarium, the hallway or the doorway to his room to keep him in touch with activity. An established routine of eating, sleeping and other daily activities also helps relieve mental confusion.

Part II – CHRONIC ILLNESS

INTRODUCTION

In 1959 a National Health Survey was conducted by the U.S. Public Health Service. The findings revealed that chronic conditions were present in 10 per cent of the population of this country. As our population increases in number as a result of the advances of medical science in treating acute illnesses and prolonging the life span, we can expect the percentage of partially or totally disabled persons to become higher. This does not mean that all persons with a chronic or long-term illness are necessarily aged. In fact, a large percentage of them are under 30 years of age.

Definition. What then is a chronic illness and how does it differ from an acute illness? An *acute* illness is usually one which has a rapid onset, lasts only a brief period of time and ends with complete recovery or death. An acute illness may develop into a chronic illness. A *chronic* illness has a more gradual beginning with vague symptoms which become progressively more severe. It requires a prolonged period of treatment and nursing care, both of which are often complicated by the presence of several diseased conditions at the same time. A chronic illness is rarely restricted to one system because of the interdependence of all systems of the body for maintenance of good health. There is also an inevitable degeneration of tissues and organs in a chronic illness and only partial recovery can ever be expected.

Patients with a chronic illness do not, however, always follow a steadily downward course. There may be times when the disease will lie dormant and present few symptoms. These times are called periods of *remission.* When the symptoms become more severe because of a flare-up of the disease, the term used is *exacerbation,* or the *acute phase,* of a chronic disease. This period may last a relatively short time and be followed by remission or it may become progressively more critical and lead to the death of the patient.

In the national survey mentioned above, the U.S. Public Health Service listed over 40 conditions as being chronic diseases. Generally these conditions fall into one of the following categories: (1) circulatory disorders, (2) metabolic disorders, (3) malignant new growths, and (4) the arthritides (plural for arthritis).[4]

Handicapped persons with nonprogressive disabilities are medically and statistically considered as having a chronic illness. These are persons who have suffered loss of vision, or have had amputation of a limb, or partial paralysis, etc., but who can adjust to life with their handicap and are not in need of continuous nursing care. For this reason we will not consider them under the heading "chronically ill" in this chapter.

NURSING CARE

Introduction. Because degeneration and inability to repair damaged tissues are common characteristics of chronic illness, some nurses may become discouraged and depressed by the prospect of nursing the chronically ill. "Death is inevitable and we know the patient can never be normal again," they say, "so why not concentrate our attention on those who can get well?"

In answer let us say: First, we agree that death of the patient is inevitable, and so it is, too, for all of us. All mortal beings will one day die. Secondly, who are we to judge which life is more worth while? The middle-aged woman, confined to a wheelchair yet managing a home as a capable wife and mother, or the young teenager admitted to the hospital with a fractured skull? It is true that sharing in the dramatic cure of an acutely ill patient is a thrilling experience for the nurse. This is a short-term goal and she can immediately see the fruits of her labors. The satisfactions in nursing the chronically ill are more difficult to gain; the rewards sometimes seen small, the effort great and the results discouraging. Try to imagine, though, how the patient must feel about his chronic illness. He depends on the nurse, the stronger of the two, for support and encouragement in his efforts, and if she is easily discouraged he will soon lose heart.

Understanding the Chronically Ill Patient. An individual's adjustment to chronic illness will depend on many factors, such as age, cultural background, type of illness and the limitations it imposes, role in the family, and emotional stability. In spite of these variances in the individual patient, in almost every case the *process* of adjustment to chronic illness and what it means to the patient's future life will be essentially the same. By understanding the stages through which the patient passes in his adaptation to his illness and disability, the practical nurse

will be better prepared to offer support and guidance.

First of all one must understand that the patient who first learns that he has a chronic illness experiences an emotional upheavel and profound grief similar to that caused by death. This is because in some ways his old "self" is indeed dead and he is faced with the task of building a new life around a new self. In order to do this he must come to the realization that his illness does exist and that it is going to make a difference in many aspects of his daily life and in his relationships with his friends and relatives. Most patients find this extremely difficult to do, and so the first step in the process of adaptation is one of denial. This denial that anything is wrong is simply a matter of self-protection. The patient feels threatened and is shocked by the fact that the illness is threatening his usual pattern of life. The nurse's reaction to such denials should be that of a quiet listener. She should not argue with him or insist that he is wrong in denying the illness; she can only allow him to express his feelings and show that she can be depended on to help him when he is able to admit that he needs her help.

Gradually the patient will begin to show that he has become aware of his predicament. He may do this by trying to place the blame for his illness on someone who cares for him or is trying to help him. During this period of anger and resentment the patient may make statements that indicate a lack of confidence in the physicians and nurses or anger toward his relatives and friends. Again the nurse must listen to the patient but she should not argue with him. Her task is to follow the details of medical attention and nursing care scrupulously, showing by her attitude and actions that she considers every phase of his treatment important and that she is sincerely interested in doing everything possible to help the patient in his illness. During this stage she may notice that the patient will become more and more dependent on her. If she can get across to him that she is available for help whenever it is needed, he will then progress to less dependence as he gains confidence in himself and the care he is receiving.

Finally, the patient must begin to reorganize his relationships with his friends and family. This is necessary because he is now a sick person with an illness that is not going to go away. Nothing can change that. Once he is able to admit that he is a different person because of his illness he will be better able to live with it.

The role of the nurse is that of a guide. She must not force or push the patient into his new way of life or try to change him so that he "fits into" the world of the chronically ill. She must offer support and guidance to the patient as he moves toward a new and different kind of existence.[6]

Phases of Chronic Illness. We may consider care of the chronically ill in three phases: (1) the acute phase, (2) the convalescent phase, and (3) the rehabilitation of the patient.

THE ACUTE PHASE. The nursing care during this phase of chronic illness will be basically the same as it would be for any acute illness, and though the nurse's main concern will be with immediate relief of the patient's symptoms and maintenance of life, she must also bear in mind the effects of the chronic condition on the patient's progress through the acute illness. Complications must be prevented so that the patient might at least recover from the acute flare-up of symptoms without suffering a setback in his chronic illness. Chapter 6 of this text describes in detail the nursing care of the critically ill patient. These same principles are applied to the care of a patient in the acute phase of a chronic illness.

THE CONVALESCENT PHASE. It is during this phase of recovery from an illness that the nurse must use all the knowledge, imagination and techniques at her disposal to keep her patient

mentally and physically able to resume his life as it was before he became ill. In a chronic illness the patient will need to make many adjustments in his life and he will need help in learning to live with his illness. The convalescent period may be somewhat prolonged and discouraging and it is possible that there will be times when the patient cannot see that he is making any progress toward recovery. He will need much encouragement and moral support from the nurses and other members of the health team in his struggle to adjust to living with a chronic illness.

There is a great overlapping of the three phases of chronic illness and the caliber and effectiveness of nursing care in one phase will determine success in the other phases. For instance, if the nursing staff allows a patient recovering from an acute exacerbation of arthritis to develop deformities from improper posture in bed and lack of exercise, the rehabilitation of this patient will be extremely difficult, if not impossible. He may also suffer from degenerative changes in the joints which would aggravate and magnify his chronic arthritis.

REHABILITATION. "Rehabilitation" is a word which first became widely used after World War I when wounded American soldiers returned home, and there was a need for finding ways to help these disabled veterans adjust to life with their handicaps. The Second World War increased the interest and scope of the problem until the present-day concept of rehabilitation includes everything which can be included under the broad statement: "*Rehabilitation helps the patient to help himself.*" All the activities concerned with reaching this goal must include many persons: doctors, nurses, physical therapists, public health workers, social workers, psychologists, and vocational counselors.

Though she is included under the title "nurses" above, the practical nurse has a more definite role in rehabilitation. Her responsibilities are threefold: (1) close cooperation with other members of the rehabilitation team, (2) continued observation of her patients with chronic or permanently disabling diseases, and prevention of complications from those diseases, and (3) helping to mold her patient's attitude toward rehabilitation.

Of these three responsibilities the most important is probably the one dealing with the patient's attitude. The desire of the patient to help himself and become as physically independent of others as possible is a vital point in determining the success of rehabilitation. There are several points on which the practical nurse should check herself in regard to this. First, is she helping her patient so much that he cannot learn to help himself? Nurses are often so much in the habit of "doing for others" that they may sometimes forget there is a time when others need to "do" for themselves. On the other hand, some patients readily agree that their case is hopeless. They must be watched for signs of an unnecessary willingness to let others take all responsibility for their intimate care, even to the point of refusing to feed and dress themselves, though they may be perfectly able to do so. Remember that some do enjoy their illness. It is an attitude more to be pitied than encouraged and the practical nurse should remain alert to the effects of her influence on the patient's acceptance of rehabilitation.

Yet she must not go to the other extreme of rushing her patient and prodding him into activities beyond his ability. Nothing can be more discouraging than striving to attain a goal beyond one's reach. Short-range goals are more desirable, and certainly there is greater chance for success, even though it means a long struggle for small gains. The practical nurse is not expected to know or determine the time when her patient is ready to begin certain activities. This is the responsibility of the other members of the nursing team with whom she is expected to cooperate. She should, however, determine the wishes of the others and assist them in helping the patient realize his full potential.

Rehabilitation does not mean a total return to normal functions; it *is* a salvaging of whatever functions the patient can perform with encouragement to do more within the limits of his handicap. For example, following a stroke the patient may feel that the resulting paralysis of one side is the final outcome and nothing can be done to change that. This is not necessarily true. He may regain some use of the affected side of the body, and the more the better, even though we know he will never again be "as good as new."

It is said that rehabilitation begins with admission of the patient. This simply means that from the beginning we must keep in sight the goal of restoring the patient to his former place in the family and community. The practical nurse, in her daily contact with and continuous care of the patient, can be of great help in achieving this goal of maximum rehabilitation. She does this by realizing the danger of allowing complications to develop and by reporting her observations to those in charge. She must familiarize herself with and diligently use all the devices and techniques available. This includes simple procedures involved in moving the patient from bed to chair, the use of footboards, bed cradles for support of the weight of covers, pillows for maintainance of good body alignment, good skin care, exercises as needed, and teaching the patient to help himself. Under the supervision and direction of the doctor, nurse in charge, or physical therapist, she may assist with active and passive exercises for the patient. She must direct her patient's attention to what he *can* do rather than allow him to dwell on what he cannot do (see Fig. 7-3).

Sources of Information and Help for the Chronically Ill. There are many local and national agencies created for the purpose of assisting in prevention

Figure 7-3. Handicapped patients learn to go up and down bus steps as part of rehabilitation to prepare them for activities outside the hospital. (Courtesy of Institute for the Crippled and Disabled, New York.)

and control of chronic illnesses and rehabilitation of persons suffering from these illnesses. Nearly everyone has heard of the American Heart Association, the American Cancer Society, and the National Tuberculosis Association, but few seem to realize that these agencies are all excellent sources of information in the form of pamphlets and other publications. This material often deals with home nursing, adjustments to chronic illness, and common problems of the chronically ill. Every state department of health has a bureau of public health information, and publications from the U.S. Government Printing Office, Washington, D.C., cover aspects of health and illness too numerous to mention. Insurance companies such as the Metropolitan Life Insurance Company or John Hancock Insurance Company also are good sources of inexpensive information booklets.

These current publications are available to anyone willing to make the effort of writing for them. The practical nurse, no less than anyone else on the medical team, must realize the need for up-to-date material on methods of prevention, treatment, and nursing care. She should continuously search for newer and better ways to serve her patient, his family, and his community.

CHRONIC ILLNESS AND IMMOBILITY

Introduction. A chronic illness does not always imply total inactivity or inability of the patient to move about, but physical limitations often do accompany chronic illness, and immobility is, unfortunately, not uncommon in these patients. The reasons for the immobility may vary from despair on the part of the patient to neglect on the part of the nurses caring for the patient. Whatever the reasons for the inactivity of the patient, the practical nurse must be aware of the hazards of immobility and must do her best to avoid these hazards.

The human body is designed for motion. All internal and external organs must move about to function and these organs are interdependent. When activity of the various parts of the body is greatly decreased the bodily functions are directly affected. Since chronic illness has become the major health problem of our day, the practical nurse can and must play an important part in preventing the complications that arise from the decreased activity imposed by many chronic illnesses.

Cardiovascular System. It is now believed that the heart works harder when the body is in a resting, supine position. We can understand this when we realize that blood normally distributed in the legs when the body is in an upright position is released from gravity pressure when one lies down. This means that the blood leaves the legs and enters the total blood volume to be redistributed in other parts of the body by the pumping action of the heart. In addition, a state of immobility leads to development of blood clots within the blood vessels. This situation is aggravated by allowing the patient to lie in one position too long so that the weight of the body causes continued pressure against the blood vessels and inhibits the flow of blood. When a patient is lying on his side with the weight of one leg resting on the other, he is quite likely to develop blood clots in the leg bearing the weight.

Nursing measures that can reduce the work load of the heart and increase circulation include turning the patient frequently, passive and active exercises of the muscles and, whenever possible, elevating the head of the bed or sitting the patient in a chair.

Respiratory System. Immobility can bring about three physiological effects on the respiratory system. These are decreased movement of the respiratory muscles and diaphragm, decreased movement of secretions within the respiratory tree, and a disturbance in the balance between carbon dioxide and oxygen.

The nursing measures to avoid these developments are not complicated, but are so simple that they are often overlooked. Obviously, some steps must be taken to exercise the muscles of respiration (the intercostals and the diaphragm) and to increase the flow of secretions. These measures include helping the patient with routine deep-breathing exercises and coughing. He also must be turned frequently and, if he is able, sit up and stretch or change position often so that there can be adequate expansion of the chest. If removal of secretions in the lower respiratory tract is extremely difficult, postural drainage and chest tapping may be necessary.

Gastrointestinal Tract. The inactive patient is subject to indigestion, loss of appetite, distention, diarrhea, and constipation. The cause of these symptoms may be the stress and nervous tension produced by immobility, or they may result from poor muscle tone, absence of normal reflexes or failure of the patient to heed the defecation reflex. Constipation is a problem that may require considerable patience and individual planning to overcome. Strong laxatives and enemas are not recommended since they are often abused and do not offer a permanent solution to the patient's problem. Stool softeners and exercises to strengthen the abdominal muscles are helpful. In addition, the patient should be instructed in the process of elimination and a routine worked out on the basis of each patient's individual need.

Musculoskeletal System. The muscles, bones and skin of an immobile

Figure 7-4.   Ranges of motion. All exercises can be performed from the supine position in bed except hyperextension of the spine, hips, and shoulders and flexion of the knees, for which the person must lie prone or on his side. (From Kelly: American Journal of Nursing, October, 1966.)

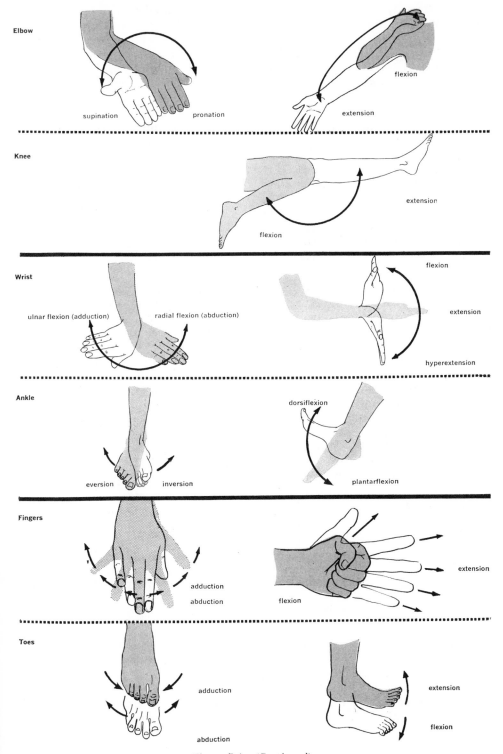

Figure 7-4. (Continued)

patient are likely to deteriorate very rapidly. Even in normal, healthy individuals a lack of activity will very soon lead to loss of muscle tone. Since about 40 per cent of the body is made up of muscle, it is imperative that some regimen of exercises be established. If the muscles are not exercised regularly, the muscle fibers lose their elasticity and their ability to contract and stretch. *Contractures* then develop and the joints become fixed in one position, making motion impossible. Proper positioning of the patient and putting the joints through their full range of motion at least once daily will help prevent these complications (see Fig. 7-4). *Osteoporosis* (porous bone) is another hazard of immobility. It is the result of demineralization of the bone and occurs when the usual stress and strain of walking and moving about is no longer placed on the bones. This stress normally stimulates the process of building bone, that is, replacing old bone cells with newer stronger ones. When activity ceases, the building process stops and the calcium, phosphorus and nitrogen that usually aid in the building process are removed from the bone. The bone then becomes soft and spongy and may easily be deformed or broken.

Decubitus ulcers (pressure sores) are a well-known problem to anyone who has cared for a bed-ridden patient. Cleanliness of the skin, frequent massage to stimulate circulation to pressure areas, and a regular routine for turning to relieve pressure on bony prominences are necessary to prevent decreased blood supply to an area and the development of necrotic tissue.

Urinary Tract. The urinary system of man functions most efficiently when the body is in an erect position. The flow of urine out of the renal pelvis and through the urinary tract is greatly reduced when physical activity ceases and one remains in a supine position for a prolonged period of time. *Urinary stasis* (decreased flow of urine) leads to the formation of urinary calculi (stones) and the development of infection.

To avoid urinary stasis and its complications one must realize the relationship between inactivity and decreased flow of urine. If at all possible the nurse should establish some routine of physical activity for the patient, utilizing both active and passive exercises. In addition, she needs to keep an accurate record of intake and output, encouraging her patient to drink sufficient fluids to keep the urine dilute and checking the patient frequently for bladder distention. With continued pressure of urine against the bladder wall, the normal reflexes may become impaired. Nursing measures to induce voiding and moderate pressure of the hand against the lower pelvis to facilitate emptying of the bladder during urination often is sufficient to prevent bladder distention. Catheterization, unless carried out under ideal conditions, tends to introduce infection into the urinary tract and is not recommended for a chronically ill patient.

The Nurse's Attitude. We have just reviewed the effects of immobility on a chronically ill patient. Earlier in this chapter we discussed a patient's painful process of adaptation to a chronic illness. But what about the nurse's attitude toward and acceptance of responsibility for the care of the chronically ill? If, after all the patient's struggling to make a new life for himself, he is allowed through inadequate nursing care to sink into the oblivion of immobility, beset by complications that are beyond his control to prevent, his nurses must face the fact that he has been denied his basic right to live as a human being. Perhaps the following description, written by a physician about an immobilized patient, will make the practical nurse more aware of her responsibilities to the chronically ill patient who must look to her for guidance and care. "What a pathetic picture he makes. The blood clotting in his veins, the lime draining from his bones, the scybala stacking up in his colon, the flesh rotting from his seat, the urine leaking from his distended bladder, and the spirit evaporating from his soul."[8]

Part III — INSTITUTIONAL CARE OF THE AGED AND CHRONICALLY ILL

INTRODUCTION

Within the past two decades there has been an increasing trend toward placing the aged and infirm in institutions instead of dismissing them from hospitals into the care of the family. For some who have no relatives or anyone else willing to take the responsibility for their care, this is apparently the only solution, but it is far from a perfect answer to the problem of what to do with those who are not acutely ill yet require some nursing care. There are many reasons given by relatives as to why they do not choose to care for these people in their own homes and it is not our intention to sit in judgment on their actions. Suffice it to say that the "best" given at the hands of strangers is never quite as good as the well-meaning attention administered by familiar and loving hands. Most individuals prefer to be and should be living at home with the family group, unless they require skilled nursing care. Yet there is a steady increase in the number of nursing homes being built today for the purpose of offering varying degrees of medical and nursing care for the aged and infirm of our country.

NURSING HOMES

In the early history of these institutions many were a disgrace to our society, and though some were worthy substitutes for the individual's own home, these were not, unfortunately, in the majority. In more recent years local, county and state health departments and federal agencies have accepted the responsibility of inspecting these institutions. The passage of laws with specific regulations and requirements for licensure of nursing homes has improved such institutions, both private and public.

Ideally, the nursing home combines the best qualities of home care and hospital care. The patient receives personal and individual care and qualified personnel are available to meet his medical and nursing needs. The "extended care facilities" that are partially paid for by the Medicare program are skilled nursing homes. By law these institutions must provide "at least one registered professional nurse or qualified licensed practical nurse who is a graduate of a state-approved school of practical nursing on duty at all times and in charge of nursing activities during each tour of duty." Under certain circumstances the regulations may be *temporarily* relaxed to allow LPN's licensed by waiver to serve as charge nurses in extended care facilities.[9]

Types of Patients. In a survey taken at a "typical" skilled nursing home the average age of the patient was 78 to 80 years. There were some patients in their

30's and some who had lived over a century. The great majority of the patients suffered from some type of chronic illness such as heart diseases or diabetes, and less than half of them were physically able to take care of themselves to a substantial degree. Between 75 and 80 per cent demonstrated some abnormal behavioral traits such as confusion, disorientation, marked agitation, paranoia, delusions, deficient memory or impaired judgment. These conditions require maintenance of physical safety conditions and constant nursing supervision to avoid accidental injury. The survey also showed that at least two thirds of the patients' families were not aware of the degree of their relative's disability. A few of the patients had no family ties and were homeless. It was concluded through the survey that most of the patients could be helped toward improvement or at least could maintain their status quo if they received skilled nursing care.[10]

Nursing Responsibilities. There are many satisfactions in store for the practical nurse who chooses this type of nursing. All the principles involved in nursing care of the acutely and chronically ill may be needed at various times. She will need to learn well the philosophy and psychology of caring for the chronically ill and aged. She will need experience in a wide variety of nursing skills and will find there is much for her to learn as she works in this particular field of nursing. Many of the points mentioned in this text under rehabili-

Figure 7-5. After supervision by public health nurse, home health aide can give foot soak. (From Rasmussen: Nursing Outlook, June, 1966.)

tation and recreation will become more meaningful and useful when applied to patients living in these "homes."

They will need attention to clothing, meals, recreation, and companionship there as they would in their own homes. Arrangements should be made to assure them some privacy and a homelike atmosphere. Since it is not always possible to have private rooms for everyone in these homes, some effort and imagination may be necessary in providing a specific place for each individual to call his own, and into which others may not trespass unless asked to do so. A corner of a ward may be all the patient has but everyone should respect his right to call it his own domain and allow him to keep there the few personal belongings he may treasure.

With the development of the Medicare program a new service has been provided for elderly and chronically ill persons who are being cared for at home. This service utilizes home health aides who go into the patient's home and assist with personal care of the patient, meal preparation, routine housekeeping and light laundry. These aides work under the supervision of a registered professional nurse (see Fig. 7-5).

The purpose of the service is to prevent or delay hospitalization by providing adequate care at home, and to allow early discharge for those already in nursing homes or hospitals.[5] The home health aide is given some training in simple nursing procedures and other aspects of caring for the aged and chronically ill. The Medicare program pays for up to 100 visits by the home health aide to the home of a person eligible for its benefits.

Part IV – HOME NURSING

INTRODUCTION

From a practical standpoint and for obvious reasons, hospitalization is necessary in many cases of illness. Ideally the best place for a person who is ill is home. This is particularly true of the aged and chronically ill. At home they feel more secure, are less concerned about their infirmities and incapacities, and can lead more normal lives in spite of their handicaps. The elderly and others suffering from long-term illnesses are not the only types of patients who might require the services of a practical nurse in the home. These two groups do, however, constitute the largest percentage. Many times the family is capable of caring for the patient in the home, but in some instances in which more skilled nursing care is necessary, a practical nurse may be employed.

RESPONSIBILITIES IN HOME NURSING

The nurse accepting a case in the home has responsibilities to her patient, to the doctor, and to the family. Her first responsibility in home nursing, as in any situation, is her patient. She must concern herself with every aspect of the patient's care and will probably have a better chance to give total care there than in any other type of nursing she might choose. She will attend to the cleanliness of her patient and his environment, administer medications and treatments ordered (including the therapeutic diet if indicated) and will give her patient emotional and moral support during his illness. She will be working for the most part without close supervision except for occasional visits by the doctor, or in some cases the public health nurse or other member of the health team. This demands integrity and absolute honesty in her actions with a constant awareness of her limitations as a practical nurse.

The doctor will depend on the home nurse to make accurate observations and report to him changes which may require his attention. He will expect to be notified immediately when a change for the worse occurs in the patient's condition. The nurse must remain calm and in control in any emergency in the home, for at times she will find that hers is the only level head in the household.

If the doctor has ordered special medications or treatments for the patient the home nurse must be as accurate in the administration and recording of these as in the hospital. Since there will not be a chart like that used in hospitals a small notebook can be used for record keeping. Any untoward reaction to a medication or treatment will be reported to the doctor. If he cannot be reached immediately the drug or treatment should be discontinued until further orders are obtained.

It is a good idea for the nurse to write down questions she might wish to ask or special problems she may need to discuss with the doctor when he visits or phones about the patient. This will eliminate unnecessary and annoying calls to his office or home.

Whether the patient is aged or incompetent or the young mother of a large family, the practical nurse must remember that she has been employed by the family and that it is their home in which she is working. Good manners and consideration of the feelings of others are as necessary in the home situation as in any other. Usually the patient and family will accept the nurse in the same manner in which she ac-

cepts them. If she is kind and thoughtful the family will respond to her warmth by doing their best to treat her in the same way. She should not make any unnecessary demands of them nor expect them to inconvenience themselves because of her presence in their home. It is best to work in a quiet and unassuming manner, showing by her efficiency and competence that whatever she does is in the best interest of the patient.

Sometimes the nurse may notice that the home situation is far from ideal, with the family making no secret of their irritation with the problems involved in having someone ill in their midst. This reaction may stem from many causes beyond the control of the nurse. Her only course, then, is to use every opportunity to help them adjust to the situation. She can do this by creating as little change in their daily routines as possible and by helping them to understand the nature of the patient's illness. Often she can enlist their aid, making them feel more useful and giving them something constructive to do. Perhaps they are irritated by the sheer frustration of facing a problem which at first seems utterly hopeless, especially if the patient is very old or severely incapacitated.

One member of the family may show some interest in the special therapeutic diet the patient requires, thus giving the nurse an opportunity to teach that person simple ways to modify a regular diet so that it is prepared according to the doctor's orders. Another member of the family may prove to be imaginative and handy with tools. His talents could be used to design and make special gadgets and equipment useful in teaching the patient how to become less dependent on others. Someone else in the home may have a special hobby interesting to the patient, which the nurse might ask him to share with the patient.

The nurse should bear in mind that one of the purposes of the patient's being in the home is to allow him to share in the joys and companionship of family life. It will be to her advantage to encourage the family to accept the patient as he is and to give freely of the love and attention he so desperately needs.

DUTIES OF THE NURSE IN THE HOME

Housekeeping and Laundry. The practical nurse in the home is responsible for the cleanliness of the patient's room and the bathroom used by the patient. She also should care for the patient's dishes and linen. Home conditions may change this somewhat. In a home where there is a maid who launders the clothes and also cooks for the family the practical nurse may serve the patient's meals and promptly return the dishes to the kitchen where they will be washed with the rest after the family's meal. If there is no one else in the home during the noon meal the nurse is expected to prepare the meal, wash the dishes and leave the kitchen as she found it. The patient's linen may be laundered with the rest of the family's unless, as in incontinent cases, large amounts of linen will require an outside laundry service.

The practical nurse should not take on so many other household duties that her patient is neglected. She is expected to be helpful whenever she can to the rest of the family. But if things get out of hand and she feels she is being overburdened with extra work or taken advantage of, her only choice is to talk the problem over with the head of the family and enlist his aid in finding a solution. It is assumed that she will use good judgment in this matter, making sure that she has done all that is normally expected of her in regard to the patient.

Cooking. Special therapeutic diets must be prepared, or the preparation supervised, by the practical nurse. The diet is considered part of the treatment and is the nurse's responsibility. There is usually no need to purchase special foods for these diets. Most family meals, if they are adequate and well planned, can be modified by different methods of cooking and seasoning. Thus the patient's portion may be taken out and prepared at the same time the family food is cooked. Whenever possible the patient should be taken to the dining room to eat his meals with the rest of the family. Eating together is an important part of family life.

When the family is very small or consists of only an elderly couple the practical nurse may need to help with the preparation of their meals even though only one of them may actually be ill.

CLOTHING FOR THE PATIENT

In thinking about her patient's participation in family living the practical nurse should consider the clothing he wears at home. Unless the patient is on absolute bed rest by doctor's orders he should be encouraged to dress in street clothes during the day. It doesn't matter that the patient might not go outside the house. If one is dressed like an invalid one tends to act more like an invalid and be treated as such by others. Visitors, neighbors and the family who see the patient dressed in something besides pajamas or a gown will react toward the patient in a more normal way, conversation will be easier, and a more optimistic view of the situation will develop in both the patient and the family. This may seem a simple point but proper clothing and development of different attitudes toward the illness will often bring surprising results.

It is possible to design articles of clothing with some imagination and attention to a patient's individual needs and limitations. The pictures in Figure 7-6 show some of the minor adaptations that can help a patient achieve some degree of self-help and independence.

Figure 7-6. *A*, Patients with hemiparesis like front closing bras fastened with Velcro; all like elastic straps. Such bras are commercially available. Pettipants make slips unnecessary, are comfortable in wheelchairs, and keep a urinal bag concealed even when a skirt hikes up during a transfer from car to wheelchair. *B*, Patients who have restricted shoulder movement find front-zippered slips convenient. *C*, Back-wrap skirts can be folded to the front when the patient sits in her wheelchair, avoiding pressure from folds of material. *D*, Halter made from half a pair of suspenders holds up the trousers adequately, lessens the danger of a patient's tripping when he raises his trousers after toilet. Velcro can replace the zipper as a fly fastening when necessary.

Figure 7-6 (cont'd.)   *E,* Drop seat makes it possible to air skin over the sacral area without the patient's having to disrobe. *F,* A cape or coat, with large armholes is just long enough to keep the patient's back warm, too short to create bulky folds under the buttocks. The front, like the waist band of the skirt above is fastened with Velcro, manageable when buttons are a problem. *G,* Ambulant patients with limited hand dexterity like full skirts with a deeply overlapping placket that needs no zipper, just a small amount of Velcro fastening at the waistband. *H,* Side zipper from ankle to waist permits applying or removing leg brace or urinal bags without disrobing. Terry top, fastened with ties, Velcro, snap fasteners, grippers, or whatever, is machine washable, needs no ironing. (From Smith: American Journal of Nursing, June, 1966.)

RECREATION FOR THE PATIENT IN THE HOME

Mental and emotional health experts encourage us to develop hobbies and avocations during our leisure time with a forward look to the days of retirement when these sidelines will become a more important part of our lives. Those who lived and worked 50 years ago did not have as much leisure time as we have. In the reputedly "good old days" a working day was from 10 to 12 hours long, an average work week 50 to 60 hours or more, and vacations were not automatically received for each year's service. The result is that today those who worked and lived during that period do not have a variety of interests and hobbies they might develop more fully now that they are no longer employed. And many times the nurse is faced with the problem of "starting from scratch" in finding something for her patient to do with his time.

First she must learn all she can about her patient. She must take into consideration his age, his disability and potential for increased activity, his interests and particular talents.

It would be ridiculous to consider a throwing game with a foam rubber ball to a man 86 years old and cruel to suggest such a thing to a patient who is paralyzed in the upper extremities. However, if the patient is young and the objective is to strengthen the shoulder and arm muscles, this would be an ideal way to accomplish that objective.

Recreation should be aimed at getting the patient interested in things outside himself. Clubs for "senior citizens" and other group activities for persons with physical problems in common have been extremely successful. If the patient cannot get out of the house for this type of activity, many persons who are bedridden enjoy corresponding by letter with others in distant cities or countries.

Witnessing the development of life and the growth of living things can be a thrilling experience. Perhaps that is why gardening is so dear to the hearts of so many. Most patients, no matter how handicapped, can enjoy this activity with an indoor or outdoor garden. There is great pleasure in thumbing through seed catalogues, "shopping" for just the right plants. Then there is the happy anticipation of waiting for the order to arrive, followed by planning the location of the plants. Those who are able to get out of doors and supervise the gardening, if not take an active part in it, will find time slipping away rather than hanging heavy on their hands. "Tomorrow" can be a dreaded word for the aged or chronically ill. If it is going to be the same as today and yesterday what is the point of looking forward to it? But if tomorrow is the day to pull weeds, finish the watercolor painting, learn a new pattern in knitting, sand down the tabletop before the next coat of varnish, get the fishing gear ready for a sunny day, or do anything at all that is interesting, enjoyable, or creative, then *that* tomorrow is worth living for.

The practical nurse must be patient in her search for something the patient enjoys doing. Not everything she suggests will be interesting to him and she should try a variety of things, encouraging the patient to share her enthusiasm for the new project. Naturally she mustn't exhaust her patient with activity, but rest does come more quickly and easily after some physical and mental exertion. The public library is a good source for books on hobbies and recreation, and any other special problems the practical nurse may meet in this area.

HOURS OF DUTY AND PAYMENTS FOR SERVICES IN THE HOME

The number of hours the nurse is to be on duty in the home will depend on arrangements made with a responsible member of the family before she accepts the case. These hours vary with the kind of care required by the patient and the number of nurses to be employed. All arrangements as to working hours and payment for nursing services rendered should be clearly understood in advance and plans should be made which are agreeable to both employer and employee. This includes the hours per day the nurse will be expected to be on duty, days off during the week, arrangements for weekly church services the nurse may wish to attend, and might also cover holidays and vacation time if she is to be employed for an indefinite period of time. The amount and regularity of payment should also be established. If the nurse expects her employer to withhold taxes from her paycheck she must provide him with her social security number and request that he withhold taxes. It is not mercenary to discuss money at appropriate times. Clear and definite arrangements with full knowledge of what is expected of all concerned in a working situation will eliminate unnecessary friction and unpleasantness.

CLINICAL CASE PROBLEMS

1.   Mrs. Dalton, age 78, is admitted to the hospital for treatment of a fractured femur. After surgical fixation of the fracture she becomes very confused and is incontinent of feces and urine. She also refuses to eat or to try to help herself in any way. Her husband is still living and they had managed to care for one another in their farm home before Mrs. Dalton's accident. They have only one child, a son who is married and lives in another city about 80 miles away. He is a successful lawyer and the father of four children. He comes to see his mother occasionally while she is in the hospital and would like to have his parents come to live with him but his wife does not feel there is room in their home for the elderly couple.

What nursing problems can you see for Mrs. Dalton while she is in the hospital?
What factors will influence Mrs. Dalton's reaction to her accident?
What other problems aside from nursing have been created by her accident? How can they be solved? What resources might be available for help for the elderly couple?

2.   You and two members of your class are assigned to four weeks of duty in a skilled nursing home. You have never even visited in such a home and have had little personal experience with elderly people.

What type of patient do you expect to find there?
What safety precautions do you think will be necessary in an institution of this kind?
Can you plan an imaginary day of caring for four of the patients in the home?
If there were few recreational and occupational therapy projects available at the home, can you think of some that might appeal to these patients?
One of these patients is 47 years of age and chronically ill and refuses to indulge in any physical activity, although she could if she had the will to do so. What kind of complications might develop as a result of her immobility? How would you go about trying to motivate her toward more physical activity?

3.   Miss Atkins is an invalid who suffered from a stroke when she was only 40 years old. For the past 15 years since the stroke she has lived in the home of a widowed sister and has been cared for by her. The sister also has two children living in the home, a boy 15 and a girl 13.
Miss Atkin's sister has decided to take a job outside the home and wishes to employ a practical nurse to take care of her sister between the hours of 9:00 A.M. and 5:00 P.M. The practical nurse on taking the assignment finds that the dietary habits and general attitude of the family leave much to be desired. She also learns that the patient has suffered from a lack of skilled care in the home and that Miss Atkins does not understand the need for any change in the daily routine or planning and preparation of meals. The patient prefaces every statement with "My sister always does it this way."

What problems is the practical nurse confronted with in this situation? What must she avoid in attempting changes?

What resources might be available to the practical nurse in solving these problems?

What are the opportunities for teaching in this situation?

REFERENCES

1. Amburgey, P. I.: "Environmental Aids for the Aged Patient." Am. Journ. Nurs., Sept., 1966, p. 2017.
2. Austin, C. L.: "The Basic Six Needs of the Aging." Nurs. Outlook, March, 1959, p. 138.
3. Beland, I. L.: *Clinical Nursing: Pathophysical and Psychosocial Approaches.* New York, The Macmillan Co., 1965.
4. Brown, A. F.: *Medical Nursing,* 3rd edition. Philadelphia, W. B. Saunders Co., 1957.
5. Butler, R. N.: "The Crises of Old Age." RN, Oct., 1967, p. 47.
6. Crate, M.: "Nursing Function in Adaptation to Chronic Illness." Am. Journ. Nurs., Oct., 1965, p. 72.
7. Homberger, F.: *The Medical Care of the Aged and Chronically Ill.* Boston, Mass., Little, Brown, and Co., 1955.
8. Johnson, J. B., Thompson, L. F., et al.: "The Hazards of Immobility." Am. Journ. Nurs., April, 1967, p. 781.
9. McKneely, T. B.: "Medicare and the Nursing Home." Journ. Pract. Nurs., April, 1967, p. 36.
10. Miller, M. B., et al.: "Nursing in a Skilled Nursing Home." Am. Journ. Nurs., Feb., 1966, p. 321.
11. Newton, K.: *Geriatric Nursing,* 3rd edition. St. Louis, Mo., C. V. Mosby Co., 1960.
12. Rasmussen, S.: "Medicare and the Licensed Practical Nurse." Nurs. Outlook, June, 1966, p. 62.
13. Schwarz, D.: "Problems of Self-care and Travel among Elderly Ambulatory Patients." Am. Journ. Nurs., Dec., 1966, p. 2678.
14. Sellew, G.: *Sociology and Its Use in Nursing Service,* 5th edition. Philadelphia, W. B. Saunders Co., 1962.
15. Shafer, K. N., Sawyer, J. R., et al.: *Medical-Surgical Nursing,* 3rd edition. St. Louis, Mo., C. V. Mosby Co., 1965.
16. Smith, E. G.: "Albianna Fashions — Wardrobe with a Purpose." Am. Journ. Nurs., June, 1966, p. 1320.
17. Sorensen, K. M., and Amis, D. B.: "Understanding the World of the Chronically Ill." Am. Journ. Nurs., April, 1967, p. 811.
18. Tierney, T. M.: "The Continuing Partnership." Nurs. Outlook, Jan., 1968, p. 22.
19. Verwoerdt, A.: "Psychological Factors in Geriatric Nursing Care." Journ. Pract. Nurs., Feb., 1967, p. 24.

SUGGESTED STUDENT READING

1. Abramson, J.: "Which One Is Mr. Jones?" Am. Journ. Nurs., April, 1962, p. 87.
2. Artwein, C.: "Geriatric Nursing Is Rewarding." Practical Nursing, April, 1962, p. 19.
3. Calloway, A. B.: "Social Needs of Geriatric Patients." Journ. Pract. Nurs., March, 1968, p. 34.
4. Carney, R. G.: "The Aging Skin." Am. Journ. Nurs., June, 1963, p. 110.
5. Davenport, R. R.: "Tube-feeding for Long-term Patients." Am. Journ. Nurs., Jan., 1964, p. 121.
6. Drake, M.: "Rehabilitation." Am. Journ. Nurs., April 1962, p. 87.
7. Henly, B. M.: "Helping the Elderly Find Community Resources." Am. Journ. Nurs., April, 1963, p. 89.
8. Masserman, J. H.: "Adages for the Aging." Today's Health, Nov., 1962, p. 20.
9. Rasmussen, S.: "Medicare and the Practical Nurse." Nurs. Outlook, June, 1966, p. 62.
10. "Rehabilitation: A Seminar for Licensed Practical Nurses." Journ. Pract. Nurs., Oct., 1964, p. 33.
11. Stokes, A.: "Institutional Care of the Aged." Journ. Pract. Nurs., Oct., 1967, p. 27.
12. "The LPN in Chronic Disease Nursing." Journ. Pract. Nurs., May, 1964, p. 24.
13. Verwoerdt, A.: "Psychological Factors in Geriatric Nursing Care." Journ. Pract. Nurs., Feb., 1967, p. 24.
14. Volpe, A., and Kastenbaum, R.: "Beer and TLC." Am. Journ. Nurs., Jan., 1967, p. 100.

OUTLINE FOR CHAPTER 7

Part I — The Aged

I. Age

A. Aging process varies with each individual. The term "aged" usually means persons 65 years or older.
  B. Terms used:
    1. Geriatrics — care of and service to the elderly.
    2. Gerontology — study of the elderly and the process of aging.
    3. Senile — having grown old. Does not necessarily imply mental deterioration.

II. Understanding the Aged

A. Attitude toward elderly persons and the nurse's own feelings about growing old have a profound effect on her ability to understand the aged.

B. Basic needs of elderly—"somewhere to live, something to do, someone to care."

C. Patient is to be motivated toward appropriate activity and self-care.

III. Physical Changes in the Aging Are a "Gradual Wearing Out"

IV. Nursing Care

A. Care of the skin is aimed at preservation of the integrity of the skin and prevention of its breakdown.

B. Keep patient's hair and nails clean and neat.

C. Cosmetics are not contraindicated and should be encouraged.

V. Diet and Nutrition

A. Adequate nutrition may be a problem because of poor life-long eating habits, difficulty with chewing and economic, cultural and emotional factors.

B. Anemia often is present.

C. Proper feeding technique for helpless patients is essential to good digestion and adequate intake of and interest in food.

VI. Other Considerations

A. Hearing may or may not be impaired. Speak clearly and distinctly.

B. Dimness of vision or "tunnel vision" may create a safety hazard.

C. Bones are often porous and are easily broken.

D. Sleep and recreation are geared to individual patient's needs. Patterns of rest and activity will vary.

E. Constipation is frequently due to inactivity and poor eating habits. It should be relieved by stool softeners, soft bulk and occasional mild laxatives.

F. Incontinence usually can be controlled through thoughtful planning and an established routine of elimination.

VII. Mental Changes

A. Older persons can "stay young mentally" by having a variety of interests, feeling needed and wanted and enjoying the companionship of others.

B. The nurse must learn to be a good listener when caring for an elderly patient.

C. Hospitalization sometimes causes a temporary mental confusion in the elderly person. The nurse should help him become oriented in his new environment, communicate with him frequently and avoid isolating him from others.

Part II—Chronic Illness

I. Chronic Illness

A. One that progresses slowly, sometimes with periods of remission, but always with a prognosis of only partial recovery.

B. Generally the chronic illnesses include circulatory disorders, metabolic disorders, cancer, and some forms of arthritis.

II. Nursing Care

A. Requires patience and an ability to be satisfied with the achievement of short-range goals.

B. Patient's adjustment to chronic illness depends on many factors and is a slow process through which the nurse guides rather than pushes the patient toward a new and different kind of existence.

C. Phases of chronic illness—acute, convalescent, and rehabilitative.

1. Rehabilitation must begin as soon as the disease is diagnosed.

2. The nurse directs her patient toward goals of self-help and as much independence as possible.

D. Chronic illness need not always be accompanied by immobility. The hazards of immobility must be understood by the nurse so that she can prevent its serious effects and complications.

1. Cardiovascular effects of immobility include increased strain on the heart and blood clot formation. Exercises and proper positioning are essential for prevention of both.

2. Respiratory effects include decreased activity of respiratory muscles, accumulation of bronchial secretions, and disturbances in oxygen-carbon dioxide balance. Nursing measures include frequent turning, deep-breathing exercises, encouraging the patient to cough and postural drainage when necessary.

3. Gastrointestinal effects include constipation, diarrhea and loss of con-

trol of bowel movements. Stool softeners, routine for elimination and adequate instruction of the patient in the process of elimination are the nursing measures used.

4. Musculoskeletal effects include contractures, osteoporosis and decubitus ulcers. Nursing measures include proper positioning, frequent turning, getting patient up if possible, exercises and good skin care.

5. Urinary tract complications are a result of urinary stasis, which leads to formation of stones and development of infection. Nursing measures include adequate fluid intake to keep the urine dilute, providing physical activity, and measures to induce voiding so that the bladder is emptied properly.

Part IV — Home Nursing

A. Licensed practical nurses are sometimes employed to give skilled nursing care in a patient's home.

B. Medicare provides for payment of home health aides.

C. Nurse who works in the home has a responsibility to her patient, the physician and the patient's family.

D. Duties of the nurse in the home may include housekeeping, laundry, cooking and serving the patient's meals and assisting with recreation for the patient.

Chapter 8

CARE OF THE PATIENT WITH AN INFECTIOUS DISEASE

VOCABULARY

Asepsis
Disinfectant
Immunity
Pathogenic
Susceptible

INTRODUCTION

In Chapter 2 we discussed infectious agents as possible causes of disease. These agents include bacteria, viruses, fungi, helminths (worms), protozoa and rickettsia. As one might suspect, the list of diseases that can be caused by these agents is quite lengthy and varied, but they all can be classified as *infectious diseases* (that is, those that are caused by specific pathogenic microorganisms). A *communicable disease* is one that can be transferred directly from one person to another or transmitted indirectly from an infected person or animal to a susceptible host. Some of the terms with which the nurse should be familiar are the following:

Contamination—the presence or possible presence of living pathogenic microorganisms in or on an article, a person or matter.

Carrier—an apparently healthy person who still harbors living pathogenic microorganisms and can spread them to others.

Disinfection—killing of infectious agents by chemical or physical means.

Concurrent disinfection is the immediate destruction of microorganisms as they leave the body or immediately after they have contaminated objects in the infected person's environment. *Terminal* disinfection is the destruction of infectious agents that remain in the patient's environment after he is no longer considered a source of infection.

Epidemic—a temporary and significant increase in the occurrence of disease in a specific area at any given time.

Endemic—a disease of low incidence that is constantly present in a community.

GENERAL PRINCIPLES OF NURSING CARE

Although the environment of man is well populated with disease-producing microorganisms, there are definite methods of control that can be used to prevent their multiplication and their spreading to susceptible persons. The best method of control for each disease will depend on the specific infectious agent involved and the ways in which it enters and leaves the body of an in-

129

Table 9.　*Incubation Periods of Communicable Diseases**

I. Incubation Period. Usually about 0 to 7 Days

DISEASE	INCUBATION PERIOD (AVG. and/or RANGE)		ISOLATION	IMMUNIZATION
Anthrax	1-4	(1-7)	'Clean' technique	
Bacillary dysentery	2-4	(1-7)	Till stool neg.	
Chancroid	3-5	(1-12)	From sexual contact	
Cholera	3	(1-5)	Till stool neg. (quarantine)	
Dengue	5-6	(3-15)	Screen	
Diphtheria	2-5		Till nose & throat neg.	Toxoid/antitoxin
Epidemic diarrhea of newborn	6-7	(2-21)	Yes (quarantine)	
Erysipelas	0-2		'Clean' technique	
Food poisoning				
Staphylococcus	2-4	(1-6) hrs.	From food handling	Antitoxin
Salmonella	12	(6-48 hrs.		
Botulinus	18-24	(2-48) hrs.		
Gonorrhea	3-5	(1-14)	From sexual contact and children	
Impetigo contagiosa	<5		From child contacts	
Infectious keratoconjunctivitis	5-7			
Influenza	1-3		Acute stage	Formalin virus
Meningitis, meningococcic	<7	(2-10)	24 hrs., if treated	
Paratyphoid	1-10		Till stool & urine neg.	Vaccine
Plague	3-6		Till well	Formalin vaccine
Pneumonia, bacterial	1-3		Respiratory precautions	
Puerperal infection	1-3		Till well	

*From Smith Kline & French Laboratories: Pocket Book of Medical Tables, 17th revised edition, 1968.

Table 9. *Incubation Periods of Communicable Diseases** (Continued)*

I. Incubation Period. Usually about 0 to 7 Days

DISEASE	INCUBATION PERIOD (AVG. and/or RANGE)	ISOLATION	IMMUNIZATION
Relapsing fever tick	3-6 (2-12)		
Rocky Mountain spotted fever	3-10		Yolk-sac vaccine
Scabies	1-2	From school	
Scarlet fever	2-5	Respiratory precautions	
Tularemia	3 (1-10)		
Yellow fever	3-6	Screen	Modified virus

II. Incubation Periods. Usually about 7 to 14 Days

DISEASE	INCUBATION PERIOD (AVG. and/or RANGE)	ISOLATION	IMMUNIZATION
Coccidioidomycosis	10-15 (7-21)	Till sputum neg.	
Equine encephalitis			
Infectious mononucleosis	11 (7-15)	Respiratory precautions	
Leptospirosis	9-10 (4-19)		
Lymphocytic choriomeningitis	8-13		
Measles	9-14	Till 5 days after rash	Vaccine
Pertussis	5-9 (2-21)	From school & susceptibles	Vaccine
Poliomyelitis	7-14 (3-35)	First 2 weeks	Vaccine
Primary atypical pneumonia	11 (7-21)	Respiratory precautions	
Psittacosis	6-15	Till afebrile	
Relapsing fever louse	7 (5-12)	To delouse	
Scrub typhus	7-10 (7-14)		
Smallpox	12 (7-21)	Till scabs off (quarantine)	Vaccinia
Trichinosis	9 (2-28)		
Typhoid fever	7-14 (3-38)	Till stool & urine neg.	Vaccine
Typhus fever	12 (6-15)	To delouse (quarantine)	Vaccine

*From Smith Kline & French Laboratories: Pocket Book of Medical Tables, 17th revised edition, 1968.

(Table continued on page 132.)

Table 9. *Incubation Periods of Communicable Diseases** (Continued)

III. Incubation Periods Usually over 14 Days

DISEASE	INCUBATION PERIOD (AVG. AND/OR RANGE)	ISOLATION	IMMUNIZATION
Amebic dysentery	21-28 (8-90)	From food handling	
Brucellosis	14 (6-30+)		
Chickenpox	14 (12-21)	Till skin clear	
German measles	16-18 (10-21)	First week	
Granuloma inguinale	10-90	From sexual contact	
Hepatitis, infectious	25 (15-35)	Stool disinfection for 3 weeks	Immune globulin
Hepatitis, serum	80-100 (60-180)		
Lymphogranuloma venereum	7-28	From sexual contact	
Malaria	10-17 (to 35+)	Screen	
Mumps	18 (12-26)	Till glands down	Vaccine
Q fever	14-21		Vaccine
Rabies	14-42 (10-180)	Aseptic technique	Attenuated vaccine
Rickettsialpox	10-24		
Syphilis	21 (10-90)	From sexual contact and children	
Tetanus	4-21		Toxoid
Tuberculosis	Variable	'Open' cases	BCG vaccine
Yaws	30-90	Desirable till treated	

*From Smith Kline & French Laboratories: Pocket Book of Medical Tables, 17th revised edition, 1968.

fected person. The nurse should know something about these factors if she is to be effective in preventing the spread of infections and reducing the incidence of infectious diseases. She also must conscientiously carry out all procedures and practices that are established for the protection of the patient and all others concerned. This will include adherence to basic principles of cleanliness as well as a thorough knowledge of isolation technique, which is discussed later in this chapter.

In addition, she must understand disinfection and the most effective means for destroying pathogenic microorganisms. Since resistance to infection is important in preventing the development of or speeding the recovery from an infectious disease, nursing care is also aimed at improving the patient's general state of health so that he will be less susceptible to infection and reinfection.

Immunization. For a review of immunity and how it provides protection against some diseases the reader is referred to Chapter 4. Within the past few decades we have seen improvements in existing vaccines and the development of new vaccines, both of which have greatly reduced the number of cases of a variety of communicable diseases in this country. The diseases most affected by such vaccines are smallpox, diphtheria, tetanus, whooping cough, typhoid fever, poliomyelitis, measles, mumps and influenza. This is quite an impressive list but we still, after more than one hundred years of immunization procedures, cannot consider any of these diseases completely eradicated.

Nurses must always encourage immunization whenever the opportunity presents itself. Unfortunately, the availability of a specific vaccine is not immediately followed by prompt removal of the disease. There remains a considerable gap between *application* of effective immunization and the rapid advances made in disease prevention. The nurse is in an excellent position to encourage immunization so that no person will needlessly suffer from an illness because of ignorance, poverty or lack of concern.

Although some infectious diseases are virtually disappearing, others are emerging as major health problems. For example, hepatitis is one of the more serious communicable diseases at the present time in the United States. In fact, viral infections of all types seem to be destined to play a major role in morbidity and mortality statistics in the future.[5]

Because of the nature of viruses, particularly their ability to change characteristics so readily, immunization against viral diseases is not so easily accomplished. It is hoped that with continued research we will eventually be able to provide immunity against a greater number of viral infections.

Another type of infection that became notorious during the 1950's was that due to staphylococci—the dread "staph infection" that received so much publicity at the time. During the mid-1960's staphylococcal infections have become less troublesome and we are now faced with a variety of gram-negative bacteria which, according to the National Communicable Disease Center, account for over 60 per cent of all hospital-acquired infections. Since infections acquired within a hospital are due in some degree to the carelessness of the hospital staff, the nurse should be particularly aware of her responsibility to avoid the spread of such infections. Studies have shown that, in some hospitals, up to 20 per cent of the patients who die there have an infection acquired in the hospital. Although these infections were not necessarily the direct cause of death, they have materially contributed to the death of the patient.[5]

Spread of Infectious Diseases. The route by which a pathogen leaves the body is called its *portal of exit;* the route by which it enters the body to establish an infection is called the *portal of entry.* An example of a portal of exit is the intestinal tract through which the typhoid bacillus leaves in the patient's feces. The digestive tract also serves as a portal of entry when one eats contaminated food or drinks water that contains pathogens. Another portal of both exit and entry is the respiratory tract, which can admit and pass on a large number of different pathogens that cause diseases ranging from measles and mumps to tuberculosis and pneumonia. The skin and mucous membranes also can serve as portals of entry and exit, as in the transmission of syphilis, gonorrhea and many different kinds of skin disorders.

Sources of infection can be any person or object that harbors an infectious agent. Patients themselves probably are the most important source of infection in hospitals and clinics. That is why the nurse is admonished over and over again to wash her hands after each contact with a patient, regardless of his diagnosis. All newly admitted patients should be observed for signs of infection such as boils, infected wounds or fever, and if there is a sign of infection this should be reported immediately so that proper precautions can be taken. Visitors and hospital personnel also can serve as sources of infection. And surely every student nurse knows that hospital dust, insects, and vermin are all extremely likely to carry microorganisms capable of causing disease. She must not, however, let familiarity breed complacency so that she becomes careless in maintaining an environment of cleanliness and order for her patients and herself.

Modes of transfer of pathogens include the following: (1) *direct personal contact* with body excreta or drainage from an ulcer, infected wound, boil or chancre, (2) *indirect contact* with inanimate objects (called *fomites*) such as contaminated needles and syringes, drinking and eating utensils, dressings and hospital equipment, (3) *vectors*, such as fleas, flies, mosquitoes and other insects that harbor infectious agents pathogenic to man, (4) *droplet infection*, or contamination by the aerial route through sneezing and coughing, and (5) an *endogenous* spread of infection from one part of a person's body to another.

A group of student nurses investigated cross infection hazards in the medical unit of a typical modern hospital. Their study was published in the October, 1967 issue of the American Journal of Nursing. Excerpts from their findings are quoted below.

Inadequate handwashing was the most serious error discovered. In the room of a patient on reverse isolation,* students

*Reverse isolation refers to isolation of the patient to protect him from infectious agents.

counted eight people who entered in a one-and-one-half-hour period. Although all persons wore masks, dust was seen on the television set, newspapers, and boxes. Soot entered through an open window, and a vacuum cleaner stirred floor dust. The laboratory technician did not wash her hands before working with the patient, and a nurse handled the medicine tray and cards which were used for all patients on the floor and then gave medicines to the isolated patient without washing her hands. Bed linen touched the floor.

Among the housekeeping personnel, a maid pushed down garbage with her bare hands in the utility room and then traveled down the hall touching various items without washing her hands. The vacuum cleaner, whose gusty exhaust blew floor dust about, was dragged from room to room including that of the patient on reverse isolation. The porter did not wash his hands throughout the morning as he performed his various tasks, and handled many items including the doctor's bag.

Utility room surveillance disclosed that when a bedpan was put into the flusher, it was considered contaminated and was replaced with a sterilized pan. However, rectal tubes did not appear to be cared for properly: an aide emptied a bedpan, helped make a bed, and then washed her hands; and trash cans were overflowing.

Nurses making a similar survey in their own hospital units might find that they can do more than they thought possible to protect their patients and themselves from needless contamination.

Disinfection. Disinfecting and sterilizing agents should be among the first subjects with which a nurse becomes familiar. In the care of a patient with an infectious disease the nurse must be especially careful in carrying out all practices in disinfecting for which she may be responsible. Autoclaving is considered the most effective means of killing bacteria. All living organisms can be destroyed by exposure to moist heat of at least 250° F. (121° C.) for 15 minutes. If the nurse is responsible for soaking objects in a sterilizing solution, she must always be sure that the articles are completely submerged in the solution. She also must know how strong the solution should be and the period of time recommended by its manufacturer for adequate sterilization. One should bear in mind that not every kind of disinfectant will destroy all types of microorganisms. The effectiveness of disinfection will depend on (1) the type and number of organisms, (2) whether or not there is organic material such as mucus present on the object to be disinfected, (3) the type and strength of disinfectant, and (4) the length of time the microorganisms are exposed to the disinfectant.[8]

SPECIFIC NURSING MEASURES TO CONTROL THE SPREAD OF AN INFECTIOUS DISEASE

Isolation. The term *isolation* probably is not the best to use in reference to the practice of separating the patient from others so that he will not continue to spread his infection. The word isolation has several psychological disadvantages for the patient and his family. A newer term, *barrier technique*, has been suggested because it does not imply that the patient is dirty or unacceptable to others.[8] Whichever term is used by the hospital staff, one must be very careful not to give the patient the impression that he is being isolated because he is a nuisance or a social or moral threat to others. His physical separation is quite a burden to him too, and he will need more than the usual amount of explanation about the nature of his disease and a good bit of emotional support and psychological bolstering while he is isolated from others.

If the nursing staff has advance warning that a patient with an infectious disease is to be admitted, all unnecessary equipment and upholstered furniture should be removed from his unit before he enters the room. Once he has entered the room everything in his immediate environment must be considered contaminated and will require either concurrent or terminal disinfection. He should have his own thermometer, tray for food, eating utensils, water pitcher and drinking glass.

Visitors are restricted to members of the family and designated friends approved by the physician, and all persons entering or leaving the patient's unit must follow the procedure outlined by the hospital to prevent the spread of disease.

While giving nursing care to the patient in isolation, the nurse must remember that whenever possible she should touch only "clean to clean" and "contaminated to contaminated." This means, for example, that she uses clean paper towels as "technic papers" to handle objects when her hands are contaminated. Once a clean object has come in contact with a contaminated article, both must be considered contaminated. A student nurse once remarked that she felt less likely to contaminate her hands if she imagined herself wearing spotless white gloves while in the isolation unit. The nurse must be careful not to spread infectious agents through careless use of her hands.

Handwashing. The term *medical asepsis* refers to the destruction of microorganisms *after they leave* the body of the patient. This is in contrast to *surgical asepsis*, which refers to destruction of microorganisms *before they enter* the body of the patient. This distinction is important to handwashing technique when one is caring for a patient with an infectious disease because in this situation the nurse must consider part of herself contaminated and part of herself clean. Her hands contain microorganisms that must be destroyed after they have left the patient's body. She must therefore be very careful to wash her hands thoroughly after each contact with the patient and even during the immediate care of the patient when she realizes that her hands are grossly contaminated. It also means that during the handwashing procedure she must keep her hands *below the level* of

Figure 8-1. During a handwash for medical asepsis, the hands are kept lower than the elbows to keep microorganisms away from the elbows. (From Kozier and DuGas: *Fundamentals of Patient Care*, W. B. Saunders Co., Philadelphia.)

her elbows (see Fig. 8-1). The hands should be washed under running water for at least one full minute. Friction between the hands is necessary to remove microorganisms from the lines and crevices of the skin. The fingernails should be given careful attention and be well lathered and rinsed. If bar soap is used it is kept in the hands throughout the entire handwashing until the final rinsing of the hands. It is best to use foot pedals to control the flow of water, but if these are not available a paper towel is used to turn off the water because the faucet handles are considered contaminated.

Using a Gown. When there is a possibility that the nurse's uniform may become contaminated while she is attending the patient with an infectious

disease, she must wear an isolation gown for protection. The gown should have long sleeves and a high neck and should tie at the back of the neck and waist. It should be long enough to cover the nurse's uniform completely. The gown is kept in the patient's room and should not be worn outside the room. If it is worn only once and discarded there is no special procedure for donning and removing the gown. If it is to be worn again, it must be put on and taken off in a certain way because the outside is considered to be contaminated and the inside clean. Figure 8-2 shows how this is to be done.

Using a Face Mask. The face mask is of most benefit when the infectious disease can be transmitted via the respiratory tract. There is a distinction between a surgical mask and a mask used for medical asepsis. During surgical procedures the nurse wears a mask primarily for the patient's protection. In medical asepsis she wears it for her own protection.

There is a variety of masks available for use and each has its advantages and disadvantages. The disposable masks are probably the most widely used in medical asepsis because they are relatively inexpensive and require no handling by persons other than the ones wearing them. The mask should fit snugly and cover both the nose and the mouth. It should be worn for no longer than one hour because it becomes contaminated in that period of time and it is not effective once it becomes wet. When the mask is removed only the ties are handled, as they are the least contaminated part of the mask. The hands are washed *before* the mask is removed so that the wearer's hair and neck will not be contaminated by the hands when the ties are untied.

Care of Equipment. Dishes, trays and eating utensils are kept in the patient's room for reuse unless they are disposable. The patient's food and liquids are transferred from the "clean" tray held at the door by a "clean" nurse to the

Figure 8-2. *A*, When taking off a contaminated gown that is to be discarded, the nurse keeps her "dirty" hands and the contaminated side of the gown away from her. *B*, When reusing a contaminated gown, the nurse slips her clean hands inside without contaminating herself with the gown. (From Kozier and DuGas: *Fundamentals of Patient Care*, W. B. Saunders Co., Philadelphia.)

patient's tray that is kept in his room. Solid left-over food may be wrapped in newspaper and discarded in the incinerator. Liquids may be flushed down the toilet in the patient's room. Disposable equipment and soiled dressings are also wrapped in paper and placed in a specially marked bag that is taken to the hospital incinerator and burned.

Medicine glasses, syringes and other nondisposable equipment should be soaked in a disinfectant solution and then autoclaved after use. Linen from the patient's unit is placed in a special laundry bag marked "contaminated" or "isolation" and it is autoclaved before it is sent to the laundry. Other equipment such as furniture, bedding and suction machines are left in the patient's room until he is discharged. His room is then closed tightly and the area is "fogged" with a fine mist of disinfectant.

Disposal of Excreta. The disposal of excreta such as feces and vomitus usually can be accomplished by flushing them down the hopper. In some communities where sewage treatment is not considered adequate for destruction of certain infectious agents the excreta must be disinfected with chlorinated lime before it is discarded in the hopper.

Diagnosis of Infectious Diseases. Every nurse should be aware of the importance of good and intelligent observation as a function of nursing. Whether she is observing a newly admitted patient, one who has been in the hospital awhile or a relative or friend of a patient, the nurse should be alert for signs of infection or early symptoms of a communicable disease. These signs include fever, elevated pulse and respiratory rate and a general malaise. Other symptoms, such as rash or skin eruption, are more specific, and it is in this area that the nurse can be most helpful in reporting her observation and helping to provide early treatment.

Diagnostic procedures such as those that involve the collection of specimens for culture and bacteriologic studies are discussed in Chapter 4. The student should be familiar with the proper technique for collecting these specimens so as to avoid spreading infection. She also must be aware of the need for particular care in handling needles and syringes that may be contaminated by an infected person's blood or body fluids, both of which can be highly infectious.

There are some diagnostic tests that are useful in certain infectious diseases. The *Schick* test is done for detecting susceptibility to diphtheria; the *Dick* test for scarlet fever. A small amount of toxoid is administered intradermally on the inner aspect of the forearm. If a red, swollen area appears in 24 to 48 hours the reaction is considered positive, and this indicates susceptibility or lack of immunity. Some patients do not exhibit a positive reaction until 3 to 5 days. For this reason they should be instructed to return for a repeat reading if they notice the area becoming red or swollen.

A tuberculin test is done in a similar manner. A reaction indicates only that the individual has been exposed to the tubercle bacillus some time in the past but it does *not* indicate that he has an active case of tuberculosis. An exception is children under two years of age. In them a positive reaction can indicate active tuberculosis.

CLINICAL CASE PROBLEMS

1. A friend of yours who lives in a rural area has a daughter who has infectious hepatitis. Her physician has said that hospitalization will not be necessary if the mother feels that she can safely care for the child at home. They live in a house with three bedrooms and one and a half baths. They use well water and a septic tank. There are three other children in the family.

　　How could you help this mother plan for the care of her daughter so that the other members of the family would not become infected with the virus?

What special precautions would be necessary in regard to dishes, linen and disposal of excreta?

2. Mrs. Chambers, age 44, is admitted to the hospital for a hemorrhoidectomy. During the admission procedure you notice a large, draining boil in the patient's axilla. She also has a temperature of 100° F. and tells you that she has not felt well for the past few days.

What would be your course of action following this discovery?
If Mrs. Chambers was found to be infectious because of a possible staphylococcal infection, what precautions would be necessary?
How would you go about explaining to Mrs. Chambers the need for such precautions?

REFERENCES

1. Ager, E. A.: "Current Concepts in Immunization." Am. Journ. Nurs., Sept., 1966, p. 2004.
2. Beland, I. L.: *Clinical Nursing.* New York, The Macmillan Co., 1965.
3. French, J. G.: "Students Study Cross-contamination." Am. Journ. Nurs., Oct., 1967, p. 2104.
4. Gallivan, G. J., and Tovey, J. D.: "Isolation for Possible and Proved Staph." Am. Journ. Nurs., July, 1967, p. 1048.
5. Gregg, M. B.: "Communicable Disease Trends in the United States." Am. Journ. Nurs., Jan., 1968, p. 88.
6. Keane, C. B.: *Saunders Review for Practical Nurses.* Philadelphia, W. B. Saunders Co., 1966.
7. Kline, P. A.: "Isolating Patients with Staphylococcal Infections." Am. Journ. Nurs., Jan., 1965, p. 102.
8. Kozier, B. B., and DuGas, B. W.: *Fundamentals of Patient Care.* Philadelphia, W. B. Saunders Co., 1967.
9. Shafer, K. N., Sawyer, J. R., et al.: *Medical-Surgical Nursing,* 4th edition. St. Louis, C. V. Mosby Co., 1967.
10. Smith, D. W., and Gips, C. D.: *Care of the Adult Patient,* 2nd edition. Philadelphia, J. B. Lippincott Co., 1966.

SUGGESTED STUDENT READING

1. Ager, E. A.: "Current Concepts in Immunization." Am. Journ. Nurs., Sept., 1966, p. 2004.
2. French, J. G.: "Students Study Cross-contamination." Am. Journ. Nurs., Oct., 1967, p. 2104.
3. Gregg, M. B.: "Communicable Disease Trends in the United States." Am. Journ. Nurs., Jan., 1968, p. 88.

OUTLINE FOR CHAPTER 8

I. Introduction

A. Infectious disease—one caused by a specific pathogenic microorganism.

B. Communicable disease—one that can be transmitted to another person.

II. General Principles of Nursing Care

A. Nurse's role in control and prevention of infectious disease:
 1. Must know about portals of entry and exit for infectious diseases.
 2. Carries out all procedures and practices established for the protection of patient and others, including strict adherence to principles of cleanliness and good hygiene.
 3. Must understand disinfection and the most effective means of destroying infectious agents.
 4. Must work to keep her patients in optimal good health to build resistance to infections.

B. Immunization important in reducing incidence of infectious diseases.
 1. Nurses must encourage immunization although public ignorance and apathy prevent many from taking advantage of the immunizations.
 2. Effective vaccines for viral infections are particularly difficult to prepare.
 3. Hospital acquired infections are still a problem for which the nursing staff must bear some responsibility.

C. Ways in which infectious diseases are spread:
 1. Patients, visitors, and hospital personnel are all possible sources of infection within a hospital.
 2. Modes of transfer include by *direct contact* with infected person, by *indirect contact* with inanimate objects (fomites), by *vectors* (insects that harbor infectious agents pathogenic to man), by *droplet infection* (aerial route through sneezing and coughing), and by *endogenous spread*

from one part of a person's body to another.
3. Inadequate handwashing probably one of the most frequent causes of spread of infection.
D. Disinfection—destruction of living microorganisms.
1. Moist heat is most effective means.
2. If objects are to be soaked in a disinfectant, use proper strength, completely cover the articles, and soak for length of time recommended by manufacturer of disinfectant.
3. Effectiveness of disinfection will depend on: (a) type and number of organisms, (b) whether or not there is organic material on the object to be disinfected, (c) type and strength of disinfectant, and (d) length of time microorganisms are exposed to disinfectant.

III. Specific Nursing Measures

A. Isolation—separation of the patient from others until he is no longer considered a source of infection.
1. Has psychological disadvantages of which the nurse should be aware so that she can reassure the patient and family.
2. Once patient has entered the unit all equipment in the unit must be considered contaminated and will require concurrent or terminal disinfection.
3. Visitors are restricted. All persons entering and leaving the room must follow hospital procedures.
4. Once a contaminated object has come in contact with a clean object both are considered contaminated, so one should touch only "clean to clean" and "contaminated to contaminated" objects.
B. Handwashing.
1. Hands are held under running water and washed for one full minute, keeping them below elbow level.
2. Bar of soap is held in the hands

throughout procedure until final rinsing.
3. If foot pedals are not available use paper towel to turn off water faucet.
C. Gown—used to protect nurse's uniform from contamination.
1. Kept in patient's room and should not be worn outside the room.
2. If to be worn again it must be hung so that outside is exposed. Inside is considered clean and should be handled so that it does not become contaminated.
D. Face mask—worn for the nurse's protection against pathogens.
1. Should fit face snugly and cover both nose and mouth.
2. Should not be worn for more than an hour at which time it is discarded and a new one put on. A wet mask is considered contaminated.
3. Wash hands before removing mask.
E. Care of equipment.
1. Disposable objects are wrapped and burned.
2. Some objects can be soaked in a disinfectant; others are autoclaved.
3. Liquid waste may be flushed down hopper.
4. Laundry is placed in specially marked bag and autoclaved before laundering.
5. During terminal disinfection equipment that cannot be disinfected in any other way is left in patient's room and "fogged."
F. Disposal of excreta.
1. May be flushed down hopper if local sewage treatment is adequate; if not, excreta must be treated with chlorinated lime before disposal.

III. Diagnosis of Infectious Diseases

A. Nurse must use caution in collection of specimens for culture and bacteriologic studies as equipment for diagnostic tests can spread infection.
B. Special diagnostic tests include Schick test for diphtheria, Dick test for scarlet fever and tuberculin test for tuberculosis.

Chapter 9

THE CANCER PATIENT

VOCABULARY

Diffusion
Excision
Lymphatic
Penetration
Synthesis
Therapeutic

INTRODUCTION

Cancer is not new; it has been with us since the beginning of time. We hear about so many cases of cancer today because diagnostic tests are more accurate now than formerly and as a result more correct diagnoses are being made. We must also remember that cancer is primarily a disease of the older age group and is more likely to develop in persons over 50 years of age, and since more persons now reach this age group we can expect the incidence of cancer to increase.

In spite of the wealth of information distributed to the public on the subject of cancer, there are still many persons who associate malignant growths with severe pain and inevitable death. The practical nurse and all the other members of the health team have an obligation to assist in public health education about cancer. It is important that lay people understand that cancer is not hopeless, that malignancies are curable in the early stages, and that prolonged suffering and death are not inevitable companions of cancer.

According to the American Cancer Society, persons cured of cancer are those who "are without evidence of the disease at least five years after diagnosis and completion of treatment." In "The Hopeful Side of Cancer," a booklet published by the American Cancer Society, it is stated that over 1,300,000 Americans have been cured of cancer, and 183,000 patients are saved each year. An additional 700,000 cancer patients diagnosed and treated within the last five years will live to join the ranks of those considered to be cured. Progress is being made in the fight against this disease.

Cancer is a neoplastic disease, which means that it is characterized by the reproduction and growth of new cells. We know that the human body is continously manufacturing new cells for the maintenance of life and the repair of damage done by illness and injury. Most of the time this process of reproduction goes on in a normal fashion and healing takes place without incident. Sometimes, however, the new cells become abnormal in their structure and they cannot function properly. They grow too rapidly so that there is not sufficient nutrition for them, they cannot perform the work expected of them,

141

and eventually they become extremely wild and disorganized. These pathological changes in the cells occur in the beginning stages of cancer.

Later, if the new growths are not destroyed completely, they become necrotic in the center because they are starved for nutrition and the cells in the outer edge of the mass break off and begin to spread through the body. This spreading of the malignant cells is called *metastasis*.

There are five routes by which malignant cells may be transferred from the original site of the tumor to other parts of the body: (1) by direct extension, (2) by growing along the lymphatic vessel, (3) by embolism through the lymphatic stream to the lymph nodes, (4) by embolism in the blood vessels, and (5) by invasion of the fluid within a body cavity, especially the abdomen and chest. Figure 9-1 illustrates these five routes of metastasis.

Cancer spreads by several routes:

1. By direct extension into neighboring tissue

2. By permeation along lymphatic vessels

3. By embolism via lymphatic vessels to the lymph nodes

4. By embolism via blood vessels

5. By invasion of a body cavity by diffusion

Figure 9-1.   Routes by which cancer is spread to other parts of the body. (Modified from *A Cancer Source Book for Nurses,* American Cancer Society.)

CAUSES OF CANCER

We do not yet know the exact reason the body should begin to manufacture cells which change their size, shape and structure, and begin to behave in a malignant way, invading and destroying neighboring tissues. There has been extensive research on cancer, however, and we do have some important and definite clues about the conditions which predispose the human body to the development of cancer.

Predisposing Causes. The predisposing or secondary causes of cancer are generally classified under three headings:

1. Conditions of long-continued and chronic irritations. For example; irritation of a mole by clothing, exposure of the skin to strong sunlight over a period of time, or chronic cervicitis with erosion of the cervical tissues.

2. Industrial cancer due to prolonged exposure to certain irritating agents such as aniline dyes or coal tars.

3. Benign tumors, such as polyps and cysts, which have a tendency to become malignant and are therefore called "precancerous."

Other predisposing causes of cancer such as race, sex, age, and an inherited tendency to develop cancer must also be considered.

Search for Specific Causes. The primary causes of cancer are not yet fully understood and it is generally agreed among scientists that there is no *single* specific cause. It is felt that cancer results from a combination of several factors.

There has been renewed interest in the possibility of a virus, or viruses, causing some forms of cancer in human beings. Leukemia has been considered to be among the forms of malignancy which apparently are related in some way to viruses. It is also believed that some other forms of cancer may be the result of toxic damage to cells from certain chemical compounds. It is extremely difficult for research teams to draw any definite conclusions, however, because the characteristics of cell growths and development have often proven to be different in each form of cancer.

Until the primary causes are discovered and successful means are found whereby the malignant cells may be destroyed without damaging normal cells, there can be no guarantee that any treatment will permanently rid the body of cancer. This does not in any way imply a hopeless situation for the cancer patient. Insulin does not "cure" diabetes, yet many diabetics are leading useful lives and living to a ripe old age. By the same token, most cancer patients may also look forward to years of active living if they have treatment begun in the early stages of the disease.

SYMPTOMS OF CANCER

Cancer begins very quietly and is capable of stealthily creeping up on an unsuspecting individual. It can cause considerable damage in the body before its victim is aware he has been attacked. Because the disease is so insidious, no one can afford to ignore the early symptoms of cancer, nor is it sensible to put off seeking expert advice from the physician when there is the slightest suspicion that cancer is present.

Cancer is sometimes called the "great masquerader" because it is capable of imitating the symptoms of a great variety of diseases. Since it may strike any part of the body and spread to any other organ (sometimes far removed from the original site), cancer is capable of producing an untold number and variety of symptoms in its later stages. Our main interest in the symptoms of cancer lies in the very early signs. They are included here for the purpose of reminding the practical nurse that they are extremely important and that she should be able to recite them from memory.

1. Any sore that does not heal.
2. A lump or thickening in the breast or elsewhere.
3. Unusual bleeding or discharge.
4. Any change in a wart or mole.
5. Persistent indigestion or difficulty in swallowing.
6. Any change in normal bowel habits.
7. Persistent hoarseness or cough.

DIAGNOSIS OF CANCER

Physical Examination. Fortunately, the diagnosis of cancer is usually not difficult. The problem is getting the general public educated to the importance of regular physical examinations so that early cancer can be detected and treatment begun. New growths located near the surface of the body can very easily be felt by palpation. It is reported that whenever the movie, "Self-examination of the Breast" (distributed by the American Cancer Society), is shown to a group of women, several women in the audience visit their physicians within a few days because they have discovered nodules in their breast tissue. In many cases these nodules prove to be early malignancies and the patient has an excellent chance of being cured of the cancer.

Skin cancer is easily seen by the naked eye, and with special instruments such as the vaginal speculum or proctoscope, cancer of the cervix or rectum can be seen by the examining physician. Other internal growths may be visualized with x-rays.

Biopsy. When the physician discovers a new growth he immediately sets out to determine whether the growth is benign or malignant. This is done by biopsy, which is the removal of a sample of living cells from the growth. The cells may be removed by surgical excision of a small part of the tumor, or by aspiration of the cells through a needle introduced into the growth (see Fig. 9-2). The specimen is sent to a specially trained pathologist who ex-

Figure 9-2. Aspiration biopsy set. *A*, 5 cc. hypodermic syringe with short and long needles for Novocain infiltration. *B*, Sterile medicine glass for Novocain solution. *C*, Scalpel with No. 11 Bard-Parker blade. *D*, 20 cc. Record syringe. *E*, 18 gauge needle with obturator. *F*, Instrument for raking out tissue from barrel of syringe. *G*, Glass slides for smears of aspirated material. (From Wolf: *Nursing Clinics of North America*, December, 1967.)

amines the cells and determines the type of growth they represent. Because of the danger of spreading the malignancy when a biopsy is taken, most surgeons prepare their patients for extensive surgery at the time the biopsy is done. Then if the growth proves to be malignant immediate steps may be taken to remove all traces of the growth.

Papanicolaou Smear. At the very beginning of the development of cancerous growths it is possible to find cancer cells in the secretions from the body tissues adjacent to the site of the malignant growth. A physician, Dr. Papanicolaou, developed a technique for collecting samples of body secretions and examining them for malignant cells, thereby detecting the presence of cancer long before any other symptoms appear. This technique has saved the lives of countless people who have had Papanicolaou smears done as a routine diagnostic test at the time of regular physical examinations. Many cases of cancer of the cervix have been cured because of the ability to detect the disease in the early stages through the use of the "Pap" smear.

TREATMENT OF CANCER

At the present time there are several different forms of treatment for cancer. These include (1) surgery, (2) radiation therapy, and (3) chemotherapy.

Because these methods may be used singly or together, there may sometimes be confusion in the minds of cancer patients as to which form of treatment will produce the best results. Actually, no one method is better or more effective than another except in relation to the location and type of malignancy present and the reaction of the particular type of growth to treatment. The physician chooses the method of treatment on the basis of many factors and in the best interest of the individual patient.

Surgery. Surgical removal of growths is the oldest method of treatment. It works very well for tumors which are readily accessible and located in areas where adjacent tissues, such as muscles, lymph nodes and lymph vessels, may also be excised. This radical cutting away of apparently normal tissue may seem unnecessarily drastic and mutilating to the lay person who does not fully understand the metastasis of cancer cells, but it has been proven that simple excision of the malignant tumor alone will not eliminate rapid spread and recurrence of the growth in adjacent tissues.

Radiation Therapy. This is a type of treatment that utilizes penetrating rays or emissions from an x-ray machine or radioactive substances. There are many types of radiations in our environment, for example, ultraviolet rays from the sun, light rays that we can see, radio waves that we can hear and infrared or heat rays that we can feel. The types of rays used for therapeutic purposes are alpha, beta, and gamma rays and x-rays. These rays vary markedly in their composition and in their ability to penetrate matter. *Alpha rays* are composed of large particles which are highly charged and thus are not capable of traveling long distances or penetrating very deeply. *Beta rays* are smaller with less electric charge and have a longer range, making them capable of deeper penetration. *Gamma rays* have no mass and no charge. Like *x-rays*, they can travel long distances in the air and can completely penetrate the tissues of the body.

Radiation is harmful to living tissue and when delivered externally in comparatively large doses can cause disturbances in cell functions and interfere with growth and reproduction. When determining the "radiation dose" for each individual patient, the radiologist takes into account the age and general condition of the patient, his response to treatment, the size, location and depth of the tumor and the type of radiation that is available.[18]

The aim of radiotherapy is permanent destruction of the malignant cells in the growth. Unfortunately, there is nearly always some degree of damage to normal tissue in the process of reaching the underlying abnormal tissue. In addition, the patient may suffer from radiation sickness or a local reaction, either of which can interfere with the administration of an effective dose.

The damage to normal tissue can be kept at a minimum in x-ray therapy through accurate adjustment of dosage or degree of penetration and by aiming the rays from several different angles. The technique of using a variety of "ports" for entry of the rays into the body increases the concentration of the rays in the area of the tumor with a minimum of damage to overlying tissues. This is called the rotation method and can be applied with both x-ray therapy and teletherapy. In this technique the patient or the apparatus revolves slowly while the rays are aimed at the tumor (see Fig. 9-3).

METHODS OF RADIATION THERAPY. The methods that may be used in therapeutic radiation include x-ray therapy, teletherapy, and interstitial therapy. *X-ray therapy* is administered by an x-ray machine that is of a higher voltage than the kind usually used for diagnostic procedures. The x-ray beam is aimed directly at the tumor and is delivered in a series of treatments planned for each individual patient.

Figure 9-3. Rotation method of radiation therapy. (Modified from *A Cancer Source Book for Nurses*, American Cancer Society.)

Teletherapy is a procedure in which the source of radiation is a radioactive element that is housed in a shielded unit and located at a distance from the patient (see Fig. 9-4). The beam of radiation is controlled and directed by heavy shutters or special shielding that localizes the area of radiation. It should be remembered that gamma rays from a radioactive substance cannot be entirely absorbed by the shield and there is no way to "turn off" a teletherapy unit; therefore one should spend as little time as possible in the teletherapy room with a patient.[18]

Interstitial therapy involves placement or implantation of a radioactive substance directly into the tissues of a malignant growth. The element used may be radium, cobalt-60, cesium-137, iridium-192, gold-198, or iodine-125. Radium is naturally radioactive; the other elements are isotopes of normally stable atoms that have been made unstable (radioactive) in a nuclear reactor. All of these radioactive elements emit gamma rays that are capable of penetrating tissue and destroying cells. There is a variety of forms of radioactive materials for implantation; they may be implanted as needles, tubes, seeds, wires, or capsules.

RADIATION PROTECTION. Those who work with patients receiving radiation therapy must become familiar with the hazards of each type and source of radiation. Alpha and beta rays, being low in penetration, present primarily internal hazards when they are accidentally ingested, inhaled or otherwise taken into the body. Gamma rays and x-rays can readily penetrate the tissues of the body, so they present external hazards.

The effects of radiation may be divided into short-term and long-term effects. Short-term effects result from relatively large doses received for a short period of time and include localized skin burns, fever, hemorrhage due to destruction of bone marrow, diarrhea, fluid loss, and central nervous

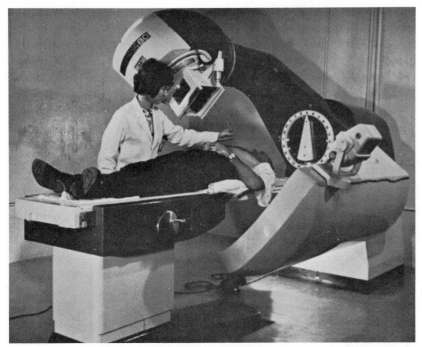

Figure 9-4. Patient treated with cobalt-60 teletherapy. (From Walker: *Nursing Clinics of North America*, March, 1967.)

system effects. The long-term effects may appear years after exposure and usually occur in individuals who have received small doses over a long period of time. These effects include shortening of the life span, predisposition toward leukemia and other malignancies, and development of cataracts; when the radiation is directed at the gonads, genetic mutations may arise.[5, 13]

When considering the hazards and effects of radiation one must avoid the extremes of complacency and total panic or paralyzing fright. After all, man has always been exposed to radiation in his environment. We are constantly being bombarded with cosmic rays from outer space and there are naturally occurring radioactive materials in the earth and therefore in the foods we eat and the water we drink. This does not mean we should be content with poor protection from radiation or complacent about the hazards when radiation is used therapeutically. Nurses simply must put these dangers

in their proper perspective. We know that oxygen supports combustion and creates a fire hazard when it is administered to a patient, but we take the necessary precautions during oxygen therapy so that the patient may enjoy its benefits.

In general, the amount of radiation a nurse might receive while caring for a patient being treated with radioactive elements depends on three factors: (1) the distance between the nurse and the patient, (2) the amount of time spent in actual proximity to the patient, and (3) the degree of shielding provided.[9]

Distance is an important factor in reducing exposure to radiation. By doubling one's distance from a radioactive element or x-ray beam the exposure is reduced by one fourth and tripling the distance reduces it by one ninth (see Fig. 9-5).[15]

Time spent near the source of radiation can be controlled by the nurse who plans her nursing care carefully so that she can spend less time with the patient

200 mr/hr   50 mr/hr   12.5 mr/hr

2'

4'

8'

Figure 9-5. The nurse nearest the source of radioactivity (the patient) is more exposed; at 2 feet, exposure is almost 15 times that at 8 feet. (From Boeker: American Journal of Nursing, April, 1965.)

without sacrificing the quality of care given. The occasions for application of this principle will most often be those in which the patient is hospitalized for implantation of a radioactive element.

Shielding from radiation exposure must take into account the type of rays being emitted. The more dense the shielding material, the less the possibility of penetration by the rays and the better the protection. A lead shield that is 1 cm. thick offers the same amount of protection as 5 cm. of concrete or 30 cm. of wood (see Fig. 9-6). Portable lead shields can be used to provide some protection for the nurse caring for a patient who is confined to bed for implantation therapy (see Fig. 9-7). Lead aprons give protection from diagnostic x-rays but do not provide adequate protection from the gamma rays emitted by radium, cesium-137 or cobalt-60.

If the nurse understands good isolation technique in the care of a patient with an infectious disease, she will have no difficulty in avoiding contamination from radioactive isotopes used therapeutically. Dressings, bed linens and other articles that may be contaminated by solutions containing radioisotopes or excreta from the patient's body are treated as radioactive waste and their disposal is carried out according to the policies of the institution in which the nurse is working. Since radioactive isotopes vary in their degree of penetration and the ways in which they can present internal and external hazards to nursing personnel, all persons concerned with the care of patients receiving radioisotopes as therapy should know exactly what precautions are necessary for each individual patient and how these precautions are to be carried out.

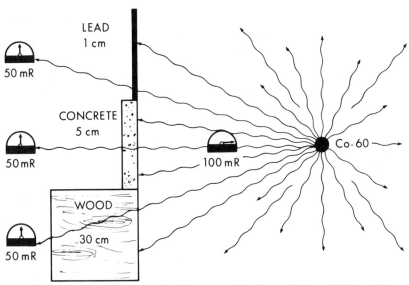

Figure 9-6. Comparison of efficacy of various materials for radiation shielding. (From Boeker: *Nursing Clinics of North America*, March, 1967.)

Figure 9-7. An improvised shield—lead drapes over a bedside table—will reduce personnel exposure. (From Boeker: American Journal of Nursing, April, 1965.)

RADIATION SICKNESS. Patients who have received large doses of therapeutic radiation sometimes suffer from a generalized systemic reaction known as radiation sickness. Symptoms of the reaction may vary from mild discomfort and malaise to severe nausea, vomiting and headache. Nursing measures that may help relieve these symptoms include providing adequate rest, encouraging the patient to eat small, nutritious and easily digested meals, and reassurance that such a reaction is temporary and will subside when the treatments have been completed. If the patient understands that such a reaction is a temporary discomfort similar in some ways to that experienced after surgery, he may accept the situation more readily and with less apprehension. Since most people associate radiation sickness or any other reaction to radiation with nuclear bombs and other destructive situations, the nurse must try to explain that radiation sickness is not unusual and will not permanently harm the patient.

Chemotherapy. Chemotherapy is the use of chemicals for the treatment of a disorder. Chemotherapy for treatment of cancer is comparatively new and has only recently come into use as an accepted measure. Some types of drugs may be used for local treatment of an accessible tumor, but most often anticancer drugs are utilized when the malignancy is not localized.

The drugs used in the treatment of cancer may be administered (1) directly into the tumor, (2) into the systemic circulation by the intravenous route, (3) orally, and (4) intra-arterially. These chemicals act in a number of ways. Some are cellular poisons (toxins), such as nitrogen mustard *(Mustargen)*, cyclophosphamide *(Cytoxan)* or chlorambucil *(Leukeran)*. Others interfere with the synthesis of essential cell components and stop the process of cellular growth and development by substituting false building blocks for the cells. These include methotrexate (5FU) and the fluoropyrimides (5FUDR). In some types of tumors that are "hormone-sensitive," hormone injections such as the male and female sex hormones and adrenal cortical hormones may be given in therapeutic doses. There are also some highly potent and toxic antibiotics such as actinomycin D and mitomycin C that show promise in the destruction of certain types of malignant cells.[6]

NURSING CARE OF THE CANCER PATIENT

Physical Aspects of Cancer Nursing. Malignant growths reproduce cells so rapidly they soon use up all available nutrition. As they continue to multiply, many of the cells cannot be supported by the body and they die, bringing about ulceration and necrosis of the cells within the growth. The area is then susceptible to hemorrhage and secondary infections. These characteristics are common to all types of cancerous growths and require continued and conscientious nursing care in order to ensure as much comfort for the patient as is possible under the circumstances.

Many of the discomforts, obnoxious "sores," and "odors," commonly believed to be a necessary part of cancer, can be eliminated by dedicated application of the basic principles of cleanliness and medical asepsis. Any ulcer, regardless of its cause, will exude unpleasant odors and drain purulent material, and make the patient very uncomfortable if he is not properly cared for. The basic treatment for elimination of these side effects of necrosis is regular and frequent irrigations. According to authorities, "The liberal use of wet dressings and irrigations is more important than what is put into the water." Thus we can see that continuous care and diligent cleansing of the area, with frequent changing ·of the dressings as needed, will greatly add to the comfort of the patient and make him feel more acceptable to others.

Hemorrhage does not occur very often, even in untreated cancer, unless the growth extends into the wall of a large blood vessel. Hemorrhage following surgery or radiotherapy is quite possible, however, and does occur occasionally. The symptoms and treatment for this type of hemorrhage are the same as for bleeding from other causes. The situation calls for close observation and prompt reporting of any signs that hemorrhage is occurring.

Emotional Aspects.   Regardless of the type of cancer involved or its location in the body, the patient suffering from this disease has some emotional problems that other patients do not have. There often is fear of incapacitating surgery and prolonged treatments, expensive hospitalization, and eventually a slow and painful death. The fact that none of these necessarily accompany cancer is not known to him and he is frequently depressed and despondent to the point of total despair. The practical nurse must be aware of these problems, and prepare herself for them so that she is able to offer comfort and moral support to the patient and the family without giving them false hopes. She must evaluate her own attitudes and feelings toward cancer, and continue to study and learn the new treatments which can offer cancer patients relief from symptoms and a longer life expectancy.

Any nurse who has close contact with a cancer patient must know whether or not the *patient knows* he has cancer. Some patients suspect that they have cancer but they do not want to be told, and the doctor will, of course, respect their wishes. In this case the nurse must also avoid a discussion of cancer in the presence of the patient and under no circumstances is she to take it upon herself to "set him straight" about his diagnosis. Other patients know that they have cancer but refuse even to discuss the disease or any aspect of the treatments necessary. These too must be treated according to their wishes. The fact that the patient cannot discuss his illness frankly and face it squarely should indicate to the nurse how very frightened the patient is and how much he will need her sympathy and understanding.

There are some deeply religious and well-adjusted individuals who can accept their illness and will strive to learn to live with it. Just because these patients are less demanding of the doctors' and nurses' time does not mean that they are less in need of reassurance and support than those who cannot, or will not, adjust to the emotional shock suffered when they learn they have cancer. *All* patients with such a serious illness need and deserve continued encouragement and help in solving their many problems.

The Surgical Patient.   The patient having surgery for the treatment of cancer is in many ways no different from a patient having surgery for any other reason. The preoperative and postoperative care of the patient having a gastrectomy requires certain procedures and nursing measures regardless of whether the operation is done to relieve the symptoms of a gastric ulcer or to remove a malignant growth. In addition to these basic principles of surgical nursing there are certain special aspects of nursing care which must be considered in the care of the cancer patient who has surgery.

Usually the preoperative preparation of the patient with cancer includes detailed instruction of the patient and planning for his rehabilitation after surgery. The type of extensive surgery demanded by cancerous growths frequently involves permanent alteration of some of the usual functions of the various organs of the body and requires full explanation of the type of prosthesis or appliance the patient must adjust to after surgery.

The patient who has his larynx removed must be prepared for the use of the laryngectomy tube. During the postoperative period he will receive special instructions in learning to talk without his larynx. This may be accomplished through "esophageal speech" or the patient may be fitted with an artificial larynx.

The patient who has a permanent colostomy, or the patient having a mastectomy, will also need preparation for his postoperative period and plans must be made for rehabilitation and his return to society.

In general, the postoperative period for a cancer patient is longer than is expected for other conditions of illness because of his need for adjustment to his physical limitations. The practical nurse is not expected to accept the responsibility of teaching the patient everything he will need to know in order to return to his former life. She will, however, need an understanding of the problems he is facing in his struggle for a normal life and she must assist him in any way she can through sympathetic understanding and encouragement.

Nursing Care of Patients Having X-ray Therapy. We know that use of x-rays for the destruction of malignant cells must necessarily be accompanied by some degree of damage to normal overlying tissues. It is, therefore, extremely unwise for the nurse to use the terms "x-ray burn" or "radiation burn" when speaking of reactions to radiation of the area involved. These terms imply a careless overdose or an amateurish handling of the case. In addition to the local reaction from radiotherapy there is also usually a general feeling of malaise, nausea, and loss of appetite (see Radiation Sickness above). These side effects from the use of x-ray are only temporary and much of the patient's discomfort can be relieved by good basic nursing care.

The following outline is included in order to help the practical nurse understand the need for special care of patients receiving x-ray therapy. Most hospitals have their own procedures written specifically for the care of such patients and these must be followed very carefully.

1. Preparation of the skin before the series of treatments is begun includes thorough washing of the area with soap and water to remove any ointments or dressings. This is followed by an alcohol rub.

2. The "ports" or areas of entry for the roentgen rays, are marked on the skin by the radiologist, and care must be taken that these marks are not washed off once the treatments are begun.

3. During the course of treatments these "ports" are not washed nor rubbed with alcohol. Any pressure or friction of the skin will increase the irritation. Thus the patient is instructed not to lie on the area and his clothing should be loose. The skin of these "ports" is very fragile and will break easily. Dusting with starch instead of powder will help relieve the itching.

4. If the skin becomes very irritated and dry before the treatments are completed, permission may be obtained from the physician to apply lanolin or petroleum jelly to the area. It is important that no other powders or ointments containing metals, such as zinc, be used because these absorb the rays and increase the damage to the skin.

5. Should blistering become severe during the treatments, the application of any dressing or medication must be done only on the order of the physician.

6. The internal mucosa reacts in much the same way as the skin when exposed to radiation. The treatments used consist of hourly irrigations of the mouth and gargles with a saline-bicarbonate solution when this is the area affected. It is helpful if the irrigations are followed with mineral oil as a mouth rinse to relieve drying and cracking of the mucosa.

7. The diet in such cases is usually a high-caloric liquid diet. If swallowing is impossible, the diet may be administered by gavage.

the only all-new nursing encyclopedia in 20 years –

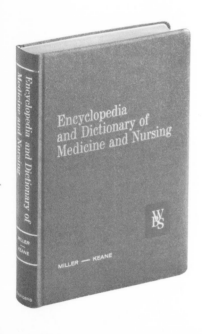

Convenient Definitions and tables are where you would naturally look for them — not where some arbitrary rule dictates.

Authoritative Written by highly qualified authors, experienced in both teaching and writing.

Up to date Completed in 1972. Every word newly chosen; every fact newly checked.

Colorful Sixteen pages of illustrations in brilliant full color.

Broad Includes latest research findings in chemistry, physics, and biochemistry as well as the newest diagnostic and therapeutic procedures.

Helpful Full pronunciation for most entries. Extensive cross references. Tables placed in their alphabetical positions, where you can find them easily.

Nursing Care of Patients Receiving Interstitial Therapy. The practical nurse who is in any way concerned with the care of the patient who has had radium or radioactive cobalt substances injected into a malignant growth must first familiarize herself thoroughly with the special precautions and policies of the institution in which she is working. Aside from the fact that radium is very expensive, it must be remembered that radioactive substances are also potentially dangerous to the patient and to those who come in direct contact with the patient. The radiologist usually assumes the responsibility for insertion, removal and storage of these substances. These materials must never be touched with the bare hands.

A few of the precautions used in the care of these patients are listed below. It cannot be emphasized too strongly that extreme care and strict observance of the rules of the hospital in regard to these patients must be scrupulously followed.

1. All linens, dressings, bedpans, or emesis basins are routinely checked before they are taken from the patient's room to see if the radium containers have been accidentally lost from the tissues.

2. Most of these patients are placed on bed rest and instructed to remain in certain positions so that emanations from radium will reach the desired area.

3. The patients are usually allowed no visitors. If visits are allowed they should be limited to five minutes.

4. The nurses caring for the patient should not remain in the patient's room any longer than necessary at one time.

Care of the Patient with Terminal Cancer. In the treatment of a patient in the last stages of cancer good nursing is of primary importance. The doctor's orders are usually limited to medications for the control of pain and the main burden of care rests on the shoulders of the nurse. It is difficult to state exactly what specific procedures are required for these patients because each patient will react in a different way to his illness. Generally it can be said that the primary concern of the nurse is the physical comfort and emotional support of the patient when the diagnosis is terminal cancer.

Rest and conservation of the strength of the patient must be regulated according to the wishes of the patient. He should be encouraged to be as active as his condition will allow and to participate in recreational activities as much as possible.

Adequate nutrition may be extremely difficult if the upper digestive tract is

Figure 9-8. Lead container (pig), radium needles, forceps, and caution sign, for use with radium therapy. (From Boeker: *Nursing Clinics of North America*, March, 1967.)

affected, and in some cases tube feedings may be necessary. Loss of appetite is aggravated by unpleasant odors or "bad taste" in the patient's mouth. Good oral hygiene and frequent mouthwashes with a mild, pleasant-tasting, antiseptic solution can eliminate this difficulty. Small feedings, properly spaced and attractively served, can provide adequate nutrition and are more likely to be accepted by the patient than large meals prepared without consideration of the patient's preference and tastes.

The *skin* must receive extra care because there is always danger of secondary infection and impaired healing in the cancer patient. Massage with lotions containing lanolin and frequent turning of the patient help to prevent pressure sores as well as adding to the general comfort of the patient.

The *control of pain* is one factor which concerns many lay people when they think of cancer. As stated before, uncontrollable pain does not necessarily accompany cancer and is, in fact, very unusual. It is best for the nurse to try simple comfort measures and mild sedatives rather than to administer large doses of drugs which can have undesirable side effects. The heavily sedated patient is likely to have little appetite and is inclined to develop incontinence and hypostatic pneumonia. If powerful drugs are administered early in the disease they may lose their effectiveness by the time they are needed.

The nurse must bear in mind that the patient and his family will face many problems as they adjust to the fact that death is approaching. She must remain sympathetic and understanding even though their demands on her time and energy may sometimes seem unreasonable.

Because the patient with terminal cancer often presents such a hopeless picture, one who nurses these patients must find deep within herself a personal philosophy and attitude that can serve as a source of strength for herself and her patients. Dr. Cecily Saunders in an article printed in the American Journal of Nursing has written:

"It seems to me that the way to find a philosophy that gives confidence and permits a positive approach to death and dying is to look continually at the patients, not at their need but at their courage, not at their dependence but at their dignity. Doctors and nurses who have fought hard to save life or relieve dying rightly comfort themselves with the knowledge that they have done all they could. But those who realize how well the patient himself played his part can find consolation for loss and courage to face the future."[14]

CLINICAL CASE PROBLEMS

1. An aquaintance tells you that she has had a mole on her back for several years and it appears to be getting larger and darker. She admits that it could be malignant, but she argues that there is no point in going to a physician because there is nothing to be done for cancer and she does not want to burden her family with doctor bills and hospital bills which will not accomplish anything.

> What is your obligation as a practical nurse in regard to encouraging this person to see a physician at once? What is your own attitude toward cancer and the treatment of the disease?

2. Mrs. Allgood went to her physician for a regular physical checkup and was found to have malignant cells in the cervical secretions obtained for a Papanicolaou smear. She was admitted to the hospital for a biopsy of the cervix and this too proved to contain malignant cells. Radium was implanted in the cervix and Mrs. Allgood was kept isolated during the treatment.

> If you were assigned to give A.M. care to this patient, what special precautions should you take? What special observations should you make?

3. You have been assigned to the care of Mr. Long, a 50-year-old man with terminal cancer of the throat. The treatment is chiefly symptomatic because the disease

was in the advanced stage before Mr. Long sought medical advice. The lesions of the throat and mouth are necrotic and draining. Mr. Long refuses foods by mouth and must be tube-fed.

What nursing measures can be used to eliminate some of Mr. Long's symptoms?

Why do you think Mr. Long waited so long to seek medical advice even though he suspected that he had cancer for some time?

REFERENCES

1. American Cancer Society: *A Cancer Source Book for Nurses.* New York, 1957.
2. American Cancer Society: *A Cancer Guide for Practical Nurses.* New York, 1961.
3. Barnett, M.: "The Nature of Radiation and Its Effect on Man." *Nursing Clinics of North America,* vol. 2, no. 1. Philadelphia, W. B. Saunders Co., March, 1967.
4. Boeker, E. H.: "Radiation Safety." Am. Journ. Nurs., April, 1965, p. 111.
5. Ferguson, L. K., and Sholtis, L. A.: *Eliason's Surgical Nursing,* 11th edition. Philadelphia, J. B. Lippincott Co., 1961.
6. Fox, S. A., and Bernhardt, L.: "Chemotherapy Via Intra-arterial Infusion." Am. Journ. Nurs., Sept., 1966, p. 1966.
7. Golby, R. B.: "Chemotherapy of Cancer." Am. Journ. Nurs., April, 1960, p. 521.
8. Hilkemeyer, R.: "Nursing Care in Radium Therapy." *Nursing Clinics of North America,* vol. 2, no. 1. Philadelphia, W. B. Saunders Co., March, 1967.
9. Horgan, P. D.: "What You Need to Know about Radium." RN, Nov., 1962, p. 61.
10. Kendall, E. B.: "Care of Patients Treated with Sealed Sources of Radioisotopes." *Nursing Clinics of North America,* vol. 2, no. 1. Philadelphia, W. B. Saunders Co., March, 1967.
11. Moore, G. C.: "Cancer 100 Different Diseases." Am. Journ. Nurs., April, 1966, p. 749.
12. Nowalk, P. A.: "Inservice Education in Radiation Health." *Nursing Clinics of North America,* vol. 2, no. 1. Philadelphia, W. B. Saunders Co., March, 1967.
13. Rodman, M. J.: "Radioactive Drugs." RN, Oct., 1959, p. 63.
14. Saunders, C.: "The Last Stages of Life." Am. Journ. Nurs., March, 1965, p. 70.
15. Sellers, J. H.: "Special Nursing Care of Patients Receiving Liquid Radioisotopes." *Nursing Clinics of North America,* vol. 2, no. 1. Philadelphia, W. B. Saunders Co., March, 1967.
16. Shafer, K. N., Sawyer, J. R., et al.: *Medical-Surgical Nursing,* 3rd edition. St. Louis, Mo., C. V. Mosby Co., 1966.
17. Thomas, D. A.: "The Nurse's Contribution in a Radiation Therapy Outpatient Department." *Nursing Clinics of North America,* vol. 2, no. 1. Philadelphia, W. B. Saunders Co., March, 1967.
18. Walker, E.: "Responsibilities of the Hospital Nurse in the Clinical Use of Radiation." *Nursing Clinics of North America,* vol. 2, no. 1. Philadelphia, W. B. Saunders Co., March, 1967.
19. Welsh, M. S.: "Comfort Measures During Radiation Therapy." Am. Journ. Nurs., Sept., 1967, p. 1880.

SUGGESTED STUDENT READING

1. American Cancer Society: *A Cancer Guide for Practical Nurses.* New York, 1961.
2. Fox, J. E.: "Reflections on Cancer Nursing." Am. Journ. Nurs., June, 1966, p. 1317.
3. Horgan, P. D.: "What You Need to Know about Radium." RN, Nov., 1962, p. 61.
4. Kautz, H. D., et al.: "Radioactive Drugs." Am. Journ. Nurs., Jan., 1964, p. 124.
5. Korsos, R. C.: "Nursing Care of the Patient with Radiation Sickness." Journ. Pract. Nurs., Oct., 1964, p. 24.
6. Saunders, C.: "The Last Stages of Life." Am. Journ. Nurs., March, 1965, p. 70.

OUTLINE FOR CHAPTER 9

I. Introduction

A. Improved diagnostic techniques have found more cases of cancer; it is not a new disease.

B. A cancer patient is considered cured if there is no evidence of the disease at least five years after diagnosis and completion of treatment.

C. Metastasis (spreading of malignant cells to other parts of the body) occurs:
   1. By direct extension.
   2. By growing along lymphatic vessels.
   3. By embolism through lymphatic system.
   4. By embolism through blood vessels.
   5. By invasion of the fluid within a body cavity.

II. Causes of Cancer

A. Predisposing causes include chronic irritation, prolonged exposure to irritating substances, and precancerous benign tumors. Others are race, sex, age and an inherited tendency toward the disease.

B. Specific causes not yet determined. Viruses are considered important in the development of certain cancers.

III. Symptoms

A. Capable of producing a great variety of symptoms.
  B. Seven danger signals:
   1. Any sore that does not heal.
   2. A lump or thickening in the breast or elsewhere.
   3. Unusual bleeding or discharge.
   4. Any change in a wart or mole.
   5. Persistent indigestion or difficulty in swallowing.
   6. Any change in normal bowel habits.
   7. Persistent hoarseness or coughing.

IV. Diagnosis of Cancer

A. Physical examination.
  B. Biopsy—removal of a sampling of cells for microscopic study.
  C. Papanicolaou smear—a technique for collecting samples of body secretions or fluids and examining them for malignant cells.

V. Treatment of Cancer

A. Surgical excision of malignant growth and adjacent tissue.
  B. Radiation therapy—use of radiation to penetrate and destroy malignant tissue.
   1. Methods of radiation therapy.
     a. X-ray therapy: the x-ray beam is aimed directly at the tumor in a series of treatments.
     b. Teletherapy: a radioactive element is housed in a shielded unit that is located at a distance from the patient.
     c. Interstitial therapy: placement of a radioactive substance directly into the tissues of a malignant growth.
   2. Radiation protection.
     a. Short-term effects of radiation exposure include localized skin burns, fever, hemorrhage due to destruction of bone marrow, diarrhea and central nervous system disorders.
     b. Long-term effects (appear years after exposure) include shortening of the life span, predisposition to leukemia and other malignancies and development of cataracts. When the radiation is directed at the gonads, genetic mutations may arise.

   c. Amount of radiation that a nurse might receive will depend on (1) distance between nurse and patient, (2) amount of time spent in actual proximity to the patient, and (3) degree of shielding provided.
   3. Radiation sickness—a generalized systemic reaction to radiation.
     a. Symptoms are temporary and may vary from mild discomfort and malaise to severe nausea, vomiting and headache.
     b. Nursing measures include providing adequate rest, encouraging small, frequent feedings rather than large meals, and reassurance that the condition is temporary.
  C. Chemotherapy—use of drugs for the treatment of cancer.
   1. May be administered (a) directly into the tumor, (b) into the systemic circulation by intravenous route, (c) orally, and (d) intra-arterially.
   2. Some are cellular poisons, others interfere with the synthesis of essential cell components and stop the process of cellular growth. For tumors that are "hormone-sensitive" the hormones may be given.

VI. Nursing Care

A. Frequent irrigations can relieve unpleasant odors from discharges that are present in some forms of cancer. Frequent changing of dressings may be necessary. Patient should be observed for signs of hemorrhage.
  B. Emotional aspects of malignancy should be considered and the patient's wishes in regard to discussing his condition accepted.
  C. Surgical patient will require general nursing care as for any surgical patient and often needs rehabilitation.
  D. Patient having x-ray therapy will require special attention to skin and mucous membranes to avoid a breakdown and introduction of infection.
   1. Do not wash off markings made for identifying "port of entry" for x-rays.
   2. Never use powders or ointments containing zinc or other metals and always have written orders for lotions, alcohol, or other medications used on the patient's skin.
   3. Instruct patient not to lie on inflamed area.

4. A high-caloric liquid diet may be necessary if patient has irritated lips and mouth.

E. Patients with implants of a radioactive element can serve as sources of radiation to those in close contact with them. Nurse must know and strictly adhere to rules and regulations of the hospital or clinic in regard to care of these patients.

VII. Terminal Cancer

A. Care of the patient involves attention to the emotional aspects of the disease and requires maturity and mental stability on the part of the nurse.

B. Physical aspects include adequate rest and conservation of the patient's strength, adequate nutrition, good skin care, and control of pain.

Chapter 10

NURSING CARE OF PATIENTS WITH DISORDERS OF THE SKIN

VOCABULARY

Debilitated
Eschar
Exudate
Necrotic
Nodular
Transmitted

INTRODUCTION

The skin that covers our bodies is actually an organ, and like the liver or heart it is one of the most essential for the maintenance of life and good health. The skin functions very much like a built-in suit of armor and is our first line of defense against invasion by the hordes of pathogenic bacteria living in our environment. The skin also protects us against loss of body heat by acting as a layer of insulation against changes in the temperature of our environment, and as a cooling system that reduces the body temperature through the process of evaporation of moisture from the skin's surface. In addition, the skin functions as a container for body fluids and helps in the disposal of some of the body's waste products.

When an area of the skin is destroyed by disease or trauma, its protective functions are immediately impaired and the body is susceptible to infection. If very large areas of skin are

158

destroyed, as in an extensive burn, there is a disturbance in the water and electrolyte balance and loss of body heat.

DIAGNOSTIC TESTS AND EXAMINATIONS

Visual Examination. The physician must make his initial diagnosis of a skin disease by visual examination of the skin. This is not quite as easy as it would seem and requires much experience and training because there is such a wide variety of skin diseases and types of lesions. In addition to examining the lesions under a strong light, the physician also palpates the lesions to determine whether they are raised or nodular. He must also determine the subjective symptoms the patient has experienced, such as pain, itching (pruritus), burning, or loss of sensitivity to heat and cold.

The diagnosis may be even more difficult if the patient has tried to treat himself with patent medicines or home-made remedies before finally consulting a doctor. These treatments may completely change the appearance of the skin lesions. Many chronic diseases of the skin could have been prevented if only the individual had sought the aid of a physician when the skin lesions first appeared.

Nurses are often asked by friends and neighbors to diagnose skin conditions and are expected to suggest some simple remedy. This is a very dangerous situation and one best handled by advising the inquirer to see his doctor at once. The list of skin lesions presented in Table 10 is given as a guide to nurses who may be expected to observe and accurately report skin lesions to the physician in charge.

History. In the diagnosis of allergic skin diseases, contact dermatitis, or infectious diseases of the skin the history of the patient is of great importance to the physician making the diagnosis. He will need to know when the individual first noticed a change in the skin, where the lesions first appeared on the body, and whether or not the patient has ever had these lesions before. If the lesions have occurred in the past the doctor will want to know under what conditions the lesions appeared. An example is the development of a rash every time a certain soap is used, or perhaps there may be a relationship between certain foods eaten and the appearance of skin lesions. The cooperation of the patient and his family are very important in the type of detective work necessary for the correct diagnosis of many skin diseases.

Skin Tests. There are two methods of testing for individual sensitivity to specific substances. The skin may be scratched slightly so that no blood appears and a sampling of pollen, food, or bacterial proteins is applied to the scratch. In the other method, the sam-

Table 10. *Classification of Skin Lesions*

NAME OF LESION	EXAMPLE	DESCRIPTION
Macule	Freckle, purpura	A discolored spot or patch on the skin. Usually is not elevated or depressed and cannot be felt.
Papule	Present in measles	A solid elevation of skin. May vary from size of a pinhead to that of a pea. Usually red, resembling small pimples without pus.
Pustule	Acne, smallpox	A small elevation of the skin or pimple filled with pus.
Vesicle	Blister	A small sac containing serous fluid.
Bleb	Common in pemphigus	A large elevation of the skin filled with fluid.
Excoriation	Friction burn, chemical burn	An injury caused by scraping or rubbing away a portion of the skin.
Wheal	Insect sting, hives, nettle rash	An area of local swelling usually accompanied by itching.

Figure 10-1. Positive skin tests. Positive reactions are characterized by a wheal surrounded by erythema. The severity of the reaction frequently is described as ranging from 1+ to 4+.

pling is injected just below the first layer of skin. In a positive reaction a small, dime-sized wheal appears at the site of contact with the sampling. This would indicate that the specific substance used in the test may be causing the disease. To prove the skin test further, the patient may be exposed to large amounts of the substance suspected and then watched carefully for the development of the skin disease.

Elimination Diets. This type of test involves simply eliminating from the diet certain substances suspected of causing the skin disease. It is essential that the patient cooperate fully with the doctor in this test, making sure that he has completely removed the substance from his diet.

Cultures and Sensitivity Tests. In the case of infectious diseases, especially boils and carbuncles, the physician may need to know the causative organism. A sampling of exudate is taken directly from the lesion and sent to the laboratory for culture. Once the organism has been isolated and identified it may then be tested for sensitivity to certain antibiotic drugs. These tests take the guesswork out of treating the skin disease and very quickly establish the antibiotic which will most effectively destroy the organism causing the trouble.

PREVENTION OF SKIN DISEASE

Cleanliness. The ritual of the daily bath is almost an obsession with the average American, and nurses are perhaps guiltier than most in their insistence on good, strong soap and plenty of hot water. No one will quarrel with the value of cleanliness, but it can be overdone and the method of cleansing the skin deserves some thought and consideration.

First, we must recognize that there are various skin types. Some individuals have very delicate skin which requires special care to prevent drying and irritation. These are usually blondes and redheads. On the other hand brunettes usually have skin that is considerably more oily and less susceptible to excessive drying and irritation.

If the skin appears dry and scaly, frequent bathing with strong soaps and water will only aggravate the condition. There are several oils and creams available which will cleanse the skin quite effectively and help replace the natural oils at the same time. The individual with oily skin will need to clean the skin frequently, using a liberal amount of soap and water and avoiding the application of additional oils to the skin.

Diet. Adequate intake of vitamins and minerals is essential to the maintenance of healthy skin. Even border-line deficiencies in these nutritious elements will cause the skin to take on a sallow and dull appearance. Severe deficiencies lead to a breakdown of the skin and the development of sores and ulcers. Many teen-agers who are so concerned with their physical appearance that they refuse to eat properly for fear of gaining weight fail to realize that they are robbing themselves of one of the sources of real beauty; that is, a healthy and radiant complexion.

Age. Young people are not the only ones who should be concerned with the care of their skin, however. As we grow older our skin undergoes certain changes which easily lead to irritation and breakdown of the skin if proper

Figure 10-2. Irritants that cause or complicate dermatitis. (From Goldman: American Journal of Nursing, March, 1964.)

care is not given. The oil and sweat glands become less active as age advances and the skin has a tendency to become dry and scaly. It also loses some of its tone, making it less elastic and more fragile. Frequent cleansing of the skin becomes unnecessary as the skin ages, and alcohol and other drying agents must be used sparingly if at all. As we grow older we should establish a regular routine of massaging oils, creams, or oily lotions into the skin, if not for the sake of vanity, at least for the sake of preserving a very important organ of our bodies.

Environment. There are several factors in the environment of an individual which may have a direct effect on the health of the skin. These include prolonged exposure to chemicals, excessive drying of the skin from repeated immersions in water or contact with soap, and excessive burning of the skin by strong sunlight. Some of these factors are occupational hazards and may necessitate changing jobs to eliminate the causative factor (see Fig. 10-2).

The current fad of acquiring a "tan" by deliberately exposing the skin to strong sunlight for long periods of time is foolish when carried to extremes because it does lead to excessive drying of the skin if not actually burning it. The parts of the body exposed become wrinkled and age much more rapidly than those parts which are shielded from the sun. We must also remember that the incidence of skin cancer is highest among those who must work out in the sun (for example, farmers), and is usually located on the neck and face where exposure is greatest.

GENERAL NURSING CARE

The word "dermatology" refers to the specialized study of diseases of the skin. A *dermatologist* is one who specializes in the treatment of disorders of the skin. Many dermatologists have some standing orders or written instructions they wish followed in the care of their patients who have been admitted to the hospital. If there are no specific instructions to follow, however, the nurse must use caution until she determines the wishes of the physician. Some general rules in the care of the patient with skin disease may be helpful as a guide until specific orders are obtained. These are as follows:

1. Bathing with soap and water is usually contraindicated in all inflammatory conditions of the skin.

2. Dressing covering the lesions should not be removed when the patient is admitted unless there are specific orders to do so.

3. Do not attempt to remove scales, crusts, or other exudates on the skin lesions until the physician has had an opportunity to examine the patient.

4. Observe the skin very carefully at the time of the patient's admission and record your observations on the chart or report them to the nurse in charge.

5. Avoid excessive handling or rubbing of the skin against the sheets and bedclothes when changing the bed.

6. Lotions and alcohol generally used in the hospital for back rubs, etc., are never applied to the skin of these patients without permission from the dermatologists.

7. If you are not sure about any part of the nursing care considered to be routine for all patients, ask before you act.

Once the physician has determined the type of lesions present, he will order specific treatments to relieve the patient's symptoms and promote healing. The two most commonly used treatments are special colloid baths and wet compresses or dressings. In addition there may be lotions, salves, or ointments to be applied locally at frequent intervals.

Colloid Baths. These are special baths prepared by adding soothing agents to the bath water. These may include starch, oatmeal or other cereals, and sodium bicarbonate. The substances to be added will depend on the type of skin disease to be treated. For procedures in the preparation of a colloid bath the reader is referred to a textbook in basic nursing.

During the bath the patient must be protected from chilling because the bath usually lasts from 30 minutes to an hour and also because most patients with skin diseases have less resistance to cold. When the patient is removed from the tub the skin is dried by patting rather than by rubbing. If medication it to be applied locally it should be put on as soon as the bath is completed so as to keep pruritus at a minimum.

The medicated bath has a very soothing and relaxing effect on the patient and also helps relieve the itching and burning so commonly associated with skin diseases. The nurse should encourage her patient to rest in bed and perhaps take a short nap after each bath.

The bed linens and gowns used for patients with severe skin diseases may need special laundering to eliminate all traces of soap. In the hospital this requires specific instructions to the personnel in the laundry and careful labeling of the linen to be used for the patient. If the patient is to be cared for in the home, vinegar may be added to the rinse water to neutralize the soap. The proportions used are one tablespoon of vinegar to each quart of water.

Wet Compresses or Dressings. There are various ways in which wet dressings may be applied to the skin but the two general types are *open dressings* and *closed dressings.* In the open type the compresses must be changed constantly and are never allowed to dry. These are used in certain diseases in which the dermatologist wishes to have air circulating to the skin lesions. In

Figure 10-3.   Plastic "mitt" and "sock," which may be used to hold "closed" wet dressings in place and maintain adequate degree of moisture to dressings. These may be improvised from plastic bags or the plastic wrapping available in most stores. (From Stryker and Grindon: J.A.M.A., July 13, 1940.)

the closed type the dressings are thoroughly soaked with the prescribed solution and then wrapped in an air-tight, waterproof material (see Fig. 10-3). It is recommended that the nurse obtain specific instructions from the dermatologist before applying wet dressings to any lesions of the skin.

HERPES SIMPLEX

Definition. Herpes simplex is the medical term used for fever blisters or cold sores. These lesions are caused by a virus and may occur alone or with other systemic diseases such as pneumonia, influenza, and meningitis.

Symptoms. The vesicles of herpes simplex are found on the lips and inside the mouth. Sometimes the lesions may be found on the genitalia. Usually the lesions themselves are not considered to be serious, even though they may cause some discomfort and slight disfigurement.

Treatment. The symptoms of burning and itching which accompany herpes simplex may be relieved by the application of warm compresses to the sores, followed by the local application of tincture of benzoin or spirits of camphor to aid in drying and healing the lesions. Antiseptic mouthwashes have been used with success in treating some mild cases.

For persistent cases in which there is frequent recurrence of the lesions, herpes simplex may be treated with smallpox vaccinations. This treatment is based on the fact that the virus that causes smallpox has some relationship to the one causing herpes simplex.

Some authorities feel that there may be some connection between certain foods eaten and the development of the lesions. Large amounts of orange juice or chocolate have been known to cause the development of these lesions on the lips and mouth.

HERPES ZOSTER

Definition. Another name for herpes zoster is shingles, probably because the scaly appearance of the skin does bear some resemblance to the material used to cover roofs. Herpes zoster is a viral disease of the skin and the peripheral sensory nerves that lie just below the surface of the skin.

Shingles is caused by a virus similar to the one that causes chickenpox and is usually found in older persons who had chickenpox in their childhood.

Symptoms. Herpes zoster begins with vague symptoms of chills and low-grade fever, and possibly a gastrointestinal disturbance. About 3 to 5 days later small groups of vesicles appear on the skin in the area of the spinal cord. The vesicles increase in number and spread around the trunk of the body, following the nerve pathways that lead from the spinal cord to the skin. The skin lesions change from small blisters to a scaly appearance and there is pain and itching in the area. The skin lesions usually occur only on one side of the body; rarely is there involvement of both sides, and there is no foundation for the superstitious belief that the patient will die if the shingles "meet" as they progress around the body.

Pain is an outstanding symptom of shingles and may be quite severe, persisting for several days after the skin lesions are completely healed.

Treatment and Nursing Care. There is no specific treatment to cure herpes zoster and the condition may continue for several months, especially in older and debilitated patients. One attack usually confers immunity.

The symptoms may be relieved by medication to reduce pain and antibiotic drugs to prevent bacterial infection of the skin lesions. If pain is severe and difficult to control with drugs, deep x-ray therapy may be of some benefit.

Fortunately, even though herpes zoster may seem to be very difficult to cope with while it is running its course, there are rarely any serious complications from the disease. In the rare cases that are very severe the patient may suffer from extreme exhaustion and death can occur as a result.

IMPETIGO CONTAGIOSA

Definition. Impetigo contagiosa is, as its name implies, a highly contagious disease of the skin. It is a very common skin disease occurring most often in infants and small children and may rapidly spread through an entire nursery or family. It is caused by a form of staphylococcus or streptococcus.

Symptoms. The disease begins with small vesicles which rupture and exude a pustular, honey-colored material that dries and forms a crust over the lesion. Impetigo is often mistaken for ringworm because of the round patches it forms (see Fig. 10-4).

The itching that accompanies impetigo brings about scratching and contamination of the hands with the exudate from the lesions. The exudate is a source of infection and thus the disease is spread to other parts of the body or to other persons.

Treatment and Nursing Care. Because the exudate is a source of infection, the crusts should be removed daily and the lesions thoroughly cleansed. An antibiotic ointment may be applied locally on the lesions several times a day; however, antibiotics by mouth are more effective. The patient or his family, in the case of small children, must be cautioned against spreading the disease by careless use of equipment used to cleanse the sores or failure to wash the hands thoroughly after each treatment.

CONTACT DERMATITIS (ALLERGIC ECZEMA)

Definition. Dermatitis is an inflammation of the skin. A contact dermatitis is an inflammation of the skin resulting from exposure to, or contact with, some substance in the individual's environment. The substance may be animal, mineral or vegetable in origin and must be a substance to which the individual has developed a

Figure 10-4. Impetigo contagiosa. Circular lesions are covered with dried crusts. Other lesions in early stages at hairline show blisters before they have ruptured. (From Top: *Communicable and Infectious Diseases,* 4th Ed., C. V. Mosby Co., St. Louis.)

sensitivity. In other words, contact dermatitis is an allergic reaction (see Fig. 10-5).

The word "eczema" is generally used to describe an external reaction to an allergen and is most often found in children who will eventually outgrow the eczema only to develop hay fever or asthma.

Symptoms. The inflammation of the skin usually begins with patches of redness on the skin followed by the formation of small vesicles which rupture and become scaly. Pruritus is very common in contact dermatitis.

Examples of contact dermatitis are reactions to poison ivy, poison oak or sumac, cosmetics, or drugs.

Treatment and Nursing Care. The basis of treatment is the determination of the specific allergens causing the dermatitis and removal of the offending substance from the patient's environment. In persistent cases the doctor may "desensitize" the individual by exposing him to small amounts of the substance until he has built up an immunity.

The symptoms may be relieved by colloid baths to soothe the inflamed skin and lotions to reduce the occurrence of scaling and peeling. Antihistamines may be given to help control the itching.

Emotional factors play an important role in the development of skin disorders, especially those related to the allergies. The patient's anxiety and restlessness, aggravated by itching and the constant sight of his physical condition, make this type of illness a challenge to the nursing staff. There is a need for sustained reassurance of the patient and extreme patience and perseverance in carrying out the long list of treatments and nursing care necessary every hour or so.

ACNE

Definition. Acne is a disorder of the skin characterized by eruption of papules and pustules over the face, back and shoulders at puberty (see Fig. 10-6). There are two kinds of acne: *acne vulgaris* and *acne rosacea.* Of the two,

Figure 10-5. Dermatitis caused by allergy to the dye in a hat band. (Courtesy of Medichrome–Clay-Adams, Inc., New York.)

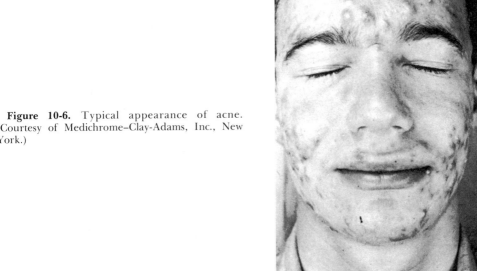

Figure 10-6. Typical appearance of acne. (Courtesy of Medichrome–Clay-Adams, Inc., New York.)

acne vulgaris is probably the most common and it has been estimated that nine out of ten adolescents have this skin disease to some degree.

Acne rosacea usually affects persons over 25 years of age and may be more difficult to contend with because there is often some deep seated emotional problem associated with the disease and there is also little possibility of the patient's outgrowing the disease. The term "rosacea" is used to designate this type of acne because the skin around the pustules is very red.

Symptoms. The symptoms of acne vulgaris are familiar to most of us. We have observed the large blackheads (*comedones*), raised pustules, and eventual pitted scarring that so frequently signals the onset of puberty and the beginning stages of adulthood. The relationship between the development of the disease and the adolescent phase is a result of the increase in hormonal activity which occurs at this time of life. The hormones apparently have some effect on the pores of the skin,

blocking the flow of secretions through the pores and setting the stage for the formation of blackheads. The blackheads become infected with bacteria and thus lead to the development of pustules on the skin. It is believed that the hormonal activity varies among individuals and this accounts for the fact that some persons are more likely to develop acne than others.

Treatment and Nursing Care. There is no specific treatment that will guarantee a cure for acne. Each patient must be treated on an individual basis because each case will react differently to certain medications or treatments. It is very important to instruct the patient about the nature of acne and the need for faithful adherence to the prescribed treatment. He should understand that treatment not only controls unsightly blemishes while the disease is active but also prevents permanent pitting and scarring of the skin.

An adequate diet with well-balanced meals has been shown to be very important in the management of acne, and while it does not guarantee absolute prevention of the development of the skin lesions, it does have some effect on the severity of the disease.

Cleanliness also plays an important role in controlling acne; however, there is no basis for the belief that acne is actually caused by improper cleansing of the skin. The purpose of frequent washing of the face and hands is to remove accumulated secretions and prevent secondary infection from bacteria that collect on the skin. The soap used should be a mild face soap and the method of cleansing restricted to gentle application. "Scrubbing" the skin must be avoided because it frequently damages the skin and causes greater irritation and inflammation. The hands are carriers of bacteria and not only must they be kept scrupulously clean, but the patient must be instructed to keep his hands away from his face.

The pricking and squeezing of pustules seems to be a common temptation for the patient with acne and he must be warned of the danger involved in such practices. There is serious danger of spreading the infection on the face and even getting the bacteria into the blood stream. It is also likely that squeezing and pressing the skin cause more scarring than necessary because the underlying tissues are damaged.

Blackheads that are not infected may be removed if they are soaked with hot compresses for 15 minutes and then removed with a specially designed instrument. The dermatologist usually wishes to instruct the patient thoroughly before allowing him to remove his own blackheads.

It is unfortunate that acne occurs during adolescence because the patient is already undergoing some emotional strain during this period of adjustment without the added burden of a disfiguring skin disease. The nurse and the family of the patient must do all they can to offer moral support and understanding to the young person with acne.

PSORIASIS

Definition. Psoriasis is a chronic and recurring skin disorder that is characterized by papules covered with adherent silvery scales that produce pinpoint bleeding when they are removed. Its exact cause is unknown but it is a relatively common condition. For some unknown reason it tends to subside and then flare up again. In some cases the skin eruptions are accompanied by rheumatoid arthritis in the fingers and toes (see Fig. 10-7).

Treatment. Treatment may be both topical and systemic depending on the severity of the symptoms. There is no known cure for psoriasis. However, by using the old reliable remedies such as mercury and coal tar ointments and the newer drugs such as the corticosteroids the condition can be kept under control.

FUNGAL INFECTIONS

Introduction. Fungal infections of the skin are called *mycoses*; systemic fungal infections of the lungs and other internal organs are systemic mycoses. Relatively few fungi are pathogenic to man, and such infections are rarely fatal if they involve the superficial tissues; nevertheless, mycotic infections are exasperating because they progress slowly, are difficult to diagnose and are often resistant to treatment.

The most common types of fungal infections involving the skin are *epidermophytosis* (athlete's foot or dermatophytosis), *tinea of the scalp* (commonly known as ringworm) and *tinea barbae* (barber's itch). *Moniliasis* (thrush) is a fungal infection that can attack the mucous membranes of the mouth, rectum and vagina. All surface fungal infections produce itching, some swelling and a breakdown of tissue. Since fungi thrive in warm, moist places, a tropical climate or other environmental factors that produce prolonged heat

Figure 10-7. *A*, Classical lesion in psoriasis is the silvery scaling plaque found most frequently over the extensors of the extremities. The scalp is another commonly affected site. *B*, Rheumatoid changes in the distal interphalangeal joints may occur in association with psoriasis. Nails also show changes. (From Wechsler: American Journal of Nursing, April, 1965.)

and moisture can encourage the development of fungal infections.

EPIDERMOPHYTOSIS. Epidermophytosis most often affects the feet, particularly in the areas between the toes. The infection may spread and cause blistering, peeling, cracking and itching of the entire foot. If it continues unchecked it can spread to other parts of the body. The condition can be complicated by a severe bacterial infection.

Treatment of epidermophytosis consists of keeping the area dry, clean, and exposed to the air and sunlight as much as possible. Clean cotton stockings should be worn every day and the affected areas between the toes should be separated by gauze or cotton. There are some medicated powders such as Desenex which work to keep the feet dry and also help control growth of the fungi. Other medications called *antifungals* or *fungicides* are effective in treating this condition.

Since most cases are contracted and spread in swimming pools, showers and other public facilities of this type, one should be careful to wash one's feet and dry them thoroughly after using such facilities. It is difficult to destroy the fungi causing athlete's foot by any method other than by boiling contaminated articles or by use of a strong disinfectant such as 0.1 bichloride of mercury or 0.2 creosol.

RINGWORM. The term *ringworm* is often used to designate tinea of the scalp and beard. Actually, ringworm is incorrect and confusing. The skin lesions do not necessarily appear in rings and they very definitely are not caused by a worm. If the infection is located on the scalp *(tinea capitis)* the hair falls out in patches and there are small, reddish lesions of the skin. Tinea capitis primarily affects children. Because it is highly infectious, any child with this condition should be kept from school until he is no longer a source of infection. His contaminated clothing should be boiled or destroyed to prevent the spread of the infection and he should wear a stocking cap or surgical cap to protect his scalp during treatment.

Tinea barbae is called barber's itch because it affects the area on the face where the beard grows and it is most often spread by carelessness in sanitary measures in a barber shop. The lesions produce a boggy swelling of the skin, soften the hairs of the beard and involve the lymph glands.

In both types of tinea the infected hairs are removed by the tedious process of pulling them out one by one or by deep x-ray therapy performed by a skilled technician. *Griseofulvin* (fulvicin or Grifulvin) is the fungistatic antibiotic that is most often used in the control of ringworm of the scalp and face.

CANCER OF THE SKIN

Introduction. Skin cancer is often neglected because there is no pain associated with it and patients often fear that treatment will involve extensive or mutilating surgery. It has been estimated that each year 68,000 persons discover they have skin cancer and 4000 of these cases are fatal because of inadequate treatment. Almost all of these deaths could have been averted through early diagnosis and treatment.[4]

Causes and Susceptibility. There are several factors that predispose one to the development of skin cancer. Among these are internal changes within the cells themselves that may be due to hereditary factors, and external influences such as chronic exposure to chemicals or other irritants in the environment. Since children tend to inherit their skin characteristics from their parents, susceptibility to skin cancer tends to run in families. Blue-eyed blondes seem to be most susceptible, probably because they lack sufficient pigment to protect the skin cells from outside irritants. The incidence of skin cancer in Negroes is very low.

Figure 10-8. *A*, Precancerous keratoses such as this one on the temple are caused by chemical irritants and should be destroyed when they appear. *B*, Precancerous leukoplakia, white patch on the floor of this 26-year-old woman's mouth, developed after eight years of heavy smoking. *C* and *D*, Basal cell epitheliomas had been present on both these patients from 1½ to 2 years; were removed by local surgery; did not recur. *E*, Squamous cell epithelioma behind ear, a typical site. Local surgery destroyed it. *F*, Melanoma, here on ankle, metastasizes rapidly; starts as tiny dark papule or nodule. (From Cipallaro: American Journal of Nursing, October, 1966.)

Irritants that can lead to the development of skin cancer include industrial dyes and chemicals, ultraviolet rays as from the sun and radiations from x-ray machines or radioactive elements. Repeated irritation of a mole, ulcer or other precancerous lesion also can lead to malignant changes within the lesion.

Treatment. Removal of cancerous skin tissue will depend on the type of malignancy present. In all but the most extensive growths, treatment is relatively simple and completely successful. Although benign precancerous lesions do not inevitably develop into malignancies, the most advisable course of action is to remove them when they are first diagnosed, before they become malignant. The nurse often is in a position to notice these lesions in their early stages and she should do her best to persuade the individual with such a lesion to seek prompt medical attention.

The three main types of skin malignancy are basal cell epithelioma, squamous cell epithelioma, and melanocarcinoma.

Basal cell epithelioma usually appears first as a small, scaly area that tends to become larger as it progresses. It occurs most often on the faces and trunks of adults. As the scales shed there will be a small amount of bleeding and the formation of a scab. As the scab is shed the affected area becomes wider and it is bordered by a waxy, translucent raised area. This process of spreading may continue very gradually over a period of several months or years. Even though these malignancies do not metastasize, they can invade underlying tissues, and death can result from complications such as infection, hemorrhage, or exhaustion. Smaller lesions can be removed under local anesthesia in a doctor's office. Larger lesions respond well to x-ray or radiation therapy.

Squamous cell epithelioma usually begins on the mucous membranes and can metastasize to other areas of the body. The tumor begins as a small nodule with rapid development of ulceration. Treatment must begin early if the condition is to be relieved before extensive damage is done. Surgical procedures must involve total removal or destruction of the lesions and surrounding tissues that have been invaded. Radiation therapy is advised for patients who are poor surgical risks or who are fearful of surgery.

Melanocarcinomas often originate in moles that have been subjected to repeated irritation or which have been incompletely removed. This type of skin cancer is highly malignant and requires radical treatment, especially if it is not treated in its earliest stages. The course of treatment depends on the stage of malignancy and the extent to which it involves other areas.

BURNS

Definition and Classification. Burns are injuries to the skin caused by exposure to extreme heat, electrical agents, strong chemicals, or radiation. The classification of burns is based on the *depth* of the lesion and the *extent* of the body surface that has been burned.

Depth of burns is classified as first degree, second degree, and third degree. A *first degree burn* involves only the outer layer of skin (epidermis); the underlying tissues are not injured. There is redness, tenderness, pain, and some edema but no blistering with a first degree burn.

A *second degree burn* is deeper and involves both the upper and lower layers of the skin. In addition to the symptoms of redness and pain, there is blistering with a second degree burn. There is usually complete regeneration of the layers of the skin and little or no scarring.

A *third degree burn* is much deeper with destruction of both the epidermis and dermis and some damage to the underlying tissues. There is no blistering, and after the initial severe pain, the patient usually does not complain of pain in the area of a third degree burn because the nerve endings have been destroyed. The surface of the skin may appear charred or it may be white and lifeless in appearance.

The extent of a burn is calculated by the doctor according to the "Rule of Nines" (see Table 11). The depth of the burn is more difficult to determine because there are various gradations of injury in a major burn. The physician must make an estimate of some kind as to depth, however, because the patient's systemic illness and his prognosis are directly related to the amount of tissue destroyed. Since third degree burns destroy all layers of the skin, there can be no epithelialization. This means that eventual grafting will be necessary for adequate coverage of the area.

Emergency Treatment. All burns should be considered potentially dangerous and even the most minor ones should be cared for as aseptically as possible. Most authorities now recommend submerging the burned area in ice water or applying cold compresses as emergency first aid for less extensive burns. This helps to relieve pain and reduce edema. Under no circumstances should salves or ointments be applied to a burned area if there is any doubt as to the depth and extent of the burn. The removal of greasy substances is very painful and the patient will suffer unnecessarily because of haste or poor judgment on the part of the person who gave improper emergency care.

(First aid for major and minor burns is discussed in Chapter 20 of this text.)

As soon as the physician evaluates the depth and extent of the burn he begins treatment aimed at combating shock and preventing infection.

The two most important measures used to combat profound shock in a burn patient are replacement of lost fluids and electrolytes and the relief of pain and mental anxiety. The loss of fluids and electrolytes is a result of the sudden shifting of the blood plasma and tissue fluids from their normal site to the area of the burn. The fluids are then lost by seepage through the open wounds where the skin has been destroyed by burns.

It is necessary to replace these fluids immediately; otherwise there will be collapse of the blood vessels and a resulting profound shock which may be fatal to the patient. Plasma, fluids and electrolytes are given intravenously, often through an incision into a vein because there will be a need for continuous replacement of fluids until a normal fluid and electrolyte balance is established. In a severely burned individual, intravenous therapy may be necessary for several days or longer.

Measures to relieve pain include the administration of morphine or Demerol as soon as possible after the burn has occurred. Later the physician may choose to order other pain-relieving drugs which are less likely to lead to addiction because of the long period of recovery which usually is associated with severe burns.

Table 11. *Rule of Nines*

AREA OF BODY	PERCENTAGE OF BODY SURFACE
Head and neck	9
Anterior trunk	18
Posterior trunk	18
Upper limbs	18
Lower limbs	36
Genitalia and perineum	1

Table 12. *Guides for Estimating Depth of Injury**

FACTOR	SECOND-DEGREE BURN (partial thickness)	THIRD-DEGREE BURN (full thickness)
Cause	hot liqids, flashes, flames	flames, electricity, chemicals
Skin		
Color	pink or mild red	pearly white or charred
Surface	vesicles are weeping	dry
Palpation	soft	leathery
Response to pin prick	painful	anesthetic
Layers involved	dermis	the fat or subcutaneous tissue

*From Larson and Gaston: American Journal of Nursing, February, 1967. Reprinted with permission.

The nurse must use gentleness and care in handling the patient as she turns him or administers other treatments. Not only does this reduce the amount of pain the patient must suffer, but the less the patient is handled the less danger there is of contaminating the wounds.

Even though there is not usually much pain involved with third degree burns, most patients who have such burns also have areas of second degree burns which are very painful long after the initial pain at the time of the accident. Added to this extreme discomfort is the patient's realization that he has been badly injured and is in serious condition. He no doubt thinks of all the horrifying sights and smells associated with burned flesh and suffers much emotional shock from such an experience.

The nurse assisting in the emergency care of the burn victim in the hospital should assemble the equipment that she can expect the physician to need. This equipment usually includes the following:

1. Intravenous fluids and apparatus for administering fluids and whole blood.

2. A catheterization tray and a No. 18 Foley catheter with tubing and drainage bottle. Specimen cup for urine specimen.

3. A tray containing equipment for withdrawing a blood sample and appropriate test tubes for blood typing, crossmatching, blood count and electrolyte analysis.

4. A tracheostomy tray.

5. A cutdown set with No. 16 tubing, suture material and skin antiseptic.

6. An instrument set and special dressings such as small gauze flats, gauze rolls, Ace bandages, adhesive tape, towels, gloves and sterile vaseline gauze.

7. Surgical gowns and masks for those attending the patient during emergency care.

The nurse should also be prepared to administer tetanus antitoxin and one or more antibiotics as ordered by the physician. Since some preparation should be made on the unit to which the patient is to be admitted, the nurse should notify the unit of his impending admission and inform them of the need for a Stryker frame or circo-lectric bed if the physician prefers one of these to a regular hospital bed for his patient.

General Treatment and Nursing Care

Treating the Wound. Although much attention must be paid to the patient's systemic reaction to the burn, one must realize that the burned area itself is the ultimate concern in good care of a burned patient. Two general ways to treat the burn are the *open* method and the *closed* method. In the open method the burned area is left uncovered and exposed to the air. In the closed method the area is covered with bulky dressings consisting of many layers and then wrapped snugly with Ace bandages.

In most burn centers today therapists usually agree that since there are advantages and disadvantages to each of the two methods it is best to use a combination of the two in most cases. For example, third degree burns of the hand may be covered with a greased layer of gauze followed by bulky dressings and then wrapped in an Ace bandage (see Fig. 10-9). Burns on the arm and chest areas may be left without a dressing and silver nitrate soaks or an antibiotic ointment such as gentamicin sulfate (Garamycin) can be applied. The use of a 0.5 per cent silver nitrate solution for soaks in the treatment of burns has gained widespread interest since it was first used in 1964 at Barnes Hospital in St. Louis. The physicians who advocate its use believe that silver nitrate soaks reduce the incidence of infection, promote prompt healing of deep second-degree burns and prevent the development of fever (see Fig. 10-10).[15]

OPEN METHOD. When this method of treatment is used the nurse must guard constantly against infection. Usually the serous fluid which exudes from the burns will harden and cover most of the burned area, but there are cracks in this exudate through which bacteria may enter. The bed linen is sterile and a bed cradle or some other device is used to support the weight of the top covers and keep them off the burned areas. Those in attendance usually wear sterile caps and gowns and gloves while caring for the patient. In recent years some hospitals have set aside special units in which burned patients are treated by the open method. These units are staffed with personnel specially trained in the care

of the burned patient. For further details the reader is referred to reference 6 under Suggested Student Reading at the end of this chapter.

Aside from preventing infection the nurse must also provide additional warmth when the open method of treatment is used. Much body heat is lost through the parts of the body where the skin has been destroyed and the patient is chilled easily. Heat lamps or small electric bulbs installed under the device used to hold up the top covers will usually provide the extra warmth needed.

Wet compresses or soaks to cleanse the area and remove excess exudate and drainage must be done with extreme care and under sterile conditions in order to minimize the danger of infecting the wound. An exception is in the silver nitrate method in which it is usually not considered necessary for the attendants to follow rigid isolation technique with masking and gowning.[15]

CLOSED METHOD. The closed method of treating burns presents fewer problems for the nursing staff because there is less danger of infection. There is also the added advantage of having the burned areas covered so that the patient does not have a constant visual reminder of his injuries. It is also true that patients who have pressure dressings are freer to move about and do things for themselves than those who do not have their wounds covered. The main disadvantage of the closed method is the need for frequent changing of the dressings which may require administration of a general anesthetic and also involves some trauma to the regenerating tissue each time the dressings are removed. Other disadvantages of bulky dressings are that they provide a culture medium for the growth of bacteria, are difficult to apply properly to areas such as the face and perineum, may increase fluid loss and heat retention, and can mask hidden bleeding.

Debridement and Grafting. Debridement involves removal of the

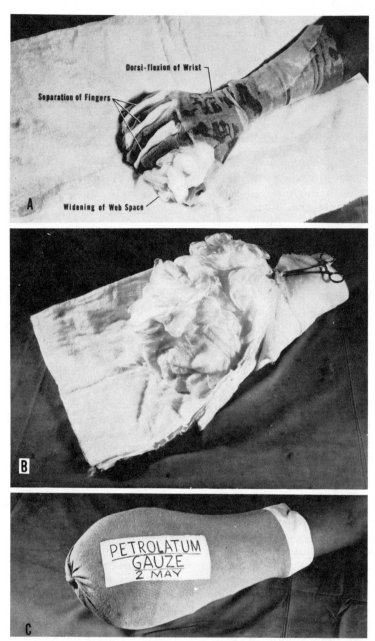

Figure 10-9. *A*, Initial step in applying an occlusive dressing to a burned hand. A layer of lightly impregnated gauze is placed over the burned area. The hand and forearm are put on two large abdominal pads. Fluffed gauze is placed on the palm of the hand in such a way that there is dorsiflexion of the wrist and acute flexion of metacarpophalangeal joints. The fingers are separated with gauze and special attention is given to maintaining the width of the webbed space between the index finger and the thumb. *B*, Additional fluffed gauze is placed over the hand to make a large, absorptive dressing. It may or may not be necessary to put a plaster splint in the dressing to maintain dorsiflexion of the wrist. *C*, The entire dressing is wrapped with even compression by means of an elastic bandage. Stockinette is placed over the dressing. Then the type of treatment and date applied are noted on the dressing. (From Artz and Moncrief: *The Treatment of Burns*, 2nd Ed., W. B. Saunders Co., Philadelphia.)

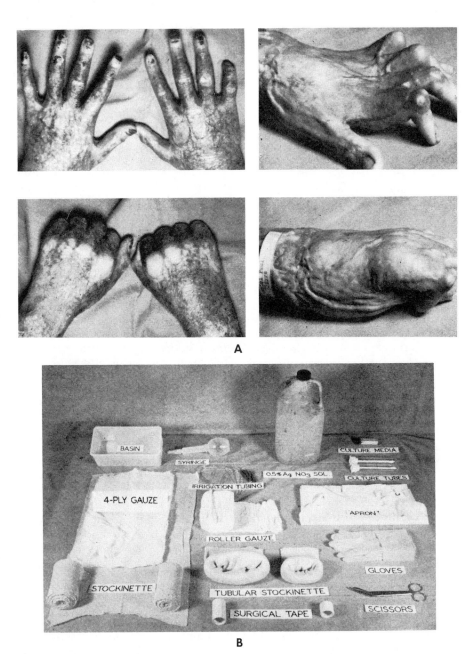

Figure 10-10. *A*, New and old treatments contrasted. The hands at the right were not treated with silver nitrate and have poor function after five skin grafts and 417 days. The hands at the left were burned so deeply that the extensor mechanisms were bared. Silver nitrate treatment was given and skin grafts were laid on the bare tendons. All tendons now glide freely and the only restricted motion is in the distal joint of the right fifth finger. *B*, Equipment necessary for changing a silver nitrate burn dressing. Thick dressings are essential to hold moisture and heat. The four-ply gauze is fan-folded to make 40 layers. (From Woods et al.: American Journal of Nursing, March, 1966.)

eschar and necrotic material from underlying tissues. This must be done with great care so that bleeding is kept at a minimum and healthy tissues are disturbed as little as possible. Some physicians prefer the method of soaking off eschar by placing the patient in a tub containing a temperature controlled balanced salt solution. The bath water is gently agitated to facilitate the debridement process. Patients do not object to the bath as they do to other methods of debridement because the bath is soothing and relaxing, less painful for them, and they can exercise more freely in the water.

Grafting of skin is done as early after the initial injury as possible. The physician usually waits until granulations have begun to form and there is no gross necrotic tissue on the surface of the wound. The donor skin is best taken from the patient (*autogenous skin graft*), but when this is not possible the skin of another person can be used (*homograft*). For further information on skin grafts the reader is referred to Student Reading Reference No. 3.

Record of Intake and Output. This
is one of the most important aspects of nursing a patient with burns. We know that many fluids and essential minerals are lost through the burned areas of skin and these must be replaced so that a normal fluid and electrolyte balance is maintained. This loss of fluids results in a decrease in the amount of blood flowing through the kidneys, which may in turn lead to damage of the cells of the kidney.

The physician will depend on the nursing staff to keep an accurate record of the patient's intake and output of fluids and will use this information to determine the need for additional fluids or minerals. He may also order frequent laboratory tests of the blood to determine its electrolyte content.

In addition to keeping a careful record on the intake and output the nurse must also observe the urine carefully for color and concentration. Blood in the urine may indicate damage to the kidneys; therefore, any unusually dark or abnormally colored urine should be reported. A large amount of very light colored urine frequently indicates overhydration and possible loss of essential minerals through the urine, while concentrated urine usually indicates dehydration.

Diet. During the period of healing
and convalescence from the burn the patient's diet is very important. The protein content is usually increased to several times that of a regular diet in order to assist the body as it rebuilds tissue. Dietary supplements for the severely burned patients usually include vitamins, especially vitamin C, minerals, such as iron, and electrolytes such as sodium, chloride and potassium.

The odor of the burn and the patient's despondency over his predicament may greatly contribute to a loss of appetite. Every device and trick known must be used to encourage the patient to eat all the meals and between-meal feedings prepared for him.

Emotional Aspects. We have mentioned
the emotional shock of a severe burn and the understandable depression of the patient once he realizes what has happened to him. The nurse can surely understand that she must give the burn patient moral support and at the same time avoid having him become too dependent on the nursing staff. As is true in most long-term illnesses, there is a danger of complete boredom and apathy with a loss of the will to live unless diversional and occupational therapy are provided.

There is also a possibility of overdependence on drugs to relieve pain and anxiety if the nursing staff does not or will not attempt to make the patient comfortable through the use of simple nursing measures before administering drugs. The nurse must realize that a "p.r.n." order for a narcotic or sedative means the administration of the drug only as a last resort after all nursing measures have failed to make the patient comfortable.

Complications of Burns. Aside from the complications of pulmonary disease and circulatory stasis which are hazards for all patients confined to bed over a period of time, the burn patient must also be protected from the complications of infection of the wounds and contractures.

Of all the functions of the skin, that of protection from pathogenic organisms is the most important. The patient with a serious burn no longer has that protection and so all exposure to possible sources of infection must be kept at a minimum. It is not possible to keep the environment completely free of bacteria, but ordinary precautions may greatly reduce the possibility of contaminating the wounds. These precautions include frequent and thorough washing of the hands, keeping all pressure dressings dry and clean, and handling the dressings or open wounds as little as possible.

Another complication to be avoided in the severely burned patient is the development of *contractures*. These are a shortening of muscle tissue with loss of elasticity and resistance to stretching, leading to loss of motion in the affected part.

The development of contractures may be traced directly to improper positioning of the patient and lack of attention to exercises for the patient confined to bed. Burn patients are particularly susceptible to contractures because motion is often painful and they tend to guard against this pain by staying in a fixed position unless encouraged to do otherwise.

If pressure dressings are used the nurse must see to it that parts which cannot be moved because of the dressings are at least kept in a position of optimum function so that foot drop and wrist drop are prevented. The parts of the body which can be moved must be exercised regularly. This is extremely difficult to accomplish if the nurse is overly sympathetic or the patient is insistent in his demands to be left alone. A common-sense approach must be used to solve the problem. Both the nursing staff and the patient must be fully aware of the crippling and permanent deformities which may result if the joints are not kept in motion and muscle tone is not maintained.

Rehabilitation should never be postponed until after the deformities occur. The long-range view must be taken so that the deformities are prevented rather than treated. Painful as the motion may be, the muscles must be gently stretched and used every day if they are to be kept in a good state of tone and functioning normally.

CLINICAL CASE PROBLEMS

1. As you are bathing a child in the pediatric ward one day you observe some small blisters on her legs. Some of these blisters appear to have burst and there is a honey-colored crust over them. These skin lesions were not reported to you when you assumed care of the child that morning and there is no record of there having been any lesions present when she was admitted a week ago.

> What are your responsibilities in regard to your observations?
> If these lesions are diagnosed by the physician as impetigo contagiosa, what special nursing care will this child require while she is in the pediatric ward?

2. Mrs. Nation, age 32, is admitted to the ward with a diagnosis of severe contact dermatitis. Both her legs and arms are covered with a rash which causes much itching and burning.

> What nursing measures can you use to help relieve her discomfort?
> What effect will you expect the patient's mental attitude to have on her physical condition?
> How can you help her to relax?

3. Martha M. is a 12-year-old child who was badly burned when her clothing caught fire while she was helping her mother cook hamburgers on an outdoor grill. She has

second and third degree burns over her abdomen and chest and down the front of both of her legs. When you are assigned to care for Martha she has been in the hospital for two weeks and has received much attention from her family and friends. She has become somewhat spoiled by all this attention and is very uncooperative when you attempt to do anything for her. In spite of the fact that she has no pressure dressings on her lower legs she refuses to sit up and help herself in any way. She has refused most of her diet and prefers the soft drinks, candy bars and fruit that have been showered on her since her accident.

How can you help this child without arousing resentment and without offending her well-meaning family and friends?

REFERENCES

1. Andrews, G. C., and Domonkos, A. N.: *Diseases of the Skin,* 5th edition. Philadelphia, W. B. Saunders Co., 1963.
2. Bennett, H. J.: "Burns, First Aid and Emergency Care." Am. Journ. Nurs., Oct., 1962, p. 96.
3. Brunner, L. S., et al.: *Textbook of Medical-Surgical Nursing.* Philadelphia, J. B. Lippincott Co., 1964.
4. "Cipollaro, A. J.: "Cancer of the Skin." Am. Journ. Nurs., Oct., 1966, p. 2231.
5. Conway, H.: "Those Skin Blemishes: Harmless or Dangerous?" RN, Sept., 1960, p. 55.
6. Conway, H., and Nayer, D.: "Skin Grafts: The Techniques, the Patient." Am. Journ. Nurs., Nov., 1964, p. 94.
7. Cooper, S. S.: "Applying Medication to the Skin or Mucosa." RN, Aug., 1960, p. 61.
8. Goldman, L.: Prevention and Treatment of Eczema." Am. Journ. Nurs., March, 1964, p. 114.
9. Larson, D., and Gaston, R.: "Current Trends in the Care of Burned Patients." Am. Journ. Nurs., Feb., 1967, p. 319.
10. Rose, L. J.: "Medical Features of Severe Burns." Tomorrow's Nurse, June–July, 1962, p. 17.
11. Samitz, M. H.: "The Industrial Dermatoses." Am. Journ. Nurs., Jan., 1965, p. 79.
12. Shafer, K. N., Sawyer, J. R., *et al.: Medical-Surgical Nursing,* 4th edition. St. Louis, C. V. Mosby Co., 1967.
13. Smith, D. W., and Gips, C. D.: *Care of the Adult Patient,* 2nd edition. Philadelphia, J. B. Lippincott Co., 1966.
14. Wechsler, H. L.: "Psoriasis." Am. Journ. Nurs., April, 1965, p. 85.
15. Wood, M., et al.: "Silver Nitrate Treatment of Burns." Am. Journ. Nurs., March, 1966, p. 518.

SUGGESTED STUDENT READING

1. Baker, T. J.: "Open Technique in the Management of Burns." Am. Journ. Nurs., Sept., 1959, p. 1262.
2. Cahn, M. M.: "The Skin from Infancy to Old Age." Am. Journ. Nurs., July, 1960, p. 993.
3. Conway, H., and Nayer, D.: "Skin Grafts: The Techniques, the Patient." Am. Journ. Nurs., Nov., 1964, p. 94.
4. Cooper, S. S.: "Applying Medication to the Skin or Mucosa." RN, Aug., 1960, p. 61.
5. Henderson, J.: "An Odd Name for Odious Pain." Practical Nursing, Dec., 1962, p. 30.
6. Horgan, P. D.: "How They Battle to Save the Badly Burned." RN, Feb., 1963, p. 46.
7. "Taming the Sun." Practical Nursing, April, 1963, p. 37.

OUTLINE FOR CHAPTER 10

I. Introduction

A. Skin protects against invasion of bacteria in the environment.

B. Helps regulate body temperature.

C. Holds in body fluids.

II. Diagnostic Tests and Examinations

A. Visual examination.

B. History—allergies, familial tendencies and environmental factors are important in determining cause of skin disorders.

C. Skin tests to determine an individual's sensitivity to specific substances.

D. Elimination diets—removal of foods that are suspected of causing the skin disease.

E. Cultures and sensitivity tests to determine pathogen causing a skin infection and to find an effective drug against it.

III. Factors in Prevention of Skin Disease

A. Cleanliness.

B. Good nutrition.

C. Age (older persons suffer from dryness of skin and loss of elasticity).

D. Environment—irritants such as chemicals and strong sunlight and other forms of radiation can lead to breakdown of skin.

IV. General Nursing Care

A. Rules for care include intelligent observation, careful handling of the skin and avoidance of alcohol, lotions or other skin applications not specifically ordered by the dermatologist.

B. Colloid baths — those in which soothing agents are added to the bath water. Avoid chilling the patient. *Pat, do not rub,* the skin dry after the bath.

C. Bed linens may require special laundering to remove all traces of soap.

D. Wet compresses or dressings are often used.

V. Herpes Simplex

A. Cold sores or fever blisters.

B. Caused by a virus similar to the one causing smallpox.

VI. Herpes Zoster ("Shingles")

A. A viral disease of the skin and peripheral sensory nerves.

B. Symptoms include blistering followed by scaling of the skin, skin lesions along nerve pathways, severe pain and itching in the affected area.

VII. Impetigo Contagiosa

A. A highly contagious bacterial infection of the skin.

B. Treatment consists of removal of crusts, thorough cleaning of the lesions and application of antibiotic ointments or administration of oral antibiotics.

VIII. Contact Dermatitis

A. An allergic eczema resulting from hypersensitivity to a substance that has come in contact with the skin.

B. Treatment includes removal of the antigen from contact with the skin, colloid baths and lotions to soothe the skin and dry the weeping lesions and antihistamines to control itching.

IX. Acne

A. A skin disorder characterized by papules and pustules occurring at puberty.

B. No specific treatment.

X. Psoriasis

A. A chronic and recurring disorder characterized by papules and adherent silvery scales that produce pinpoint bleeding when removed.

B. There is no known cure, but coal tar and mercury remedies used in conjunction with cortisone can keep the condition under control.

XI. Fungal Infections (Mycoses)

A. Examples are epidermophytosis (athlete's foot), tinea of the scalp (ringworm) or face (barber's itch) and moniliasis (thrush). All produce some itching and breakdown of the skin.

B. Fungistatic drugs such as griseofulvin are most helpful in the control of fungal infections.

XII. Cancer of the Skin

A. Almost all cases can be treated successfully if they are caught early.

B. Causes are unknown but hereditary factors and environmental influences such as chronic irritation can increase susceptibility to skin cancer.

C. Treatment consists of surgical removal or radiation therapy.

D. Types include (1) basal cell epithelioma, (2) squamous cell epithelioma, and (3) melanocarcinoma.

XIII. Burns

A. Caused by exposure to heat, electrical agents, strong chemicals or radiation.

B. Classified as first degree, second degree or third degree.

C. Emergency treatment:
    1. All burns should be considered potentially dangerous.
    2. Salves or ointments should not be used without a physician's order.
    3. Immersion in ice water or cold compresses applied to the burn help relieve and reduce edema.
    4. Dangers are shock, infection and fluid loss.
    5. Nurse should anticipate the needs of the physician and have necessary equipment and medications prepared.

D. Treatment of the wound.
    1. Open method (wound is cleansed and then left uncovered). There may be more danger of infection, but soaks, compresses and other treatments are more easily carried out.
    2. Closed method. Wound is cleansed, covered with lubricated gauze followed by several layers of absorbent, fluffy gauze. Finally Ace bandages are wrapped snugly around the dressings.

a. Main disadvantages are that the dressings can serve as culture medium for bacteria and that they must be changed often; this can be traumatic to regenerating tissue. Other disadvantages are increased body temperature and loss of body fluids.

3. Silver nitrate soaks using a 0.5 per cent solution are now being used more extensively. They reduce infection, promote prompt healing and prevent the development of fever.

4. Debridement and grafting often necessary.

E. Record of intake and output essential for aiding physician in restoring and maintaining a normal fluid and electrolyte balance. Also important for determination of kidney damage that can occur in severe burns.

F. Diet—usually high protein with supplements of vitamins and minerals.

G. Emotional aspects must be considered because the patient may have permanent physical handicaps or cosmetic difficulties.

H. Complications of burns.

1. Infection due to improper handling of burned area or equipment used for patient, or greatly lowered resistance of patient.

2. Contractures as a result of improper positioning and inadequate exercise.

Chapter 11

NURSING CARE OF PATIENTS WITH DISORDERS OF THE MUSCULOSKELETAL SYSTEM

VOCABULARY

Abduction	Flexion
Adduction	Hyperpnea
Exacerbation	Placebo
Extension	Remission

INTRODUCTION

The special branch of medical science concerned with the preservation and restoration of the functions of the skeletal system is called *orthopedics*. We cannot confine orthopedic nursing to patients with diseases and deformities of bones and joints, however, because the basic principles of orthopedic nursing are applicable to the nursing care of all patients, and most especially to those confined to bed. Whatever the diagnosis may be, attention to the musculoskeletal functions of the patient is essential to his general well-being and continued activity.

The three main functions of the musculoskeletal system are *motion, support*, and *protection*. Of these three, the preservation of motion is probably the most important consideration as far as the practical nurse is concerned. It is the long bones of the limbs which give the body support and provide motion by acting as levers to which the muscles are attached. Joint motion is a result of the shortening and stretching of opposing sets of muscles. For example,

when the flexor muscles of the leg contract and shorten the opposing extensors must relax and lengthen. Disuse or undue strain on these muscles can lead to permanent disabilities and loss of motion.

If we follow the development of bones within an individual from conception to old age we can see that the bony tissues of the infant differ greatly from those of the adult. That is because all bone cells do not follow the same pattern of development from the embryonic stage to full maturity. There are two distinct groups of bone cells. Some of them are designed so that they are immediately transformed into mature cells. The normal newborn infant will have this type of firm bone cells in his skull and shoulder bones. In the second group the bone cells form cartilage first and then are gradually replaced by mature bone cells as the individual grows older. Thus, the bones of an infant are really mostly cartilage. *Ossification*, or replacement of cartilage by more solid bony tissue, is not completed throughout the body until 20 to 25 years of age.

183

Because the bony structure of the infant and young child is softer and more pliable, there is less danger of their breaking bones during the time of life when they are learning to walk and run and are therefore more likely to have frequent falls. If a fracture does occur, however, it will heal more rapidly in a very young person because growth is still taking place within the bone.

On the other hand, the bones of elderly persons are brittle and less compact, breaking easily. In addition, they do not heal readily when a fracture is sustained because the physiological exchange of minerals has decreased with advancing age, making the process of repair much slower.

In studying the process of bone development and repair it must be remembered that *bone is a living tissue*, with a complex system of canals through which blood and lymph vessels pass. This system allows for the adequate transportation of nutrients to the bone cells and removal of wastes. There is also a continuous depositing of, storing, and removing from the bony tissues certain minerals which are essential to the normal functioning of bones.

Muscles compose one third to one half of the body's entire bulk. In this chapter we will be concerned only with the skeletal muscles which are instrumental in moving the various parts of the body. Involuntary muscles and cardiac muscle tissues will be discussed in appropriate chapters.

DIAGNOSTIC TESTS

X-ray Films. X-ray is the diagnostic aid most often used by the orthopedic surgeon. Through the use of roentgen rays, which are capable of penetrating structures less dense than bone, thereby presenting an outline of bony structures in the body, the physician is able to discover abnormal changes in the contour, size, and density of bones.

Cultures. Samples of infected bone tissues are sometimes taken for the purpose of growing cultures in the laboratory. These cultures make it possible for the physician to determine the specific organism causing the infection and the appropriate drug to be used in the treatment of the infection.

Biopsy. In the case of bone tumors, the surgical removal of samples of the cells within the growth (biopsy) is an important diagnostic aid in determining the type of tumor present.

GENERAL NURSING CARE

Lifting and Turning the Patient. There are special skills necessary for the proper care of a patient with musculoskeletal disorders, particularly in regard to moving the patient and changing his linens.

First, the nurse must use good body mechanics herself so that she can safely and correctly use her strength to the greatest advantage. An awkward posture or failure to use the correct methods of lifting and moving the patient will often cause him unnecessary discomfort and apprehension about being moved, and will also lead to painful muscle strain for the nurse.

Secondly, all movements must be *gentle* and *firm*. When moving or turning the patient there should be sufficient help from adequately trained personnel. Each person involved, including the patient, should understand exactly what is going to be done and the steps to take in accomplishing the move. If the patient can help without danger to the diseased joint or limb he should be encouraged to do so. If he is not able to help, the nurse explains the procedure to him and asks him to cooperate by relaxing completely during the procedure. Many times the patient is afraid that moving and turning will cause him pain. It is then necessary to help him understand the reasons for frequent changing of the position and gain his confidence and cooperation so that he will not make the task more difficult by resisting all efforts to turn him.

Nurses are sometimes tempted to allow their patient the privilege of assuming any position and remaining in that position as long as he appears comfortable. They reason that it seems unkind and unnecessary to force the patient to move about when he is apparently resting and does not wish to be disturbed. This is actually not a kindness and could be considered as nothing short of neglect when we know the terrible consequences of poor body posture.

The nurse might also take the time to find a reason for the patient's assuming certain postures in bed. It is possible that the patient is curled up in a fetal position becuase he is trying to keep warm. Older patients and those with poor circulation instinctively huddle their shoulders and tuck their limbs close to their bodies when they are chilly. It is also possible that the patient is flexing his knees, hips and back because he is attempting to relieve pain in his abdomen or lower legs. These possibilities should always be considered and they should make the nurse even more aware of her responsibility in performing sensible and practical nursing measures for the comfort of her patient.

Orthopedic Bed Making. When a patient has traction applied to an upper or lower limb, or when he is in a large body cast, it is not always convenient to arrange the bed linens in the conventional manner. Some institutions in which there are large orthopedic units provide specially made linens which have been designed so that bed making and changing of linen is much easier for the nurse and less disturbing to the orthopedically handicapped patient. If there is such linen available the practical nurse should seek specific instructions in its use.

In institutions in which there is no such linen available, the practical nurse must improvise with the materials she has at hand. This requires some ingenuity and imagination but it can be done. For example, two draw sheets may be used for the foundation of the bed in lieu of one large bottom sheet. This would be useful in instances in which the patient's lower limb is in a traction apparatus which uses a frame resting on the mattress rather than suspended from an overhead frame. Obviously there will be a good bit of disturbance of the frame and the traction if the large bottom sheet must be changed each time it becomes soiled. When two draw sheets are used, however, only the draw sheet under the patient's body need be changed and the frame will not be disturbed at all. Top covers may be folded so that the limb in traction is not covered. If extra warmth is needed for the affected limb it can be covered with a small baby blanket.

One important point to remember in changing the linen is avoidance of pulling sheets from under the patient and causing friction against the skin. The patient confined to bed for a long period of time must have his skin preserved at all costs. He must be gently turned on and off the sheets being changed; sheets are never pulled from under him.

Prevention of Deformities. The nurse must constantly bear in mind her responsibilities in the prevention of deformities for *all* of her patients. Maintenance of good body position, preservation of muscle tone, and continued joint motion are no less important for the patient with a stroke or the burned patient than they are for the patient with an orthopedic disorder. No matter what the diagnosis, the patient confined to bed over a prolonged period of time will need proper positioning of the joints and adequate exercising of the limbs in order to prevent irreparable damage and deformities. According to an article by Madden and Affeldt (see No. 6 on Student Reading List), "Nursing care that will prevent deformities and helplessness requires no written order of the physician. It should be routinely and consistently provided by all nursing personnel at all times."

The deformities most commonly associated with poor positioning and lack of exercise are *contractures, loss of muscle tone,* and *ankylosis.* The first two are directly concerned with the muscles; ankylosis affects the bones.

CONTRACTURES. When skeletal muscles are not regularly stretched and contracted to their normal limits, they attempt to adapt themselves to this limited use by becoming shorter and less elastic. This "adaptive shortening" is referred to as a contracture. The most frequent contractures occurring in patients confined to bed for long periods of time are "foot drop," knee and hip flexion contractures, "wrist drop," and contractures of the arm (see Fig. 11-1).

LOSS OF MUSCLE TONE. We know that joint motion is a result of the shortening and stretching of opposing muscles. That is, when the flexor muscles of the leg contract and shorten, the opposing extensor muscles must relax and lengthen. Muscle tone is defined as the readiness of the muscles to go to work, to contract and relax as needed. If a muscle is not stimulated to action

regularly, or if it is stretched beyond its normal limits for an extended period of time, it will lose its ability to work. An example is "foot drop," in which the calf muscles are shortened and the opposing flexor muscles are stretched so that they lose their "tone."

ANKYLOSIS. Ankylosis is a permanent fixation of a joint and is the result of a disease or injury in which the tissues of the joint are replaced by a bony overgrowth which completely obliterates the joint. Sometimes this process cannot be prevented, as for example in some types of arthritis. In these cases the physician braces the joint in the position that will be most useful to the patient, even though there is no motion in the joint. Imagine your wrist locked in a position in which the palm and fingers are dangling at right angles to the lower arm. Now imagine your wrist locked in a position in which the wrist is slightly flexed. If you had your choice of positions you would choose the one in which your wrist was slightly flexed because this would allow you to perform many of your daily activities. The term used for these positions of choice is "positions of optimum use" or "positions of maximum function."

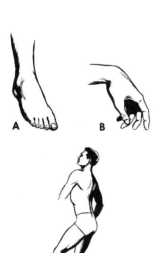

Figure 11-1. *A,* Foot drop resulting from improper support of the feet while patient is confined to bed. A simple footboard could easily prevent this deformity. *B,* Wrist drop resulting from improper support of the hand. *C,* Flexion contracture of knee and hip force this patient to walk on tiptoe on the affected side. If both legs are involved, walking is impossible.

In her daily care of patients who have their joints braced in positions of this kind, the practical nurse must use care that the limb is in the position established by the physician.

Nursing Care in Prevention of Deformities. We have stated that good body position and exercises are necessary for prevention of the type of deformities defined above. It is important then that the nurse fully understand her role in the prevention of such deformities.

Good body position for the patient simply means good posture for the patient confined to the bed or wheelchair. The nurse can judge whether her patient has good posture in bed by observing him to see if his position conforms to the following rules:

1. The back is straight with the normal curves of the spine unexaggerated.

2. The legs are *slightly flexed* to relieve

Figure 11-2. *A*, Patient lying on back. Blanket roll or footboard and pillows may be used to keep feet in correct position. Note support of patient's back with pillows. *B*, Patient lying on side. Pillow is placed under knee to maintain good alignment of back. *C*, Patient lying in prone position. Small pillow is placed under abdomen and under lower legs. Alternate position of feet may be used to maintain correct position of feet. (A and B, from Todd and Freeman: *Health Care of the Family.* C, from Montag and Swenson: *Fundamentals in Nursing Care,* 3rd Ed., W. B. Saunders Co., Philadelphia.)

the strain on the lumbar spine, the abdomen, and the legs.

3. The ribs are elevated and the rib cage supported so that constriction is prevented.

4. The legs are supported so that the weight of one does not fall on the other.

5. Excessive ankle extension is prevented.[7]

Figure 11-2 illustrates the correct positioning and support of the patient according to the above rules. Since any position is tiring if maintained too long, it is also necessary for the nurse to assist the patient in changing his position at least every two hours.

Even though it is well understood by the nurse that changing the body positions from supine to side to prone will prevent decubitus ulcers, ciculatory stasis, and respiratory and urinary complications, she may not fully appreciate the fact that *changing of the body's position will not guarantee freedom from orthopedic deformities. It is also necessary to change joint positions.* Figure 11-3 illustrates this very important point. In order to prevent ankylosis of the joints and contractures of the muscles the nurse must remember to flex and extend the limbs alternately when she changes the patient's position.

Another important point in the prevention of orthopedic deformities is the matter of exercise. Physiotherapists tell us that all joints should be put through their full range of motion at least once daily, preferably more often. If the patient is not able to do the exercises, the nurse or physiotherapist must carry out *passive exercises* for him. If the patient is able to perform the exercises under the guidance of the nurse or physiotherapist, the term used is *active exercises.*

The responsibility of the practical nurse in regard to these exercises lies in her obligation to familiarize herself with the exercises necessary for each individual patient and to carry out these exercises as ordered. She will find that in some cases it will not be possible to exercise all of the joints because of traction to a limb or a cast

Figure 11-3. In these illustrations the patient's body position has been changed four times and yet the positions of the joints at the knees, hips, elbows, and neck have been changed very little or not at all.

covering certain parts of the body. In other instances the more complicated exercises will require the attention of the physiotherapist. The ideal time for the administration of passive exercises to the limbs so that each joint is put through its full range of motion is during the morning bath. They take so little time and they could easily be made a part of the routine morning care.

Emotional Aspects of Orthopedic Disorders. Unfortunately, many orthopedic conditions require prolonged periods of confinement to bed, or, at best, immobilization of a part of the body and restricted physical activities. This leads to frustration and a feeling of hopelessness and despair on the part of the patient so confined. When the patient is young and unaccustomed to dependence on others for his personal care he may react with anger and bitterness toward his plight. If the patient is a wage-earner or an active member of the family, and one upon whom others are dependent, he has the additional burden of financial and social problems.

Immobilization and some degree of helplessness can greatly affect an individual's personality. Some never cease to rebel against the situation, while others become "institutionalized" and do not wish to return to their former lives and responsibilities. The nurse must understand that the long convalescent period filled with tedious hours of waiting for the bone to heal and the surrounding tissues to mend is a very difficult time for the patient. She will need much tact and patience as well as a lively imagination to help him spend his time happily and busily. Occupational therapy is available in most institutions and should be used to the fullest for the orthopedic patient. Suggestions offered in Chapter 7 of this text may be of help to the practical nurse in her efforts to provide recreation for the orthopedically handicapped.

NURSING CARE OF THE PATIENT IN A CAST

Casts are used for the purpose of immobilizing a certain part of the body so that it is firmly supported and completely at rest in a specific position.

Types of Casts. Leg and arm casts may cover all or part of the limb. These are called *long-leg* or *short-leg* casts, depending on how much of the leg they cover. A *walking cast* is a leg cast with extra material added to the sole for weight bearing. This is most often a metal bar ("walking iron") covered with rubber. A *spica* cast covers the trunk of the body and one or both extremities. There are long-leg and short-leg spicas, which cover one or both legs, and shoulder spicas which include the trunk and one arm.

The material most commonly used for casts is plaster of paris. This material is used because it is cheap, durable, fairly easy to apply, and readily available. Plaster of paris is gypsum from which the water has been removed. Strips of crinoline are impregnated with this plaster and are available in various widths. When they are to be used, these strips are soaked in water and applied wet. When the material dries there is a firm shell of plaster molded to the exact shape of the part of the body to which it has been applied.

Preparation for Application of a Cast. The mattress and pillows of the patient with a cast should be protected with a waterproof material until the cast is completely dry. Most orthopedic surgeons prefer a firm cotton mattress with steel or wooden slats underneath to prevent sagging of the mattress, resulting in improper support of the cast.

Before a cast is applied the patient's skin is thoroughly cleaned with soap and water and any breaks in the skin are reported to the doctor if he is not aware of them. Shaving is not done unless surgery is to be performed before application of the cast. In this case a special orthopedic surgical preparation according to the hospital procedure is necessary.

In emergencies, a thorough explanation of what is going to be done is not always possible. In all other cases, however, it is best if the patient is prepared for the type of cast that will be applied, the precautions that must be taken while the cast is drying, and any special devices that may be put on his bed to help him turn and move about in the bed. An example is the trapeze bar attached to an overhead frame which allows the patient to lift himself and turn without strain on the affected part.

Care of the Fresh Plaster Cast. The newly applied cast is usually not dry for a period of time, most often 48 hours, depending on the type of cast. While the plaster is damp its shape can be changed by careless handling or improper support. It follows, then, that extreme care must be used in moving the patient or the cast during this time.

When transferring the patient from the stretcher to the bed there must be enough help available so that the patient is not "tumbled" into bed. Pillows for support should be placed on the bed *before* moving the patient onto them. For large casts, pillows are used to support the curves of the cast so that there will be no cracking or flattening of the cast by the weight of the body (see Fig. 11-4).

The patient in a body cast or spica is more comfortable if pillows are not put under the head and shoulders because they push the chest and abdomen against the front of the cast, causing an uncomfortable crushing sensation and dyspnea.

While a cast is still damp it should not be grasped by the fingers in the process of lifting or moving it. An effort should be made to use only the palms of the hands or the flat surface of the extended fingers. The reason for this is apparent when we realize that fingertips can sink into the damp plaster and make impressions through the thickness of the cast, thus pressing mounds of plaster against the tissues under the cast. These can harden and will in time lead to pressure sores.

Drying the Cast. The speed with which a plaster cast will dry is directly affected by (1) the humidity of the atmosphere around the cast, and (2) circulation of air around the cast.

Thick body casts sometimes take several days to dry out completely. Others, such as the thin casts for clubfoot or long-leg casts, may dry within a few hours. A cast dryer, similar in principle to a hair dryer, may be used to speed up the evaporation of moisture from the cast. The advantage of using the dryer is the increased circulation of air around the cast, NOT the application of heat. The use of heat is dangerous because it may easily lead to burns under the cast. It is also possible that heat exhaustion and excessive loss of body fluids from perspiration will

Figure 11-4. Proper support of cast so that weight of body does not flatten curves in cast. (From Wiebe: *Orthopedics in Nursing*, W. B. Saunders Co., Philadelphia.)

occur. A dryer should not be used without a written order.

Frequent turning of the patient helps the cast dry evenly and prevents prolonged pressure and flattening of one side of the cast. The patient should always be turned onto his "good side," i.e., with the fractured limb uppermost, while the cast is drying.

Bed cradles are not advisable, as they trap the moisture and increase the humidity around the cast. The patient in a cast may experience chilling from the dampness. He should be covered adequately with blankets but the cast must remain uncovered until it is thoroughly dry.

It is not possible to determine whether a cast is dry simply by feeling its surface; therefore, it should be handled very carefully for the first few days or until the physician states specifically that the cast is dry. A dry cast is white, has a shiny surface, and will resound when tapped. A wet cast is grayish and dull in appearance and will give a dull thud when tapped.

Complications to Be Watched for. Gangrene and/or paralysis can result from swelling under the cast or pressure on an area that is not properly supported. It is the responsibility of the nurse to make frequent and intelligent observations of her patient and to report any unusual events promptly and accurately. The following statements will serve as a guide for the nurse caring for the patient in a cast.

1. *Listen to the patient's complaints.* If he complains of numbness, a tingling sensation, or sharp localized pain due to pressure of the cast, report it immediately. Do not attempt to judge whether his complaints are justifiable. A dull throbbing pain can sometimes be relieved by elevating the limb. If not, this should also be reported.

2. *Observe the fingers or toes protruding from a cast for signs of impaired circulation.* These signs include a bluish-gray discoloration of the skin, coldness to the touch, or slow return of color to the skin after pressure by a finger.

3. *A sudden, unexplained elevation of temperature or unusual odor may indicate infection.* Either of these signs should be brought to the attention of the nurse in charge or the physician.

4. *Check frequently to see if the cast is properly supported or if there is undue pressure on any one part of the body.*

Daily Care. After the cast is thoroughly dry and the initial swelling under the cast has subsided, the practical nurse must concern herself with the cleanliness of the patient and the cast. The problems involved will vary according to the type of cast and the area it covers. All parts of the body not included in the cast should be bathed daily, using care not to wet the cast with bath water. The skin around the edges of the cast should receive special attention, including massage with alcohol or lotion and close observation for signs of pressure or breaks in the skin. The edges of plaster casts tend to crumble, with bits of plaster dropping down inside the cast and causing the patient discomfort and skin irritation. This can be avoided by covering the rims of the cast with stockinette or tape.

Wetting a cast will cause it to disintegrate rapidly. After it has been thoroughly dried a cast can be painted with shellac or varnish which allows for cleaning of the surface and removal of stains without damage to the cast.

The patient in a long-leg cast or a spica can very easily soil the cast when attempting to use the bedpan. The problem of protecting the cast is even more difficult when the patient is a very young child who is not yet toilet trained, or an older patient who is incontinent. To avoid soiling, the perineal area of the cast can be covered with a waterproof material, such as the waxed paper or plastic wrapping used to keep refrigerated foods airtight. The material should be applied so that it covers the outside edge of the cast and extends down inside the cast for a few inches. This covering may be changed as often as necessary and also gives the added advantage of allowing for thorough cleaning of the buttocks and perineal area without danger of wetting the cast with bath water.

When a bedpan is used by the patient in a spica there is the possibility of a backward flow of urine under the cast unless the head of the bed is slightly elevated. Since the patient cannot bend at the hips to sit up on the pan the head of the bed should be elevated on shock blocks or some other device and the lumbar area of the cast supported to prevent cracking it.

Itching is a common complaint of the patient in a cast. Patients must be instructed not to use sharp objects such as pencils or rulers to scratch under the cast. These can, of course, tear the skin, leaving an open break for the entrance of bacteria. A coat hanger, bent so there is a safe round edge to use for scratching, will help the patient who is determined to scratch. This can be suggested, but may be done only with the approval of the physician.

When a cast is removed the underlying skin is usually dry and scaly. Cleaning of these areas should be done under the direction of the physician since the type of care to be given will depend on whether or not another cast is to be applied. In any case, over-enthusiastic scrubbing of the area must be avoided so as to prevent damage to the deeper layers of skin.

NURSING CARE OF THE PATIENT IN TRACTION

Types and Uses of Traction. Traction is the application of a mechanical *pull* to a part of the body for the purpose of extending and holding that part in a certain position. Through a system of ropes and pulleys, weights are attached to a fixed point below the area of injury or disease. The apparatus is rigged so that the weights on one end and the weight of the patient's body on the other will pull the affected part in opposite directions, thus straightening and holding that part in the desired position. There are several ways of accomplishing this. The two general types of traction are *skeletal* and *skin traction.* In skeletal traction the surgeon inserts pins, wires, or tongs directly through the bone at a point distal to the fracture so that the force of pull from the weights is exerted directly on the bone. With skin traction a bandage such as moleskin or ace-adherent is applied to the limb below the site of fracture and the pull is exerted on the limb in this manner. For cervical traction, either method may be used. Crutchfield tongs are inserted directly into the skull for skeletal traction, or a cloth head halter may be applied for skin traction (Fig. 11-5).

The most common types of traction apparatus used are Bryant's traction for small children, Russell traction, and the Thomas splint with Pearson attachment (see Fig. 11-6).

Traction is used in the treatment of fractures and contracture deformities and to relieve the muscle spasm of severe back pain.

Most traction patients must lie on their backs with a limited amount of turning on either side. This is not an excuse for neglect of the patient's back. He still must be kept clean and comfortable and free of pressure sores. Special back care, particularly in the sacral region where pressure is greatest, must be given every hour. This includes a gentle massaging of the area with lotion, use of a rubber ring at intervals to relocate the area of pressure, and careful attention to keeping the bottom sheet clean, dry, and free of wrinkles.

The bottom sheets are always changed *starting with the unaffected side.* This decreases the number of times the affected side is disturbed. To provide adequate covering of the patient two sets of top linen may be used if specially made fracture linen is not available. One set covers the upper half of the body and the other set covers the lower half and the unaffected limb. A small

Figure 11-5. *A*, Skeletal traction of the cervical vertebrae, using tongs. *B*, Halter traction, applying straight pull on the cervical vertebrae. (From Wiebe: *Orthopedics in Nursing*, W. B. Saunders Co., Philadelphia.)

Figure 11-6. Various types of traction. (From Wiebe: *Orthopedics in Nursing*, W. B. Saunders Co., Philadelphia.)

cotton baby blanket may be used to cover the limb in traction.

If the physician will not permit turning the patient far enough to allow for adequate back care the patient may use a trapeze bar to lift himself so that back care can be given and the bottom sheet changed or tightened. The patient should be instructed to lift himself straight up so that the amount of pull exerted on the limb in traction will not be altered. This same manuever can be used when the patient is placed on a bedpan (see Fig. 11-7). A small, child-size bedpan should be used and the lower back supported by a small pillow or folded blanket.

Frequent observations of both the patient and the traction apparatus should include the following:

1. *Be sure the weights are hanging free.* If the weights are resting on or against any support such as the foot of the bed or the floor, the purpose of the traction is lost. Be careful not to bump against the weights when walking around the foot of the bed. This can be painful to the patient and may cause damage to the diseased bone. It is not necessary to lift the weights when pulling the patient up in bed. The amount of pull on the limb will remain the same as long as the weights are hanging free.

2. *Check the position of the patient, making sure his body weight is counteracting the pull of the weights.* Should the patient slip down in bed so that his feet are resting against the footboard, there will be a loss of force exerted on the limb.

3. Observe all bony prominences for signs of impaired circulation and tissue necrosis.

4. Observe the patient's posture in bed and position of joints for proper alignment.

CARE OF THE PATIENT ON A FRAME

There are times when the nursing care of a patient with an orthopedic condition is extremely difficult if the patient is lying on a conventional hospital bed. To solve the nursing problems brought about by these conditions there are specially designed frames or orthopedic beds available. The Stryker frame and Foster bed are examples of these frames. They are used (1) to facilitate the nursing care and frequent turning of patients who are helpless, (2) to aid in immobilizing the spine as a means of treating spinal fractures and other diseases of the spine, and (3) to provide a means of keeping clean and dry those patients who cannot be moved for placement of a bedpan, or those who are incontinent.

There are several modifications of the frames but the basic structure consists of two metal frames covered with

Figure 11-7. Patient lifts body straight up by pushing down with one or both feet and pulling up on trapeze. Small of back is supported by nurse's hand. After patient is on bedpan, a folded towel may be used to support the lumbar curve of spine. (From Wiebe: *Orthopedics in Nursing*, W. B. Saunders Co., Philadelphia.)

a heavy duck or canvas material. One of the frames is designed so that there is a perineal opening under the buttocks and this frame is used when the patient is lying on his back. The second frame is covered so that it matches its mate and is used when the patient is lying in a prone position. The position of the patient may be alternated from back to abdomen by using alternate frames. In the prone position the head of the patient is supported with a strap across the forehead so that the face is uncovered, allowing for eating, reading, or any other simple recreational activity. In addition to the frames there are detachable supports for the arms, and a footboard attachment for proper positioning of the patient's feet.

Since turning the patient is a comparatively easy procedure when these frames are used, many complications caused by the patient's lying in one position too long can be avoided. It must be remembered, however, that these patients are *more likely to develop decubitus ulcers* than those in a conventional bed unless they are turned at least every two hours.

Turning the Patient. The practical nurse caring for a patient on a frame must seek instruction in the use of these frames before accepting any responsibility for such a task. Unless the patient is turned quickly and smoothly and is adequately strapped onto the frame, there is danger of injury to the patient and disturbance of the body alignment desired by the physician. It is strongly recommended that the practical nurse observe and assist with the use of the frame before attempting to care for the patient on a frame (see Fig. 11-8).

Daily Care. When bathing the patient on a frame, the usual procedure for a bed bath must be altered. The anterior portion of the patient's body is washed while the patient is lying on the posterior frame. He is then turned onto the matching frame while the remaining portions of the body are bathed.

There should be adequate support of

Figure 11-8. The Stryker turning frame. (Courtesy of the Orthopedic Frame Company, Kalamazoo, Michigan.)

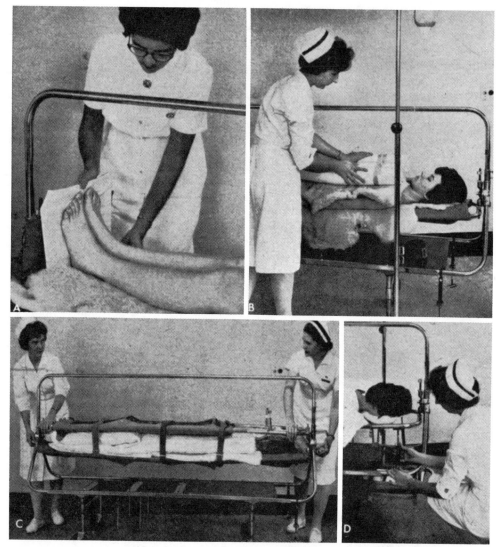

Figure 11-9. *A*, Foot support, taken from the posterior frame, is used to prevent foot drop. *B*, Rolls of foam rubber and pillow supports prevent pressure on patient's chest and upper abdomen. *C*, The anterior frame is securely strapped and screwed into position prior to turning the patient. Nurses stand at head and at foot of frame to execute the turn. *D*, The turn accomplished, the posterior frame is removed and the arm boards and the utility board are positioned. (From Dalton: *American Journal of Nursing*, February, 1964.)

the buttocks over the perineal opening of the frame while the patient is on his back, or there will be a disturbance of alignment of the spine and added pressure on the sacral region. When the patient wishes to use the bedpan, the perineal or buttock strap is removed and the pan is placed on the rack beneath the opening. A piece of waterproof material may be tucked up under the buttocks and the other end placed in the bedpan to direct the flow of urine into the bedpan. Before replacing the supporting strap under the buttocks, the perineum and buttocks are thoroughly cleaned, dried and powdered.

CRUTCH WALKING

Introduction. For the convalescent patient or one who may always need support while walking, crutches can mean the difference between freedom to move about and confinement to one location. Before attempting to walk with crutches one should have sufficient instruction in their use and

Figure 11-10. Above, the tripod position. All gaits begin from this stance. Below, the four-point alternate gait, the slowest and safest crutch gait. It offers maximum balance and support because there are always three points of contact with the ground. The right crutch is brought forward, then the left foot. The left crutch comes forward and then the right foot. *(Continued on following pages.)*

Figure 11-10 *continued.* This three-point gait, used by patients who can bear a little weight on their injured leg or foot, begins from the tripod position. Both crutches and the affected leg are brought forward at the same time. The patient must then rest lightly on the crutches while she moves forward the unaffected limb.

Figure 11-10 *continued.* This three-point is used by patients who cannot bear any weight on the affected leg or foot. It begins from the tripod position. Then both crutches are brought forward and the uninjured leg is swung through the crutches. The affected leg is kept off the ground. *(Continued on next page.)*

Figure 11-10 *continued.* The swing-through gait is used mainly by paraplegics and severe arthritics who have good balance and muscle power in the arms and hands. From the tripod position, both crutches are brought forward. The patient bears down on the handpieces, lifts the body, and swings it through crutches into a reversed tripod position. To maintain balance in this gait, pelvis moves first, then shoulders and head.

Figure 11-10 *continued.* The swing-to gait is slower than the swing-through gait. From the tripod position, the patient places both crutches forward and then swings his body ahead into a tripod position. The crutches and feet must never be even or patient loses stability. In the drag-to gait, the feet are slid along the ground and not raised. (From: *The Modern Medical Encyclopedia*, Vol. 3, Western Publishing Co., Ind., Racine, Wisconsin.)

manipulation so that they can be handled safely and effectively. The ease with which some persons apparently handle themselves on crutches is the result of patience and hard work to learn the proper use of crutches.

The type of crutch to be used will depend on the amount of disability or paralysis present and the patient's ability to bear weight and keep his balance on his feet. If the crutches are too short or too long they can create problems of lifting and moving about for the patient. In regard to this one must bear in mind that the muscles of the arms, shoulders, back and chest are all used in the manipulation of crutches. Since this is true, many physical therapists start the patient on special exercises to strengthen these muscles several weeks before the patient begins to use the crutches.

Gaits. The patient usually learns at least two gaits if he is to be using the crutches for an extended period of time. Usually he learns one for rapid movement and one for walking in crowded conditions or close quarters.

The gaits described in Fig. 11-10 are those most often used. The term "point" indicates the number of points of contact with the ground. A three-point gait, for example, uses two crutches and one foot; a four-point gait uses both feet and two crutches.

FRACTURES

Definition. A fracture is a break or interruption in the continuity of a bone. The amount of injury to the neighboring tissues varies according to the type of fracture, but at the site of injury there is always some degree of tissue destruction, interference with the blood supply, and disturbance of muscle activity in that area.

Types of Fractures. *Complete fracture* is the breaking of a bone into two parts with complete separation of the two broken ends. An *incomplete fracture* is the breaking of a bone into two parts but the two fragments are not completely separated.

A *comminuted* fracture is one in which the bone is broken and shattered into more than two fragments.

A *closed (simple) fracture* is one in which there is no break in the skin.

An *open (compound) fracture* is one in which there is a break in the skin through which the fragments of broken bone protrude.

A *greenstick fracture*, commonly found in children, is one in which the bone is partially bent and partially broken. Other types of fracture may be classified according to their appearance on x-ray (see Fig. 11-11).

Treatment. The primary aim in the treatment of fractures is the establish-

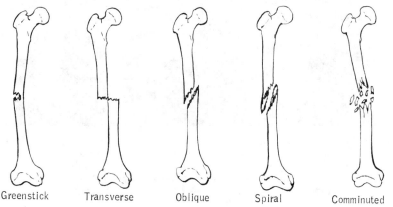

Greenstick   Transverse   Oblique   Spiral   Comminuted

Figure 11-11. Types of fractures classified according to their appearance on x-ray. (From Wiebe: *Orthopedics in Nursing*, W. B. Saunders Co., Philadelphia.)

ment of a sturdy union between the broken ends of bone so that the bone can be restored to its former state of continuity. The healing and repair of a fracture begins immediately after the bone is broken and goes through four stages:

1. Blood oozing from the torn blood vessels in the area of the fracture clots and begins to form a hematoma between the two broken ends of bone.

2. Other tissue cells enter the clot and granulation tissue is formed. This tissue is interlaced with capillaries, and it gradually becomes firm and forms a bridge between the two ends of broken bone.

3. Young bone cells enter the area and form a tissue called "woven bone." At this stage the ends of the broken bone are beginning to "knit" together.

4. The immature bone cells are gradually replaced by mature bone cells and the tissue takes on the characteristics of typical bone structure.

It is hoped that a thorough understanding of these stages of healing in the process of bone repair will make the practical nurse more aware of the need for gentle handling of a fractured bone while it is in the process of healing.

To facilitate the process of repair and insure proper healing of the bone without deformity or loss of function, the surgeon must bring the two broken ends together in proper alignment and then immobilize the affected part until healing is complete. The procedure for bringing the two fragments of bone into proper alignment is called *reduction of the fracture* (see Fig. 11-12).

There are three methods of reducing a fracture: (1) closed reduction, (2) open reduction, and (3) internal fixation.

Closed reduction is done by manual manipulation of the bone without making a surgical incision into the skin. A general anesthetic may be given before the fracture is reduced.

An *open reduction* is done after a surgical incision is made through the skin and down to the bone at the site of the fracture. In cases of open (compound) fractures, or comminuted fractures, an open reduction is always necessary so

Figure 11-12. Illustrations of various methods of internal fixation, using plates, pins, nails, or screws to hold fragments of bone in place. (From Wiebe: *Orthopedics in Nursing*, W. B. Saunders Co., Philadelphia.)

that adequate cleansing of the area and removal of bone fragments can be done.

When a fracture cannot be properly reduced by either open or closed reduction, and it is impossible to guarantee adequate union of the bone fragments, the physician must perform a procedure called *internal fixation* of the bone. This means that pins, nails, screws, or metal plates must be used to stabilize the position of the two broken ends. This type of operation is particularly useful in the treatment of fractures in elderly patients whose bones are brittle and will not heal properly (see Fig. 11-13).

In elderly patients who have suffered a fracture of the head of the femur the surgeon may choose to take out the broken head fragments and replace it with a prosthesis. This device is designed so that it has a ball to replace the head of the femur and is shaped so that it can be fitted into or onto the shaft of the femur in such a way that the patient can bear weight on it. Although a prosthesis is not as good as a normal hip joint, many patients who have such a prosthesis are able to walk again and use the limb effectively.[11]

Nursing Care. The emergency treatment and nursing care of fractures consist of preventing shock and hemorrhage and the immediate immobilization of the part to avoid unnecessary damage to the soft tissues adjacent to the fracture. For the emergency care of a possible fracture the reader is referred to Chapter 20.

After an x-ray picture of the injured part has been made and the type of fracture and extent of damage established, the physician will decide which method to use in reducing the fracture and providing immobilization. There is always some degree of pain with a fracture because of muscle spasm, but after proper reduction this pain should be relieved. A constant unrelenting pain in the area may indicate nonunion and improper reduction and should be reported to the physician.

Since an open fracture is very easily infected, the nurse must use extreme care in changing the dressings and caring for the wound. Any rise in temperature, foul odor, or purulent discharge should be reported immediately.

The nursing care of the patient in traction or a cast has been discussed earlier in this chapter (see pp. 189-192).

AMPUTATION

Definition. An amputation is the surgical removal of a limb or part of a limb. It is a very serious operation and brings about many emotional, physical and sometimes financial problems for the patient and his family.

Indications for Amputation. Severe physical trauma, malignancy and gan-

Figure 11-13. Reduction of a fractured bone. A gradual pull is exerted on the distal (lower) fragment of the bone until it is in alignment with the proximal fragment. (From Wiebe: *Orthopedics in Nursing*, W. B. Saunders Co., Philadelphia.)

grene are the most common indications for an amputation. When the surgeon removes a limb he cuts away only the damaged tissue and always tries to leave enough of a stump so that a prosthesis (artificial limb) may be properly fitted. For some patients two or more surgical procedures may be necessary before the stump is in condition to receive a prosthesis. During the time before complete closure of the wound, the stump is kept in traction (see Fig. 11-14). This is done to prevent flexion contracture in the remaining part of the limb.

Preoperative Nursing Care. Unless the amputation is an emergency procedure following severe trauma, the physician will tell the patient that removal of the limb is necessary and assist him in plans for rehabilitation, including fitting and use of the prosthesis. Additional plans for rehabilitation of the patient give him something to look forward to. This will be a very difficult time for the patient as he awaits a surgical procedure that will undoubtably leave him handicapped. He will need sympathetic understanding and a great deal of encouragement from the nursing staff to help him over this period of adjustment.

Physical preparation of the surgical area includes shaving and thorough cleaning of the affected limb. If the surgeon wishes additional preparation with special antiseptics and wrapping of the part in sterile towels he will give a written order to that effect.

Postoperative Nursing Care. Immediately after surgery the stump is elevated on a pillow. There will be some oozing of blood and serum, so the pillow should be protected with some waterproof material. The drainage must be watched carefully and any large or sudden increase in amount or change in its color to a bright red, indicating fresh bleeding, must be reported immediately. Since sudden hemorrhage may occur with any amputation, a large tourniquet must be kept at the bedside at all times during the postoperative period. In order to prevent hip flexion contractures while the amputee is confined to bed he should be encouraged to lie on his abdomen as much as possible, especially when he is sleeping. The nurse also must be careful to support the limb and hip (if it is not in traction) with a blanket roll or pillow so that external rotation and abduction of the limb are avoided.

Exercises are usually begun soon after the amputation so that the patient may

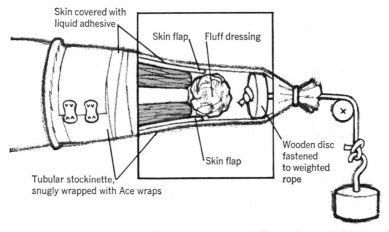

Figure 11-14. Prior to closure, stump is kept in traction. Fluff dressing soaked in Betadine covers open end of stump; tubular stockinette is held in place with liquid adhesive, Ace wrap. (From Kirkpatrick: American Journal of Nursing, May, 1968.)

begin to strengthen the muscles he will use most while wearing an artificial limb. When a lower limb has been removed the patient must learn how to balance himself on one leg, how to stoop and bend over without losing his balance and how to use his back muscles to maintain good posture while wearing an artificial limb. The use of crutches and fitting and applying an artificial limb are best supervised by a physical therapist.

Sensations referred to as "phantom sensations" or "ghost pains" in the limb which has been removed are not unusual. The patient may insist he has pain in his toes or cramps in his foot after his foot or leg has been removed. These sensations are very real and are not the result of superstition or an overactive imagination. The patient actually experiences these sensations because the nerves which formerly led to the foot or lower leg are still functioning and therefore carrying impulses to the brain. The nerve ending in the stump may be compared to a "live" electric wire; that is, the wire may have been shortened but it still carries electrical charges. The nerves may have been shortened but they are still in the remainder of the limb and their endings are sensitive and capable of transmitting impulses. Early ambulation and early weight bearing on the stump are often helpful in reducing phantom sensations. It is sometimes necessary for the surgeon to reopen the stump and remove more nerve tissue, but this is not always successful, as there are still some nerve endings left and they can continue to transmit sensations of discomfort.

Emotional Aspects and Rehabilitation. Unless there are complicating factors that will prevent early ambulation, most surgeons agree that the most important factor in successful rehabilitation of the amputee is early ambulation so that the patient can see for himself that he can eventually become independent once again. The elderly and chronically ill can benefit from a positive yet realistic approach to their problems. The nurse must, of course, avoid giving false hopes or unreal assurances that everything is going to be all right. It is insulting to the patient to tell him that he will be "just like new again" when he obviously can't be restored to his former state of health. On the other hand, tears and a long face won't do much toward giving him courage to face his problems and work toward a solution. By helping her patient find short-range goals that can be accomplished without great difficulty and that indicate progress toward independence the nurse can be of real help to the amputee. For example, she can guide him toward devising ways in which he can meet his own personal needs such as bathing and shaving. Later, he can be encouraged to sit up, exercise his other limbs and assist with changing his dressing. Finally, she can set for him the goal of wearing a prosthesis successfully and walking without assistance.

SPRAIN

A sprain involves the stretching of the ligaments around a joint so that there is a rupture of the fibers. This leads to an inflammation and some small hemorrhages in the area. The result is pain, bruising, and swelling with loss of function. Sprain is treated with rest, support of the joint and ligaments with an elastic bandage, elevation of the part to reduce the swelling, and local applications of heat and cold.

DISLOCATION

Definition. A dislocation involves stretching and tearing of the ligaments around a joint with complete separation of the bones which make up the joint. Dislocation occurs most frequently at the shoulder joint, knee joint, and the jaw. The symptoms are severe pain aggravated by motion of the joint, muscle spasm, and an abnormal appearance of the joint.

Figure 11-15. A young Marine wheels to parallel bars, gingerly puts his weight on temporary prosthesis, and takes his first step. (From Kirkpatrick: Anerican Journal of Nursing, May, 1968.)

Treatment. As soon as possible, a dislocated joint must be reduced, that is, returned to its normal position. If reduction is delayed certain pathological changes will take place within the joint, making reduction and future normal motion of the joint very difficult to accomplish. After reduction the joint is immobilized by a bandage or cast.

OSTEOMYELITIS

Definition. Osteomyelitis is a bacterial infection of the bone. The causative organism is most often *Staphylococcus aureus,* which enters the blood stream from a distant focus of infection such as a boil or furuncle, or from an open wound as in an open (compound) fracture. It occurs most often in children under the age of 15, and is usually found in the tibia or fibula.

Symptoms. Osteomyelitis has a sudden onset with severe pain and marked tenderness at the site, high fever with chills, swelling of adjacent soft parts, headache, and malaise.

Diagnosis. Diagnosis is made on the basis of (1) laboratory findings indicating an acute infection, e.g., high sedimentation rate and white cell count, (2) x-rays, which may show bone destruction 7 to 10 days after onset of the disease, (3) history of injury to the part, open fracture, boils, furuncles or other infections, and (4) biopsy, in which the bone sample exhibits signs of necrosis.

Treatment and Nursing Care. The earlier the condition is diagnosed and treatment is begun the better the prognosis. General treatment and nursing care are aimed at improving and maintaining the physicial condition of the patient through adequate fluid, mineral, and vitamin intake. Specific treatment includes elimination of the infection through the use of antibiotics and immobilization and absolute rest of the affected limb. In some unusually stubborn infections this treatment is not adequate and surgical incision for drainage of the abscess and removal of dead bone and debris from the site of infection is necessary.

The problem of keeping a formerly active and alert child quiet and content during the weeks of immobilization of the affected bone is a challenge to the nursing team. The parents should be informed of the purpose of the immobilization so that they may cooperate with the physician and nurses in their efforts to limit the child's activities. Attractive meals and menus planned with some consideration for the child's preferences will help to maintain adequate nutrition during the time he cannot be active and will not have much appetite or interest in food. It is also important that the child be protected from other infections during the acute and convalescent phases of the disease. After dismissal from the hospital both the child and the parents should be cautioned against his participation in strenuous games and activities which may lead to injury of the affected limb.

ARTHRITIS

Definition. The term "arthritis" is used to cover all inflammatory diseases of the joints. Actually, research has shown there are approximately 100 different types of arthritis, but all are capable of producing disability and most are generally treated in the same manner. For classification of arthritis and rheumatism see Table 13.

Etiology. The exact cause of arthritis is not yet known; however, there are some definitely established predisposing factors. These include:

1. Infection, the most common being with streptococcus, staphylococcus and gonococcus.
2. Trauma, overweight, and/or poor posture.
3. Prolonged physical stress and strain (see Fig. 11-16).
4. Emotional disturbances.
5. Metabolic disorders (gout)
6. Heredity.

Table 13. *Classification of Arthritis and Rheumatism**

    I. Polyarthritis of unknown etiology
        A. Rheumatoid arthritis
        B. Juvenile rheumatoid arthritis (Still's disease)

   II. "Connective tissue" disorders
        A. Systemic lupus erythematosus
        B. Polyarteritis nodosa
        C. Scleroderma
        D. Polymyositis and dermatomyositis

  III. Rheumatic fever

  IV. Degenerative joint disease
        Primary/secondary osteoarthritis, osteoarthrosis

   V. Nonarticular rheumatism
        A. Myositis
        B. Tenosynovitis

  VI. Associated with known infectious agents

 VII. Traumatic or neurogenic disorders.

VIII. Allergy and drug reactions

  IX. Miscellaneous and associated diseases

*From Marmor, et al.: American Journal of Nursing, July, 1967. Reprinted with permission.

7 STEPS IN TIME

Case histories of women crippled by arthritis usually show long hours of hard work, in the home or outside, with little rest or relaxation.

With this in mind doctors urge women to take steps to prevent arthritis. They have special advice for housewives and mothers:

1	Relax your housekeeping standards a bit
2	Don't do all your ironing in one batch Rest at the half way mark
3	Do your major house cleaning by installments; rest a day between bouts
4	Take it easier with the children.
5	Keep rested, relaxed and well nourished, but not overweight.
6	Protect yourself against cold and dampness and get sunshine when possible
7	Avoid strain, fatigue and worry and you will lessen your chances of suffering from arthritis

Figure 11-16. Steps to prevent arthritis in women. (From a pamphlet published by the Arthritis and Rheumatism Foundation, 10 Columbus Circle, New York.)

Symptoms. In most cases the onset of arthritis is slow and gradual with weight loss, malaise, and pain in the joints. In the less common acute form of arthritis the symptoms occur more rapidly and are extreme in nature with a high temperature, severe joint pain, elevated white cell count and prostration of the individual.

Rheumatoid Arthritis

Introduction. The most crippling and one of the most common types of arthritis is rheumatoid arthritis. It is a disease of connective tissue and may affect not only the joints, but the nerves, tendons, muscles and blood vessels as well. Rheumatoid arthritis is second only to heart disease as a cause of permanent disability.

According to the handbook for patients, "Home Care in Arthritis," issued by the Arthritis and Rheumatism Foundation, the progressive changes that occur as a result of rheumatoid arthritis are as follows:

As the disease progresses, structures in and around joints become thickened and shortened, with consequent limitation of motion. Pain itself becomes a very important factor in the limitation of joint motion. In good health there is a happy balance between the opposing sets of muscles, but in rheumatoid arthritis there develops an imbalance, which gradually bends fingers, arms, legs, and even the spine, making it difficult to keep full motion in a joint. One finds it increasingly difficult to straighten out his fingers, or perhaps his knee. Muscles become tight in an effort to protect a joint from the pain resulting from motion to the joint. All these changes tend to limit motion.*

Treatment and Nursing Care. Because rheumatoid arthritis can be such a crippling disease if left untreated, treatment is aimed at relief of discomfort, prevention of deformity, rehabilitation of the patient, and physical and emotional support.

RELIEF OF PAIN. The relief of joint

---

*See Student Reading No. 1.

pain in arthritis is most often achieved by use of the salicylates. These would include aspirin, Empirin, and sodium salicylate. The amount prescribed is quite large and averages about 12 tablets of 5 grains each per day, or a total of 60 grains daily. These drugs are preferred for most patients because they are relatively safe and inexpensive and they tend to retard the inflammatory process in the joints as well as provide relief from pain. The nurse should be aware, however, that these drugs can produce side effects such as gastrointestinal irritation and bleeding, ringing in the ears, hearing loss and hyperpnea. Codeine and other narcotics for relief of pain are used with great caution because of the danger of addiction, which can be a real threat when it is necessary to control pain in a chronic disease.

Other drugs used in the treatment of arthritis include *antimalarial compounds* such as chloroquine phosphate and gold sodium thiosulfate; the *corticosteroids* such as prednisone and hydrocortisone; and the *phenylbutazones* such as Butazolidin and Tandearil. It should be emphasized that no drug will cure arthritis and that those available for relief of symptoms can produce serious and sometimes irreversible side effects. This is especially true of the phenylbutazones, which are highly toxic. For this reason they are prescribed with caution and on an individual basis. The effectiveness of these various drugs is extremely difficult to evaluate because arthritis tends to subside and then flare up again for no apparent reason, and if a patient is taking a drug at the time his symptoms subside he may readily, and perhaps falsely, conclude that the drug was the cause of the remission. Another factor is the hope of the patient that the drug will work. Studies have shown that as a group arthritics respond more favorably to placebo medications than other patients. This probably is one reason that fraudulent cures and quackery are so successful in their appeal to many victims of arthritis.

Application of heat is often recommended for temporary relief of pain and reduction of joint stiffness and swelling. Some patients receive hot soaks and paraffin baths on an outpatient basis at a clinic or receive deep heat through short-wave diathermy under the supervision of a physical therapist. The patient also may obtain some relief at home by submerging the painful joint in a tub or pan of water heated to about 100° F. Or, if the joint cannot be submerged with ease, the patient may apply hot towels for 10-minute periods several times a day.

PREVENTION OF DEFORMITY. A regimen of *rest and exercise* is recommended for the arthritic patient. It is important to realize that neither alone will do the job of preventing deformities. To guard against fixation of the joints, contractures or atrophy of the muscles, prescribed exercises are necessary. Because motion can cause pain, both the nurse and the patient must realize the danger of allowing a joint to remain in one position for long periods of time. The exercises should be carried out slowly and carefully and strictly according to the directions

Table 14. *General Exercises**

Back Lying

_____Times Hands together, bring arms overhead—elbows as close to ears as possible—stretch but stop at point of pain.

_____Times Hands together—make big circles—*OUT UP AND OVER*. May use stick or wand.

_____Times Shoulders and elbows at right angles—roll arms forward and backward.

_____Times Elbows at right angles—roll forearms so that palms face you and face away from you.

_____Times Bring alternate knees to chest. (You should keep other knee and hip bent about 45 degrees if comfortable.)

_____Times Straight leg raising with other knee bent at 45 to 90 degrees if comfortable.

_____Times Ankle circling—both directions.

_____Times Roll legs in and then out.

_____Times One at a time, spread legs apart, then bring back to the midline.

Face Lying

_____Times Arms at sides—raise arms up, bring shoulder blades together.

_____Times Arms at sides—raise head and shoulders.

_____Times Bend alternate knees.

_____Times Pinch buttocks together.

_____Times Raise legs alternately from hips—keep knees straight.

Sitting or Lying

_____Times Make fist.

_____Times Straighten fingers completely—assist with other hand if necessary.

_____Times Keeping hand flat, bring each finger toward thumb (use powder or finger paints if helpful).

_____Times Oppose each finger and thumb (ball of digits),

*From Marmor, et al.: American Journal of Nursing, July, 1967. Reprinted with permission.

of the physician or physical therapist. Overstretching of the muscles and tendons or overuse of the joint can be more harmful than helpful. Exercises do not necessarily need to hurt to be effective in maintaining motion.

Rest is also an essential part of the arthritic patient's treatment. It reduces inflammation and relieves some of the emotional strain, tension, fatigue and worry that are frequently associated with an exacerbation of the patient's symptoms.

Good positioning of the body is essential at all times, whether the patient is lying, sitting or standing. Earlier in this chapter we discussed the various methods of changing body positions as well as maintaining proper joint positions. These must be diligently applied when caring for an arthritic patient, particularly one who is confined to bed for a period of time. When the ambulatory patient is resting he should understand and follow the principles of good posture in a bed or chair.

ORTHOPEDIC DEVICES. In the early stages of rheumatoid arthritis severe muscle spasms and accompanying pain can rapidly lead to serious deformities, particularly of the upper and lower extremities. There are specially designed splints and braces that hold the joint in a position of maximum function and provide rest. These corrective devices are also designed in such a way that they can increase joint function and relieve pain.

When arthritic changes involve the joints of the feet there are special orthopedic shoes that the patient can wear to prevent deformities. These shoes also can redistribute weight-bearing stresses on the foot so that pain and injury to the joints are lessened.

SURGERY. In recent years there has been an increased use of surgical procedures in the treatment of arthritis. Formerly, surgery was a kind of "last ditch" measure to be used when all other measures had failed and the patient was severely handicapped with serious deformities. It is now considered feasible in some cases to use surgical intervention as a means of preventing such deformities, relieving pain and arresting the progress of the disease.[9]

The type of surgery done will depend on the joint involved and the specific kind of deformity present. For example, if the synovium of the joint is diseased, a synovectomy (removal of the synovium and repair of the tendons) is done. If the muscles and tendons are involved, causing a tightness of the extensor mechanism, these muscles and tendons will also require surgical correction. It is believed that surgical treatment of arthritic joints is fast becoming accepted as another useful tool in the hands of those who are working toward relief of symptoms and prevention of disability in the arthritic patient.

DIET. There is no special diet that will cure or relieve arthritis, in spite of many fraudulent claims to the contrary. The patient should eat an average, well-balanced diet with no excess or limitations in amount or types of foods. Obesity can contribute to additional stress on the weight-bearing joints and aggravate the arthritic condition. This should be explained to the patient who has a tendency to be overweight so he can be properly motivated and encouraged to lose weight and continue to keep his weight within normal limits.

EMOTIONAL FACTORS. It is now believed that joint diseases such as rheumatoid arthritis are definitely related in some way to personality and emotional factors. Obviously, any disease that hampers physical activity and produces pain, that often results in an unattractive appearance, and that can greatly alter one's everyday life will bring about some unpleasant emotional response in its victims. Whether the emotional upheaval is the cause of the disease or vice versa is a matter of speculation.

There is evidence that response to treatment of arthritis can vary greatly in individuals even though they may have the same amount of joint involvement and are receiving the same treatment. The patients who respond poorly are usually suffering from some emotional problems stemming from feelings of insecurity and lack of confidence in themselves. Those who respond more favorably to treatment are for the most part well-adjusted persons who think well of themselves and believe themselves to be accepted by society. One must realize, of course, that the individual's state of mind can be a result of the successful treatment rather than a cause or contributing factor. There is no doubt, however, that psychological and emotional factors do play an important role in the etiology and progress of arthritic changes in the joints. There are many instances in which emotional traumas resulting from unpleasant and uncontrollable events in a person's life have led to the development of arthritis, or to a flare-up of symptoms in a person who has a chronic form of the disease.

It is important, then, for the nurse to recognize the relationship between the patient's emotional state and his physical symptoms. She must strive to help the patient achieve serenity and peace of mind; and she should always avoid creating, by her words or actions, a situation in which she could add further to the patient's emotional problems and feelings of insecurity.[15]

Education of the Patient. As in all chronic diseases, the arthritic patient's understanding of his illness and his ability to cooperate with the physician in the treatment of his illness will go a long way toward the success of the treatment. The Arthritis and Rheumatism Foundation issues several excellent booklets for the express purpose of helping the patient and his family understand arthritis. These publications are sold for 10 cents and 15 cents and may be obtained from the local chapter of the Foundation or by writing to the Foundation at 10 Columbus Circle, New York 10019.

Osteoarthritis

Definition. Another common type of arthritis is osteoarthritis. In this type of arthritis there is a gradual "wearing out" or degeneration of the joint rather than an acute inflammatory type of process. Osteoarthritis is one of the less serious types of arthritis and rarely leads to crippling. Most persons suffering from this disease are over 40 years of age, and have only mild pain and stiffness of the joints.

The joints of the fingers are often affected, particularly in women. These fingers then take on the characteristic appearance commonly associated with this type of arthritis (see Fig. 11-17).

Treatment and Nursing Care. Since this type of arthritis is basically a process of degeneration little can be done to reverse the disease process itself. However, much can be done to eliminate the obesity, poor posture, or physical strain which may have predisposed the

Figure 11-17. Joint deformities commonly associated with osteoarthritis.

joints to the disease. The joints should also be protected from injury by accidental falls or twisting of the joints. The application of mild heat gives some relief when the discomfort becomes severe. Exercises as prescribed by the physician or physiotherapist also keep the joints active and help maintain good muscle tone. The physician may order salicylates for the relief of pain, and in some cases of poor posture or orthopedic disability he may prescribe certain orthopedic appliances. For the rare cases of severe disability, joint debridement may be necessary.

COLLAGEN DISEASES

The collagen diseases affect connective tissue. Although each collagen disease presents a distinct clinical picture, all affect various organs, cause inflammation of the connective tissue and deposit fiber-like material in the ground substance of the tissue. It is not surprising that one or more organs can be involved in a collagen disease since some type of connective tissue can be found in all organs or the body.

The cause of collagen diseases is not clearly understood, but they are believed to be related in some way to an autoimmune reaction. This means that the individual develops antibodies that are specific against his own body tissues.

Diseases that are included in the collagen group include scleroderma, systemic lupus erythematosus, polyarteritis and arthritis. Scleroderma involves the skin, joints, and blood vessels. It often is confused in its early stage with arthritis and Reynaud's disease because of the symptoms it presents. The skin gradually loses its elasticity and pigmentation and becomes hardened and mummy-like. Bodily motion is greatly restricted by the fixation of the skin and underlying tissues and involvement of the muscles and soft tissues of the joints. Systemic lupus erythematosus involves skin, blood vessels and serous and synovial membranes. It occurs in both acute and chronic form and is now known to be fairly common, occurring most often in young women.

Treatment for the collagen diseases is limited to the administration of adrenocorticosteroids for the relief of symptoms and measures to keep the patient as healthy as possible under the circumstances. The antimalarial compounds are often successful in relieving the symptoms of lupus erythematosus.

GOUT

Introduction. Gout is not a type of arthritis, but a metabolic disease. It is the result of a defect in the metabolism of purines, which are products of the digestion of proteins. This faulty metabolism results in an accumulation of uric acid in the blood, and eventually there are deposits of sodium urate crystals in the joints, kidneys, cartilage of the ear and sometimes in the heart or other internal organs. Subcutaneous deposits of urea crystals are called *tophi* and they appear in about one third of the patients who have gout.

Cause and Incidence. The cause of gout is not known. It is considered a familial disease and about 95 per cent of its victims are men. Contrary to popular belief, gout is not a rich man's disease resulting from "high living" or overindulgence in expensive and highly seasoned foods. In fact, the disease occurs most often in individuals who are in the middle and low income groups.

Symptoms. Arthritic changes with tenderness, swelling, and pain in the joints are characteristic of the acute phase of gout. The joints most often affected are those of the great toe, ankle, instep, knee, and elbow. With repeated attacks there can be permanent damage and deformity of the joint. Renal failure can occur as a result of attacks that produce urea deposits in the kidneys and thereby damage renal cells.

Treatment. Colchicine is usually used in treating gout. It helps increase the uric acid output and thereby prevents and controls acute attacks of gout. Allopurinol is a drug that acts to interfere with the formation of uric acid. It is often used in the treatment of gouty arthritis. Aspirin also may be given regularly to help increase uric acid excretions and prevent attacks. Probenecid (Benemid) is another drug used with some success.

The diet of the patient usually is slightly limited so that foods high in purines are kept at a minimum. These foods include brains, kidneys and sweetbreads. The patient also should avoid alcohol and large amounts of fat. Alkaline-ash foods such as fruit juices, vegetables and milk are helpful in inhibiting the precipitation of uric acid. Fluids are forced to help flush uric acid crystals from the kidneys.

Early treatment can help prevent serious deformities and other complications of gout. One of the first symptoms is pain in the foot at night, and although this does not necessarily indicate gout, one should be aware of the need to bring such a symptom to the attention of a physician. Once gout has been diagnosed the patient should be given a thorough explanation of the disorder with explicit instructions in the ways in which he can avoid precipitating an acute attack.

CLINICAL CASE PROBLEMS

1. Mrs. Wilkins, age 38, weight 210 pounds, has been admitted to the hospital with a diagnosis of fracture of the right femur. You have been told that when the patient returns from the cast room she will have on a hip spica. This cast will cover all the right leg and foot except the toes, and the left leg will be covered down to the knee. The body section of the cast will stop at the waistline. You have been assigned to assist in the care of Mrs. Wilkins when she returns from the cast room.

How will you prepare the bed for the patient's return?
What equipment will you anticipate needing?
How can you support the cast while it is drying?
How is the patient to be transferred from the stretcher to the bed?
What provision can be made for drying the cast?
List the observations you must make while the cast is drying.
If the doctor orders a trapeze bar installed over the patient's bed, how would you plan the procedure for getting Mrs. Wilkins on and off the bedpan?

2. Mr. Moss is a young man, age 33, who has been injured in a fall from a building on which he was working. When you are assigned to the care of this patient you are told that he has a fracture of the tibia and fibula of the left leg. These fractures were reduced under anesthesia, after which pins were inserted for skeletal traction. The accident occurred three days ago and now you are assigned to give A.M. care to this patient.

What nursing problems will skeletal traction present?
What special observations must you make?

3. Mrs. Carter, age 50, is a very obese woman who comes to the orthopedic clinic for treatment of arthritis of the knees and ankles. She has great difficulty walking and would use a wheel chair if she could afford one. Her daughter states that the patient is becoming more and more inactive and, though her mother says that she does not want to become an invalid, that she refuses to move about and do things for herself. Mrs. Carter lives alone and prefers not to live with her daughter because the grandchildren make her nervous. In fact, she prefers to be left alone because she feels that she cannot be of any use to anyone in her condition. Her daughter feels that her mother could find many useful things to do in her neighborhood if she would only try.

What problems can you see in this situation? How could proper instruction help Mrs. Carter in her illness? What effects could Mrs. Carter's attitude have on her physical condition?

4. Mrs. Lewis, age 52, has been told she has osteoarthritis. She is a very nervous individual and extremely apprehensive about her condition. While you are bathing her one morning she tells you that she knows she will be helpless and completely useless as a wife and mother within a few months because she has arthritis and she knows what a crippling disease this is. She is very depressed and refuses to help herself during the bath and changing of the bed linen, saying, "I know I will soon be an invalid and I might just as well get used to having others do everything for me."

How can you help this patient understand the type of arthritis she has and the ways in which she can prevent deformity and crippling?

REFERENCES

1. American College of Surgeons, Committee on Trauma: *The Management of Fractures and Soft Tissue Injuries.* Philadelphia, W. B. Saunders Co., 1961.
2. Arje, F. B.: "How to Teach Crutch Walking." RN, March, 1961, p. 38.
3. Beland, I.: *Clinical Nursing.* New York, The Macmillan Co., 1965.
4. Brunner, L. S., et al.: *Medical-Surgical Nursing.* Philadelphia, J. B. Lippincott Co., 1964.
5. Dalton, A.: "Using a Stryker Frame." Am. Journ. Nurs., Feb., 1964, p. 100.
6. Guyton, A. C.: *Textbook of Medical Physiology,* 3rd edition. Philadelphia, W. B. Saunders Co., 1966.
7. Harmer, B., and Henderson, V.: *Textbook of the Principles and Practice of Nursing,* 5th edition. New York, The Macmillan Co., 1960.
8. Kerr, A.: *Orthopedic Nursing Procedures.* New York, Springer Pub. Co., 1960.
9. Marmor, L., Walike, B. C., and Upshaw, M. J.: "Rheumatoid Arthritis – Surgical Intervention." Am. Journ. Nurs., July, 1967, p. 1430.
10. *Modern Medical Encyclopedia,* vol. 3. New York, Golden Press, 1965.
11. Neufeld, A. J.: "Surgical Treatment of Hip Injuries." Am. Journ. Nurs., March, 1965, p. 80.
12. Rodman, M. J.: "Drug Treatment of Gouty Arthritis." RN, Dec., 1960, p. 33.
13. Shafer, K. N., Sawyer, J. R., et al.: *Medical-Surgical Nursing,* 4th edition. St. Louis, C. V. Mosby Co., 1967.
14. Smith, D. W., and Gips, C. D.: *Care of the Adult Patient,* 2nd edition. Philadelphia, J. B. Lippincott Co., 1966.
15. Walike, B. C.: "Rheumatoid Arthritis – Personality Factors." Am. Journ. Nurs. July, 1967, p. 1427.
16. Walike, B. C., Marmor, L., and Upshaw, M. J.: "Rheumatoid Arthritis." Am. Journ Nurs., July, 1967, p. 1420.
17. Weibe, A. M.: *Orthopedics in Nursing.* Philadelphia, W. B. Saunders Co., 1961.

SUGGESTED STUDENT READING

1. Arthritis and Rheumatism Foundation (pamphlets): "Rheumatoid Arthritis," "Home Care in Arthritis," "Osteoarthritis," "Questions and Answers on Arthritis" and "About Gout."
2. "Arthritis: The Nation's No. 1 Crippler." RN, Sept., 1962, p. 65.
3. Arje, F. B.: "How to Teach Crutch Walking." RN, March, 1961, p. 38.
4. Cameron, B. M.: "Whiplash Injuries." Am. Journ. Nurs., Nov., 1962, p. 72.
5. Kirkpatrick, S.: "Battle Casualty: Amputee." Am. Journ. Nurs., May, 1968, p. 998.
6. Madden, B. W., and Affeldt, J. E.: "To Prevent Helplessness and Deformities." Am. Journ. Nurs., Dec., 1962, p. 59.
7. Magee, K. R.: "Myasthenia Gravis." Journ. Pract. Nurs., Nov., 1965, p. 23.
8. Mendelson, J. A.: "Sprains and Strains." Am. Journ. Nurs., June, 1961, p. 45.
9. Skinner, G.: "Head Traction and the Stryker Frame." Am. Journ. Nurs., June, 1952, p. 694.

OUTLINE FOR CHAPTER 11

I. Introduction

A. Orthopedics – concerned with the preservation and restoration of the functions of the skeletal system (motion, support and protection).

II. Diagnostic Tests

A. X-ray films aid in diagnosis of abnormal changes in the contour, size and density of bones.

B. Cultures aid in diagnosing infections of the bone.

C. Biopsy – samplings of cells taken from bone tumors.

III. General Nursing Care

A. Lifting and turning. Nurse must maintain good body posture of the patient.

B. Orthopedic bed making. Make the bed

with a minimum of disturbance to the limb in traction and to the skin.

C. Prevention of deformities.
1. Contractures—adaptive shortening of the muscles when they are not used and are poorly positioned.
2. Loss of muscle tone from lack of exercise.
3. Ankylosis—permanent fixation of a joint.

D. Good body posture of patient, with frequent changes of position.

E. Exercises, active or passive. Each joint should be put through its full range of motion at least once daily.

IV. Care of the Patient in a Cast

A. Cast is used to immobilize a certain part of the body so that it is firmly supported and completely at rest.

B. Preparation for application of a cast includes proper washing of the skin with soap and water and shaving if surgery is to be done.

C. Care of the fresh plaster cast: patient should be handled gently. Wet cast is picked up only with the palms of the hand. Pillows to support the cast to prevent flattening should be waterproofed. Patient must be turned frequently to avoid misshaping the cast.

D. Drying the cast: use of heat is dangerous. Circulating air is best method.

E. Complications: gangrene or paralysis can result from a cast that is too tight. Nurse must check for signs of impaired circulation, numbness or tingling, sudden or unexplained increase in temperature or unusual odor.

F. Daily care.
1. Use care not to wet cast when patient is bathed or uses bedpan.
2. Observe condition of skin at edge of cast.

V. Nursing Care of the Patient in Traction

A. Traction extends and holds part of the body in a certain position by mechanical pull. Skeletal traction exerts pull on the bone; skin traction exerts pull on the skin.

B. Nursing care.
1. Special and diligent back care.
2. Bed is made so that traction apparatus is disturbed as little as possible.
3. Weights must be hanging free, and patient positioned so that his body weight is counteracting the pull of the weights. Check bony promi-

nences frequently for signs of impaired circulation. Patient must be kept in good body alignment.

VI. Care of the Patient on a Frame

A. Stryker frame or Foster bed is used to (1) facilitate nursing care and frequent turning, (2) immobilize the spine as a means of treating fractures and other disorders of the spinal column, and (3) provide a means of keeping clean and dry for those patients who cannot be moved with ease.

VII. Crutch Walking

A. Type of crutch will depend on amount of disability and the patient's ability to bear weight and keep his balance on his feet.

B. Gaits include three-point, four-point, swing-to and swing-through gait.

VIII. Fractures

A. A break or interruption in the continuity of a bone.

B. Types.
1. Comminuted—the bone is shattered.
2. Closed (simple)—no break in the skin.
3. Open (compound)—there is a break in the skin through which fragments of broken bone protrude.
4. Greenstick—the bone is partially bent and partially broken.

C. Treatment—to establish a sturdy union between the broken ends of bone.
1. Closed reduction is done by manual manipulation without a surgical incision.
2. Open reduction—a surgical incision is made and the exposed bone is aligned.
3. Internal fixation—pins, plates or screws are used to stabilize the position of the broken ends of bone.

IX. Amputation

A. Surgical removal of a limb or part of a limb because of severe physical trauma, malignancy or gangrene.

B. Preoperative care includes thorough cleaning and shaving of the limb.

C. Postoperative care.
1. Observe for signs of hemorrhage.
2. Encourage patient to lie on his abdomen as much as possible, keeping stump in good alignment to prevent flexion contractures. Exercises are

done to keep joints from ankylosing and to prepare limb for fitting of prosthesis.

3. Phantom sensations often can be relieved by pressure on the stump.

D. Emotional aspects and rehabilitation. Early ambulation is important for improving patient's morale and helping him achieve independence. Nurse should have positive, hopeful attitude, provide her patient with short-range goals, and avoid giving false hopes.

X. *Sprain*

A. Stretching of the ligaments around a joint so that there is rupture of some of the fibers.

B. Treatment: Rest, support of the joint, elevation to relieve edema, and local applications of heat and cold.

XI. *Dislocation*

A. A stretching and tearing of the ligaments around a joint with complete separation of the bones that make up the joint.

B. Treatment: Reduction of dislocation so that joint is returned to its normal position. Immobilization accomplished by bandage or cast.

XII. *Osteomyelitis*

A. A bacterial infection of the bone.

B. Symptoms: Sudden onset with severe pain and marked tenderness at site of infection, fever, and swelling of adjacent parts.

C. Treatment: rest, antibiotics and measures to improve the general health of the patient. Surgical incision for drainage of abscess and debridement of infected bone if necessary.

XIII. *Arthritis*

A. Inflammatory diseases of the joints.

B. Exact cause unknown. Predisposing factors may include trauma, emotional disturbances and metabolic disorders.

C. Symptoms: weight loss, malaise, pain, swelling of the joints, and loss of motion.

D. Two main types:

1. Rheumatoid arthritis.
   a. Can cause permanent disability.
   b. Treatment and nursing care aimed at relief of pain, prevention of deformity, rehabilitation of the patient and physical and emotional support.
2. Osteoarthritis.
   a. Gradual wearing out and degeneration of the joint.
   b. Rarely leads to crippling.
   c. Treatment aimed at eliminating factors that may aggravate the condition.

XIV. *Collagen Diseases*

A. A group of little understood diseases that affect various organs, cause inflammation of the connective tissue and deposit fibrous material in the ground substance of such tissue.

B. Includes scleroderma, systemic lupus erythematosus, polyarteritis, and arthritis.

C. Treatment varies but the corticosteroids offer some relief from symptoms in almost all these diseases.

XV. *Gout*

A. A metabolic defect in which purines are not completely metabolized, allowing uric acid to accumulate in the blood and sodium urate crystals to be deposited.

B. Cause is unknown.

C. Symptoms include pain and swelling of the joints, especially those of the great toe, ankle, instep and knee. Renal failure can occur as a result of sodium urate crystals in the kidney.

D. Treatment includes administration of colchicine, aspirin or probenecid. Diet should be low in purines and high in alkaline-ash.

E. Early diagnosis and treatment can prevent serious deformities.

Chapter 12

NURSING CARE OF PATIENTS WITH DISORDERS OF THE CARDIOVASCULAR SYSTEM

VOCABULARY

Amino acids
Autoimmunity
Avitaminosis
Diastole
Filtration

Globulin
Platelet
Resorption
Systole
Thromboplastin

Part I — NURSING CARE OF PATIENTS WITH DISORDERS OF THE BLOOD

INTRODUCTION

The blood is actually a tissue. A little more than half of it is liquid and the remainder is composed of cells. These cells carry on some of the most important functions in the body; and since their life span is comparatively short, (a red blood cell only lives two or three months) new ones must be manufactured by the bone marrow, lymph nodes, and spleen in order to assure the body of a plentiful supply.

The white cells aid in the body's defenses against infection and the platelets assist in the clotting of blood. The red cells (erythrocytes) carry on the vital functions of transporting nutrients to all the other tissues of the body, exchanging these nutrients for waste products, and then carrying the waste to specific organs for disposal. The erythrocytes contain a pigmented protein called hemoglobin. Without hemo-

globin the red cells would not be red, nor would they be able to transport oxygen, because it is the hemoglobin which absorbs oxygen and carbon dioxide and releases them when they have reached their destinations. We can see, then, that a deficiency of hemoglobin as well as well as a substantial decrease in the number of erythrocytes can lead to serious difficulties for the other cells of the body.

The blood cells are suspended in a liquid. This liquid is called *plasma.* Plasma is a complex fluid containing antibodies, hormones and some nutritive elements and waste products. Plasma also contains *fibrinogen,* a chemical which plays an important part in the clotting of blood. When fibrinogen is removed from plasma through the formation of a clot the remaining liquid is spoken of as *serum.* Both plasma and cells contain minerals such as calcium, sodium and potassium, the electrolytes

217

so essential to the health of an individual.

The total volume of blood in the body varies from 4 to 6 quarts in a healthy adult, but it is not always the amount that matters so much as it is the quality of the blood itself. The rapid loss of a quart or more may result in death. However, a gradual loss of blood over a period of time will seriously deplete the number of red cells and lead to a serious anemia.

BLOOD DYSCRASIAS

Definition and Types. A blood dyscrasia is an abnormal or pathological condition of the blood, especially one that involves some imbalance in its elements. In general there are two types of blood dyscrasias—those present at birth *(congenital)* and those *acquired* after birth. Most congenital blood dyscrasias are a result of the body's inability to produce blood elements that are primarily concerned with the formation of blood clots. The individual who has such a condition maintains most normal physiological functions, but if there is any damage to the blood vessels he has a tendency to bleed freely because his blood will not clot normally. One of the best known examples of this type of blood dyscrasia that is present at birth is hemophilia.

Blood dyscrasias that are acquired are usually a result of some imbalance between production and destruction of certain blood elements, particularly the red blood cells. Whether production of erythrocytes is decreased or their destruction is increased, there is inevitably a deficiency of these elements. Since erythrocytes are vital to the transportation of oxygen, the body cells, which must have oxygen to carry on the metabolism that is necessary for their existence and functions, will be seriously affected by any deficiency of red blood cells. It can readily be understood, then, that a blood dyscrasia can be extremely serious and even fatal if the imbalance between supply and demand is not cor-

rected. The acquired blood dyscrasias include a number of diseases such as the various anemias, the leukemias and hemolytic jaundice.[12]

Symptoms. Although the congenital and acquired blood dyscrasias vary widely in their specific pathology, they have many symptoms in common. One of these symptoms is fatigue. This is a result of inadequate transportation of oxygen, which must be present for the body cells to transform nutrients into energy. Another symptom is dyspnea, and it too is brought about by inadequate transportation of oxygen. As the body attempts to compensate for the oxygen deficiency the heart beats faster. This will produce the symptom of increased pulse rate and the patient may be aware of palpitations of the heart. Another compensatory mechanism is the shifting of blood from the peripheral vessels to the more vital internal organs. The body does this by constricting the peripheral blood vessels so that the flow of blood through them is decreased. This produces the milder symptoms of shock and also impairs proper distribution of body heat so that the patient becomes chilled very easily.

In some dyscrasias the blood elements necessary for clotting of blood are in short supply. These elements, such as platelets, are obviously essential, and when they are lacking the patient will suffer from a tendency to bleed and is in danger of hemorrhage from the slightest injury. When blood cells such as white blood cells are lacking in sufficient numbers or behaving abnormally, as in leukemia, the patient has a greatly lowered resistance to infection and has difficulty establishing an immunity to infectious diseases.

Since the blood dyscrasias have many symptoms in common, they will also have certain principles of nursing care in common. In many instances nursing measures are governed by the patient's symptoms and the needs arising from such symptoms. To avoid repetition we have presented most of the nursing care under anemia, which is present in almost all blood dyscrasias. The reader should bear in mind that these basic principles of care can be applied to any patient with a blood dyscrasia that presents similar symptoms.

ANEMIA

Definition and Classification. "Anemia" is a term used to designate an abnormal reduction in the number of red blood cells circulating in the blood. In a healthy person there is an even balance between the production of new red cells and the disposal of old "worn-out" red cells. When something happens to upset the normal balance, anemia results. Thus, anemia is really a symptom rather than a disease.

There are various types of anemia but they may be classified into three general groups: (1) anemia from blood loss, (2) anemia resulting from a failure in blood cell production, and (3) anemia associated with an excessive destruction of red cells.

Loss of blood leading to anemia may result from severe trauma to the blood vessels and massive hemorrhage, or it may be the result of a more gradual loss of blood, as in a small, bleeding, peptic ulcer.

The type of anemia caused by a failure in cell production is the result of a deficiency of certain substances necessary for the formation of red blood cells. Examples of this type of anemia are nutritional anemia in which there is an inadequate intake of foods containing proteins and iron, or pernicious anemia in which there is faulty absorption of specific nutrients such as vitamin B_{12} and iron.

Anemias associated with excessive destruction of red blood cells are exceedingly rare. They are known as *hemolytic anemias* ("hemolysis" means the destruction of red blood cells). Some of the hemolytic anemias are inherited while others are caused by exposure of the erythrocytes to poisonous agents such as chemicals or certain bacterial toxins.

Diagnosis. The diagnosis of anemia is easily established by a red cell count and hemoglobin evaluation. However, the determination of the specific type of anemia present is more difficult and requires a more thorough microscopic examination of the blood because the size and color of the erythrocytes vary in the different types of anemia. For example, the red cells are larger than normal when pernicious anemia is the diagnosis, while in an iron-deficiency anemia they are smaller than normal and contain less hemoglobin.

Sternal Puncture. Since most erythrocytes are manufactured in the red bone marrow there is much information to be gained from an examination of a specimen from the bone marrow. The sternum, being a flat, thin bone and readily accessible for an aspiration biopsy, is usually the site selected for removal of cells from the bone marrow. The procedure is referred to as a *sternal puncture*. It is often used in the diagnosis of several types of blood disease in which impaired production of blood cells is suspected.

Symptoms. The patient suffering from chronic anemia presents a typical picture of poor health. The skin is pale and the mucous membranes of the mouth and conjunctiva are noticeably lacking in color. He may complain of being easily fatigued or "tired all the time." Headache, dizziness, shortness of breath following slight exertion, and digestive disturbances are usually present. If the patient is an adult female there may be menstrual difficulties.

In an acute anemia the blood pressure falls rapidly, and dyspnea and restlessness appear. Symptoms of shock become apparent and emergency treatment must be used.

General Treatment and Nursing Care. The treatment of anemia logically begins with determination of its cause.

The doctor may order extensive diagnostic tests to aid him in his search for the etiologic factor present. Most physicians feel that treatments which alter the patient's blood picture by increasing the number of erythrocytes or changing their appearance will only confuse the issue. They prefer to order simple hygienic measures to improve the general health of the patient until a definite diagnosis has been made. The nurse may need to explain this to the patient should he complain that nothing is being done to cure him of his disease. Anemia is most often a chronic disease, which means that nursing measures are aimed at conserving the strength of the patient as much as possible over an extended period of time. It also means that these patients will need encouragement and emotional support during their long illness.

REST. It is only in the acute stages of anemia that absolute bed rest will be necessary. If the patient is ambulatory he should be encouraged to indulge in mild forms of exercise followed by short periods of rest. He must be warned never to exert himself to the point of exhaustion because of the unnecessary strain this puts on the heart and lungs.

Those who have anemia are suffering from a diminished supply of oxygen to the tissues of the body. When the brain is deprived of a small amount of oxygen dizziness will occur, and if the supply of oxygen is greatly diminished, as in a severe anemia, a loss of consciousness will occur. Because the patient may easily injure himself during attacks of dizziness or fainting he should be instructed to lie down when he first begins to feel faint. The best position is flat in bed without a pillow and with the feet slightly elevated. It is often helpful if the ambulatory patient will lie down in this position several times a day to improve the blood flow to the brain, thereby relieving the cause of dizziness.

WARMTH. Other tissues suffer not only from a decreased supply of oxygen but also from a lack of the warmth which adequate circulation provides. Thus, the anemic patient nearly always feels chilly and suffers from the cold. Caution should be used to avoid drafts when providing adequate ventilation in his room, and extra blankets and warm sleeping clothes will make him more comfortable. Care must also be used in the application of hot water bottles or electric heating pads because of the danger of burning the patient who has poor circulation and decreased sensitivity to heat.

DIET. The diet is an important part of the treatment of anemia. The patient is encouraged to eat foods which are rich in iron, protein, and vitamins B and C because the body uses all of these in the manufacture of new red blood cells. It is not unusual for the anemic patient to have a poor appetite. Factors which contribute to the anorexia are fatigue, weakness, and soreness of the tongue and gums. Patients with nutritional anemia usually have very poor eating habits because of ignorance or indifference to the nutritional values of food.

Before attempting to force any kind of diet on the patient the nurse should try to determine why he does not eat properly. If she will take a few minutes to discuss the diet with the patient she may find an excellent opportunity to teach him the value of eating a variety of foods and the kinds of food that are rich in the nutrients his condition requires. The nurse might also encourage her patient to eat as much as he can and to learn to rest a little before mealtime so that he will feel more relaxed and ready for his tray when it arrives.

If the tongue and gums are extremely tender and sore the foods must not be highly seasoned or served too hot. It is also helpful if the foods are of semi-solid consistency so that chewing is kept at a minimum.

SPECIAL MOUTH CARE. Bleeding of the gums may be among the early symptoms of anemia. As the disease progresses the gums become more tender and bleed quite freely. When this occurs brushing of the teeth must be discontinued and some form of special mouth care substituted. Crusts of dried blood may form inside the mouth, especially around the teeth. The crusts of blood may be gently removed by cotton applicators dipped in a solution of diluted hydrogen peroxide. Frequent cleansing of the mouth with cotton applicators dipped in a mild mouthwash will also keep down the odor of halitosis and make the patient feel more comfortable. The lips may be lubricated with mineral oil to prevent dryness and cracking.

VITAL SIGNS. The temperature, pulse and respiration should be checked frequently. An increase in the pulse and respiratory rate could indicate an increasing severity of the disease in which the heart and lungs are working harder in their efforts to provide oxygen to the body tissues. The body's resistance to infection is greatly reduced in all blood diseases; therefore, an elevation in the temperature may indicate that an infection is present. Any rise in the temperature of these patients should be reported immediately so that treatment may be begun before the infection becomes widespread.

SPECIAL OBSERVATIONS. It is possible for a patient to lose a small amount of blood continuously from an internal lesion without being aware of what is happening to him. The nursing staff must carefully observe all bodily excretions for signs of bleeding. When this is suspected as a cause of anemia the stools of the patient should be checked carefully for signs of fresh blood or old blood (tar-colored stools). When the physician suspects intestinal bleeding he may order a laboratory examination of the gastric contents or stools for occult (hidden) blood. The urine may also show signs of blood. Bright red blood rarely goes unnoticed but the hazy brown color caused by old blood in the urine may be considered unimportant if the nurse does not realize its significance. The practical nurse should know that any unexplained coloring of body excreta is to be reported immediately.

Blood Transfusions. The administration of whole blood to replace that which the patient has lost or is unable to produce himself is one of the most common treatments of anemia. The first record we have of such a procedure was in 1818 when an English obstetrician by the name of James Blundell began to treat successfully cases of postpartum hemorrhage with the administration of human blood. He was unaware of blood types and did not fully understand what happened when a reaction to the blood transfusion resulted in serious illness or death. It was not until 1900, when Landsteiner completed his research on blood groups, that an explanation could be given. It was he who determined that there are four main groups of human blood and that these groups cannot be mixed without disturbing the normal action of the red blood cells in the person receiving the transfusion.

BLOOD GROUPS. Landsteiner divided human blood into four main groups or "types" and labeled them A, B, AB, and O. The reactions of incompatible blood types are a result of an agglutination (clumping together) and destruction of the red cells. The reaction is brought about by a substance on the surface of the red blood cells of the person receiving the blood and is an antigen-antibody reaction. The blood cells of the donor act as *antigens* which stimulate the plasma of the recipient to produce antibodies.

In order to clarify the reactions of incompatible blood types, Figure 12-1 shows what happens when a small sample of diluted blood from one type is mixed with test sera from an incom-

Recipient

Donor	O	A	B	AB
O				
A				
B				
AB				

Figure 12-1. Horizontal letters designate blood type of recipient, vertical letters those of the donor. If types are compatible, the red blood cells remain in normal position. If types are incompatible, the red blood cells clump together, producing a reaction in the individual receiving the blood.

patible type. This clumping of the red cells can readily be seen, even with a low power microscope.

THE RH FACTOR. In 1940 Landsteiner and Weiner described yet another means of differentiating human blood. Since much of their work was done using rhesus monkeys they named the newly discovered factor Rh. This factor is an *agglutinogen*, which means that it is capable of causing a clumping together of red cells. About 85 percent of the population have this factor present in their red cells; they are typed *Rh positive*, and the remaining 15 percent who lack this factor are typed *Rh negative*. As long as Rh positive individuals receive only Rh positive blood in transfusions no problem will develop, provided they are compatible according to other groupings. But if an Rh negative individual should receive Rh positive blood he will receive the agglutinating factor into his blood and become "sensitized." If he then receives another transfusion of Rh positive blood he will suffer from a serious reaction due to the clumping of the red cells.

Besides transfusions with Rh positive blood there is another way an Rh negative individual may build up antibodies; that is, during pregnancy in which the plasma of an Rh negative mother is stimulated to build antibodies against the Rh positive fetal blood, which enter her circulatory system and become mixed with her blood. The mother's blood may become sensitized just as it would if she had received a transfusion of Rh positive blood. With subsequent pregnancies she may build up a high level of antibodies which would affect the fetus in a serious way. The condition which occurs when this happens is called "erythroblastosis fetalis" and may cause the child to be stillborn or if delivered living, it may present symptoms of a transfusion reaction.

RESPONSIBILITIES OF THE NURSE DURING TRANSFUSION OF WHOLE BLOOD. Even though the administration of whole blood is now a fairly common procedure, familiarity does not justify an attitude of complacency or indifference on the part of the nurse. Very serious, even fatal reactions can occur during the procedure, and close observation of the patient is always necessary. The following precautions are listed to remind the practical nurse of her responsibilities when caring for a patient receiving a transfusion.

1. Always be certain that the patient is receiving the blood assigned to him. Carefully check the name and blood type written on the label of the container.

2. Check frequently to see that the blood is flowing properly and at the rate

prescribed by the physician. If the practical nurse is in doubt as to the proper rate of flow she should ask the nurse or physician in charge.

3. If chills, rash, or other symptoms of a reaction occur during the transfusion stop the transfusion and notify the physician or nurse in charge immediately.

4. Observe the patient closely during and immediately after the transfusion. Check both temperature and pulse rate for evidence of a transfusion reaction.

5. Inspect the first urine specimen after a blood transfusion for signs of transfusion reaction (hemoglobinuria). The urine will be red or dark brown in color.

Iron Therapy. We know that iron is one of the substances the bone marrow uses to manufacture normal healthy red blood cells. When the body is lacking in iron, the amount of hemoglobin is decreased in the red cells, making them very small and pale in color. In a simple deficiency anemia the condition is relieved by administering iron salts. The iron preparation most often used is ferrous sulfate.

Iron salts are irritating to the gastrointestinal tract and should not be given on an empty stomach. There will be fewer gastric upsets if this medication is given in divided doses and immediately after meals. The patient should be warned that the taking of iron salts by mouth produces tarry stools and there is no cause for alarm if he notices this change in the color of his stools. Because iron salts may deposit on the teeth and gums, causing a discoloration, the liquid forms of this medication should be given through a straw. Following administration of each dose the teeth should be thoroughly cleansed and the mouth rinsed well.

Some patients suffer such severe gastric disturbances from the oral intake of iron salts that the medication must be given by another route. Other patients who are anemic because of gastric or intestinal bleeding cannot take iron by mouth because the irritation aggravates the condition. The drug of choice in these cases is Imferon, an iron preparation which is given into the muscle. These injections must not exceed 2 ml. at each site and the sites of injection should be rotated to allow for proper absorption and to minimize the hazards of a local inflammation.

Vitamin C is usually given with iron because this vitamin enhances the absorption of iron.

Vitamin B$_{12}$ and Liver Extract. The glands of the stomach secrete many different substances which help the body absorb and utilize the food which is taken in and digested. There is one specific substance (intrinsic factor) normally secreted by the stomach mucosa that is essential for the proper growth and development of normal red blood cells. In pernicious anemia the *intrinsic factor* is missing from the gastric juices so that the iron and protein taken into the stomach cannot be properly absorbed. The result is that the red cell production is decreased and those red cells which are produced are abnormal in structure and function. In order to correct this condition the physician will order the administration of vitamin B$_{12}$, or liver extract, which contains vitamin B$_{12}$.

These injections are given daily for the first few weeks and then may be spaced so that they are given weekly. As the patient improves the injections may be necessary only once a month.

In some ways the patient with pernicious anemia can be compared to a diabetic. There is no cure for the disease but the patient can lead a normal life as long as he receives adequate medication and does not indulge in excesses or dissipate his energy. Here, however, the similarity ends. The diabetic cannot neglect his daily doses of insulin or ignore his diet without soon suffering the consequences. The patient with pernicious anemia may neglect his injections of liver extract or

Vitamin B_{12} and continue to feel well for weeks or even months. The disease will progress from bad to worse in a gradual manner and eventually lead to serious mental as well as physical deterioration. This neurological damage dulls the patient's awareness of what is happening to him and thus he may not fully realize that he needs the help of his physician.

In view of these possibilities the patient and his family must be warned of the dangers involved. They should be made aware of the need for continued treatment for the rest of the patient's life, and informed of the unplesant outcome they can expect if the injections are neglected. In explaining these things to the patient the nurse must use tact and patience. The prospect of facing a lifetime of regular injections with the expense and inconvenience this involves is not a pleasant one. With sympathetic understanding and a genuine display of interest in the patient's well-being the nurse can do much to help him adjust to his illness and the treatments necessary to keep him as well as possible.

LEUKEMIA

Definition. The word "leukemia," when translated literally, means "white blood." Actually, the white blood cells would have to number one million per cubic millimeter before the blood would have a milky white appearance, and although leukemia is characterized by an increase in the number of leukocytes, they rarely rise above 500,000 per cubic millimeter. In addition to the increase in number, the leukocytes of the patient with leukemia are abnormal in appearance and do not function as normal white cells do.

The common lay term for leukemia is "cancer of the blood." The various types of leukemia are classified as progressive malignant diseases because there is a metastatic growth of leukemic cells. These cells can spread from the bone marrow or lymph nodes to the spleen, liver and other highly vascular regions. After they have invaded these organs and surrounding tissues they destroy the tissues by using the nutritive elements for their own rapid growth. Since the new cells utilize the available amino acids and vitamins at a prodigious rate, the patient with acute leukemia is very likely to suffer from severe debilitation and avitaminosis.[13]

Types. There are various types of leukemia but they are generally classified as the lymphogenous leukemias and the myelogenous leukemias. This classification is based on the origin of the malignant white blood cells. *Lymphogenous* leukemias originate in the lymphoid tissues where they proliferate and spread to other parts of the body. *Myelogenous* leukemias have their beginnings in the bone marrow.

Another way in which the leukemias can be differentiated is by their rate of progress. *Acute* leukemia develops rapidly and is more common in younger persons who are going through a rapid stage of development when all body cells are multiplying at an accelerated rate. *Chronic* leukemia occurs in older persons, usually over 45, who are not in the growth period of their lives.

ACUTE LEUKEMIA. This type of leukemia has an abrupt onset with symptoms of an upper respiratory infection, extreme pallor, ulcerations of the mouth and gums which also bleed easily, and a high fever. Later there is bleeding from all the body orifices and small hemorrhages under the skin. The disease runs a rapid course and in a short while the patient is critically ill. Death often occurs within weeks or months after the onset of the disease.

CHRONIC LEUKEMIA. As expected from its name this type of leukemia progresses more slowly. The onset is insidious with vague symptoms of fatigue and pallor; a sensation of heaviness in the abdomen, especially in the area of the spleen; and some symptoms of anemia, since there is a decrease in the red cell count and marked reduction of the platelet count. This lowering of the number of platelets accounts for the fact that these patients bleed easily and may have had a history of severe bruising from minor blows years before other symptoms appear.

Later in the disease there is swelling of the lymph nodes and enlargement of the spleen. Death may result from infection, severe anemia, or hemorrhage.

Incidence and Cause. It is estimated that in the United States there are about 14,000 deaths per year resulting from leukemia. The disease most often strikes youngsters under the age of 5 and is the major form of cancer in children aged 2 to 10. There has been an increase in the death rate from leukemia in persons over 45 years of age.[17]

As in other types of cancer, the exact cause of leukemia is not known. There are, however, some factors that are considered to be closely linked with the development of leukemia. *Ionizing radiation* in relatively large doses is one such factor. Another is *certain chemicals* that are toxic to bone marrow. The third factor is one that has been the subject of much research in the past few years. This is the theory that *tumor viruses* are in some way linked to the development of leukemia, but no one has yet been able to isolate a virus that can be identified as the specific cause of leukemia.

Treatment and Nursing Care. There is no known cure for leukemia. Treatment is aimed at: (1) slowing down the growth of the malignant blood cells; (2) maintaining a normal level of red cells, hemoglobin, and platelets; and (3) providing relief from symptoms which accompany the disease.

The use of chemotherapy as a means of slowing the progress of leukemia and producing a remission of symptoms began in 1942 with the use of nitrogen mustard. Since that time many drugs have been evaluated, and at this writing the most effective means of treatment is to use a combination of drugs from a list of the five most promising ones. For the most part these drugs, when given in combination, have an additive effect; that is, they are more effective in combination than either would be alone. It is also possible to combine a drug with a high toxicity with one that has a low toxicity, thereby increasing the destruction of leukemic cells without causing severe toxic reactions in the patient.

There are five groups of drugs that are used in the treatment of leukemia. Examples of these are presented in Table 15 with their major toxic effects.

Blood transfusions are often necessary in order to maintain a near-normal blood picture. Antibiotics may be given to control infections since the body's defense mechanisms against infection have been impaired by the leukemia.

Of the three aims listed above in the treatment of leukemia, providing relief from symptoms is the most challenging to the nursing staff. Regardless of the type of leukemia present, the nursing care of the leukemia patient is a difficult assignment, one demanding perseverance and ingenuity in solving the many problems this disease presents.

Extreme care must be used in handling these patients because of their tendency to bleed at the slightest injury. Care of the mouth and gums is similar to that described under care of the patient with anemia. If rectal temperatures are necessary, as in the case of a small child or a delirious person, it must be remembered that the mucous membranes are very fragile and injuries are easily sustained.

Protection against infection must be exercised constantly. The skin will require continued observation and special care so that no pressure sores or other breaks in the skin will occur. Pruritus (severe itching) is a very common complaint in some types of leukemia. In these cases the fingernails should be trimmed to prevent scratching and tearing the skin. Special medications may be ordered to help relieve the itching.

Table 15. *Acute Toxicity of Active Agents**

	SEVERITY AT THERAPEUTIC DOSE	MAJOR TOXIC EFFECTS
1. Prednisone	±	Hypertension, electrolyte imbalance, osteoporosis
2. Vincristine	+	Peripheral neuropathy
3. 6-Mercaptopurine	++	Marrow depression and nausea and vomiting
4. Methotrexate	+++	Stomatitis and marrow depression
5. Cyclophosphamide	++++	Marrow depression

*From Freireich, E. J., and Frei, E., in Moore, C. V., and Brown, E. B., eds.: Progress in Hematology, Volume IV. New York, Grune and Stratton, Inc., 1964.

Respiratory difficulty often accompanies leukemia when the lymph nodes of the neck become greatly enlarged. Then proper positioning of the patient for adequate breathing becomes necessary. In severe cases the physician may order the administration of oxygen.

The patient with leukemia should remain ambulatory as long as possible because of the pulmonary and circulatory complications which frequently arise from inactivity and confinement to bed. The nurse will then have the added responsibility of providing some mild forms of recreation for her patient so that time will not pass so slowly and his attention will be diverted from his illness.

It is generally believed by authorities that the leukemic patient, even if he is a child, should be told that he has leukemia. Nurses who have worked with leukemic patients have found that deception and trying to avoid direct answers to the patient's questions cause him more frustration and fear than telling him the nature of his illness. This does not mean that one should be brutally frank or morbid in answering the patient's questions. His physician should be the one to tell him his diagnosis. The nurse should encourage the patient to talk about his fears and anxieties when he seems inclined to do so. He will need much emotional and moral support, and his family may not be capable of providing enough of this support for the patient, since they too are going through an emotional upheaval. The nurse must be able to show a hopeful attitude without giving the patient and his family false hopes. She will need to understand the severity of the patient's physical and emotional state without becoming unduly depressed and morose herself.

HEMOPHILIA AND HEMOPHILIC STATES

Definition. Classical or *true* hemophilia is a rare hereditary disease that is characterized by prolonged coagulation time, which can lead to a serious or even fatal hemorrhage. It is transmitted through the female to the male. Although the female does not have the disease herself, she and all her female descendants can transmit it to their offspring.

There are other conditions, similar to hemophilia, which can occur in either sex. In one type the victim, usually an adult female, produces an autoimmune antibody which specifically affects the thromboplastin in her body. This antibody neutralizes thromboplastin, thereby rendering it ineffective in the formation of blood clots. The cause of this condition is unknown but it sometimes develops spontaneously during delivery or the postpartal period. This results in severe hemorrhage that often is fatal in spite of intensive treatment.

Treatment and Nursing Care. The patient with hemophilia or a hemophilic state must avoid injury whenever possible. If he has a nosebleed, for example, it can rapidly lead to severe blood loss. If he is to have a tooth extraction he must warn his dentist in advance so that the procedure is done in a hospital where antihemophilic globulin, blood transfusions and other treatments are readily available.

Once bleeding starts, even from the smallest cut or wound, it is very difficult to stop. Some authorities recommend as an emergency measure applying a piece of fresh meat directly on the open wound. Local applications of fibrin foam and thrombin often are helpful in the control of bleeding from external wounds.

Instruction of the patient in the ways in which he can avoid injury must be extremely detailed and it is very difficult for many patients to adjust their lives to this handicap. Every person who knows he has hemophilia should carry a card or wear some type of identification so that proper medical treatment will be obtained immediately in case of accidental injury or sudden illness.

PURPURA

Definition and Types. The word purpura refers to small hemorrhages in the skin and mucous membranes; they occur as a result of leakage from the capillaries into the tissue spaces of the subcutaneous tissues. If the hemorrhages are small, pinpoint in size, they are called *petechiae;* the larger ones which resemble bruises are called *ecchymoses.* Purpura actually is a symptom and may be secondary to a number of diseases including scurvy, liver disease with failure to utilize vitamin K and allergy to certain drugs.

Idiopathic thrombocytopenic purpura is a disease of unknown cause in which the thrombocytes (blood platelets) are destroyed before they reach maturity. It is primarily a disease of young people and is accompanied by enlargement of the spleen.

Treatment of purpura is concerned with curing the primary disease whenever possible and controlling the symptoms. Idiopathic purpura is treated by splenectomy.

Part II – NURSING CARE OF PATIENTS WITH DISORDERS OF THE HEART

INTRODUCTION

Heart disease is still the major cause of death in the United States. Circulatory diseases, which include heart disease, account for a large percentage of the chronic illnesses that disable to some degree another large segment of the population of this country.

While these facts may be somewhat sobering, they should not be interpreted to mean that all heart diseases are either fatal or totally disabling. There are many different types of heart disease and although any disease which involves the heart is a serious affair, many heart conditions are relatively minor and can be cured. Even in the case of these which cannot be cured the knowledge that one has a heart disease may actually prolong his life if he follows his doctor's orders and lives sensibly.

DIAGNOSTIC TESTS AND EXAMINATIONS

The diagnosis of heart disease is primarily based on a physical examination, accurate history, and careful evaluation of the patient's symptoms. The electrocardiogram is used almost routinely as a diagnostic aid when a heart disease is suspected and is particularly useful in the identification of disturbances in the rhythmic beats of the heart muscle. X-rays of the chest will often reveal abnormal changes in size or contour of the heart and larger blood vessels.

In addition to the diagnostic aids just mentioned there are specific procedures and laboratory tests which will help the physician determine accurately the specific type of heart disease present.

Heart Catheterization. In this procedure a small, flexible catheter is introduced into a vein of the right arm. The catheter is gently passed into the vena cava, right atrium, right ventricle, and on to the pulmonary artery. By using a special manometer the physician can measure the pressure of the blood in any of these large vessels and chambers of the heart. Samplings of blood are withdrawn from the vessels and chambers for the purpose of determining the oxygen content of the blood as it passes through each of these. The cardiac catheterization is especially useful in diagnosing congenital heart disease.

Angiocardiogram. This is a special type of x-ray examination using an opaque dye to aid in visualizing the heart and large blood vessels leading to and from the heart. The dye is injected through a catheter such as is used for cardiac catheterization. In the event the examination involves the left side of the heart the dye is sometimes injected directly into the heart chambers. Immediately after the dye is injected x-rays are taken in rapid sequence. This type of examination is done for congenital heart diseases or other structural defects of the heart, its valves, or the large blood vessels.

Radioactive Isotopes. Within recent years there has been an increasing interest in the use of radioactive isotopes for the diagnosis of heart disease. For example, structural defects within the heart itself and abnormal routing of the blood to or from the great vessels can be diagnosed by the use of a Geiger counter over the heart to locate radioactive material injected or inhaled into the circulatory system. Radioactive iodine can be used to determine the cardiac output and thereby determine the heart's ability to function as a pump.

Other information that can be obtained through radioactive isotopes include estimation of blood loss and determination of the life span of individual red blood cells.

General Nursing Care of the Cardiac Patient. The basic principles underlying the nursing care of the patient with heart disease remain essentially the same even though the diagnosis and treatments may be more specific in each case. In order to avoid repetition in this area the general nursing care is discussed first. Additional nursing responsibilities involved in specific types of heart disease are included under each disease later in the chapter.

REST. After the physician has made a definite diagnosis he decides the amount of rest demanded by the condition of the patient's heart. He may order the patient on complete bed rest or he may allow some limited activity. In less acute types of heart disease the patient may be ambulatory.

It is of extreme importance that every one on the nursing team understand exactly what is meant by *absolute* or *complete bed rest.* When either of these is ordered the physician does not want the patient to exert himself any more than is absolutely necessary. The nurse may need to interpret the doctor's orders to the patient, explaining the need for absolute rest and enlisting his cooperation. It is very difficult for a person who has always been active suddenly to find himself in a position of total dependence on others even for his most basic needs. The fact that he may feel well enough to exert himself does not alter the situation. *As long as the patient is on absolute bed rest everything involving the slightest physical effort must be done for him.* He must be fed, bathed, dressed, and his position changed by those in attendance. When turning the patient and changing his position, sudden movements and rough handling must be avoided. He should be instructed not to sit up suddenly or turn too quickly.

The clothing of the patient on bed rest should be designed to allow for changing with a minimum of effort. The hospital gown is ideal but if the patient insists on wearing something different, a gown or pajama coat which does not have to be pulled over the head is best.

It is often a helpless and lonely feeling to be confined to bed for days at a time. The patient on bed rest will need reassurance that his nurse is never very far away. He must never be left without having a call bell at his fingertips and the nurses on duty should make a special effort to answer his light immediately. A delay in getting to his room may result in undue anxiety or excitement for the patient.

We have spoken of physical rest, but the patient's emotional serenity and peace of mind are equally important. His room should be quiet, neat and orderly, and away from confusion and centers of activity such as the elevator or nurses' station and utility room. The number of visitors is usually decided by the physician or nurse in charge. If the practical nurse notices that a particular visitor leaves the patient agitated and unable to rest after a visit she must report this to the nurse in charge. It is obvious that the patient must also be protected from any startling news or other occasions of emotional excitement.

The attitude of the nurse caring for him will greatly affect the patient's acceptance of bed rest. If she performs every task willingly and with a genuine desire to be helpful, the patient will be more inclined to relax and cooperate. If, on the other hand, he is made to feel that he is a burden to the nursing staff, causing them a great inconvenience every time he asks for a glass of water or to have his position changed, he will soon start doing things for himself rather than ask for help.

DIET AND FLUIDS. There are three factors to consider in the diet and fluid intake of the cardiac patient: (1) the amount of food allowed for each meal, (2) the types of food to avoid, and (3) the restriction of sodium intake and limiting of fluids when edema is present.

We know that digestion of food requires an increased amount of blood flow to the stomach which in turn places an extra burden on the heart to supply that blood. It is also true that a full stomach may interfere with the lowering of the diaphragm and complete expansion of the lungs. In view of these facts it is evident that patients with heart disease should be fed several small meals of easily digested foods rather than three large meals a day. In the acute stages of the disease the diet may be limited to liquids and semisolid foods to prevent overtaxation of the heart.

In addition to providing small, digestible meals the diet is also planned so that highly seasoned foods and stimulants such as tea and coffee are avoided, as are all gas-forming foods which may lead to abdominal distention. Most physicians will request that extremely hot and cold foods and liquids be eliminated from the diet, especially cold drinks and iced foods because of the constriction of blood vessels brought about by cold.

In the presence of edema, sodium is restricted in the diet because of its ability to hold fluid within the tissues. The seasoning of foods with salt substitutes and other condiments may be allowed by the physician to make the diet more palatable. The limitation of fluids by mouth depends on the type of disease present and the wishes of the physician in charge. In some cases the practical nurse may find that fluids are limited to as little as 1000 or 1500 ml. within a 24-hour period. In this case *completely accurate* records must be kept and the intake of liquids scheduled so that the patient does not have to wait an unreasonable length of time before he may have something to relieve his thirst.

RELIEF OF DYSPNEA AND CYANOSIS. Normal respiration depends upon an adequate internal exchange of oxygen and carbon dioxide, as well as proper external exchange of these gases. The cardiac patient suffers from dyspnea because the heart muscle is not functioning efficiently as a pump. As a result the circulation becomes sluggish, delaying the journey of the red cells to the lungs for a fresh supply of oxygen. In an effort to compensate for this the pulse and respirations are increased and the patient appears to gasp for air. He will seek relief by sitting straight up and assuming what is called the *orthopneic* position. This is not necessarily true of all cardiacs, but the nurse may assume that if her patient refuses to lie flat in the bed because he "can't breathe," she must assist him into a position for optimal breathing and provide support so that he may rest comfortably. Use of the overbed table and pillows to properly position the patient and the use of the footboard to keep him from slipping down in the bed are discussed in Chapter 3, page 27.

CARE OF THE SKIN. The fact that the patient must not exert himself and should remain immobile presents quite a problem in the proper care of the skin and prevention of pressure sores. When edema is present the problem is even more difficult because edematous tissue breaks down more readily than normal tissue. Frequent turning of the patient must be done with adequate help so that the patient does not feel the need to exert himself in an effort to help. As stated before, sudden movements and rough handling are to be avoided. The area of the sacral bone must be given special attention, especially when the patient is in orthopneic position because of the tendency for edema to localize at the lower spine. Care of the back may be accomplished fairly easily with the patient sitting up and leaning across the overbed table padded with pillows.

MEDICATIONS. Drugs useful in the treatment of the patient with heart disease consist mainly of three types: (1) those which decrease the rate and improve the strength of the contractions of the heart muscle so that it beats more normally, (2) those which relieve edema, and (3) those which provide relief from pain. Other more specific medications are discussed later in this chapter under their related diseases.

The drug used most often to slow and strengthen the heart beat is *digitalis*. This drug is classified as a heart tonic; that is, it improves the muscular contractions of the heart, making it more effective as a pump. There are several different forms of digitalis and there are preparations which may be given by intramuscular injection as well as by mouth. In the administration of any of these preparations the pulse should be counted just before each dose is given. It is a generally accepted rule in all institutions that the medication is withheld if the pulse is below 60 per minute, and the doctor is informed of the situation.

Another drug used to control the heart beat is *quinidine*. This drug is a heart depressant. It stops the convulsive twitching of the heart muscle (fibrillation) and improves the rhythm of the heart beat. By depressing the heart's contractions quinidine allows for a more complete relaxation of the heart muscle between contractions so that the chambers may completely fill with blood. Since it is a heart depressant the pulse should also be counted before quinidine is administered.

Edema of the tissues may be relieved by the administration of drugs which increase the urinary output.

These drugs are called *diuretics*. Diuretics can be classified according to their physiological action. One type increases the rate of glomerular filtration and thereby increases urinary output. A second type affects the osmotic pressure in the tubules of the kidney and prevents reabsorption of fluid back into the blood stream so that these fluids remain in the tubules and are excreted as urine. A third group of diuretics inhibit the secretion of antidiuretic hormone (ADH). As a result of this deficiency of ADH, water is not reabsorbed into the blood stream and it is excreted in large amounts as dilute urine.[13]

Most physicians wish to have the patient receiving a diuretic weighed daily in order to estimate the amount of fluid lost from the tissues. When weighing a patient daily the nurse should schedule the procedure so that the patient is weighed at the same time each day (preferably in the morning before breakfast), on the same scales, and with the same amount of clothing. In addition to daily weighing the physician will most likely request that an accurate record be kept of the patient's intake and output of fluids. The procedure for measuring and recording intake and output varies in each hospital. The important point to be emphasized is that everyone who is in any way responsible for the care of the patient must carry out this procedure conscientiously.

Severe pain is most often associated with heart disease of an acute nature such as myocardial infarction. The drugs used most often are morphine sulfate and Demerol. As the acute phase and severe pain subside these drugs may be replaced with milder sedatives which promote relaxation and freedom from anxiety. Much of the patient's pain may be due to his nervousness and anxiety, and so the nurse can do much to help relieve his pain by providing complete physical and mental rest for him. In the scheduling of necessary procedures such as turning the patient, skin care, etc., she should use common sense so that the patient is not disturbed any more often than necessary, and most especially she should realize that medications which induce sleep and relieve pain are not given as a substitute for good nursing care.

Rehabilitation of the Patient. The amount and type of activities permitted the patient during convalescence and after discharge from the hospital are governed by the response of the heart to treatment and the amount of residual damage to the heart itself. The physician will impress on the patient the importance of following his orders so that future attacks can be avoided. The patient with a chronic heart disease must adjust his life so that no extra demands are placed on the circulatory system. Members of the health team, including the dietitian, social worker, and public health nurse, may all play an important part in teaching the patient how to live with his illness.

Prevention of Heart Disease. As a recognized member of the nursing team, the practical nurse has a responsibility in the education of the public regarding the prevention of heart disease. A few of the "facts of life" in regard to the heart diseases are presented below.

1. Obesity does not directly cause heart disease, but it does place an unnecessary strain on the heart, making it more susceptible to heart disease.

2. A diet that is habitually high in calories, total fats, saturated fats, cholesterol, refined carbohydrates and salt presents a major risk in the development of coronary heart disease.

3. Cigarette smoking increases the proneness to coronary heart disease from two- to six-fold, depending on the number of cigarettes smoked.

4. Elevated blood pressure (that is, a diastolic pressure in the range of 90 to 94 mm. Hg) is closely associated with coronary heart disease.

5. Atherosclerotic heart diseases are

closely associated with diabetes mellitus.[26]

6. Exercise does not damage the heart; in fact, light to moderate exercise is a good protective device, provided it is done regularly. Sudden bursts of strenuous exercise by a person who is not accustomed to exercise can be damaging to the heart.

7. Periodic physical examinations for children will facilitate early detection of congenital heart diseases that are not severe enough to present serious symptoms.

8. There is a definite relationship between streptococcal infections of the throat and rheumatic heart disease. The practical nurse must encourage early treatment of sore throats and other infections that could be streptococcal in origin.

SURGERY OF THE HEART

Introduction. Until the 1950's there was little that could be done in the way of surgical procedures involving the heart itself because prolonged interruption of circulation meant certain death for the patient. But with the advent of the heart-lung machine and hypothermia techniques surgeons could repair or replace damaged valves and correct many congenital heart defects.

The heart-lung machine, which has many variations in design and appearance, functions as artificial heart (pump) and lungs (oxygenator). For this reason it is sometimes called a pump-oxygenator. Since all of this is done outside the patient's body, the procedure is called extracorporeal circulation. The surgeon inserts large tubes in the venae cavae and reroutes the unoxygenated venous blood through the heart-lung machine (see Fig. 12-2). There the blood is exposed to an atmosphere of oxygen in which an exchange of gases takes place—carbon dioxide is released and oxygen is taken up— and the oxygenated blood is returned

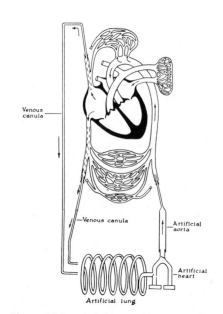

Figure 12-2. *A,* Schema of intrathoracic cannulation for extracorporeal maintenance of circulation. Systemic venous return is diverted to oxygenator by intracaval catheters. Although blood return is pictured returning from oxygenator entering aortic arch by way of the subclavian artery, the current mode of returning oxygenated blood is by extrathoracic cannulation of the femoral artery. The diagram also demonstrates the first method of elective cardiac arrest by injection of 4.5 mEq. of diluted potassium citrate into the aortic root. *B,* Diagram of artificial maintenance of circulation. Extrathoracic cannulation: Blood is sucked out of venae cavae into oxygenator and is pumped through a side-branch (femoral artery) back into the aorta. Flow in aorta is reversed. All tissues are perfused with blood coming from the aorta. (From Quinn: Journal of Practical Nursing, November, 1965.)

to the patient via the femoral artery. The blood also may be cooled so that the patient's body temperature is lowered (hypothermia), thereby reducing the body's metabolic needs during surgery.

Extracorporeal circulation and hypothermia permit the cardiac surgeon adequate time to open the heart, visu-ally inspect its internal structures and perform the necessary surgery. Congenital heart defects such as abnormal openings in the septum can be repaired fairly easily. Others that involve more than one defect and require extensive repair of the heart and one or more of the great vessels are less successful and present more of a risk to the patient.

An artificial valve such as the one shown in Figure 12-3 can be inserted as a replacement for a diseased valve that has been damaged in rheumatic heart disease or other acquired heart disorders.

Preoperative Care. Prior to surgery the patient undergoes a series of diagnostic tests and examinations such as those presented in the previous pages of this chapter. These tests are done to determine as far as possible the exact nature of the heart's structural defects. With this information the surgeon plans the type of surgical procedure he will perform to correct the condition. If the procedure seems relatively simple he will so inform the patient and his family. If the defect involves a very high risk the patient and his family must make the decision as to whether or not the surgery is to be done. The physician or some other qualified person also will instruct the patient, explaining what he can expect to be done, the kind of equipment to be used during and after surgery and the expected results of the surgical procedure. Most authorities agree that the patient should not be told so much as to confuse him and cause undue worry, nor so little that he is apprehensive and frightened when he awakens from anesthesia and finds himself in the midst of complicated machinery. The information given is tailored to each patient's individual needs, level of intelligence and apparent desire to know what is in store for him.

During the operative procedure the surgical personnel must function as a team. Each person must be thoroughly trained in his duties. Figure 12-4 shows

Figure 12-3. Hufnagel (top) and Starr-Edwards cardiac valves operate on the ball-valve principle: a ball regulates an opening by suction and by its own weight. Sound is produced by the forceful back-and-forth movement of the ball as it strikes its stationary cage. (From Slatin: American Journal of Nursing, June, 1967.)

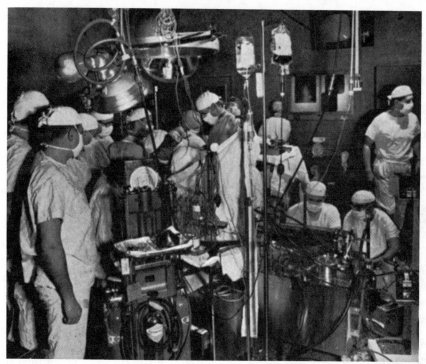

Figure 12-4. The scene in the operating room during open-heart surgery in which an artificial valve was inserted to replace a leaking aortic valve. The artificial heart-lung machine is seen in the lower right hand corner. The full "team" consists of 14 people: four surgeons, two scrub nurses, two circulating nurses, two anesthesiologists, two technicians operating the artificial heart-lung machine, one nurse operating the monitoring and recording equipment, and one cardiologist.

The electrocardiogram, arterial and venous blood pressure, and blood pressures in various chambers of the heart are recorded and visible on the large monitor screen in the upper right hand corner.

Although the maze of wires and tubing seen in this picture seems to have achieved almost nightmarish proportions, when each member of the team carries out his assigned task there is no confusion and the whole operation proceeds with quiet efficiency. (From Rogoz and Holswade: Journal of Practical Nursing, April, 1966.)

the many persons and types of equipment involved in open-heart surgery.

Postoperative Care. During the entire postoperative period intelligent observation is the primary concern of the nurse. The patient is kept in an intensive care unit where specially trained personnel and monitoring equipment are in constant attendance. After the first 48 hours the surgeon will assess the patient's condition and decide whether he can be transferred to a general surgical unit. The patient will continue to need nursing care of the most detailed kind. His vital signs must be taken and recorded at regular intervals. His intake and output must be measured and recorded at least every eight hours and his fluid intake may be restricted for a period of time. Thoracotomy tubes for drainage and proper re-expansion of the lungs will need special attention (see page 285 for details). He may be given oxygen by tent or nasal prongs.

Until the surgeon allows the patient out of bed it is necessary to encourage gentle daily exercises of the arms and legs. These are necessary to improve circulation and to maintain full range of motion in the joints, especially that of the left shoulder which the patient hesitates to move and uses as a protective splint to avoid motion in the operative area. The amount of physical activity is very gradually increased and is governed by the type of surgery done and the patient's reaction to surgery.

CONGESTIVE HEART FAILURE

Definition. Congestive heart failure is actually a complication of other cardiac conditions rather than a disease in itself; in fact, it is the chief complication in 70 per cent of all patients who have heart disease. When the heart loses its efficiency as a pump the result is congestion within the heart chambers. This may develop gradually over a period of years or it may appear suddenly following an acute disease of the heart or kidneys.

It is usually the left side of the heart that fails first in congestive failure, but eventually both sides will be affected. To understand the mechanism involved in congestive failure one must have some knowledge of the circulation of blood through a normal, well-functioning heart. Normally, the ventricles contract while the atria relax, so that with each contraction of the ventricle, blood is poured into the atrium on each side of the heart. The ventricles then relax and receive a new supply of blood. In congestive failure the contractions of the ventricles are weak, thus they cannot empty and so become engorged with blood. When the left ventricle fails, there will be a damming up of blood in the left atrium and the pulmonary veins. If the right ventricle fails, there will be a damming up of blood in the right atrium and the vena cavae.

Symptoms. The symptoms of congestive failure can readily be understood by analyzing the steps mentioned above. The key word is *congestion.* We know how our progress is slowed down when we approach a congested area of traffic while driving an automobile. So it is with the circulation of blood when congestion is present. The sluggish flow of blood through the pulmonary vessels produces dyspnea, cough, and sometimes hemoptysis (the spitting of blood). If the situation continues unchecked the serum from the blood inside the pulmonary vessels empties into the air sacs of the lung and begins to fill the lower branches of the bronchial tree. When this happens the patient is said to have *pulmonary edema.*

Congestion of the venae cavae leads to a dependent type of edema, which means that the lower parts of the body are edematous. There is also an accumulation of fluids in the liver and abdominal organs. Congestion of the kidneys may lead to impaired kidney function which only aggravates the condition of edema. Inadequate circulation of fresh blood to the brain may cause mental confusion and irritability which sometimes progresses to delirium or loss of consciousness.

Treatment and Nursing Care. REST. In providing rest for the patient with congestive failure the nurse must remember the hazard of the formation of an embolus when the circulation is so sluggish. The doctor may order passive exercises of the lower extremities and flexion of the legs several times a day to speed up the blood flow and discourage the development of clots. If these exercises are ordered it is important to explain to the patient that they are passive exercises to be done by the nurse and require no effort on his part.

The patient with mild congestive failure may be ambulatory or may be sent home with instructions to perform only light work. These patients usually must receive help and guidance from the public health nurse, social worker, visiting nurse, or other individuals and agencies concerned with the welfare of cardiac patients.

Those patients who are confined to bed with acute congestive failure should have side rails on their beds because of the mental confusion and disorientation which frequently accompanies this condition.

DIET. While the patient is in the hospital he has no responsibilities in the preparation of his meals or restriction of sodium from his diet. When he is discharged from the hospital, however, he or a member of his family must have some instruction in the preparation of meals and planning of menus within the limitations of a low-sodium diet. Although the dietitian is usually responsible for this instruction. repetition and further explanation by the nursing staff will help to impress on the patient the importance of this phase of his treatment. The physician may or may not allow substitutes for table salt. The nurse might explain to the patient and his family that there is no need for purchasing expensive foods specially prepared for low-sodium diets as long as the person preparing the food at home understands the proper way to modify the family's regular meals so that the patient's food has a low-sodium content. Seasonings such as garlic, onions, lemon juice, vinegar, and other herbs are acceptable on the low-sodium diet and help to make the food more palatable. The patient should be cautioned to read the labels on all cereals and processed foods because some of these have sodium added for preservation. He must also be warned that many patent medicines, cough syrups, and dentifrices contain sodium. And finally, though this is obvious to those who know the correct term for baking soda, sodium bicarbonate is not allowed the patient on a low-sodium diet.

MEDICATIONS. Drugs used in the treatment of congestive failure are most often diuretics and digitalis. These have been discussed earlier under general treatment and nursing care. However, it may be well to remind the reader that many persons with chronic congestive failure must continue to take digitalis daily for the rest of their lives.

Practical nurses may hear the doctor use the term "digitalized" in reference to the patient. This means that the patient has been given the drug several times a day while in the hospital until it has had the desired effect. After the patient is "digitalized" he must continue to take a maintenance dose of the medication every day so as to sustain the desired effect as long as necessary. The patient should have impressed on him the importance of faithfully continuing his medication once he has been discharged from the hospital even though he may feel that his condition has improved to the point that he does not need it any more.

Pulmonary Edema

The accumulation of fluid within the lung tissues can occur very suddenly following rapid failure of the left side of the heart or as a result of an abrupt increase in the work load of the heart. This acute condition can be fatal in a very short period of time if not relieved by emergency measures. The patient with chronic congestive heart failure involving the left side of the heart can also suffer from pulmonary edema, and though the symptoms are less dramatic in the chronic form than in the acute form, they are no less uncomfortable or frightening for the patient.

Symptoms. In *acute pulmonary edema* the patient experiences a sudden, frightening dyspnea. He cannot lie down flat in the bed because such a position only increases the edema in his lungs and aggravates his shortness of breath. He may complain of a heaviness or pressure in his chest rather than a sharp pain. He often becomes slightly cyanotic and he perspires profusely. His respiration is rapid and each time he breathes, a moist rattling sound can be heard some distance away from him. The congestion in his lungs produces a persistent hacking cough and the sputum brought up is thick at first, becoming thin, frothy and blood-tinged. The pulse rate increases and the venous pressure becomes so great that the jugular veins become distended and are easily observed. The patient becomes more and more apprehensive and begins to struggle for air, breathing more rapidly (hyperventilating) and thereby further aggravating the situation. Unless the condition is relieved, the heart weakens and begins to beat irregularly and the patient eventually loses consciousness. Finally, death occurs as the heart and lungs fail.[15]

Treatment and Nursing Care. If the nurse is the first to observe a patient in acute pulmonary edema she must realize that an emergency situation exists and that without proper treatment the patient may literally "drown" in his own secretions. She should place the patient in orthopneic position, so that he can breathe as well as possible, and summon help immediately. She also must strive to reassure the patient and keep him as calm as possible. Oxygen is administered and the patient is given a sedative such as morphine sulfate to relieve anxiety, induce rest and repress the respiratory reflexes. If the patient is not already receiving digitalis, some fast-acting form of this drug is given to slow and strengthen the heart beat.

Because of the congested state of the

Figure 12-5.   Rotation of tourniquets at 15-minute intervals.

pulmonary blood vessels, some measures must be taken to reduce the venous return of blood to the heart. One way in which this can be accomplished is by rotating tourniquets on the extremities (see Fig. 12-5). Note that the tourniquets are changed promptly every 15 minutes. This is necessary so that circulation to the extremities is not seriously impaired and blood clots do not form in the veins.

In addition to the measures given above the patient may be given a rapid-acting diuretic to speed up the elimination of body fluids and thereby reduce fluid volume in the blood vessels and tissue spaces. Of course, a very accurate record must be kept of the patient's intake and output. Weight is usually checked daily and the patient's diet restricted in fluids and sodium.

DISEASES OF THE CORONARY ARTERIES

Definition. The heart is actually a muscle and as such must have its own supply of blood to nourish it and remove waste products. The blood ves-

sels which supply blood to the heart muscle *(myocardium)* are called the coronary vessels. They were given this name because the main trunks of these vessels encircle the top of the heart like a crown and send their branches downward into the heart muscle (see Fig. 12-6). The coronary arteries are especially important because any disease involving these vessels will ultimately result in a decrease in the efficiency of the heart.

The coronary arteries may be affected by a hardening and loss of elasticity of their walls *(arteriosclerosis)* or deposits of material inside the vessel *(atherosclerosis)*. In either case the condition causes a narrowing of the lumen of the vessel and predisposes it to a complete blockage of blood flow through the artery.

Types of Coronary Disease

There are two main types of disease processes which may affect the coronary arteries once they have become narrowed. The first is a sudden occluding or closing of the artery by a blood clot. This clot may be formed within the

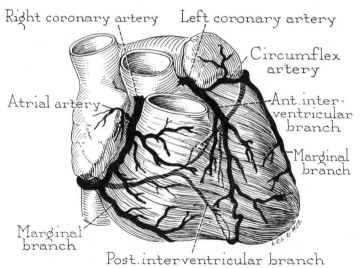

Figure 12-6. The heart, showing the coronary arteries, which encircle the top of the heart and send branches down into the muscle tissue of the heart. (From King and Showers: *Human Anatomy and Physiology*, 5th Ed., W. B. Saunders Co., Philadelphia.)

artery at the site of the occlusion (*thrombus*) or may be one which has entered the blood stream at a distant point and been carried along until it reached a vessel too small to allow its passage (*embolus*). The sudden blocking of a coronary vessel may be referred to as a *myocardial infarction, coronary occlusion*, or *coronary attack*.

In the second type of coronary artery disease the arteries become hardened or filled with layers of deposits over a period of time so that the openings inside these tubular structures gradually become more and more narrow until they are eventually closed. This disease process leads to a condition called *angina pectoris*.

Acute Myocardial Infarction. An *infarction* is an area of necrotic tissue caused by an obstruction to the flow of blood to that area (see Fig. 12-7). Myocardial means "pertaining to the heart muscle." Thus in a myocardial infarction there is an area of necrosis in the heart muscle. The prognosis of the patient who suffers an acute myocardial infarction depends to a great extent on the size of the artery plugged by a clot and the amount of heart tissue that artery had formerly supplied with blood. If a large area of the heart is affected, instant death may occur. Smaller areas may heal if treated promptly and effectively.

SYMPTOMS. The clinical picture presented by the patient with an acute myocardial infarction is one that most lay people recognize as a "heart attack." There is a sudden, severe pain in the chest, usually described as crushing or burning. Sometimes the pain is mistaken as a symptom of acute indigestion. The patient also shows symptoms of shock with pallor, profuse sweating, anxiety, and often has nausea and vomiting.

Although the above symptoms are usually present in an acute myocardial infarction they are not always so severe and in some cases the patients have described their pain as mild. The severity of the symptoms will depend on the size of the area of infarction.

Whenever there is necrotic tissue anywhere in the body the white cell count increases and the sedimentation rate is elevated. Within 24 hours of an acute attack the temperature of the patient with myocardial infarction rises and leukocytosis appears.

TREATMENT AND NURSING CARE. *Immediate care.* An acute myocardial infarction is an emergency case and requires immediate treatment to combat shock and prevent further circulatory collapse. Pain is relieved by morphine sulfate or Demerol. The first dose is often given directly into the vein by the physician. Oxygen may be necessary to relieve cyanosis and assist the heart in its efforts to circulate oxy-

Figure 12-7. Shaded area represents region of infarct resulting from obstruction to the flow of blood through vessel plugged by clot.

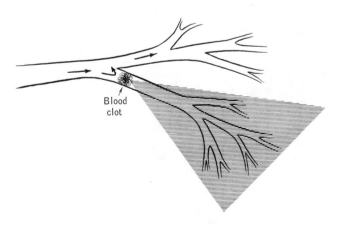

Blood clot

genated blood through the body. The patient often feels panic and expresses a sensation of approaching death. This pessimistic attitude may persist for several days after the attack. The nurse must do all that she can to convey a feeling of calm reassurance to the patient and convince him that the situation is in hand and his only concern is to relax and let the medications take effect.

Rest. Most patients who have suffered a myocardial infarction are placed on bed rest for at least one month or more to allow the heart to rest and healing to take place. The principles and practices mentioned earlier in this chapter in regard to providing rest for the cardiac patient are extremely important in the care of the patient with an acute myocardial infarction.

Sometimes the physician will order exercises of the legs to prevent the formation of a thrombus in the veins. These exercises may be done by the nurse (passive) or by the patient (active) depending on the desires of the physician. It is also important in the prevention of phlebothrombosis to avoid pressure on the back of the leg under the knee. This means that the knee rest or pillows under the knees should be used only for brief periods of time and alternated with an exercise in which the patient presses his feet against the footboard or foot of the bed.

Another common complication of acute myocardial infarction is "frozen shoulder." This is a term used to describe limited motion of the shoulder and arm. It is caused by the patient's attempt to relieve the pain in his chest by keeping his left arm immobile against his chest. To avoid this complication, massage and exercises under the doctor's orders may be done. It is also helpful if the nurse will place a pillow between the arm and chest wall to support the arm and relieve the tension of the muscles.

Medications. In addition to the digitalis mentioned under general treatment of heart diseases there is one group of drugs that is specifically used in the treatment of acute myocardial infarction. These are the *anticoagulants,* so called because they impair the clotting mechanism of the blood. These drugs are usually ordered by the physician daily as "stat" doses only after he has received a laboratory report on the patient's current prothrombin level (see p. 43).

Prevention of acute myocardial infarction. The high incidence rate of coronary heart disease in men between the ages of 40 and 60 years has prompted Dr. Robert McMillon of Winston-Salem, North Carolina, to write "A Coronary Decalogue." Some of these rules may

Figure 12-8. Some of the special equipment used in a coronary care unit to provide constant surveillance of coronary patients and immediate treatment of those who go into cardiac arrest, failure, or shock, or who show significant arrythmias. Each patient is connected to an electrocardiographic monitor with a pacemaker attachment in place for immediate activation. The monitors have an emergency alarm signal that goes off when the rate or quality of the beats changes. The ECG and pulse rate are constantly displayed on oscilloscopes at the bedside and at the nurses' station. Equipment needed for defibrillation, heart reactivation, cardiopulmonary resuscitation, and emergency drug therapy is available. (From Hazletine: American Journal of Nursing, November, 1964.)

seem a bit flippant to include in a text-book, but they are all based on sound principles and are presented with the sincere conviction that they offer an excellent guide for those who wish to avoid an acute attack of coronary heart disease.

1. Thou shalt not try to be a champion athlete after 50.
2. Thou shalt not struggle to be a perfectionist.
3. Thou shalt not fill up thy stomach with food nor engage in exercise after eating.
4. Thou shalt consider losing thy temper a luxury to be indulged in sparingly.
5. Thou shalt avoid worry—the government will probably take care of you.
6. Thou shalt keep thy alcoholic intake below the point where it may delude thee into thinking thou art a better man than thou ever were.
7. Thou shalt not smoke tobacco if possible.
8. Thou shalt take regular vacations.
9. Thou shalt avoid cold weather.
10. After a certain age thou shalt not take unto thyself a young wife, nor even a reasonable facsimile.*

Angina Pectoris. The term "angina pectoris" literally means a severe cramp-like pain in the chest; however, it is used universally to designate a serious cardiac disorder resulting from a decreased blood supply to the heart muscle. It is caused by a narrowing of the arteries due to arteriosclerosis or atherosclerosis.

Angina pectoris is similar to myocardial infarction in that it results from an inadequate oxygen supply to the myocardium. The difference is that myocardial infarction is a result of a rather sudden blockage of a coronary artery, whereas angina pectoris is a more gradual process in which the coronary vessels cannot bring sufficient blood supply (or oxygen) to the myocardium because they are occluded by atherosclerotic plaque and their walls have lost their elasticity.

*Reprinted from the *Atlanta Constitution*, Thursday, February 7, 1963.

The attacks of pain in angina pectoris vary in each individual so that an activity that precipitates an attack one day may have no effect on the patient the next day. Generally, however, there are some factors that can be considered relevant to an attack. These include sudden physical exertion, especially in the morning, cold air, eating a very heavy meal and emotional upsets.[10]

SYMPTOMS. The type of pain or discomfort may vary in individuals but in most cases it is described as a dull pain or tightness under the sternum. It may or may not radiate down one or both arms. Sometimes the patient experiences dyspnea and there may be pallor or flushing of the face and profuse perspiration.

In general it is felt that the patient with chronic but unchanging angina pectoris is not in serious trouble and his condition is not critical. However, if his condition becomes worse very suddenly, he most likely will suffer from serious damage to the heart muscle.

TREATMENT AND NURSING CARE. The treatment of angina pectoris is mostly symptomatic with emphasis on eliminating those factors which are known to precipitate an attack in the individual patient. With guidance from his physician the patient may soon learn to correlate certain activities with an attack and thereby learn to avoid them whenever possible.

Medications. The most specific type of medication used for angina pectoris are the *vasodilators*, that is, those drugs which expand the blood vessels, allowing for a more rapid flow of blood. The drug of choice is usually nitroglycerine in tablets, administered under the tongue. This drug acts almost immediately and often produces a feeling of warmth, flushing of the face, or throbbing in the head. When these patients are hospitalized it is not unusual for the physician to write an order granting permission for the patient to keep nitroglycerine tablets at his bedside to be taken as needed.

Effects of Cold. We know that cold has a direct effect on the blood vessels, causing them to contract. The patient with angina pectoris is already suffering from a narrowing of the arteries; thus, he must avoid exposure to cold, which would further aggravate the condition. He should be instructed to wear warm clothing and stay indoors when the weather is extremely cold. In the summer months some patients have suffered attacks when they entered an air-conditioned building after being out in the hot sun.

DISORDERS OF THE HEART'S CONDUCTION SYSTEM

Introduction. One can hardly read a newspaper or magazine today without becoming aware of the great strides being taken in the field of electronics and the ways in which this advancing research can be of benefit to the health and welfare of mankind. The comparatively new transistors have now been found to be useful in initiating electrical impulses in the hearts of persons suffering from disorders of the heart's electrical conduction system. Although the surgical procedure involved in inserting an artificial pacemaker cannot be termed simple, it probably will become more and more common in the years to come.

We know that the normal heart is capable of generating tiny electrical impulses that can be picked up, amplified and recorded by an electrocardiograph. These impulses are essential to normal contraction of the heart's ventricles and atria. The impulses originate in the sino-atrial (S.A.) node

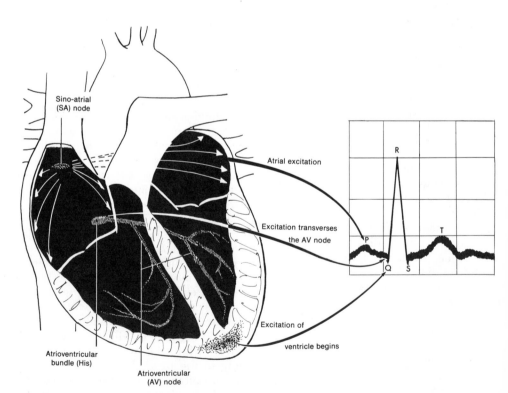

Figure 12-9. Conducting system of the heart showing source of electrical impulses produced on electrocardiogram. (After Jacob and Francone: *Structure and Function in Man*, W. B. Saunders Co., Philadelphia.)

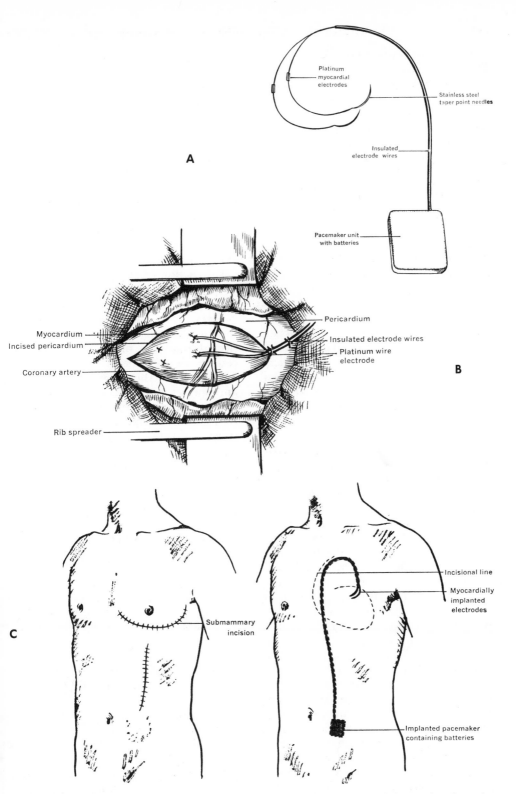

Figure 12-10. *A*, Implantable pacemaker with myocardial electrodes. *B*, Platinum wire electrodes are implanted usually in the left ventricular wall. *C*, Outward appearance of patient with abdominally implanted pacemaker. Position of implanted pacemaker and electrodes is shown at right. (From Heller: American Journal of Nursing, April, 1964.)

and the atrioventricular (A.V.) node. These are neuromuscular structures. One, the S.A. node, is located in the wall of the right atrium between the openings for the inferior and superior venae cavae. It stimulates contraction of the atria. The A.V. node is located in the septum between the atria and transmits impulses via the bundle of His and the Purkinje fibers to the ventricles, causing them to contract (see Fig. 12-9).

When the heart's electrical conduction system fails, the normal contractions of the heart that are necessary to its pumping action also fail. It is now possible to relieve this condition by implanting the electrodes of an artificial pacemaker directly into the heart muscle. These electrodes are attached to the very small pacemaker batteries which are pre-set to stimulate ventricular contractions at a rate of 70 per minute. The pacemaker batteries are implanted in the patient's body (see Fig. 12-10).

Indications for Use of the Pacemaker. There are four general disorders that may respond to the artificial pacemaker. They are: (1) Stokes-Adams disease, a condition characterized by disturbances in the rhythm of ventricular contractions. The arrhythmia interferes with normal flow of blood to the brain and produces symptoms of dizziness, unconsciousness, convulsions or death. (2) Carotid sinus syndrome, a disorder involving the carotid sinus, which works by reflex action to ensure a steady flow of blood to the brain and other parts of the body. When the carotid sinus does not function normally the patient suffers from attacks of fainting, lowered blood pressure or convulsions. Such an attack can be precipitated by slight pressure on the carotid sinus, as from turning the head quickly or wearing a tight collar. (3) Surgical injury to the heart's conduction system during corrective cardiac surgery. (4) Arteriosclerosis with atrioventricular block in some elderly patients.[14]

Nursing Care. During the preoperative period the nurse cooperates with the physician and other members of the medical team in diagnostic tests and other procedures that will be useful in determining the patient's readiness for surgery. She must be especially observant of the patient's vital signs, and if any attacks of fainting or dizziness occur, they should be reported accurately. During such an attack the patient's pulse should be taken and recorded. The nurse also should chart the duration of the attack and any aftereffects noted.

Instruction of the patient and physical preparation for surgery are approximately the same as for any major surgery. The physician will explain the artificial pacemaker and the expected outcome of the surgical procedure. The patient also should be informed of the type of equipment and special apparatus that will be used postoperatively. This includes thoracic tubes and drainage bottles, intravenous tubes, oxygen and possibly gastric suction.

After the patient recovers from surgery he will be able to return home within one to two weeks. The artificial pacemaker should cause him no discomfort and should not hamper the movement of his chest or arm. Many of these patients will be able to indulge in activities that formerly were restricted because of the danger of precipitating an attack. They can lead normal lives again without the constant fear of a serious or even fatal attack.

INFLAMMATORY DISEASES OF THE HEART

Definition. The tissues of the heart are subject to the same inflammatory conditions that may affect other parts of the body. The inflammation may be present in the inner lining (*endocarditis*), the heart muscle (*myocarditis*), or the sac surrounding the heart (*pericarditis*). The process may also involve the valves between the heart chambers or those located at the base of the major vessels leading from the heart.

Bacterial infection of the heart can result from an acute infection elsewhere in the body such as those caused by staphylococci, pneumococci, and gonococci. However, the most common occurrence is inflammation of the heart as a complication of rheumatic fever.

Unfortunately, rheumatic heart disease is the most common form of heart disease among children and the leading cause of death in individuals between the ages of 5 and 25.[4] The tragedy of the situation is compounded by the fact that so many of these cases could be prevented by early treatment of streptococcal infections, especially "strep throat." The practical nurse must realize the importance of these facts and do her part in educating the public to the danger of allowing cases of tonsillitis and sore throat to continue untreated.

Symptoms. The symptoms of rheumatic heart disease are the symptoms of a complication and therefore do not appear until after the acute stage of rheumatic fever has subsided. These symptoms will vary according to the location of the inflammation. With a myocarditis there may be changes in the rate and rhythm of the heart beat and enlargement of the heart. In an endocarditis there may be characteristic heart murmurs, hematuria, small red areas over the entire body (petechiae), and undue fatigue. In pericarditis there are the symptoms of pain in the heart region, increase in the heart rate, and dyspnea. All of these conditions may eventually lead to congestive failure.

Treatment and Nursing Care. REST. Inflammatory conditions are primarily treated with rest of the part and so it is with inflammatory diseases of the heart. The treatment consists of measures intended to decrease the work load of the heart. The length of time for con-

finement to bed may extend to months and even years. The physician uses information of the patient's current sedimentation rate to determine the progress of the disease and the amount of rest required. As the sedimentation rate is lowered he may allow more activity; if it becomes elevated, he will order the patient back to bed.

Detailed care of the patient on bed rest is discussed on page 228.

MEDICATIONS. Specific medications for the treatment of inflammatory conditions of the heart include the antibiotics, particularly penicillin, which is given in massive doses and often by a continuous intravenous drip. If the causative organism is resistant to penicillin other antibiotics may be given.

SURGERY. In recent years surgery inside the heart, or open heart surgery, has become a relatively safe and acceptable method of treating some forms of heart disease. A technique referred to as *commissurotomy* is used to restore the functions of a diseased mitral valve, or other valves which may have been affected by bacterial invasion of the heart.

If the valve is beyond repair it can be replaced by an artificial valve (see page 233).

HYPERTENSIVE HEART DISEASE

Definition. An increase in the blood pressure places an extra burden on the heart as it works harder to force the blood through the blood vessels. This brings about an increase in the size of the heart and impaired function as a result of fatigue of the heart muscle. The term used to describe this condition is "hypertensive heart disease."

Hypertension may result from chronic kidney infections or diseases of the arteries such as arteriosclerosis. It may also occur without any apparent cause, having no known relationship with any other disease. This second type is called *essential hypertension.*

Symptoms. As the heart begins to fail because of fatigue from its attempts to compensate for hypertension, the patient develops dyspnea, undue fatigue, edema of the extremities, and eventually cyanosis. Congestive failure develops rapidly if the hypertension is not relieved.

Treatment and Nursing Care. Treatment is aimed at relief of the underlying cause, when this can be determined, and measures to decrease the work load of the heart. The patient with hypertensive heart disease will need intelligent nursing care based on the needs of the individual patient. Physical and emotional rest are of great importance. The patient must learn to use moderation in everything he does, avoiding excesses in eating, drinking, smoking, exercise, and emotional excitement.

MEDICATIONS. Drugs used in the treatment of hypertensive heart disease include those that lower the blood pressure in addition to medications that improve the strength and character of the heart beat. The hypotensive drugs (those that lower the blood pressure) include reserpine (Serpasil) and hydralazine (Apresoline).

CONGENITAL HEART DISEASE

Definition. The word "congenital" means "born with" or "present at birth." Thus a congenital heart disease is actually a defect in the structure of the heart which has resulted from improper growth and development of the infant's heart, or a major blood vessel. There may be one or more defects present and they constitute abnormal openings or obstructions which impair the circulation of blood (see Fig. 12-11).

The exact cause of the improper development of the heart in a fetus is not fully understood although a virus infection in the mother (especially German measles) during the first three months of pregnancy is believed to be a causative factor.

Types. There are many different types of congenital heart disease depending on the number and kind of structural defects present and the symptoms resulting from the impaired circulation. The term "blue baby" is often used to describe any infant who has cyanosis as a result of a congenital heart defect, but it is more correctly used to describe a condition known as "tetralogy of Fallot."

This condition was given the name "tetralogy" because there are four defects present, and Fallot is added because that was the name of the French physician who first described the condition.

The four defects that make up this group are:*

1. *Ventricular septal defect*: In the wall (septum) between the two ventricles, there is an abnormal opening, causing unoxygenated blood in the right ventricle to mix with oxygenated blood in the left ventricle.
2. *Overriding aorta*: Instead of rising solely from the left ventricle, the aorta straddles both ventricles, rising from a joint just over the septal defect. Thus it receives both oxygenated and unoxygenated blood, and sends this poorly oxygenated mixture through the body.
3. *Pulmonary stenosis*: There is a narrowing in the pulmonary valve, which obstructs the flow of blood through the pulmonary artery to the lungs.
4. *Enlarged right ventricle*: Owing to the strain of pumping blood through the narrowed pulmonary valve, the right ventricle overworks, becomes enlarged, and is not able to function effectively.

The main result of this combination of defects is that the blood and the body tissues do not get enough oxygen. Since blood which is low in oxygen is a bluish red, this gives the skin a blue tinge.

---

*From the booklet "If Your Child Has a Congenital Heart Defect," published by the American Heart Association.

Figure 12-11. Congenital defects of the heart. (From Jacob and Francone: *Structure and Function in Man*, W. B. Saunders Co., Philadelphia.)

Table 16. *General Signs and Symptoms of Congenital Heart Abnormalities**

INFANTS	CHILDREN
1. Dyspnea	1. Dyspnea
2. Difficulty with feeding	2. Poor physical development
3. Stridor or choking spells	3. Decreased exercise tolerance
4. Pulse rate over 200	4. Recurrent respiratory infections
5. Recurrent respiratory infections	5. Heart murmur and thrill
6. Failure to gain weight	6. Cyanosis
7. Heart murmurs	7. Squatting
8. Cyanosis	8. Clubbing of fingers and toes
9. Cerebrovascular accidents	9. Elevated blood pressure
10. Anoxic attacks	

*From NSF Education Service, Ross Laboratories.

However, certain other defects also cause cyanosis.

Symptoms. See Table 16.

Treatment and Nursing Care. Recent advances in the techniques of open-heart surgery have provided methods of successfully treating some but not all types of congenital heart defects. In these surgical procedures attempts are made to correct the defect so that the circulation of the blood is established to a state as near to normal as possible. In order to accomplish this the surgeon may repair the defect by enlarging or tying off sections of the

Table 17. *Classification of Heart Disease*

TYPE	CAUSE	SPECIFIC TREATMENTS
Congestive heart failure	Complication of another primary heart disease or renal failure. Ventricles fail to empty properly leading to congestion of all tissues served by the venae cavae and pulmonary veins.	Rest to relieve stress and strain on the heart. Diuretics and restriction of sodium intake to relieve edema. Drugs which increase the cardiac output by improving the muscular contractions of the heart.
Coronary heart diseases	1. Arteriosclerosis, causing a narrowing of the blood vessels which serve the heart muscle. This results in a decreased supply of oxygen to the heart muscle. 2. Acute coronary occlusion. A sudden blocking of a coronary vessel by a blood clot. This leads to myocardial infarction with death of the area being deprived of its blood supply.	Vasodilator drugs. Limited activities to avoid overexertion and added strain on the heart. Avoiding sudden exposure to cold. Analgesics for relief of pain. Treatment of shock. Rest. Relief of pain. Anticoagulant drugs such as Dicumarol and Coumadin. Oxygen for dyspnea and cyanosis.

Table continued on page 249.

Table 17. *Classification of Heart Disease* (Continued)

TYPE	CAUSE	SPECIFIC TREATMENTS
Inflammatory diseases of the heart	Most often rheumatic fever following a streptococcal infection of the throat. Sometimes following acute infections such as diphtheria and typhoid fever.	Absolute bed rest. Antibiotics to treat the infection. Treatment of anemia, which is usually present. Surgery to restore proper functioning of the heart valves.
Hypertensive heart disease	Hypertension: essential, in which the cause is unknown, or secondary following chronic kidney disease or a disease of the aorta.	Drugs which lower the blood pressure. Treatment of the primary condition. Sympathectomy to block the nerve impulses to the blood vessels.
Congenital heart disease	Unknown. May be due to viral infections, especially German measles, during the first three months of pregnancy.	Surgery for types amenable to this type of treatment.

major vessels, rerouting the blood through the use of grafts, and suturing together openings in the septum.

Medical treatment with drugs may be of more benefit than surgery for some types of heart defects. In cases in which the defect cannot or need not be repaired by surgery, the patient may be kept under continuous medical supervision for observation of his progress and administration of medications to relieve his symptoms.

Part III—NURSING CARE OF PATIENTS WITH DISORDERS OF THE PERIPHERAL VASCULAR SYSTEM

INTRODUCTION

The peripheral blood vessels are those veins and arteries which are situated a distance from the heart. Diseases of the peripheral blood vessels are most often chronic in nature, affecting persons of the older age group, and associated with other diseases of the cardiovascular system or the kidneys. Diabetics are also particularly susceptible to diseases of the peripheral blood vessels.

The lower extremities, being farthest away from the center of the body's circulatory system, are often subject to diseases of the blood vessels which diminish the supply of blood to these parts. These conditions will be discussed first in this section of the chapter.

Since the blood vessels leading to and from the brain also come under the general heading of peripheral vessels, cerebrovascular diseases are presented after diseases of the extremities in this same section.

Table 18. *Conditions Causing Reduced Arterial Supply**

DISEASE	PREDISPOSING FACTORS
Buerger's disease or thromboangiitis obliterans	Unknown; suspect infection or activity of some toxic agent
Arteriosclerosis (atherosclerosis)	Diabetes, hypertension, disturbances of lipid metabolism, especially cholesterol
Arterial embolism	Heart disease—atrial fibrillation, vascular lesions, bacterial endocarditis, coronary occlusion, venous thrombosis
Arteritis	Systemic infections—syphilis, pneumonia, typhus fever, typhoid fever, influenza, septicemia, scarlet fever, cholera
Constant constriction of peripheral vessels	Pathologic overactivity of sympathetic nervous system
Spasmodic cyanosis of the fingers	Spondylitis, cervical rib
Frostbite	Exposure to cold

Table 19. *Conditions Causing Decreased Venous Flow**

DISEASE	PREDISPOSING FACTORS
Varicose veins	Familial defects of valves, pregnancy, abdominal tumors, ascites
Phlebothrombosis (noninflammatory clot formation)	Heart disease, obesity, varicosities, trauma, surgery, debility, polycythemia, certain anemias
Thrombophlebitis (inflammatory clot formation)	Local injury to endothelium by stretching or trauma, chemical irritation, infection, esp. pneumonia, influenza, typhoid fever. Prolonged bed rest during infections.

*From Fulcher: Nursing Clinics of North America, W. B. Saunders Co., March, 1966.

CIRCULATORY DISORDERS OF THE EXTREMITIES

General Treatment and Nursing Care. In order for the body to remain in a state of good health there must be an equal balance between the metabolic needs of the tissues and the supply of nutrition brought by the blood stream to meet those needs. When the supply cannot meet the demand the cells begin to degenerate from a lack of nutrition. All treatments and nursing care of the patient with a disease of the peripheral blood vessels are aimed at the establishment of good circulation so as to provide adequate nutrition and at prevention of further breakdown of the tissues.

USE OF HEAT. Whenever there is impaired circulation to the extremities over a period of time the peripheral nerves begin to degenerate. The patient then has a decreased sensitivity to all stimuli, particularly heat and cold. Since chilling causes constriction of the blood vessels (the very condition we are trying to combat), these patients must be provided with extra warmth. Their decreased sensitivity to heat rules out the practice of applying local heat in the form of hot water bottles or electric heating pads because the patient may be burned without his realizing it. In addition, local heat increases the metabolic activity of the area to which it is applied and further upsets the balance of supply and demand mentioned above.

The best means of preventing chilling and providing comfort for the patient is to raise the temperature of his environment and dress him in extra warm clothing made of flannel and wool. These will provide an even distribution of heat to the body. It is not unusual for these patients to develop the habit of huddling close to radiators, heaters, or open fires in an effort to keep warm. They must be warned that this is a dangerous practice that can easily lead to severe burns and damage to the tissues of the lower extremities.

INSTRUCTIONS TO THE PATIENT. So much can be done to prevent complications from diseases of the peripheral vascular system by properly educating the patient and his family in the special care of the lower extremities, that it might well be considered one of the most important aspects of treatment and nursing care. Many special clinics in the larger medical centers have specially printed cards or booklets to distribute to their patients. The following, taken from A. F. Brown's *Medical Nursing,* is an example of the points to be emphasized when instructing these patients.

INFORMATION FOR PATIENTS OF THE
PERIPHERAL VASCULAR CLINIC

1. Keep warm.
2. Do not use tobacco in any form.
3. Take great care that the foot is not injured. Avoid crowded places.
4. Wear wide-toed shoes which cause no pressure and have adequate support for the arches.
5. Do not wear circular garters.
6. Do not sit with the knees crossed.
7. If the weight of the bedclothes is uncomfortable, use a pillow to hold the bedclothes off the feet.
8. Soak the feet in a basin of warm soapy water for five minutes every day. Dry thoroughly, especially between the toes, by mopping, not rubbing.
9. Do not apply any medicine to the feet without directions.
10. If the feet are dry and scaly, rub with lanolin, olive oil, castor oil, or cold cream.
11. If the feet are moist, use talcum powder.
12. Before filing nails, soak feet in warm (not hot) water for five minutes to soften nails. File straight across. Do not use a razor blade or knife.
13. Proper first aid treatment is important. Consult your physician immediately for any redness, blistering, pain, or swelling.
14. Do not attempt to treat corns or calluses. Ask your physician what should be done.
15. Drink an abundance of water, at least the equivalent of 20 glasses of water in each 24-hour period.

REST AND EXERCISE. Exercises of a special type may be ordered by the physician in an effort to improve circulation in the lower extremities because much of the movement of blood through the deeper veins in the lower leg depends on muscular activity. These exercises have several contraindications however, and are to be done only on the specific orders of the physician. Periods of rest are alternated with the exercises to prevent fatigue and to allow the body time for healing and repair.

There are times when the physician advises complete rest of the affected limb and the patient is confined to bed. When this occurs the skin must receive particular attention to prevent pressure and breakdown of the tissues. Special notice must be given the heels, and weight relieved by extending the heels over the end of the mattress or placing a pillow under the lower leg. A bed cradle over the legs or footboard with pillows may be used to bear the weight of the top covers.

In using any of these measures to prevent pressure on the heels it must be remembered that relocating the pressure to another part of the lower leg may also cause difficulties. It is important, then, that these patients change position frequently to avoid pressure in any one area for too long. It is also true that sitting or lying in one position over a long period of time decreases the flow of blood and further aggravates the static condition of the circulation.

ULCERS. The starvation of any tissue will inevitably lead to degeneration and death of the tissue cells. An ulcer, or open sore, develops on the skin and erodes the underlying tissues, accompanied by suppuration and drainage of purulent material. Ulcers are quite common in peripheral vascular diseases. Treatment of this condition consists of measures to aid in draining the purulent material and removal of dead tissues so that healing can take place. Wet compresses, Furacin dressings, surgical debridement of necrotic tissue and irrigation may all be necessary to heal these ulcers. Because of the impaired circulation they heal very slowly and may require special skin grafting to replace the tissue lost by necrosis.

There are special pressure bandages or paste "boots" which are used in treating ulcers of the lower extremities. These "boots" are applied so that they cover the entire lower leg and have a threefold purpose: (1) they exert an even pressure on the blood vessels, thereby eliminating local areas of congestion, (2) they give support to the veins near the surface of the limb, and (3) they protect the ulcer from injury and infection from outside sources.

As stated before, these ulcers heal very slowly. The reason for this is that the body's mechanisms against inflammation and infection cannot function as they should when the supply of blood to an area is decreased. The patient often becomes discouraged and depressed by the lack of progress in healing and will require encouragement and constant reassurance from the nursing staff.

APPLIANCES FOR SUPPORT AND COMFORT. Even, well-distributed support of the vessels near the surface of the body will help in the return of the venous blood from the legs. To provide this type of support the physician may recommend that the patient wear an elastic bandage or fitted elastic stockings. Because of their comfort and ease of application, the stockings are more satisfactory than elastic bandages for an ambulatory patient. When these stockings are worn daily the following rules should be observed:

1. The hose should be applied early in the morning before arising from the bed. The blood vessels are less congested after a night's rest.

2. Stockings must be held up with supporters rather than with garters. Circular garters are forbidden.

3. Never roll the tops of the hose and

"knot" them as a means of holding them up.

4. Two pairs are necessary to allow for daily washing and drying of the hose.

DIET. Obesity adds an extra burden of weight and pressure on the peripheral blood vessels and further aggravates congestion of these vessels. Overweight patients must be made aware of the dangers involved in being overweight and encouraged to follow the diet recommended by the physician.

The increased intake of fluids to the equivalent of 20 glasses within a 24-hour period mentioned on page 251 is based on the belief that the removal of waste products from the blood is improved in this manner. Many physicians also agree that the intake of such large amounts of liquids will make the blood less thick and therefore more easily circulated through the vessels.

DRUGS. Medications used in the treatment of peripheral vascular diseases are of two main types: vasodilators, which enlarge the size of the blood vessels, and anticoagulants, which impair the clotting ability of the blood.

Nicotine, which is found in tobacco, has the effect of producing spasmodic narrowing of the peripheral arteries. It is obviously very dangerous for a patient to continue smoking when the peripheral arteries are affected by disease. The patient may experience some difficulty in giving up smoking if he has developed the habit, but the warning that to continue to smoke may result in gangrene and eventual loss of a limb may help him to adjust.

Arteriosclerosis of the Extremities

Definition. Sclerosis means a gradual hardening. In arteriosclerosis the walls of the arteries become hardened over a period of years and eventually lose their elasticity. This brings about a narrowing of these vessels and a decreased flow of blood. It also produces an increase in the blood pressure because of the extra force needed to push the blood through the smaller openings. Arteriosclerosis of the lower extremities is more common than that of the upper extremities, and, being farther from the heart, the lower extremities are more likely to suffer from poor circulation. Diabetics frequently have arteriosclerosis of the lower extremities, which is why amputations are so common in persons who have diabetes.

Symptoms. In the early stages of the disease the lower extremities feel cold to the touch and the patient complains of being unable to keep his feet warm. He may also experience tingling and numbness in the lower legs. Later, there develop fatigue and weakness of the muscles of the affected limb and the patient may tell of leg cramps at night which are relieved by rubbing or lowering the leg over the side of the bed. In the last stages ulcers may appear or there may be a dry gangrene which first involves the toes and then progresses up the extremity if left untreated.

Treatment and Nursing Care. Arteriosclerosis itself cannot be cured at present. Treatment, then, is aimed at relieving the symptoms and improving and maintaining adequate circulation to the extremities so that gangrene or ulcers will not develop. It is also important to avoid any breaks in the skin which may lead to an infection. Once an extremity becomes gangrenous little can be done beyond surgical amputation of the limb.

EXERCISE. Active exercising of a muscle will improve the circulation of blood to that muscle. The physician may order the patient with arteriosclerosis of the extremities to take regular exercises. He will encourage him to walk whenever possible, play golf, ride a bicycle, or perform some similar form of exercise as consistently and regularly as he would take a medication.

WARMTH. Warm clothing and adequately heated rooms are helpful in maintaining continued dilatation of the blood vessels. The reasons for avoiding extremes in temperatures are discussed under General Nursing Care, page 251.

PREVENTION ON INJURY TO THE EXTREMITIES. Arteriosclerosis of the extremities is most common in older persons, and since persons in this age group are frequently in danger of injury from falls because of poor eyesight or decreased muscular coordination, they must be protected from all safety hazards. They should also be instructed carefully in the proper care of the feet and nails mentioned under General Nursing Care. Their shoes should fit snugly enough to prevent blistering, but not so tightly that they impair circulation to the toes. Darned socks or hosiery and stockings that are too loose or too tight must also be avoided.

PHYSIOTHERAPY. Special exercises (for example, Buerger's exercises), sitz baths, and whirlpool baths are all of value in maintaining a good flow of blood to the lower extremities.

Buerger's Disease

Definition. Buerger's disease, also called thromboangiitis obliterans, is an inflammatory disease of the medium-sized vessels, particularly the arteries of the legs. It is characterized by the formation of clots within the arteries, a sharp spasmodic pain in the area, and eventual destruction (obliteration) of these vessels.

The exact cause of Buerger's disease is not known but the most outstanding predisposing factor is thought to be excessive smoking over a period of years.

Treatment. Aside from elimination of smoking and other factors that lead to constriction of blood vessels, treatment is primarily symptomatic, as in cases of arteriosclerosis of the extremities (see above).

Buerger-Allen Exercises. These specific exercises are prescribed to improve circulation to the lower extremities. The patient is taught to do these exercises at home several times a day. He also is instructed in proper care of his feet and legs to avoid aggravation of his condition (see page 251 for details). The Buerger-Allen exercises are as follows:

1. Lie down in a supine position and elevate the lower extremities at an angle of 45 to 90 degrees. Support them in this position until the skin of the extremities turns dead white.
2. Lower the feet and legs so that they are below the level of the rest of the body, being careful that there is no pressure on the back of the knees.
3. When redness appears in the lower extremities place them flat on the bed for 3 to 5 minutes.

Thrombophlebitis

Definition. A *thrombus* is a blood clot which forms inside a blood vessel and remains attached to the side of the vessel wall. This clot may continue to enlarge until it eventually closes off the flow of blood through the vessel. *Phlebitis* is an inflammation of a vein. Thus, *thrombophlebitis* is an inflammation of a vein resulting from circulatory stasis caused by a blood clot in the vessel.

In thrombophlebitis there is local inflammation of the vein and since there is decreased circulation to the area served by the vein, there is also a local inflammation of the tissues adjacent to the vein.

Aside from the local problems presented by impaired circulation there is also danger that the clot may break away from the wall of the vessel and be carried along in the blood stream until it reaches a vessel too small for it to pass through. This results in an area of infarct as described earlier in this chapter.

Many cases of thrombophlebitis are associated with postoperative or postpartum confinement to bed. That is the reason early ambulation is so important in the care of these patients.

Symptoms. Thrombophlebitis may or may not be accompanied by pain in the affected area. However, whenever a patient complains of severe pain in the calf of the leg that is aggravated by flexion of the foot, the nurse should recognize this as a sign of thrombophlebitis and notify the physician immediately. Under no circumstances should the leg be massaged because this could easily dislodge the thrombus and produce an embolism.

In addition to the pain in the leg or thigh along the course of the affected vein, the patient may also have an elevated temperature and increased pulse rate.

Treatment and Nursing Care. Treatment of thrombophlebitis is mostly symptomatic and is aimed at prevention of complications such as embolism, local cellulitis, or ulceration of the area.

Anticoagulants, such as heparin, Dicumarol, and Coumadin, are given to inhibit the clotting of the blood and thereby prevent enlargement of the thrombus.

There is some disagreement among physicians as to the amount of rest required and the type of activity allowed a patient with thrombophlebitis. Some physicians prefer to have the affected part elevated while others do not. Whatever the choice of the physician, the nurse must fully understand his wishes and carry out his orders conscientiously.

Warmth in the form of compresses, heating pads set on "low," and extra blankets are all helpful in increasing the blood supply to the area.

Patients with thrombophlebitis must not become constipated because straining at defecation may dislodge the thrombus. A seizure of coughing may have the same effect. Thus the patient must also be protected from respiratory infections.

Varicose Veins

Varicose veins are veins which have become greatly enlarged and distorted in shape. When blood is returned from the lower extremities it is kept flowing in one direction by a system of cup-shaped valves (see Fig. 12-12). These valves open to allow the upward passage of blood and then close to prevent a backward flow toward the feet. If these valves fail to function properly the vein fills with blood and becomes enlarged and tortuous.

The valves may lose their ability to function properly through injury or disease. In some cases, however, it is believed that weakness of valves in the veins is inherited by some persons, thus making them more susceptible to varicose veins.

Figure 12-12. The valves of a vein. *A*, Valve is closed and the cusps are filled with blood, thus preventing a backward flow. *B*, Valve is open and blood ascends, passing through the valve. (From King and Showers: *Human Anatomy and Physiology*, 5th Ed., W. B. Saunders Co., Philadelphia.)

Symptoms. In the early stages of development varicose veins may present mild symptoms of fatigue and a feeling of heaviness in the legs, or swelling of the ankles after prolonged standing. Later there may be a dull or sharp pain in the legs. Sometimes the patient complains of cramps in the legs after going to bed at night. Itching along the course of the vein is also very common. As varicose veins continue to enlarge there are repeated inflammations locally which lead to the formation of ulcers. These are usually found on the lower leg or ankle.

Treatment and Nursing Care. Medical management of varicose veins consists of: (1) support of the veins by the application of fitted elastic bandages, (2) removal of causative factors, such as obesity or prolonged standing or sitting in one position, and (3) a prescribed regimen of rest and exercises.

Another form of treatment is the injection of a sclerosing agent into the varicose vein. The solution hardens the vein, obstructing the flow of blood through it and thereby preventing further engorgement. This method is only a temporary measure, however, and does not cure the condition.

Surgical treatment of varicose veins may be necessary when the more conservative methods fail to relieve the symptoms. The surgery may involve a *simple ligation* in which the large saphenous vein is tied off at the upper end (at the thigh). A more common procedure and one that offers more satisfactory results is a "vein stripping." In this procedure the entire vein is actually pulled out of the subcutaneous tissue. An instrument is inserted in the upper part of the vein through an incision in the thigh. The vein is tied to the instrument and as the instrument is passed along the course of the vein and pulled out through a lower incision, the vein is "turned inside out" so to speak and removed. The surgeon then applies even pressure along the course of the vein to control bleeding. After the vein has been removed the larger, more deeply imbedded veins take over the task of draining blood from the part of the leg formerly served by the surgically removed vein.

After this surgery the patient is usually out of bed at least once during the first postoperative day so that good circulation is maintained in the lower legs. The dressings and elastic bandages must be checked frequently for signs of hemorrhage. While the patient is in the bed the limb is elevated on pillows to facilitate the flow of blood through the veins.

DISEASES OF THE CEREBRAL VESSELS

Arteriosclerosis of the Cerebral Vessels

Definition. Arteriosclerosis of the cerebral vessels is a hardening of the arteries serving the brain. The condition occurs most often after 50 years of age and increases in frequency with the advancing years.

Symptoms. The symptoms presented are a direct result of a gradual starvation of brain tissue due to a decreased blood supply. These patients manifest signs of mental deterioration with a slowing down of the mental processes and a decrease in intelligence. They often show emotional changes as well, such as being very easily upset and prone to crying and pouting as if they were children once again.

Treatment and Nursing Care. Very little can be done for these patients because arteriosclerosis is a disease of degeneration in which there is little hope of stopping or reversing the process. The nursing care mainly involves acceptance of the patient as he is, and providing a quiet and restful environment so as to avoid any emotional or physical excitement which would aggravate his condition.

Cerebrovascular Accident
(Stroke, Apoplexy)

Introduction. Research has shown that by the time we reach the age of 30, one fourth of us will have sufficient hardening of the cerebral arteries to provide the setting for a stroke at any time. By the time we reach 70 years of age the percentage increases to 80. Stroke is a common disease, more common than many of us realize, for autopsy studies have shown that nearly half the people who die from other causes have had minor strokes without ever having been aware of them. Since stroke is a disease of middle-aged and older persons, we can expect the incidence of this disease to increase as the lifespan increases.

Cause. A cerebrovascular accident may occur as a result of (1) cerebral thrombosis (blood clot forms in the cerebral vessel); (2) cerebral hemorrhage (vessel ruptures and leaks blood into brain tissue), or (3) atherosclerosis of the arteries of the neck and head. Any one of these conditions can lead to an interruption in the flow of blood to the brain tissues, thereby producing ischemia (local anemia) and destruction of the brain cells that formerly were served by the affected blood vessels. High blood pressure, endocarditis and other heart disorders and atherosclerosis are predisposing factors in the gradual blockage of the flow of blood, or in a sudden "blow-out" of an artery.

Symptoms. The symptoms of stroke are varied. They depend on the condition causing the stroke and the size and location of the area of brain tissue affected by the vascular accident (see Fig. 12-13).

The patient may have some warning that an attack is coming on even though he does not know exactly what is wrong. He may feel dizzy, have a headache or lose consciousness for a moment. When a large area of the brain is affected death may be instantaneous. The most common after-effects of a stroke are disturbances of speech and paralysis on one side of the body.

Fortunately, the cerebral arteries are capable of enlarging and eventually taking over the work of the damaged arteries. This means that there is a possibility that the patient may ultimately regain use of the affected parts of his body. In some cases there may be slight residual effects such as weakness on one side and a slight limp or dragging of the lower limb.

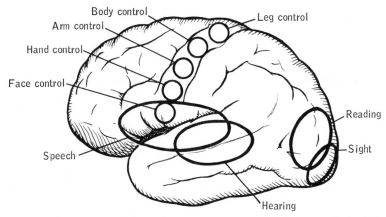

Figure 12-13. Control zones of the cerebral cortex. Nerve cells that control physical and mental activities are located in specific centers or zones of the cerebral cortex, the largest part of the human brain. The left side of the cerebral cortex with its control zones is diagrammed here. If the normal flow of blood to one of these zones is stopped, the activity controlled by the zone will be impaired. (Modified from Stokes, American Heart Association, 1958.)

Treatment and Nursing Care. Emergency treatment consists of loosening all constricting clothing, especially around the neck, and turning the victim's head to one side to prevent obstruction of the air passages. No attempts should be made to move the person until an ambulance has arrived. Never attempt to arouse a person who is unconscious from a stroke.

After the patient has been admitted to the hospital the vital signs are taken and recorded every hour for the first 24 hours. Observations are made as to the patient's apparent state of consciousness and ability to move his leg or arm, and whether or not he can speak.

During the acute phase of this illness attention must be paid to maintenance of an airway. This includes positioning of the patient for maximum respiration and suctioning whenever necessary to prevent obstruction of the trachea with mucus or saliva. As long as the patient is unconscious or unable to respond the head is kept turned to the side to facilitate drainage of mucus and saliva from the mouth.

Fluids may be given by vein until it is definitely established whether or not the stroke victim can swallow. For those who absolutely cannot handle liquids in the mouth, tube feeding may be necessary. If at all possible the patient should be placed in an upright position, at least a 45° angle, during the tube feeding. The formula should be diluted with water, usually half and half, so that diarrhea is avoided and the patient's fluid intake is adequately maintained. Vomiting and diarrhea also can be prevented by administering the formula slowly. The inconvenience to the patient and the added burden to the nurses brought about vomiting and frequent watery stools should be sufficient reason for proper administration of tube feedings. Unfortunately, this procedure often is handled in a haphazard way.

Positioning the patient who has had a stroke is of extreme importance. A stroke involves only the *control* centers of muscular activity. It does not affect the muscles themselves. It has been said that in the past, stroke patients have been rendered "tender, loving neglect" because doctors have placed these patients on bed rest and nurses have proceeded to do everything possible for the patient rather than encourage him to learn to help himself. We must remember that one of the main goals of nursing is to help restore those who are ill to a state of health. The stroke patient cannot move or position himself at first. He must depend on the nursing staff to keep his musculoskeletal system in good working order until he is able to use it once again.

The body is positioned so that the joints remain movable and the muscles maintain their tone. The patient's position is changed every hour from back, to side, to prone, and then to the back and so on. While the patient is on his back the affected arm is raised above his head and the hand tucked under the pillow. This helps prevent "frozen shoulder" so common in these patients (see Fig. 12-14).

In addition to proper positioning, the joints are put through their full range of motion at least once a day (see Fig. 7-4). This may easily be done as the daily bath is given. Other exercises for the stroke patient are given only on the order of the doctor in charge and are usually done under the supervision of a physiotherapist. If such a person is not available, however, the booklet, "Strike Back at Stroke," published by the U.S. Government Printing Office, contains excellent, well illustrated directions for these exercises recommended for the stroke patient.

There are many other little things the nurse can do to encourage her patient and strengthen his muscles as well as his will to help himself. Instead of feeding the patient every item on his tray the nurse can let him hold bread or other "finger foods," suggesting that he feed himself these while she handles the more difficult foods. Strange as it may seem, solids and semisolids are

Figure 12-14. *A,* A pillow is placed next to the body on the weak side. The weak arm is placed on the pillow. Make sure that the elbow points away from the body and that the lower arm and hand are placed alongside the body and about 12 inches away from it. A rolled napkin or small towel is placed under the weak hand to keep the fingers open. Note trochanter roll along affected side to keep hip from rotating. *B,* The affected arm is tucked under the pillow with hand flattened to prevent curling of fingers. *C,* In this side-lying position, a pillow is used to support the weak arm. Another pillow is used to support the weak leg. (From *Strike Back at Stroke,* U.S. Government Printing Office, Washington, D.C.)

easier for the patient to get down without strangling than water and juices are. Chewing will be very slow for the patient at first; he must not be hurried or allowed to chew to the point of exhaustion.

Combing and brushing the hair is good exercise for the arm and shoulder, as are brushing the teeth and washing the face. The patient may not be able to carry all of these procedures through to completion at first, but with encouragement he can gradually improve until he is able to perform much of his own personal toilet himself. This is a tremendous morale booster to one who might have formerly considered himself totally helpless.

There will be many moments of despair and depression for the stroke patient as he struggles to regain control of his muscles. He will need calm reassurance and sincere words of encouragement—not an artificially gay and hopeful kind of encouragement, but a serious understanding from his nurse that he does indeed have many problems, and her solemn, warm-hearted promise that she will do everything within her power to help him overcome those problems.

Surgical Treatment of Stroke. Until recent years there was no sugical treatment for a cerebrovascular accident. Now, however, it has been found that about one third of all strokes can be traced to obstruction of any one of the four arteries in the neck which supply blood to the brain. These arteries are readily accessible, so that the surgeon may open the artery and remove the obstruction. He then sutures the vessel wall or sews a Dacron patch over the incision, leaving the vessel larger than before. If a long section of the artery is blocked the surgeon may reroute the blood through a Dacron tube grafted onto the affected vessel (see Fig. 12-15).

These new surgical procedures are also used as means of preventing many major strokes. When the patient experiences warnings such as spells of dizziness or numbness of the limbs the doctor may suspect "little strokes" and order special x-rays of the arteries serving the brain. If the tests show an obstruction, surgical intervention will

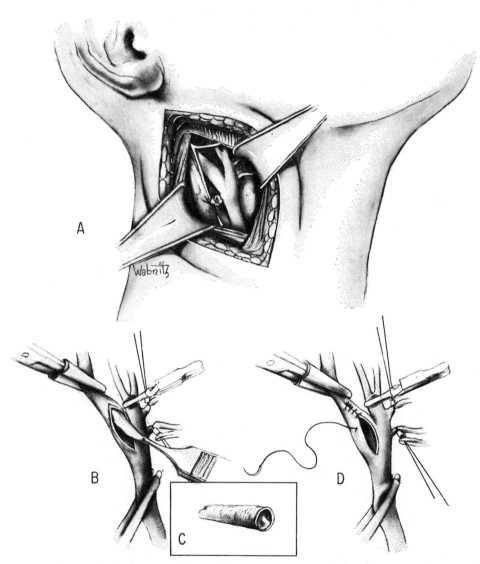

Figure 12-15. Steps in removal of atherosclerotic plaque. *A,* Carotid artery bifurcation is surgically exposed. *B,* Vessel is incised and plaque freed. *C,* Darkened area in vessel lumen is plaque's diaphragm, which further blocks artery. *D,* Vessel is sutured after removal of plaque. (From Long: American Journal of Nursing, September, 1966.)

prevent further development of the obstruction and an eventual cerebrovascular accident.

Prevention. There are measures that can be taken to prevent stroke other than the surgical procedures presented above. Now that more is known about the cause of stroke we are able to eliminate or at least keep under control some of the conditions that predispose an individual to a cerebrovascular accident.

Control of hypertension is one such factor. Another is adequate treatment of rheumatic heart disease and coronary artery disease, both of which can produce blood clots in the heart that eventually break loose and find their way into the cerebral vessels, thus causing a stroke. Individuals with diabetes, cardiac arrhythmia, atherosclerosis, hypertension and rheumatic heart disease should have periodic examinations for evidence of an impending stroke. In this way measures can be taken to avoid emotional, physical or infectious stresses that can precipitate a stroke.[28]

Hypertension

Definition. The term *hypertension* refers to a condition in which the pressure of the blood within the arteries is sustained at an elevated level. Although both the systolic and diastolic pressure may be high, an elevated diastolic pressure is considered especially significant because it indicates an increased blood pressure during the resting phase of the cardiac cycle. This means that the blood vessels are under relentless pressure at all times and the hypertensive individual is a very good candidate for heart disease or a vascular disease of some kind. The occurrence of stroke is very often associated with hypertension.

The average blood pressure range is between 100/60 and 140/90, depending on the person's age, body build and state of physical and mental rest. Although blood pressure may increase with age, and vascular diseases likewise are more likely to develop as one grows older, it is not inevitable that old age be accompanied by hypertension. It is also a fallacy that one's blood pressure should be 100 plus his age.

There are two general categories of hypertension: *essential* and *secondary*. Essential hypertension is the most common type and it occurs without any known cause. Secondary hypertension is, as its name implies, secondary to or a result of another disorder. The term *malignant hypertension* is sometimes used to describe an extremely severe form of essential hypertension that is usually fatal within one to two years after an abrupt onset.

Symptoms. The symptoms of high blood pressure may vary in individuals, but usually there is a throbbing headache, fatigue and restlessness. Complications also can cause symptoms and some of these can be quite severe and even fatal. Most of these symptoms are caused by rupture of and hemorrhage from a blood vessel or by obstruction of the blood flow within a blood vessel.

Visual disturbances or blindness can result from damage to the blood vessels of the retina. Congestive failure can occur when the heart is overworked and fatigue develops in the heart muscle. Stroke may occur as a result of increased pressure within a cerebral vessel which in turn produces rupture of the vessel wall and leakage of blood into the brain tissue. The kidneys may fail as a result of impaired circulation to the renal cells.

Treatment and Nursing Care. Prevention of the complications presented above is one of the principal aims of treatment of hypertension. Unless the basic disorder causing secondary hypertension can be eliminated, there is no possible cure for this condition. The patient should avoid obesity and emotional stresses and tensions, limit his intake of sodium and strive for moderation in everything he does.

The drugs that are used in the control of hypertension include *chlorothiazide*

(Diuril), a diuretic that also lowers blood pressure; *reserpine* (Serpasil), a hypertensive that also has a tranquilizing effect; and *mecamylamine* (Inversine) and *guanethidine sulfate* (Ismelin), two potent anti-hypertensive drugs. Sedatives such as phenobarbital are sometimes given to promote rest and relaxation, which serve to lower the blood pressure.

CLINICAL CASE PROBLEMS

1. Mr. Wilkins is admitted to the hospital with a diagnosis of myocardial infarction. He is obviously very apprehensive the first few days he is in the hospital and apparently is afraid that he is going to die.

　　After he begins to recover from his heart attack, Mr. Wilkins does not wish to stay in bed as the doctor ordered, and he demands iced coffee with his meals.

　　How can you help relieve the patient's anxiety when he is first admitted to the hospital?
　　What could you say to help Mr. Wilkins understand the need for absolute bed rest until his physician gives permission for him to be up?
　　Why is it not permissible for Mr. Wilkins to have any iced drinks or foods?

2. Mrs. Thomas is a young mother who has three small children. She is admitted to the hospital with a severe anemia. Her hemoglobin is 5 gm. and red cell count is also very low. The young mother confides in you that she has never eaten as she should, especially when she was a teen-ager, and with the added strain of having the children to care for at home she doesn't take the time to cook the meals she knows they should have because she is so tired all the time.

　　Her husband makes a fairly good salary, but Mrs. Thomas is under the impression that an adequate diet would cost more than they can afford at present.

　　How can you teach the patient the value of good food and help her with shopping practices which would provide her family with good food that is not expensive?

What could you suggest to help her with the problem of chronic fatigue?

3. Mrs. Wolffe is an acquaintance of yours who works at a check-out counter in a grocery store. She has recently complained to you about pain in her legs and the development of unsightly varicose veins. She is about 50 pounds overweight and has tried several times to lose weight on a "crash" diet, but has never been successful. She tells you that her mother also had varicose veins and so she supposes that the condition is inherited and that nothing can be done about it.

　　What advice can you give this person?
　　What treatment is used in the care of varicose veins?

4. You have been assigned to the task of teaching a patient in a peripheral vascular clinic. The patient is suffering from arteriosclerosis of the extremities and has had this condition for several years. You have been told that this is the patient's second visit to the clinic and he needs instruction in the prevention of complications and in daily care of the feet and legs.

　　What instructions would you give this patient?
　　How can you help him understand the importance of following these instructions?

REFERENCES

1. American Journal of Nursing: *The Patient with Myocardial Infarction*, supplement C. Nov., 1964, pp. 1-31.
2. American Heart Association: *If Your Child Has a Congenital Heart Defect.* New York, 1960.
3. Beland, I.: *Clinical Nursing.* New York, The Macmillan Co., 1965.
4. Brown, A. F.: *Medical Nursing*, 3rd edition. Philadelphia, W. B. Saunders Co., 1957.
5. Brunner, L. S., et al.: *Textbook of Medical-Surgical Nursing.* Philadelphia, J. B. Lippincott Co., 1964.
6. Buck, M. W.: "Adjustments during Recovery from Stroke." Am. Journ. Nurs., Oct., 1964, p. 92.
7. Davenport, R.: "Tube-feeding for Long-term Patients." Am. Journ. Nurs., Jan., 1964, p. 21.
8. Fulcher, A. J.: "The Nurse and the Patient with Peripheral Vascular Disease." *Nursing*

Clinics of North America, vol. 1, no. 1. Philadelphia, W. B. Saunders Co., 1966.

9. Goode, M.: "The Patient with a Cerebral Vascular Accident." Nurs. Outlook, March, 1966, p. 60.

10. Griep, A. H., and Sister DePaul: "Angina Pectoris." Am. Journ. Nurs., June, 1965, p. 72.

11. Grellman, A.: "Diuretics." Am. Journ. Nurs., Jan., 1965, p. 84.

12. Gurski, B. M.: "Rationale of Nursing Care for Patients with Blood Dyscrasias." *Nursing Clinics of North America*, vol. 1, no. 1. Philadelphia, W. B. Saunders Co., 1966.

13. Guyton, A. C.: *Textbook of Medical Physiology*. Philadelphia, W. B. Saunders Co., 1966.

14. Heller, A. H.: "Nursing the Patient with an Artificial Pacemaker." Am. Journ. Nurs., April, 1964, p. 87.

15. Larsen, E. L.: "The Patient with Acute Pulmonary Edema." Am. Journ. Nurs., May, 1968, p. 1019.

16. Long, J. M.: "Carotid Thromboendarterectomy." Am. Journ. Nurs., Sept., 1966, p. 1969.

17. Lunceford, J. L.: "Leukemia." *Nursing Clinics of North America*, vol. 2, no. 4, Philadelphia, W. B. Saunders Co., 1967.

18. Olwin, J. H., and Keppel, J. L.: "Anticoagulant Therapy." Am. Journ. Nurs., May, 1964, p. 107.

19. Piterak, E. F.: "Open-ended Care for the Open Heart Patient." Am. Journ. Nurs., July, 1967, p. 1452.

20. Quinn, C. A.: "LPN: Heart–Lung Technician." Journ. Pract. Nurs., Nov., 1965, p. 30.

21. Rawlings, M. S.: "Heart Disease Today." Am. Journ. Nurs., Feb., 1966, p. 303.

22. Redman, M. J.: "Drugs Used in Coronary and Cerebral Vascular Disease." RN, Sept., 1966, p. 63.

23. Rogez, B. D., and Helswade, G. R.: "Care of Patients Having Open-Heart Surgery." Journ. Pract. Nurs., April, 1966, p. 22.

24. Shafer, K. N., Sawyer, J. R., et al.: *Medical-Surgical Nursing*, 4th edition. St. Louis, C. V. Mosby Co., 1965.

25. Smith, D. W., and Gips, C. D.: *Care of the Adult Patient*, 2nd edition. Philadelphia, J. B. Lippincott, 1966.

26. Stamler, J., et al.: "Coronary Proneness and Approaches to Preventing Heart Attacks." Am. Journ. Nurs., Aug., 1966, p. 1788.

27. Ullman, M.: "Disorders of Body Image after Stroke." Am. Journ. Nurs., Oct., 1964, p. 89.

28. White, P. D.: "Strokes—Prevention, Diagnosis and Patient Care." Journ. Pract. Nurs. Oct., 1965, p. 24.

29. Wilson, S.: "Chronic Leg Ulcers; Nursing Management." Am. Journ. Nurs., Jan., 1967, p. 96.

STUDENT READING LIST

1. "Advances in Heart Research." Practical Nursing. July-August, 1962, p. 19.

2. American Heart Association (booklets): *If Your Child Has a Congenital Heart Defect, Stroke (A Guide for the Family), Strike Back at Stroke, and Varicose Veins.*

3. Callaghan, J.: "Making the Cardiac Patient's Work Easier." Am. Journ. Nurs., Aug., 1955, p. 950.

4. Declan, Sister M.: "Nursing Care After a Cerebral Accident." Practical Nursing, Feb., 1962, p. 12.

5. Elliott, F. C.: "Heart Catheterization and Angiocardiography." Am. Journ. Nurs., Oct., 1960, p. 1418.

6. Frohman, I. P.: "Digitalis and Its Derivatives." Am. Journ. Nurs., Feb., 1957, p. 172.

7. Johnson, O. C.: "Low Sodium Diet." Journ. Pract. Nurs., Sept. 1966, p. 19.

8. "Open Heart Surgery." Practical Nursing, May, 1962, p. 14.

9. Ratcliffe, J. D.: "How Science Is Saving Stroke Victims." Today's Health, March, 1962, p. 23.

10. Rogez, B. D., and Holswade, G. R.: "Care of Patients Having Open-heart Surgery." Journ. Pract. Nurs., April, 1966, p. 22.

11. Smith, R.: "Let's Dress the Disabled for Living." Nurs. Outlook, Dec., 1965, p. 59.

12. Smith, G. W.: "A Stroke Is Not the End of the World." Am. Journ. Nurs., March, 1957, p. 303.

13. White, P. D.: "Strokes—Prevention, Diagnosis, and Patient Care." Journ. Pract. Nurs., Oct., 1965. p. 24.

14. Willman, V.: "Anatomy and Physiology of the Heart in Congenital Heart Disease." Am. Journ. Nurs., Feb., 1960, p. 190.

15. Wilson, S.: "Chronic Leg Ulcers: Nursing Management." Am. Journ. Nurs., Jan., 1967, p. 96.

OUTLINE FOR CHAPTER 12

Part I — Disorders of the Blood

I. Introduction

A. Blood is a tissue composed half of cells and half of liquid.

B. Blood cells transport essential nutrients and oxygen for proper utilization of these nutrients and remove wastes. Blood is also essential to the body's protective devices.

II. Blood Dyscrasias (Abnormal Conditions of the Blood, Congential or Acquired)

A. Symptoms common to all blood dyscrasias include fatigue, dyspnea, increased pulse rate and heart beat and sensitivity to cold.

B. Anemia.
1. An abnormal reduction in the number of circulating red blood cells from blood loss, from failure in blood cell production, or from excessive destruction of red blood cells.
2. Diagnosis of anemia established by red cell count and hemoglobin evaluation. Determination of exact type of anemia much more complex.
3. General treatment and nursing care:
   a. Rest.
   b. Provision of warmth.
   c. Special mouth care.
   d. Observation of vital signs and checking for hidden blood loss.
   e. Blood transfusions.
   f. Iron therapy, vitamin B_{12} and liver extract.

C. Leukemia.
1. A progressive malignancy of the white blood cells.
2. Types: lymphogenous (originating in the lymphoid tissue) and myelogenous (originating in the bone marrow). Also, acute and chronic.
3. Incidence and cause. Occurs most often in youngsters under the age of five years. Death rate from leukemia is increasing. Factors associated with its development include ionizing radiation, certain chemicals and viruses.
4. Treatment and nursing care.
   a. Treatment to slow down growth of malignant cells and maintain a normal level of red cells and hemoglobin.
   b. Nursing care: relieve symptoms and help prevent complications, especially those of infection and hemorrhage.
   c. Patient should be told of his diagnosis.
   d. Chemotherapy involving a combination of antileukemic drugs.

D. Hemophilia.
1. Characterized by prolonged coagulation time. Patient is in danger of hemorrhage from the slightest injury and therefore must adjust his life to avoid injury.

E. Purpura.
1. Small hemorrhages in the skin and mucous membranes.
2. Symptomatic of primary diseases such as scurvy, liver disease and allergy to certain drugs.
3. Treatment aimed at control of primary disorder.

Part II – Disorders of the Heart

I. Introduction

A. Heart diseases are still a major cause of death in the United States, although not all kinds are fatal.

II. Diagnostic Tests and Examinations

A. Electrocardiogram and x-rays.
B. Heart catheterization – determines pressures within heart chambers; takes blood samples for determining oxygen content in various parts of the heart and great vessels.
C. Angiocardiogram – x-ray using dye to visualize the heart and blood vessels.
D. Radioisotopes – aid in diagnosing structural defects of the heart and great vessels. Also can determine the life span of individual red blood cells.

III. General Nursing Care

A. Physical, emotional and mental rest.
B. Diet: serve small, easily digested meals and know types of food to avoid and whether to limit intake of sodium and fluids.
C. Relief of dyspnea and cyanosis – proper positioning, administration of oxygen.
D. Care of the skin – avoid breakdown of skin during immobility of patient.
E. Medications
1. To decrease the rate and improve the strength of the contractions of the heart muscle (for example, digitalis).
2. To relieve edema (for example, diuretics).
3. Analgesics (for example, morphine sulfate and Demerol).
F. Rehabilitation – patient can lead a useful, active life within the limitations imposed by his illness.
G. Prevention – adequate exercise and avoidance of obesity, tobacco, emotional

strain and other stresses that place an added burden on the heart. Periodic examination of children for early detection of heart disorders.

IV. Surgery of the Heart

A. Introduction.
1. Development of new machinery and techniques has greatly reduced the risk of heart surgery and made open-heart surgery possible.
2. Examples include repair of structural defects and repair or replacement of diseased valves in the heart.

B. Preoperative care includes instruction of the patient and comprehensive tests and examinations to determine the type of surgery needed and the risk to the patient.

C. Immediate postoperative care is given in an intensive care unit. Nursing care includes intelligent observation of vital signs, measuring intake and output, care of thoracotomy tubes and possibly administration of oxygen. Exercise of limbs necessary to avoid circulatory and musculoskeletal complications.

V. Congestive Heart Failure

A. A complication of other cardiac conditions in which the heart loses its efficiency as a pump and the blood flow becomes congested.

B. Symptoms.
1. Left-sided failure produces congestion of the lungs and eventually pulmonary edema.
2. Right-sided failure produces edema of the lower part of the body and impaired circulation to the brain.

C. Pulmonary edema (an accumulation of fluid within the lung tissues).
1. May result from left-sided failure of the heart or an abrupt increase in the work load of the heart. Acute pulmonary edema can be fatal in a short period of time.
2. Symptoms include severe dyspnea and coughing up sputum that may be blood-tinged and frothy.
3. Treatment to relieve symptoms and reduce venous return of blood to the heart includes keeping patient calm, giving him oxygen and a sedative, and rotating tourniquets on the extremities. Diuretics aid in elimination of fluids causing pulmonary failure.

VI. Diseases of the Coronary Arteries

A. Coronary arteries provide blood supply to the heart muscle.

B. Main diseases are myocardial infarction and angina pectoris.
1. Myocardial infarction is an area of necrotic tissue in the myocardium resulting from impaired blood supply to the area.
   a. Symptoms—crushing or burning sensation in the chest, pallor, profuse perspiration, anxiety, nausea and vomiting.
   b. Immediate care—relief of pain, oxygen to relieve dyspnea and prevention of shock. Later care—rest and medication.
   c. Prevention—avoidance of predisposing factors such as obesity, high fat diet and smoking. Control of disorders such as rheumatic heart disease and atherosclerosis helps avoid formation of blood clots within the arteries.
2. Angina pectoris is pain in the chest arising from decreased blood supply to the heart muscle, caused by a narrowing or occlusion of these arteries.
   a. Symptoms—a dull pain or tightness in the chest, profuse perspiration, pallor or flushing of the face and dyspnea.
   b. Treatment—vasodilator drugs, especially nitroglycerine, and avoidance of exposure to cold, sudden physical exertion or emotional upsets that may precipitate an attack.

VII. Disorders of the Heart's Conduction System

A. If the sino-atrial node and the atrioventricular node fail to initiate the electrical impulses that stimulate contraction of the heart muscle, an artificial pacemaker can be inserted to stimulate the contractions.

B. Indications for its use include Stokes-Adams disease, carotid sinus syndrome, surgical injury to the heart's conduction system during corrective cardiac surgery, and some cases of arteriosclerosis in elderly persons who are suffering from atrioventricular block.

C. Nursing care—accurate observation of the patient prior to surgery. Reporting of any attacks that occur. Surgeon instructs the patient. Physical preparation same as for any major surgery. Special equipment may include thoracic tubes and drainage bottle, intravenous tubes, oxygen, and gastric suction.

VIII. Inflammatory Diseases of the Heart

A. Inflammatory conditions involving the heart muscle (myocarditis), the inner lining (endocarditis), or the sac surrounding the heart (pericarditis).

B. Symptoms vary according to the structure involved.

C. Treatment and nursing care—rest to reduce the work load of the heart, medication to control infection and surgery to repair or replace valves destroyed by the inflammatory process.

IX. Hypertensive Heart Disease

A. High blood pressure places an added burden on the heart and can enlarge the heart and fatigue the heart muscle.

B. Symptoms include dyspnea, fatigue, edema of the extremities and cyanosis. Congestive failure develops rapidly if the condition is not relieved.

C. Treatment aimed at relief of underlying cause and administration of hypotensive drugs to control the blood pressure.

X. Congenital Heart Disease

A. A defect in the structure of the heart that has resulted from improper growth and development during the prenatal period.

B. Exact cause is unknown but there is a definite relationship between these defects and some viral infections, particularly German measles.

C. Types include a variety of defects in the septum, position of the great vessels and chambers of the heart.

D. Symptoms include dyspnea, cyanosis, increased pulse rate, poor physical development, decreased exercise tolerance and elevated blood pressure.

E. Treatment includes correction by surgery whenever possible. Medications such as digitalis may be given.

Part III—Disorders of the Peripheral Vascular System

I. Introduction

A. Peripheral blood vessels (situated at a distance from the heart) include the cere-

bral blood vessels as well as those of the extremities.

II. Circulatory Disorders of the Extremities

A. General treatment and nursing care.

1. Provide extra warmth. Extreme heat may cause burns or increase the metabolic needs of an area already suffering from poor circulation.

2. Instruction to the patient is essential to prevention of injury and avoidance of factors that may predispose the patient to complications.

3. Ulcers, a result of tissue death due to impaired blood supply, heal slowly and can be very discouraging to the patient.

4. Appliances for support and comfort include elasticized stockings and paste "boots."

5. Low-calorie diet may be necessary to avoid obesity, which aggravates the condition. Fluid intake should be increased.

6. Drugs include vasodilators and anticoagulants.

7. Tobacco must be avoided.

B. Arteriosclerosis of the extremities.

1. Hardening and loss of elasticity in the walls of the arteries supplying the extremities.

2. Symptoms—extremities feel cold to the touch. Patient may experience numbness and tingling, fatigue, weakness of the muscles and leg cramps at night. Ulcers will develop and there may be dry gangrene.

3. Treatment and nursing care.

   a. Treatment is aimed at relief of symptoms and improving and maintaining adequate circulation. No cure.

   b. Active exercise is helpful in improving blood supply to muscles.

   c. Warmth can help maintain continued dilation of the blood vessels.

   d. Extremities must be protected from injury.

   e. Physiotherapy may include special exercises, warm baths and whirlpool baths to improve circulation.

C. Buerger's disease.

1. An inflammatory disease of the medium-sized blood vessels, particu-

larly the arteries of the legs. Definitely related to excessive smoking over several years.

2. Symptoms include severe pain, due to clots in the blood vessels, and interruption of blood flow.

3. Treatment is primarily symptomatic.

4. Buerger-Allen exercises maintain adequate circulation to the lower extremities.

D. Thrombophlebitis.

1. An inflammation of a vein resulting from a blood clot in the vessel.

2. Symptoms may or may not include pain in the affected area. Patient also may have fever and increased pulse rate.

3. Treatment aimed at prevention of complications such as embolism, local cellulitis or ulceration.

   a. Anticoagulant drugs such as heparin, Dicumarol and Coumadin may be given.

   b. Physician will prescribe amount of activity he desires patient to have.

   c. Patient should avoid physical strain until clot is dissolved.

E. Varicose veins.

1. Veins that have become greatly enlarged and distorted in shape.

2. Caused by impaired flow of venous blood. Often due to deficient valves in veins.

3. Symptoms include fatigue and feeling of heaviness in legs, cramps and itching along course of vessel. Ulcers may form after repeated inflammations.

4. Treatment and nursing care: support of the veins by elasticized stockings or bandages, removal of causative factors and a prescribed regimen of rest and exercise. Surgical correction in severe cases.

III. Diseases of the Cerebral Vessels

A. Arteriosclerosis of the cerebral vessels.

1. Hardening of the arteries serving the brain.

2. Symptoms—patients manifest signs of mental deterioration with a slowing down of mental processes and emotional changes.

3. Treatment and nursing care concerned with accepting the patient as he is and helping him live fully within the limitations imposed by his illness.

B. Cerebrovascular accident (stroke, apoplexy).

1. Caused by sudden interruption of the flow of blood to the brain. Cells served by the affected vessel eventually lose function.

2. May be caused by: (a) cerebral thrombosis, (b) cerebral hemorrhage, or (c) atherosclerosis of the arteries of the neck and head.

3. Predisposing factors may be hypertension, endocarditis and atherosclerosis.

4. Symptoms vary according to the portion of the brain that is affected. Stroke may cause some slight residual paralysis or death. Most common after-effects are speech disturbances and paralysis on one side of the body.

5. Treatment and nursing care. Primary goal is prevention of complications so that patient can return to useful and active life. Surgical treatment is effective if done early enough—if diagnostic tests or patient's "small strokes" indicate a gradual obstruction of the arteries in the neck. Little can be done surgically once a stroke has occurred.

C. Hypertension.

1. The pressure of the blood within the arteries sustained at a high level. High diastolic pressure most indicative of hypertension.

2. Types—*essential hypertension* (without known cause) and *secondary hypertension* (secondary to another disease). *Malignant hypertension*—an especially serious type of essential hypertension, usually fatal within a few years).

3. Symptoms—headache, dizziness, fatigue and restlessness.

4. Complications—visual disturbances or blindness, cardiac disorders and renal failure.

5. Treatment—keep the patient calm, free from obesity and in a state of optimal health. Sodium intake should be limited. Drugs include hypotensive agents, tranquilizers and sedatives. No cure.

Chapter 13

NURSING CARE OF
PATIENTS WITH DISEASES OF
THE RESPIRATORY SYSTEM

VOCABULARY

Atelectasis
Expiration
Inspiration
Intercostal
Mediastinum
Prophylaxis

INTRODUCTION

The respiratory system is chiefly composed of a system of hollow tubes through which we breathe. These tubes are constructed so that they resemble a tree; therefore the term "bronchial tree" is frequently used to describe the respiratory tract. The trunk of the tree is the trachea, the branches the bronchi and the twigs, or smaller branches, the bronchioles. As a breath of air travels down the bronchial tree it eventually ends its journey in tiny little air sacs called *alveoli*. These minute sacs comprise most of the tissues of the lungs. It is in the alveoli that the exchange of carbon dioxide and oxygen takes place.

Each lung is covered with a membranous sac called the pleura. There are two layers of the pleura and between these layers there is a fluid which acts as a lubricant to prevent friction when the lung expands and deflates. The pleural sac which encloses each lung is an airtight compartment. The pressure within the pleural cavity is less than that of the outside atmosphere. Thus, if the pleura is penetrated from the outside, air will rush in and collapse the lung.

While the outer surface of the lungs and bronchial tree are normally protected from contamination by outside sources, the inner lining of the respiratory tract is constantly exposed to dust, germs, and other foreign materials in the air. In defense against these substances the mucous membranes contain tiny hairlike projections called *cilia*. These tiny projections trap and help to remove small foreign particles which are inhaled. The membrane also secretes a watery substance that helps prevent infection by cleansing foreign substances from the respiratory tract. If an inflammation does occur, these secretions are automatically increased in an effort to wash away bacteria and other debris. That is why watery eyes, running nose, and cough are common to all upper respiratory infections.

Respiration is a very vital function of the body and yet we are usually unaware of performing this function. It is only when we experience difficulty in breathing that we realize how important normal respiration is to our comfort and well-being.

Diseases of the respiratory system are the most common affliction of mankind. The common cold and other undifferentiated respiratory infections account for more absenteeism from work than any other illness. It is fortunate that most of these illnesses are not of a serious nature. However, there is always the danger of a serious infection and permanent disability, or even death, as a result of complications from a seemingly minor upper respiratory disease.

GENERAL NURSING CARE

There are many symptoms common to all types of respiratory diseases. These symptoms include coughing, increased flow of secretions from the nasal and bronchial mucosa, varying degrees of respiratory difficulty, and some elevation of temperature. The nursing care necessary for relief of these symptoms will be discussed first in this chapter. Specific diseases of the respiratory system and the special treatments and nursing care required are discussed after the general nursing care.

Coughing. The act of coughing may be stimulated by any foreign substance in the respiratory tract. A cough may be dry, harsh, and *nonproductive,* in which case the patient is unable to produce any sputum; or the cough may be deep, moist and *productive* of moderate to large amounts of sputum. When a cough is productive the patient should be instructed to take deep breaths and cough up the sputum. Sputum should be expectorated, never swallowed. If coughing is painful to the patient the nurse may support his chest with the palms of her hands during the seizure of coughing, or the chest may be supported with a binder or elastic bandage.

A nonproductive cough is very irritating to the mucous membranes and exhausting for the patient. Non-narcotic cough mixtures should be given to suppress nonproductive coughing. Any person with a chronic cough should seek medical advice because this is frequently an early symptom of chronic respiratory disease.

There are several different types of cough medicines. Some decrease secretions within the bronchial tract while others actually increase the flow of these secretions, making them more easily coughed up and expectorated. The latter type are referred to as *expectorant* cough mixtures. Other preparations contain special drugs (for example codeine) which depress the cough reflex and lessen the desire to cough. These are called *sedative* cough mixtures. Cough preparations are administered in very small amounts at a time and are not followed by water.

Increased Secretions. Since the majority of respiratory diseases are caused by infectious organisms that can easily be transmitted by way of the nasal and bronchial secretions, the nurse must protect herself and others from contamination. It is far better to teach the patient the proper care of these secretions than to try to avoid contact by wearing a mask when in his presence. The patient is usually not offended if he is tactfully told to place a folded tissue over his nose and mouth while coughing and sneezing and to turn his head away from the nurse whenever close contact is necessary as during a bed bath or other procedure.

Care must be used in handling all nasal secretions and sputum. Disposable tissues should be used and discarded in a small paper bag pinned to the bedside or made readily accessible to the ambulatory patient. A used tissue should never be put in the pocket of one's clothing. If a patient has such a copious amount of sputum that tissues are not practical, he should be given a waxed sputum cup and instructed in its use.

In bacterial infections and chronic respiratory diseases the sputum is often foul-smelling and leaves a disagreeable taste in the mouth. Frequent oral hygiene is important for patients with this condition, especially before meals when the taste or odor of the sputum may directly affect the appetite.

Respiratory Distress. There are few persons living today who have not experienced the discomforts of a common cold. The annoyance of trying to breathe in spite of nasal congestion, and the discomfort of being awakened in the night with an irritating cough are familiar to all of us. The patient with a severe respiratory disease experiences these discomforts to an even greater degree. He may become physically exhausted and actually suffer from lack of oxygen because of partial obstruction of the air passages or impaired function of the lungs.

The position which best facilitates breathing is the semi-Fowler's or high Fowler's position. The shoulders and back should be supported with a pillow to allow for full expansion of the lungs and to assist in keeping the chin off the chest. The diaphragm and the intercostal muscles are responsible for the mechanical expansion of the thoracic cavity which allows the lungs to inflate with air (see Fig. 13-1). Proper positioning of the patient will allow these muscles to function at their best.

When the deficiency of oxygen is severe the physician orders administration of concentrated oxygen by mask, catheter, or tent to relieve the anoxia.

The air the patient breathes should be kept moist to prevent further irritation of the mucous membranes by drying, and to assist in the removal of secretions from the bronchial tree. Whether the air is warm or cool will depend on the wishes of the physician in charge. If warm, moist air is ordered, a vaporizer is set up in the patient's room or a croup tent is arranged. Warmth provides for relaxation of the bronchioles, thus allowing for improved inspiration of air into the lungs.

In the treatment of children with croup a *croupette* which provides a fine mist of cool, moist air has been proven to be very beneficial. The droplets provided by the croupette are so small they can reach into the smaller bronchioles that the larger droplets of steam cannot reach. The cool air is also considered to be more advantageous than warm air when the patient is suffering from a high fever.

Rest. Whenever an inflammation is present, the affected part must be allowed to rest so that the body can repair the damaged tissues. In a respiratory illness this same principle is applied. Since any undue exertion places an immediate burden on the respiratory

EXPIRATION   INSPIRATION

Figure 13-1. Schematic drawing showing action of first five ribs, sternum, and external intercostal muscles. All act to increase the diameter of the chest during inspiration of air into lungs. (From King and Showers: *Human Anatomy and Physiology,* 5th Ed., W. B. Saunders Co., Philadelphia.)

system bed rest is an important part of the treatment of respiratory diseases. Even minor infections require rest in bed if complications are to be avoided and the infection overcome in a short period of time. The nurse should explain the reasons for the needed rest and anticipate the needs of the patient so that he may be spared undue activity.

Diet. While the inflammation is acute the diet should consist of high-caloric, high-vitamin liquids. Milk and milk products are especially important because of the need for protein in the repair and rebuilding of damaged tissues.

Later as the patient progresses, the diet is changed to include soft foods and eventually a regular diet is resumed. During the convalescent period the patient will still have need for additional vitamins and proteins while his resistance to infection is low.

Medications. In addition to the expectorant and sedative cough mixtures mentioned earlier, there are several other medications used in the treatment of respiratory diseases. *Antipyretics,* or drugs which lower the temperature, may be necessary when the fever becomes dangerously high. Aspirin and pyralgin are examples of of antipyretics. Aspirin has the added advantage of relieving the headache and other general aches and pains frequently associated with respiratory infections.

Antihistamines, which help to dry up secretions of the nasal and bronchial mucosa, are quite often used. These drugs should be taken only on the order of a physician, however, because they often produce undesirable side effects.

Antispasmodics, such as aminophylline, Adrenalin, and ephedrine sulfate serve to decrease the muscular contractions of the bronchioles. They are particularly useful in the treatment of asthma.

Antibiotics are useful primarily in bacterial infections. In most viral infections they are ineffective.

Inhalation Therapy. The inhalation of certain drugs such as bronchodilators and liquefying agents can be of benefit to patients who have difficulty with proper ventilation of the lungs. The drugs are in solution, which can be reduced to a fine spray that is inhaled easily and carried to the lower portions of the respiratory tract. The methods by which inhalation therapy may be carried out include (1) by a hand operated nebulizer, (2) through a nebulizer attached to compressed air or oxygen apparatus, and (3) with an intermittent positive-pressure breathing machine.

Drugs administered by inhalation therapy usually are antibiotics, bronchodilators, liquefying agents and diluents. Bronchodilators enlarge the lumen to alleviate spasm of the bronchial tubes and to facilitate breathing for adequate ventilation of the lungs. Examples of bronchodilators are isoproterenol (Isuprel) and epinephrine hydrochloride (Vaponefrine). The liquefying agents and diluents help to thin bronchial secretions and make them more liquid and less tenacious so that they are more easily coughed up and expectorated. These liquefying agents include sodium etasulfate (Tergemist), distilled water and tyloxapol (Alevaire).

Intermittent Positive-Pressure Breathing Therapy. The patient with a chronic lung disorder such as emphysema, bronchiectasis or asthma may have partial obstruction to the air passages or damaged lung tissue or both. Every breath he takes is a great effort and often the breath he has struggled for provides him with less oxygen than he actually needs. The intermittent positive-pressure (IPPB) breathing machine, such as the Bennet respirator, provides for increased inspiration of air into the lungs by introducing air or a mixture of oxygen and air under positive pressure. The machine can be cycled to a respiratory rate set and controlled by the patient. Each time he takes a breath the machine provides a kind of "boost" that makes inspiration easier. In this way IPPB helps overcome bronchial resistance to the inward flow of air, allows for more uniform distribution of oxygen to the alveoli, aids in the removal of carbon dioxide and makes coughing easier and more effective in removing secretions that have accumulated deep in the respiratory tree.

Some patients can leave the hospital and visit a local pulmonary clinic on a regular basis for the purpose of receiving IPPB therapy. Others may purchase a machine for their own use at home. Every patient who has IPPB therapy should be instructed in the way in which the machine works and the results that are expected. Instructions of this type and further details on respirators are presented in Chapter 6 of this text.

Breathing Exercises. The mechanics of breathing can become increasingly less efficient as chronic respiratory disease progresses. The patient suffers a loss of lung elasticity, a flattened diaphragm and fixation of the rib cage as he becomes more and more dependent on the muscles of his upper chest and neck for breathing. The purpose of breathing exercises is to help correct this situation by strengthening the abdominal muscles so that they can push upward against the diaphragm and assist in the expiration of air from the lungs. These exercises also help overcome rigidity of the thorax so that the lungs can inflate and deflate more easily. Patients who follow the exercises prescribed for them often find that they can lead more active and useful lives than formerly because their exertional dyspnea is less severe. This means that they can make better use of all the muscles of their body and are less likely to develop complications that accompany immobility. They also are better able to cough up secretions that would otherwise remain in the lower bronchi and serve as a growth medium for bacteria or as a cause of atelectasis. The psychological value of being able to indulge in ordinary activities that once left the patient breathless cannot be estimated.

Figure 13-2 shows some of the breathing exercises that may be prescribed for a patient with chronic obstructive lung disease.

Postural Drainage. The term *postural drainage* refers to positioning the patient so that his thorax is lower than the rest of his body. In this way the force of gravity and ciliary activity of the small bronchial airways will move secretions to the main bronchi and trachea. Once the secretions have reached this point the patient should be able to remove them by coughing.

The exact position in which the patient should be placed depends on the area of the lung to be drained (see Fig. 13-3). The nurse who assists a patient with postural drainage should obtain specific directions from the physician or physical therapist so that she can position the patient properly. The physician also may wish to have the nurse use certain tapping, clapping and vibrating techniques during postural drainage. These measures are carried out for the purpose of dislodging mucus plugs so that they can be coughed up more easily. They must be done with precision, preferably by a physical therapist, but only by someone who has received adequate instruction in the proper technique. Improper clapping and vibrating can cause much discomfort to the patient and accomplish little more than upsetting him to the point that he refuses the treatment.[9]

Because there is likely to be some gagging during coughing episodes that take place during postural drainage, it is best to carry out the procedure before meals when the stomach is relatively empty and vomiting is less likely. If the patient is to have postural drainage only once a day it should be done in the morning when he awakens. At this time secretions that have accumulated during the night's sleep can be removed. After postural drainage is

Figure 13-2. Breathing exercises help to improve the patient's respiratory function. *A*, The physical therapist teaches patients abdominal breathing. Placing one hand on his chest and the other on his abdomen helps the patient to recognize when he is doing the exercise correctly. During abdominal breathing the movement of the abdomen is felt with each breath, whereas the chest remains quiet. *B*, Blowing out a candle at various distances. This exercise can be performed also without the chin rest by holding or placing the candle at various distances. *C*, A blow bottle like this one can be prepared easily for use at home or in the hospital. The long glass tube extends below the water and is connected to rubber tubing, through which the patient blows. By taking deep breaths and exhaling, the patient causes the water to bubble vigorously.

Figure 13-3. Postural drainage requires that the patient assume various positions to facilitate the flow of secretions from various portions of the lung into the bronchi, trachea, and throat so that they can be raised and expectorated more easily. Drawing shows the correct position to drain various portions of the lung. At the bottom of the drawing is illustrated a frequently ordered and less specific position, in which the patient lies across the bed, with his arms resting on a pillow on a chair. (From Shafer et al.: *Medical-Surgical Nursing*, 4th Ed., C. V. Mosby Co., St. Louis.)

completed the nurse must be sure to assist the patient with proper oral hygiene including tooth brushing and a refreshing mouth wash. This will help overcome the foul taste left in the mouth by the sputum.

Irrigations. In order to help the patient eliminate thick, tenacious mucus from the throat and nasal passages, the doctor may order gargles and nasal irrigations. Warm salt water (one teaspoonful of salt to a pint of water) is very good as a gargle. It helps remove the mucus and soothes the throat. When nasal irrigations are done the patient must sit upright and care must be taken never to use force. To do so may wash the infection up into the sinuses or frighten the patient into aspirating the solution into the trachea. The tip of the irrigating tube is inserted so as to allow space for the return flow of the solution.

DIAGNOSTIC TESTS

Chest X-ray. The most common diagnostic aid used for respiratory illnesses is, of course, the chest x-ray. The physician will usually order films taken from the front, back, and side of the chest (anterior, posterior, and lateral), to obtain views of the lungs from several angles. No special preparation is necessary for a chest x-ray.

Respiratory Function Tests. These tests are done to evaluate functioning capacity of the lungs and to determine specific pulmonary disorders that produce dyspnea. A test for *vital capacity* measures the greatest amount of air that an individual can exhale after he has inhaled as much air as he can. A *tidal volume* test measures the amount of air inspired *and* expired during a normal breath. *Residual volume* refers to the air that is left remaining in the lungs after an individual has exhaled normally. The *total lung capacity* can be determined by adding the vital capacity and the residual volume.

Sputum Analysis. Laboratory tests of sputum are frequently done in cases of respiratory disease. These tests include stained smears for pathogenic microorganisms or malignant cells, and gross examination for color, consistency and general characteristics of the sputum specimen.

The nurse should explain the procedure to the patient, emphasizing the need for coughing up sputum from the lower respiratory tract. If the patient is not instructed properly he may cough in a shallow and ineffective manner so that he expectorates only saliva. The sputum cup should be kept covered when the patient is not using it as it may be unpleasant for him and those who enter his room. If a specimen is collected for culture the container should have a tight-fitting lid so that the spread of the infectious agents in the sputum can be avoided.

Bronchogram. This is an x-ray of the bronchial tree. The x-ray films are taken after a radiopaque oil has been introduced into the trachea. The patient lies down and is tilted in various positions so the oil will be distributed over the bronchial tree. The oil is a special type that will not damage the mucosa of the respiratory tract and even though postural drainage may be ordered to remove some of the oil after the test, the remaining oil will not damage the lungs or bronchi.

Bronchoscopy. A bronchoscope is a special instrument designed to be inserted into the bronchi for the purpose of visualizing the inside of the trachea and bronchi *(bronchoscopy)*. The instrument is also used to remove foreign bodies from the respiratory tract or to obtain a biopsy for further study.

For both a bronchogram and a bronchoscopy the patient's throat is anesthetized so that the gag reflex is no longer present. He is not given any food or liquids for at least 2 hours after either of these examinations because in the absence of the gag reflex he is likely to aspirate the material into his trachea.

THE COMMON COLD

Definition. The common cold is an inflammation of the upper respiratory tract. It is caused by a virus. There are so many different strains of viruses which can produce the symptoms of a common cold that immunity is difficult, if not impossible, to establish. Avoiding exposure to those who have a "cold" and maintaining a state of good health and high resistance are the only ways one can avoid catching a cold.

Symptoms. The common cold usually starts with a mild sore throat or a hot, dry sensation in the nose and back of the throat. Within hours after the onset the nose becomes congested with increased secretions, the eyes begin to water, and sneezing and an irritating nonproductive cough appear. There is usually no elevation of temperature, or, if fever does develop, it is of a low-grade type.

Treatment and Nursing Care. The main purpose of treating a cold is the prevention of complications from a bacterial infection. While the mucous membranes are irritated and inflamed they are much more susceptible to invasion by bacteria. The patient should stay indoors, preferably in bed, and away from others. Fluids, especially citrus fruit juices, are given in large amounts to keep the temperature down and to help the body remove wastes. Vitamin C in the citrus fruits helps in the repair of inflamed tissues. The patient should avoid chilling and exposure to drafts or sudden changes in temperature. Aspirin are helpful in relieving the aches and pains of a cold and eliminate the headache usually present.

Nose drops of normal saline, or those containing a mild decongestant such as ephedrine, help in the removal of nasal secretions.

ACUTE BRONCHITIS

Definition. This is an acute inflammation of the bronchi. The differentiation between bronchitis, tracheobronchitis, tonsillitis, and laryngitis is somewhat difficult and not always necessary since these upper respiratory infections are generally treated in the same way.

Symptoms. Bronchitis presents approximately the same symptoms as the common cold at the outset. The cough is usually more persistent and later becomes productive of purulent sputum in fairly large amounts. The temperature is usually elevated in bronchitis and in children it can become high enough to produce febrile convulsions.

Treatment and Nursing Care. The coughing and dyspnea which accompany bronchitis are best relieved by the inhalation of moist air. A vaporizer in the room will increase the general humidity and relieve some of the coughing and dyspnea. For small children in a crib a croup tent can be improvised by placing a cotton blanket or sheet over the top and sides of the crib and adjusting the flow of steam under this covering. Extreme care must be used with all types of vaporizers in the home or the hospital. They must be placed so that the child cannot reach the vaporizer or its nozzle, and the steam must be directed away from the patient. Adult patients or others in the room may easily turn over a vaporizer which is not placed out of the way.

The patient with chronic bronchitis usually has a persistent cough and copious amounts of sputum, especially upon arising in the morning. Postural drainage is helpful in removing sputum from the lower parts of the respiratory tract. These patients should avoid exposure to cold, damp weather, and dust or smog which will further irritate the bronchi. They should maintain a sensible schedule of rest and good nutrition so that their resistance to bacterial infections is kept high.

PNEUMONIA

Definition. Pneumonia is an extensive inflammation of lung tissues. There are two general types of pneumonia: (1) *bacterial pneumonia,* which is most often caused by pneumococci; and (2) *primary atypical pneumonia,* or *viral pneumonia.* This second type of pneumonia is caused by a virus or a combination of several different organisms (mixed infection).

Symptoms. A bacterial pneumonia usually begins abruptly with severe chills and elevated temperature. The onset of atypical pneumonia is usually much more gradual. The patient complains of a severe stabbing pain in the chest or side which is aggravated by coughing or taking a deep breath. The sputum is frothy and white at first and then changes to a characteristic rust color. Cyanosis is not uncommon and the skin is moist and hot. "Fever blisters" *(herpes simplex)* frequently are present around the nose and lips. Patients with pneumonia appear exhausted and usually do not wish to be disturbed for even the most essential of nursing care. Delirium is not an uncommon occurrence in pneumonia, and demands constant attendance by the nursing staff so that the patient will not injure himself.

Treatment and Nursing Care. The aims of treatment of pneumonia include: (1) conservation of the patient's strength and energy, (2) relief of symptoms, and (3) control of the infection.

The patient is placed on absolute bed rest with medications and nursing care scheduled so that he is disturbed as little as possible. Fluids are forced to combat dehydration and help the body in eliminating wastes. Special attention to the mouth is necessary because the patient usually breathes through his mouth, which produces drying and cracking of the lips and inside of the mouth.

The patient is kept warm and away from drafts. Bedclothes, dampened by perspiration, should be changed as often as necessary to keep the patient dry and comfortable. The patient must be protected from chilling during the bed bath and change of linens.

Since pneumonia is an infectious disease and easily transmitted by droplet infection, the patient is isolated and extreme care is taken with nasal secretions and sputum.

Abdominal distention frequently accompanies pneumonia. The measures used to relieve this condition include rectal tubes and low enemas as ordered by the physician.

The vital signs of the patient must be observed closely and checked frequently. Any change in the pulse rate, falling blood pressure, or difficult respiration must be reported immediately. Other signs of danger to be reported include increasing cyanosis, restlessness, or delirium.

Complications following pneumonia are not uncommon, especially if the patient does not exercise caution during the convalescent period. Pneumonia is a dangerous disease. It is very exhausting and depletes the body's reserve of energy, thus lowering the resistance to infections. Empyema is a common complication of pneumonia (see p. 280). Congestive heart failure may also occur as a complication of pneumonia.

BRONCHIECTASIS

Definition. Bronchiectasis is a chronic disease of the respiratory system characterized by permanent dilatation of the bronchi. This condition may follow pneumonia and other respiratory infections or it may be the result of a congenital defect in the alveoli. These small sacs are not as elastic as they should be and they fill with secretions. Because the bronchioles are enlarged and unable to remove the secretions the sputum collects and becomes stagnant.

Symptoms. The most outstanding

symptom of bronchiectasis is severe attacks of coughing in which the patient brings up large amounts of thick, foul-smelling sputum. The coughing is most noticeable in the morning when the patient first gets out of bed. In addition to the coughing attacks the patient may complain of fatigue and loss of weight. The majority of individuals with true bronchiectasis begin having symptoms by the time they are 20 years of age. As the disease progresses they develop clubbing of the fingers, which is characteristic of many chronic respiratory diseases (see Fig. 13-4).

Treatment and Nursing Care. There is, unfortunately, no cure for bronchiectasis other than surgical removal of the affected part. If the involved area is so extensive that surgery is not possible, the patient's prognosis is very poor.

Other measures to aid in the removal of mucus plugs from the bronchioles include expectorant drugs, removal by way of a bronchoscope, and inhalation or aerosol therapy. Antibiotics may be given during acute attacks to prevent further infection of the lungs. They also help in decreasing the amount of sputum produced.

General measures of good nutrition and adequate rest are necessary to conserve the strength of the patient and prevent the development of complications.

CANCER OF THE LUNG

Introduction. In 1930 the lung cancer death rate for males was 3.6 per 100,000 population; in 1960 the rate had increased to approximately 32.5 per 100,000. Today, while death rates from other forms of cancer are decreasing or remaining stable, lung cancer has become a leading cause of death in white males. Factors that contribute to this increase include increasing air pollution, the increase of cigarette smoking by young persons and the increasing numbers of older persons in the population. The condition is found most often in men 40 years of age or older.

Symptoms. Most lung tumors begin in the epithelial lining of the bronchi. There are few symptoms at first, usually only a cough and some wheezing. As the tumor grows larger, the patient may have some pain or discomfort in the chest, exertional dyspnea, and expectoration of blood-streaked sputum. Diagnosis is confirmed by an x-ray showing a definite

Figure 13-4. Clubbed fingers of patient with chronic respiratory difficulties and cyanosis. (From brown: *Medical Nursing*, 3rd Ed., W. B. Saunders Co., Philadelphia.)

mass or by removal of malignant cells during bronchoscopy.

Treatment. The only possible cure for cancer of the lung at this time is by surgical removal. The type of surgery, lobectomy or pneumonectomy, depends on the size and location of the malignant growth. Radiation therapy and chemotherapy may help in some cases to retard growth of the tumor and provide some relief from symptoms.

ASTHMA

Definition. Bronchial asthma is an allergic reaction characterized by swelling of the mucous membranes of the respiratory tract and increased production of secretions within the bronchioles. These conditions produce dyspnea and wheezing because they obstruct the flow of air through the respiratory passages.

Symptoms. Most patients with asthma are free from symptoms between attacks. During an attack, which is usually brought on by exposure to one or more antigens, the patient has itching and watering of the eyes, cough and a wheezing type of dyspnea. Respirations may be so difficult that the individual uses all accessory muscles of respiration, such as the chest and abdominal muscles, in an effort to breathe. The patient cannot lie down and may sit up all night struggling for breath during the attack.

Treatment and Nursing Care. The treatment of asthma begins with determination of the substances to which the individual is allergic. Once these allergens have been determined every effort is made to avoid them. Dust is a very common offender in adults, while foods such as eggs, wheat and milk are common causes of asthmatic attacks in children.

Emotional factors also play an important role in precipitating attacks of asthma. The patient and his family will need help in understanding the relationship between emotional anxiety and attacks of asthma. In some cases professional counseling for the patient and family can help in removing sources of tension for the patient.

Other factors which may contribute to an attack of asthma are sudden changes in termperature, physical exhaustion, contact with animal dander, and overeating.[1] Teaching the patient to look for situations which lead to an attack so that he might avoid them in the future will help in reducing the number of attacks.

Drugs used in the treatment of asthma are given primarily to relieve the symptoms. They do not cure the condition. Bronchodilators such as epinephrine and aminophylline are frequently used in the treatment of asthma. Aerosol therapy with *Isuprel* also is used. Expectorants such as *potassium iodide* and *ammonium chloride* assist the patient in raising sputum by thinning the secretions, thus making them more easily coughed out of the bronchioles.

Sometimes an acute attack of asthma does not respond to treatment and the symptoms persist for days. When this happens the patient is said to have *status asthmaticus.* In this situation the patient is very seriously ill and death may occur from excessive strain on the heart. The nursing care includes providing a quiet and restful environment for the patient. All possible sources of dust, pollen and other allergens are removed from the patient's room and a special air filter may be installed in the window. The patient is placed in Fowler's position to faciltate breathing. Oxygen is usually administered, for these patients often have severe cyanosis. The nurse must anticipate the needs of the patient and do everything possible for him so that he will not exert himself. The patient must be protected from too many visitors and all other sources of emotional excitement.

PLEURISY

Definition. Pleurisy is an inflammation of the pleural membranes surrounding the lungs. In *pleurisy with effusion* there is also an increase in the amount of serous fluid within the pleural cavity.

Symptoms. The most outstanding symptom of pleurisy is a sharp, stabbing pain in the chest. The pain is aggravated by taking a deep breath. Pleurisy may occur alone or in conjunction with another disease of the respiratory system.

Treatment and Nursing Care. The patient is placed on bed rest and observed carefully for signs of the development of an infection in the respiratory tract. The chest may be supported by strapping with adhesive tape. This offers some relief of the pain.

When pleurisy is accompanied by effusion of serous fluid the physician may remove this fluid from the thorax for diagnostic tests or relief of symptoms. The procedure for removal of fluid from the pleural cavity is called a *thoracentesis.* It is not uncommon for as much as 500 ml. to be removed at one time during a thoracentesis.

EMPYEMA

Definition. When the fluid within the pleural cavity becomes infected, the exudate becomes thick and purulent and the patient is said to have empyema. The organisms causing the infection may be the staphylococcus, streptococcus, or pneumococcus.

Treatment and Nursing Care. Empyema is treated by eliminating the infection through the use of specific antibiotics and the removal of the excess fluid from the pleural cavity. The physician may order that a sampling of the fluid collected during a thoracentesis be sent to the laboratory and a *sensitivity test* done. This test determines the exact antibiotic which will most effec-tively destroy the organism causing the infection.

PULMONARY EMPHYSEMA

Definition. This is a chronic respiratory disease that results from a long-standing inflammation of the bronchi as in chronic bronchitis, asthma and bronchiectasis. The small bronchioles at the end of the respiratory tree become plugged with infectious material which prevents normal expansion and contraction of the air sacs (alveoli) of the lung. Air becomes trapped in the alveoli causing them to become distended, and eventually the alveolar walls thicken and become less elastic. The damaged alveoli then cannot be emptied completely during expiration and so the lungs remain partially expanded at all times. The patient cannot rid his lungs of stale air to make room for oxygenated air.

One patient who has had emphysema for more than 26 years suggests that a healthy person can get some idea of the effects of emphysema by doing the following: Take a deep breath and then exhale only about one third of the air you have breathed in. Continue trying to breathe while retaining the two thirds of that original breath.[7] If you should try this you would find that it is little wonder that emphysema often is called the "living death."

Cause and Incidence. Although there is no one specific causative factor in all cases of emphysema, many authorities believe that cigarette smoking is the leading cause of chronic bronchitis which eventually leads to emphysema. Other contributing factors include asthma, chronic upper respiratory infections, congenital defects in the respiratory tract and continued irritation of the bronchi by polluted air.[3]

According to the U.S. Public Health Service emphysema is a major health problem that is second only to heart disease as a cause of disability. It is more widespread than lung cancer and tuberculosis combined, disabling one out of every 14 wage earners over the age of 45.

Symptoms. The first symptom usually is a chronic or recurring cough that often is ignored by the patient. He finds it distressing but does not consider it serious. As the disease gradually progresses the individual notices a shortness of breath every time he exerts himself *(exertional dyspnea)*. This can continue for quite a number of months or years and the patient may not be inconvenienced enough to seek medical treatment. If he chooses to continue to ignore his symptoms he eventually finds that breathing is becoming more and more difficult, especially during the expiratory phase. He coughs continuously—a moist, wheezing cough—but he is not able to clear his respiratory tract satisfactorily. He then becomes less and less active; his thorax becomes fixed and assumes a barrel shape and there are large spaces between the ribs. If x-rays are taken they will show inflated lungs, a flattened diaphragm and abnormal heart shadows.[11] The appearance of the emphysematous patient is usually quite characteristic and one can almost diagnose his condition by looking at him. He wears an anxious and strained facial expression. He cannot lie down flat in bed, but sits up on the edge of his bed or chair leaning forward and using his abdominal muscles to exhale. He makes an obvious effort to exhale with each breath and often puffs out his cheeks on expiration. He must speak quickly and in short sentences because he has so little breath.

Treatment and Nursing Care. Unfortunately, by the time a patient manifests the severe symptoms mentioned above there is nothing that can be done to reverse the pathologic changes responsible for such symptoms. There are, however, some therapeutic measures that can help relieve the symptoms. If the disease is detected early and treatment and rehabilitation plans are carried through, it is possible to help these patients maintain adequate ventilation and continue to lead a fairly comfortable and moderately active life.

Treatment usually consists of administration of medications to prevent infections, bronchial obstruction and chronic inflammation. These drugs include antibiotics, bronchodilators and corticosteroids. Also, the patient must learn to avoid conditions that further aggravate his condition. This includes not smoking, avoiding cold air, dust or other irritants that can bring spasm and constriction of the bronchioles, regulation of physical activity so that he does not overexert himself, avoiding emotional upsets and stressful situations that increase breathing difficulties, and maintaining adequate nutrition and other measures that will maintain a resistance to infection.

Exercises such as these described on page 272 are of benefit to some patients who do not have severe dyspnea or are otherwise greatly debilitated. These exercises improve ventilation of the lungs by strengthening the abdominal muscles and other accessory muscles of respiration so that they can be used efficiently in breathing.

Intermittent positive-pressure breathing also can be of benefit in proper ventilation of the lungs and "stretching" of the respiratory muscles so that there can be adequate removal of carbon dioxide from the lungs. This treatment also allows for administration of aerosol drugs which facilitate coughing and bronchial expansion for removal of accumulated secretions.

Complications. The most common complications of emphysema are infection, respiratory acidosis and a heart condition called *cor pulmonale.* One should bear in mind that cor pulmonale is cardiac failure produced by a lung disease rather than a result of some disorder of the heart itself. It is generally agreed that cor pulmonale occurs because of hypertension within the pulmonary artery. This hypertension places a tremendous burden on the right ventricle because it must work doubly hard to overcome the pressure within the pulmonary artery. Eventually the ventricle enlarges and becomes fatigued. Then the patient has right-sided failure with symptoms arising from accumulation of fluid in the abdominal cavity, in the peripheral tissues and in the thoracic cavity. The liver becomes enlarged as a result of congestion in the portal circulation. Treatment for cor pulmonale is the same as for other types of cardiac failure; that is, digitalization, use of diuretics and restriction of sodium and fluid intake.

Treatment and Nursing Care. The patient with emphysema is usually treated at home unless he is suffering from acute respiratory distress. His activities are regulated so that he has frequent periods of rest and all undue physical exertion is avoided.

Special exercises which increase the contracting ability of the diaphragm and thereby help in deflating the lungs are of some benefit. Abdominal support with elastic bandages or girdles also assist in maintaining good contraction and elevation of the diaphragm.

Aerosol therapy is especially beneficial to the patient with emphysema.

PULMONARY TUBERCULOSIS

Definition. Pulmonary tuberculosis is an infectious disease of the lung characterized by lesions within the lung tissue. The lesions may continue to degenerate and become necrotic or they may heal by fibrosis and calcification. The causative organism is the tubercle bacillus.

Incidence. The widespread use of anti-tuberculotic drugs has brought about some changes in the distribution of tuberculosis in the United States. In the mid 1940's tuberculosis could be found in almost all communities and in all social and ethnic groups. Today it is primarily found in nonwhite males; nonwhite females rank second and all individuals in the age group of 65 years or older run a close third. Crowded urban areas show a much higher rate than do rural areas.[10]

Diagnosis. Early detection of tuberculosis is of great importance, because the anti-tuberculotic drugs are more effective in the early stages of the disease, the period of disability is much shorter and the complications are fewer.

A tuberculin test such as the Mantoux intradermal test or the Heaf multiple puncture skin test are valuable in ruling out tuberculosis. If the skin test is positive it indicates a need for further testing by x-ray and a complete physical examination.

X-ray examination of the chest also is useful in detecting tubercular lesions of the lungs. The Public Health Department and other health agencies such as the state Tuberculosis and Health Associations offer free x-ray films from a mobile unit that visits neighborhoods. In this way cases of tuberculosis can be detected in individuals who might not otherwise be tested for lung disease. These x-ray programs have been especially effective in communities known to have a high tuberculosis rate.

Analysis of sputum for the presence of the tubercle bacillus is another diagnostic test that is used. If the bacilli are present a diagnosis of tuberculosis is very definitely established. Since individuals are quite likely to swallow sputum rather than expectorate it, a sample of the stomach contents can be examined for the presence of tubercle bacilli.

Symptoms. The symptoms of tuberculosis include cough, low-grade fever in the afternoon, loss of weight, night sweats, and sometimes *hemoptysis* (spitting of blood).

Treatment and Nursing Care. All of the general principles essential to the proper care of a patient with a respiratory disease are applied to the nursing care of a patient with pulmonary tuberculosis. Rest, good nutrition, proper handling of secretions from the respiratory tract, and control of coughing are all important aspects to be considered. Of these, rest is probably most important. For the specific procedures and methods of isolation of the patient and destruction of the tubercle bacillus the student is referred to a text on communicable diseases.

Tuberculosis is more a chronic disease than acute in nature and has a prolonged period of convalescence. Because the patient is confined to an institution or his home for months or even years, some provision must be made for occupational therapy and other diversional activities. The student is referred to Chapter 7 of this text for further information on the care of the chronically ill.

Drugs used in the treatment of tuberculosis are usually given in combination; that is, two drugs are chosen and given simultaneously for maximum effect. The most common drugs used are *streptomycin, para-amino-salicylic acid (PAS),* and *isoniazid (INH).* These drugs have a specific action against the tubercle bacillus and have greatly facilitated arrest of the disease.

The patient must receive these injections over such an extended period of time that it is extremely important that the sites of injection are rotated faithfully. The patient often becomes discouraged by the number of painful injections necessary and the nurse must help him understand the need for uninterrupted administration of the medication. When drugs are not administered regularly the bacilli become resistant and the drugs are no longer effective.

Surgery is also used in the treatment of tuberculosis. Surgical removal of a diseased lobe of the lung is referred to as a *lobectomy.* A *pneumonectomy* is surgical removal of the entire lung. A *thoracoplasty* is removal of several ribs for the purpose of collapsing the lung. *Artificial pneumothorax* is the injection of air into the pleural cavity for the purpose of collapsing the lung. Both a thoracoplasty and an artificial pneumothorax are done so that the collapsed lung may be in a state of complete rest, thereby aiding in the healing of the tuberculous lesion.

Prevention. Tuberculosis is an infectious disease that is contracted by inhaling the tubercle bacillus. This microorganism is capable of surviving for long periods of time in dark, damp places. It cannot survive more than two hours of direct sunlight and also can be killed by boiling for a full five minutes. Autoclaving is the most efficient method of killing the tubercle bacillus.

The best way in which the spread of tuberculosis can be controlled is through adequate detection and treatment of active cases and through education of the public about the disease. Once a person is diagnosed as tubercular he should be taught the ways in which the disease can be spread and his responsibility in following directions so that he does not contaminate others. He must learn to cover his nose and mouth with a disposable tissue each time he clears his throat, coughs or sneezes. The contaminated tissues should be flushed down a toilet or wrapped in paper and burned. Ordinary face masks are not effective in screening out the tubercle bacillus and should not be relied upon by the nurse as protection from the patient who cannot or will not cover his nose and mouth. There are some specially made masks that are effective barriers against the bacilli and they should be used when a patient is unable to cooperate.

Strict isolation of the tubercular patient is not considered necessary. He and his family should understand, however, exactly how the disease is spread and what precautions they should take when the patient is staying at home. Since small children and infants are particularly susceptible to the disease, special precautions must be taken to protect them from contamination.

There is available a vaccine made from living, attenuated bacilli. It is called BCG (bacille Calmette Guérin) and is capable of offering some protection but cannot be depended upon to provide complete immunity to tuberculosis. The BCG vaccine has the disadvantage of causing a positive reaction to the tuberculin test and this interferes somewhat with the usefulness of tuberculin testing programs. Public health officials in this country advise the administration of BCG vaccine only to those persons who live in communities that have a very high rate of tuberculosis. In New York City, for example, every child entering the seventh grade is offered the vaccine. In rural areas where the tuberculosis rate is low the vaccine is not recommended.

If during the tuberculin testing program an individual shows a positive reaction within six months after a negative reaction, some authorities recommend that he receive isoniazid as a prophylaxis. The drug is given for one full year. It also may be given as a preventive medication to individuals with silicosis because they are more susceptible than usual to tuberculosis.

EXTRAPULMONARY TUBERCULOSIS

Definition. It is possible for the tubercle bacillus to attack and damage parts of the body other than the lungs. This is called extrapulmonary tuberculosis. The areas most frequently affected are the bones, meninges, urinary tract and reproductive system.

Tuberculous meningitis involves infection of the meninges which line the brain and spinal cord. This disease can be fatal unless it is promptly treated with anti-tuberculotic drugs. The symptoms of this disorder are essentially the same as those in other types of meningitis.

Tuberculous infection of the bone is now less common than it formerly was because of better methods of detecting pulmonary tuberculosis and elimination of contaminated milk as a source of infection. Because of extensive bone destruction in a tubercular infection there can be serious orthopedic deformities in thise disease. Tuberculosis of the spine, called Pott's disease, is now quite rare in the United States. The deformity most commonly seen in Pott's disease is kyphosis or "hunchback,"

NURSING CARE OF THE PATIENT HAVING CHEST SURGERY

Preoperative Care. The preoperative period is somewhat longer when chest surgery is done because the breathing capacity of the patient will be greatly diminished during the immediate postoperative period and the patient will need to be in the best possible health to withstand the strain. Special exercises may be done under the supervision of a physiotherapist. These exercises are planned so that the chest and shoulder muscles and the muscles of respiration will be able to provide the maximum respiration possible after surgery.

The patient may have extensive diagnostic tests including a bronchoscopy and sputum examination immediately before surgery. Postural drainage and expectorant drugs are given to remove as much sputum from the bronchi as possible.

Postoperative Care. When the patient returns from surgery he will require close observation for signs of respiratory distress. Dyspnea, cyanosis, or sudden severe pain in the chest must be reported immediately because these may indicate a collapse of the lung due to a leakage of air into the pleural cavity. The vital signs of the patient are checked frequently and recorded. Oxygen is usually administered for the first few postoperative days.

The position of the patient once he has recovered from the anesthesia will depend on the type of surgery performed and the orders of the surgeon. The patient is turned every 2 hours or more often as ordered. Before attempting to turn the patient the practical nurse must ascertain whether or not the surgeon wishes to allow the patient to lie on the *unoperative* side. Many surgeons do not allow the patient to lie on the unoperative side because this position diminishes the expansion of the good lung and thereby adds to respiratory distress. There is also danger of infection of the good lung by drainage from the affected lung when the patient lies with the operative side up. When the patient has a tube inserted for drainage from the operative site, lying on the operative side facilitates the flow of drainage. Unless contraindicated the most comfortable position is semi-Fowler's. After the vital signs have become stable the head of the bed may be elevated to a 45° angle. In this position the diaphragm stays down and there is more room for lung expansion.

Coughing is encouraged during the postoperative period so that secretions will be removed from the bronchial tree and complications thereby avoided. The nurse must realize that coughing is painful for the patient and he will need support of the chest during a seizure of coughing.

It is not unusual for the patient who has had chest surgery to return from the operating room with a tube inserted through the surgical incision in his chest. This tube provides *closed drainage* of the fluids which accumulate in the pleural cavity during and after surgery.

SPECIAL POINTS IN THE CARE OF A CLOSED DRAINAGE SYSTEM

1. Remember that the pleural cavity is an airtight compartment. The apparatus for closed drainage must also remain airtight *at all times*.

2. Never raise the drainage bottles from a thoracotomy tube above the level of the surgical incision. It is best to keep the bottles on the floor at all times.

3. Never disconnect the tubing from the bottle. If the tubing becomes disconnected accidentally, pinch the tubing leading to the patient's chest and summon help immediately.

4. Do not allow the tubing to become kinked or obstructed by the weight of the patient.

5. Never pin the tubing to the bedclothes.

6. Do not empty a thoracotomy drainage bottle. The surgeon usually prefers to do this himself. If the bottle becomes filled with fluid notify the nurse in charge. The surgeon will want to know immediately if the patient is having that much drainage.

7. Dressings may be reinforced but are never changed by the practical nurse as long as closed drainage is being used.

8. If the patient has two thoracotomy tubes, each one must be connected to its own water-seal drainage bottle. The purpose of the two tubes is to provide drainage of air and fluid from the pleural space (see Fig. 13-5).

9. Check tubing at least once every two hours to be sure that there is no obstruction to the flow of drainage. If the tube is open and unobstructed the saline in the drainage bottle will rise and fall with each inspiration and expiration. Blood clots that are obstructing the tubing can be removed by gently "milking" the tube in the direction of the bottle.

PNEUMOTHORAX

Definition. The term pneumothorax refers to an accumulation of air or gas in the pleural cavity. Normally the pleural space is an airtight compartment with a negative pressure that allows for expansion of the lungs. If any

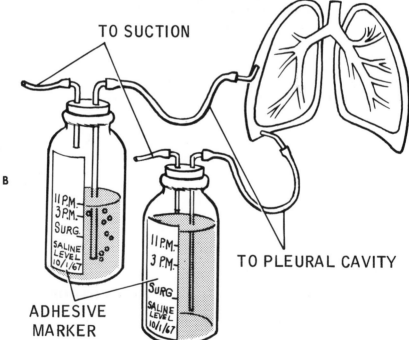

Figure 13-5. *A*, Unwilling but able, patient walks q4h trailing drainage bottles with rope. Kelly hemostats clamped to pajamas prevent pull on tubes. *B*, Underwater drainage bottles act as one-way valves, permitting air and blood to escape from, but not to return to, pleural cavity. Escaping air causes saline to bubble. Rising fluid level in bottles is marked to indicate amount and rapidity of blood loss. (From Dittbrenner and Herbert: American Journal of Nursing, October, 1967.)

external or internal chest injury causes a break in the wall of the pleural space, air will rush into the cavity and collapse the lung. This also will cause a shift of the heart and mediastinum toward the affected side.

Spontaneous pneumothorax can occur during the course of a pulmonary disease or it may follow a perforating injury to the external chest wall. *Artificial pneumothorax* is a surgical procedure sometimes used in the treatment of tuberculosis in order to collapse the lung and give it rest.

Symptoms. Spontaneous pneumothorax is characterized by severe dyspnea, a sudden, sharp pain in the chest with cessation of normal chest movement on the affected side, and a fall in blood pressure with a weak, rapid pulse.

Treatment and Nursing Care. Spontaneous pneumothorax usually is treated conservatively with bed rest until the lung is reinflated and the administration of oxygen when needed to relieve dyspnea. If the internal lesion causing the leak of air into the pleural cavity eventually seals off and air becomes trapped in the pleural cavity, a thoracentesis may be necessary to remove the air and allow the lung to inflate.

Traumatic pneumothorax may involve more extensive surgery to repair the chest wall and other damaged internal structures. If air continues to leak from a defect in the lung surface or from an outside wound, tubes are inserted and attached to a closed water-seal drainage apparatus. These tubes are removed when the lung expands and the wounds heal. The patient is allowed up and about as soon as lung expansion is complete.

CLINICAL CASE PROBLEMS

1. You are assigned to the care of a 16-year-old girl who has pneumococcal pneumonia. She is receiving oxygen by mask to relieve her dyspnea and cyanosis. The doctor has placed her on absolute bed rest, and though the girl appears exhausted, she does not wish to have others do anything for her. She appears to be delirious at times and when you check her temperature you find that it is 104.6° rectally.

> What nursing problems do you see in this situation?
> How can you help this patient be more comfortable without further exhausting her?
> What special observations must you make?
> What nursing measures may be used for the high temperature?

2. Mr. Cook, age 45, is admitted to the hospital with the diagnosis of cancer of the lung. The surgeon has scheduled Mr. Cook for a pneumonectomy 10 days after admission. What preoperative care would you expect this patient to receive? When Mr. Cook returns from surgery he has a thoracotomy tube in place. The surgeon attaches this tube to a water-seal apparatus in the patient's room. You are assigned to assist in the care of this patient on his second postoperative day.

> What position would be best and most comfortable for this patient?
> What are your responsibilities in regard to the thoracotomy tube and drainage apparatus?

3. Mr. Brown, age 69, is assigned to your care. He has chronic bronchitis with an acute flare-up of symptoms. He also is an arthritic and has great difficulty moving about. One of the treatments ordered for Mr. Brown is postural drainage.

> When would you give the patient postural drainage?
> What problems will you have with this procedure? How can you overcome them?
> Why is postural drainage ordered for this patient?

4. Mr. Warner is a 59-year-old man who has a moderate amount of dyspnea from emphysema. He was admitted to the hospital for a foot infection and while there his emphysema was diagnosed. Mr. Warner

is not a very agreeable person. He complains about the temperature of his room and the treatment prescribed for his emphysema (which he feels is a very minor thing compared to his foot infection), and he is especially upset about the restriction on smoking that has been imposed on him by his physician. One day while you are applying warm soaks to Mr. Warner's foot he asks you, "Just what is emphysema anyway? What will happen if I don't follow my doctor's orders?"

How would you answer Mr. Warner's questions?
How could you motivate him toward taking sensible precautions against aggravating his condition?
What are some of those precautions?
How would you explain intermittent positive-pressure breathing to Mr. Warner?

REFERENCES

1. Brown, A. F.: *Medical Nursing*, 3rd edition. Philadelphia, W. B. Saunders Co., 1957.
2. Brunner, L. S.: et al.: *Textbook of Medical-Surgical Nursing*. Philadelphia, J. B. Lippincott Co., 1966.
3. Chuan, H.: "Impaired Pulmonary Circulation Due to Pulmonary Emphysema." *Nursing Clinics of North America*, vol. 1, no. 1. Philadelphia, W. B. Saunders Co., 1966.
4. Dittbrenner, M., Sr., and Hebert, W. H.: "Regimen for a Thoracotomy Patient." Am. Journ. Nurs., Oct., 1967, p. 2072.
5. Hadley, F., and Berdicks, K. J.: "When a Patient Has a Respiratory Difficulty." Am. Journ. Nurs. Oct., 1962, p. 64.
6. Johansen, J. L.: "Taking the Mystery out of Water-sealed Chest Drainage." RN, Jan., 1960, p. 40.
7. Jones, W. R.: "Living with Emphysema." Nurs. Outlook, Sept., 1967, p. 53.
8. Kinney, M.: "Rehabilitation of Patients with C.O.L.D." Journ. Nurs., Dec., 1967, p. 2528.
9. Kurihara, M.: "Postural Drainage, Clapping and Vibrating." Am. Journ. Nurs., Nov., 1965, p. 76.
10. Mushlin, I., and Amberson, J. B.: "Tracking down Tuberculosis." Am. Journ. Nurs., Dec., 1965, p. 91.
11. Secor, J.: "The Patient with Emphysema." Am. Journ. Nurs., July, 1965, p. 74.
12. Shafer, K. N., Sawyer, J. R., et al.: *Medical-Surgical Nursing*, 4th edition. St. Louis, C. V. Mosby Co., 1967.
13. Smith, D. W., and Gips, C. D.: *Care of the Adult Patient*. Philadelphia, J. B. Lippincott Co., 1966.

SUGGESTED STUDENT READING

1. Fontana, V. J., and Rappaport, I.: "Asthma." Journ. Pract. Nurs., Dec., 1965, p. 24.
2. Frenay, M. A. C., Sr.: "Drugs in Tuberculosis Control." Am. Journ. Nurs., April, 1961, p. 82.
3. Isler, C.: "Pneumonia: The Still Present Killer." RN, Feb., 1962, p. 63.
4. Isler, C.: "What's the Score on TB Treatment and Control?" RN, May, 1963, p. 60.
5. Johansen, J. L.: "Taking the Mystery out of Water-Sealed Chest Drainage." RN, Jan., 1960, p. 40.
6. MacVicar, J.: "Exercises Before and After Thoracic Surgery." Am. Journ. Nurs., Jan., 1962, p. 61.
7. Steele, J. D.: "These Mysterious Drainage Bottles." Am. Journ. Nurs., Nov., 1955, p. 1358.

OUTLINE FOR CHAPTER 13

I. Introduction

A. Respiratory organs take the form of a tree. Alveoli are small air sacs through which the oxygen and carbon dioxide are exchanged.

B. Diseases of the respiratory tract are the most common afflictions of mankind.

II. General Nursing Care

A. Concerned with relief of symptoms and prevention of complications.

1. Coughing—stimulated by a foreign substance in the respiratory tract. Nonproductive cough—no sputum brought up. Productive cough—varying amounts of sputum brought up.

2. Increased secretions—body attempts to rid itself of irritating and infectious agents. Secretions can spread infection if not handled with care.

3. Respiratory distress. A very disturbing and frightening symptom. Proper positioning can give relief. If distress is severe the physician may order concentrated oxygen by mask, nasal prongs or catheter. Warm, moist air can provide relief in cases of croup and less severe respiratory disorders.

4. Rest reduces the need for oxygen and prevents exhaustion.
5. Diet should be high-caloric, high-vitamin liquids for patients with acute diseases of the upper respiratory tract. All patients should have a well-balanced diet to provide resistance to infection.
6. Medications.
   a. Expectorant and sedative cough mixtures.
   b. Antipyretics.
   c. Antihistamines to dry up secretions.
   d. Antispasmodics and bronchodilators.
   e. Antibiotics.
7. Irrigations help remove thick mucus from the nose and throat.
8. Inhalation therapy — administration of drugs as a very fine spray that can be inhaled deep into the respiratory tract. Drugs may include antibiotics, bronchodilators and liquefying agents. These drugs combat infection, enlarge the lumen of the air passages and liquefy mucus so that it is thinner and more easily coughed up.
9. Intermittent positive-pressure breathing therapy — use of a respirator to increase the amount of air inhaled into the lungs. This allows for more uniform distribution of air to the alveoli, aids in the removal of carbon dioxide and makes coughing easier and more productive of sputum.
10. Breathing exercises strengthen the abdominal muscles and increase the patient's tolerance to physical exertion.
11. Postural drainage — patient is positioned so that the force of gravity and ciliary action of the bronchioles will move secretions to the main bronchi and trachea so they can be coughed up. Position depends on the area of the lesion in the lung.

III. Diagnostic Tests

A. Chest x-ray.
B. Respiratory function tests — vital capacity, tidal volume, residual volume and total lung capacity.
C. Sputum analysis for microorganisms, malignant cells, blood, etc.

D. Bronchogram — an x-ray of the bronchial tree using a radiopaque dye.
E. Bronchoscopy — visual examination of the bronchi by utilizing an endoscope.

IV. The Common Cold

A. Caused by many different strains of viruses.
B. There is no cure but one can increase his resistance to a cold.
C. Purpose of treatment is to prevent complications such as bacterial infection or development of a chronic bronchitis.

V. Acute Bronchitis

A. An acute inflammation of the bronchi.
B. Symptoms similar to those of the common cold but usually there is a more persistent cough that is productive of purulent sputum.
C. Treatment includes rest, humidifier and antibiotics. Can develop into chronic bronchitis if not completely relieved and patient continues to be exposed to irritants that inflame the bronchi.

VI. Pneumonia

A. An extensive inflammation of the lungs.
B. Two general types are bacterial and primary atypical or viral pneumonia.
C. Symptoms include chills, elevated temperature, cough and severe stabbing pain in the chest or side that is aggravated by coughing or taking a deep breath.
D. Treatment and nursing care concerned with conservation of the patient's strength and energy, relief of symptoms and control of infection.

VII. Bronchiectasis

A. A chronic disease of the respiratory system characterized by permanent dilatation of the bronchi.
B. May follow pneumonia or other respiratory infections or result from a congenital defect in the alveoli.
C. Most outstanding symptom is severe attacks of coughing during which the patient brings up large amounts of foul-smelling sputum.
D. Treatment and nursing care are aimed at relief of symptoms. No cure. Postural drainage helps remove stagnant sputum from the lower bronchi.

VIII. Cancer of the Lung

A. Leading cause of death in white males.

B. Tumors usually begin in epithelial lining of bronchi. Symptoms include coughing and wheezing and, later, pain and bloody sputum.

C. Surgical removal only possible cure. Radiation and chemotherapy may help retard tumor growth.

IX. Asthma

A. An allergic reaction characterized by swelling of the bronchial mucosa and increased production of sputum in the bronchioles, causing wheezing.

B. Symptoms include cough, wheezing, dyspnea and watering of the eyes.

C. Treatment is aimed at removal of the offending allergen and avoidance of emotional upsets or other situations that may precipitate an attack.

X. Pleurisy

A. An inflammation of the pleural membranes surrounding the lungs. Pleurisy with effusion is accompanied by an increase in serous fluid in the pleural cavity.

B. Symptoms—sharp, stabbing pain in the chest.

C. Treatment includes bed rest and measures to prevent infection. Thoracentesis may be necessary in pleurisy with effusion.

XI. Empyema

A. The presence of thick and purulent fluid within the pleural cavity.

B. Treated by antibiotics and removal of fluid from the pleural cavity.

XII. Pulmonary Emphysema

A. A chronic respiratory disease that results from chronic inflammation of the bronchi.

B. The alveoli lose their elasticity and become distended with air. The patient cannot exhale stale air so as to make room for oxygenated air.

C. Symptoms include exertional dyspnea, persistent cough that does not effectively clear the respiratory passages, fixation of the rib cage and a barrel shaped chest.

D. Treatment is aimed at preventing complications and improving ventilation of the lungs. If the disease is detected early the pathologic changes can be halted and the patient can be rehabilitated to lead a moderately active life. Medications include antibiotics, bronchodilators and the corticosteroids.

XIII. Pulmonary Tuberculosis

A. An infectious disease of the lung caused by tubercle bacillus.

B. Characterized by lesions that may continue to degenerate and become necrotic or may heal by fibrosis and calcification.

C. Symptoms include cough, low-grade fever in the afternoon, loss of weight, night sweats and hemoptysis.

D. Diagnostic tests include tuberculin skin tests, x-ray examination, analysis of sputum and examination of gastric contents for tubercle bacilli.

E. Treatment includes rest, good nutrition, proper handling of secretions from the respiratory tract and control of coughing. Specific anti-tuberculotic drugs are streptomycin, para-aminosalicylic acid (PAS) and isoniazid (INH).

F. Surgical treatment may involve removal of part or all of the affected lung.

XIV. Extrapulmonary Tuberculosis

A. Tubercle bacillus infects parts of the body other than the lungs, like the bones, meninges, urinary tract or reproductive system.

B. Tuberculous meningitis is treated with the specific anti-tuberculotic drugs.

C. Involvement of the bone can cause serious orthopedic deformities.

XV. Nursing Care of the Patient Having Chest Surgery

A. Preoperative care involves diagnostic tests, measures to remove as much mucus from the respiratory tract as possible and special exercises to strengthen the muscles of respiration.

B. Postoperative care involves careful attention to drainage tubes that remove air and fluid from the pleural space. Collapse of the lung is possible.

C. Special points in the care of a closed-drainage apparatus:

1. Keep the drainage bottle below the level of the chest at all times.
2. Keep all connections airtight.
3. Observe the tubes to be sure they remain unobstructed.
4. Observe thoracotomy bottles to determine amount of drainage. Do not empty these bottles.

Chapter 14

NURSING CARE OF PATIENTS WITH DISEASES OF THE DIGESTIVE SYSTEM

VOCABULARY

Decompression
Duct
Enzyme
Hemolytic
Sinus

INTRODUCTION

The main portion of the digestive system is actually one long tube which extends from the mouth to the rectum. This tube is known as the *alimentary tract* or *intestinal tract*. For the sake of clarity the various sections of this tract are considered as organs. Thus, the large bulge just below the esophagus is known as a separate organ, the stomach, even though it is only a continuation of the same tube that forms the esophagus above it and the small intestine below it.

As food enters the alimentary tract by way of the mouth, it immediately begins to undergo physical and chemical changes; that is, it is not only changed in appearance but new substances are formed from the original material. These changes are the first stages of *digestion*. The food is propelled downward through the alimentary tract by wavelike motions of involuntary muscles within the walls of the alimentary tract. This rhythmic squeezing action is called peristalsis. As the food passes down the digestive tube it continues to

undergo changes until it reaches a liquid state and can then be taken into the blood stream. The transfer of nutrients from the intestines into the blood is referred to as *absorption*. Substances such as cellulose which are not digested and absorbed continue through the tube and are eventually eliminated through the anus. The conversion of the food elements into energy and production of body tissues is called *metabolism*.

The accessory organs of digestion are those organs outside the alimentary tract which are directly concerned with digestion. They include the liver, which manufactures bile, and the gallbladder, which stores the bile until it is needed to help in the digestion of fats. The pancreas is also an accessory organ of digestion. The cells of the pancreas secrete pancreatic juice which contains six enzymes. These enzymes are special substances necessary for the chemical breakdown of foods. Ducts leading from the liver, gallbladder and pancreas empty their secretions directly into the small intestine where all digestion is completed (see Fig. 14-1).

In this chapter the diseases of the

291

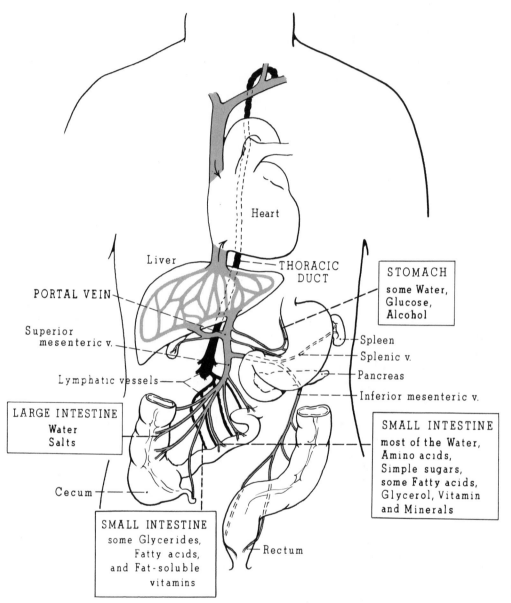

Figure 14-1. Products of digestion are absorbed in the stomach and small and large intestines. (From Jacob and Francone: *Structure and Function in Man,* W. B. Saunders Co., Philadelphia.)

digestive tract and diseases of the accessory organs will be considered separately. It must be remembered, however, that the two groups of organs are closely related and diseases which primarily affect the accessory organs will inevitably affect the function of digestion.

Part I—NURSING CARE OF PATIENTS WITH DISEASES OF THE DIGESTIVE TRACT

DIAGNOSTIC TESTS

X-ray Examination. Special x-ray examinations of the digestive tract should include a *gastrointestinal series* and a *barium enema.* In a gastrointestinal series the patient drinks a barium suspension. This substance is radiopaque and therefore outlines the hollow organs as it passes through them. The filling and emptying of the esophagus, stomach, and duodenum may be observed by the radiologist through a fluoroscope. Films of the stomach are taken after the patient drinks the barium and again 6 hours after the fluoroscopy to determine how much barium has passed through the stomach. The gastrointestinal series is useful in diagnosing obstructions, ulcerations and growths within the esophagus, stomach, or duodenum.

In preparation for a gastrointestinal series the patient is not allowed food or fluids for at least 6 to 8 hours before the examination.

The x-ray examination of the lower digestive tract using a radiopaque substance is called a *barium enema.* As the name implies, the barium suspension is instilled through a rectal tube. The barium must be retained by the patient while x-ray films are taken, thus allowing for visualization of the lower bowel. The barium enema is useful in the diagnosis of ulcerations, tumors, obstructions, and other abnormalities in the structure of the walls of the lower intestine.

Preparation of the patient for a barium enema usually includes the administration of laxatives and enemas the night before and again on the morning of the examination. The responsibilities of the nurse in preparing a patient for these special x-ray examinations are discussed more fully on pages 50 and 51.

Gastroscopy and Esophagoscopy. In both of these examinations the physician is actually able to see the inner lining of the stomach or esophagus. He does this by inserting a special instrument through the mouth and into the esophagus (see Fig. 14-2). The instrument may be passed further down into the stomach if a gastroscopy is done. Foods and liquids are withheld 6 to 8 hours before the examination. The patient is sedated lightly and the procedure explained so that he may be more cooperative during the examination. While there is no actual pain associated with the procedure, it is uncomfortable for the patient.

Proctoscopy and Sigmoidoscopy. These examinations are similar in principle to the gastroscopy. They are done for the purpose of visualizing the inner lining of the anus, rectum, and sigmoid colon (see Fig. 14-3).

The patient is prepared for the examination with enemas until the return solution is clear. According to Brown, "By clear returns one means that there is no solid matter in the returns. No more than three enemas should ever be given without consulting the doctor." Other methods of cleansing the lower bowel depend on the individual wishes of the examining physician.

The position of the patient during

Figure 14-2.   Fiber optic gastroscope. (Courtesy American Cystoscope Makers, Inc., Pelham Manor, N.Y.)

the examination is usually the knee-chest position unless a special examination table which breaks in the middle is available.

Gastric Analysis.   In this test a tube is passed into the stomach and samples of the gastric contents are withdrawn. The first specimen taken is called the "fasting specimen." Other specimens are taken after a substance is given to stimulate the flow of gastric juices. The specimens are then taken to the laboratory where they are tested for the amount of hydrochloric acid present.

A *tubeless gastric analysis* may be done when the physician wishes to know whether or not there is any hydrochloric acid in the gastric contents. A tubeless gastric analysis cannot give information on the exact amount of hydrochloric acid present.

As the name implies, there is no need to insert a tube into the stomach for a tubeless gastric analysis. Instead, the patient is given special granules to drink in 240 ml. of water. At prescribed intervals urine specimens are collected. If hydrochloric acid is present the urine will be blue; if none is present

Figure 14-3.   Fiber optic proctoscope with obturator. (Courtesy American Cystoscope Makers, Inc., Pelham Manor, N.Y.)

in the stomach the urine will remain straw-colored.

Stool Examination. The stool may be examined for: (1) presence of blood, (2) presence of specific bacteria, and (3) cysts, ova, and parasites.

When the stool is examined for *occult* (hidden) blood, the patient must abstain from red meat for 48 to 70 hours before a specimen is collected. If an examination for amebas is ordered, the specimen must be kept warm and taken to the laboratory immediately after it is collected.

STOMATITIS

Definition and Symptoms. The term stomatitis refers to a generalized inflammation of the mucous membranes of the mouth. It may be caused by certain drugs, trauma from ill-fitting dentures or malocclusion of the teeth, other mechanical irritants in the mouth, nutritional deficiencies, pathogenic organisms and excessive smoking or drinking. Poor oral hygiene can be a major factor in the development of stomatitis.

General symptoms include pain and swelling of the oral mucosa, increased salivation, severe halitosis and sometimes fever. More specific symptoms will depend on the type of inflammation or infection present.

Aphthous Stomatitis. This is commonly called "canker sores" and is characterized by small, white, crater-like ulcers in the mouth. They are quite uncomfortable and frequently interfere with eating because of the discomfort they cause. The exact cause of aphthous stomatitis is unknown but it is probably a viral infection to which certain individuals are highly susceptible. There is no specific treatment or cure for this disorder.

Vincent's Angina. Another name for this inflammation of the mouth is "trench mouth" because it was quite common during the first World War. It is believed to be caused by a combination of two organisms—a fusiform bacillus and a spirochete. The characteristic lesions are shallow ulcers that are covered with a grayish membrane. These are painful and can interfere with eating. Treatment consists of mouthwashes using sodium perborate and antibiotics.

GASTRITIS

Definition. Gastritis is an inflammation of the mucous membrane lining of the stomach. It may be acute or chronic in nature.

The main causes of acute gastritis are overeating, drinking an excessive amount of alcohol, eating contaminated food, or the ingestion of a poisonous drug or chemical.

Chronic gastritis usually follows ingestion of highly spiced food or excessive amounts of alcohol over an extended length of time.

Symptoms. In both acute and chronic gastritis the main symptoms are nausea, vomiting, pain, and tenderness in the stomach region, and sometimes diarrhea. The patient with chronic gastritis may also have massive hemorrhage from the stomach.

Treatment and Nursing Care. Acute gastritis is usually of very short duration. Treatment consists of withholding all foods by mouth and administration of drugs which slow down the peristaltic action of the alimentary tract. If severe dehydration occurs, fluids may be given intravenously. The nursing care of a patient having nausea, vomiting and diarrhea is discussed more fully in Chapter 3, pages 31 and 32.

Chronic gastritis is not as easily treated as acute gastritis. Diet therapy is of primary importance in chronic gastritis because the patient frequently admits to indiscretion in his dietary and drinking habits and finds it difficult to change. The diet for these patients is basically a bland diet in which all strong seasonings and roughage are avoided. Frequent small feedings are recommended to prevent overloading of the stomach and unnecessary stimulation of the flow of gastric juices. It is always difficult to change one's eating habits of long standing and the nurse must use tact and patience in encouraging the patient to follow the prescribed diet faithfully.

Medications which coat the gastric mucosa also help prevent ulceration of the stomach lining. Examples of this type of drug are *bismuth* and *barium.* Since the patient frequently suffers from painful spasmodic contractions of the stomach, antispasmodic drugs are also used.

ULCERATIVE COLITIS

Definition. Ulcerative colitis is an inflammation, with the formation of ulcers in the mucosa of the colon. It is often a chronic disease and the patient is usually free from symptoms between acute flare-ups.

The exact cause of ulcerative colitis is not known. Acute infections and emotional tension frequently bring about acute attacks.

Symptoms. The chief symptom is diarrhea. The stools are frequent and watery, containing shreds of mucus, blood, and pus. Nausea and vomiting, or loss of appetite without actually vomiting, are also common symptoms. The loss of body fluids soon brings about dehydration and malnutrition.

Treatment and Nursing Care. Treatment for this condition is difficult and the prognosis is poor. Supportive measures, such as blood transfusions, and a diet high in proteins, vitamins, and calories must be used. Rest and freedom from anxiety help in the relief of the symptoms. *Antidiarrheic* drugs containing paregoric and kaolin are also of some benefit in the control of the diarrhea.

In caring for the patient with ulcer-ative colitis the nurse must bear in mind the importance of the patient's individual personality. These patients are often tense and nervous individuals who are easily offended by the remarks of others. They keep their anxieties well hidden, however, and may give a false impression of serenity and resignation to their illness. Yet these are the very patients who are most in need of small, extra attentions and encouragement.

The stools must be carefully observed and their number and character reported to the nurse in charge or written on the patient's chart. For further information on the nursing care of a patient with diarrhea see page 32.

APPENDICITIS

Definition. Appendicitis is an inflammation of the vermiform appendix. It is called vermiform because it is wormlike, and appendix because it is an appendage of the cecum. The appendix is a blind pouch and is therefore easily infected by bacteria passing through the intestinal tract.

Symptoms. Pain in the lower right side, halfway between the umbilicus and the crest of the ileum is the best known symptom of appendicitis. However, the location of the pain may and often does vary with individuals. An elevated temperature, nausea and vomiting, and an increase in the white cell count are also characteristic of appendicitis.

Treatment and Nursing Care. Treatment is surgical removal of the appendix *(appendectomy).* Before surgery the patient is allowed nothing by mouth and an ice bag may be placed on the abdomen to slow down localization of the inflammation and thus avoid rupture of the swollen and inflamed appendix. Under no circumstances should laxatives be given when appendicitis is suspected. Hot water bottles to relieve abdominal pain are also forbidden.

The patient is usually allowed out of bed the day after surgery if no complications are present. The convalescent period is most often uneventful and the patient may return to his former activities within two to three weeks.

PERITONITIS

Definition. The peritoneum is a serous sac that lines the abdominal cavity and encloses the intestines, stomach, liver and spleen and partially encloses the uterus and uterine tubes. Peritonitis is an inflammation of the peritoneum. It usually occurs when one of the organs it encloses ruptures or is perforated so that the organ's contents (including bacteria) are spilled into the abdominal cavity. Examples of common causes of peritonitis are ruptured appendix, perforated duodenal or gastric ulcer, ruptured ectopic (tubal) pregnancy and traumatic rupture of the spleen or liver.

Symptoms. As the peritoneum becomes inflamed there is local redness and swelling of the membrane with production of serous fluid that becomes more and more purulent as the bacteria multiply. Normal peristaltic action of the intestines slows or ceases altogether and the symptoms of intestinal obstruction occur. The patient experiences nausea, vomiting, severe abdominal pain and distention, high fever, tachycardia, pallor and other symptoms of shock. Unless the patient is treated promptly and successfully, peritonitis can be fatal.

Treatment and Nursing Care. Antibiotics are given in massive doses to combat infection, fluids and electrolytes are administered to restore a normal balance, and gastric or intestinal suction is instigated to relieve distention. Surgical procedures such as those done to repair a ruptured organ are done as soon as the patient's condition will permit.

Nursing care is primarily concerned with close, intelligent observation of the patient and prompt and accurate reporting of unexpected changes in his condition. He is usually placed in semi-Fowler's position to facilitate breathing, prevent respiratory complications and aid in localizing the purulent material in the lower abdomen or pelvis. His vital signs are noted and recorded every four hours during the critical stage. If he is nauseated and vomits, the characteristics and amount of vomitus are noted. The emesis of fecal material indicates complete intestinal obstruction. If the patient passes flatus or feces rectally this should be recorded on his chart as it indicates return of peristalsis. Because of the high fever and toxicity that accompany peritonitis the patient may be delirious or disoriented and he must be protected from self-injury. This includes putting side rails on the bed and supervising the patient at all times. High fever and the presence of the gastric tube demand frequent mouth care to protect the lips and prevent halitosis and a foul taste in the mouth. The patient should be turned *very gently* and moved in the bed with care because of the extreme tenderness in his abdominal region.

PEPTIC ULCER

Definition. A peptic ulcer is an open lesion on the mucosa of the stomach or small intestine. When the ulcer is located in the stomach it is called a *gastric ulcer* (see Fig. 14-4); if it is located in the upper third of the small intestine it is called a *duodenal ulcer.*

The ulcerated area is actually the result of digestion of the membranous lining of the stomach or small intestine by the gastric juices secreted by glands in the stomach. The exact reason that an ulcer should develop is not known; however, there are many predisposing factors. They include: (1) a particular type of personality characterized by the expression of constant anxiety and inner tensions; (2) poor eating habits

Figure 14-4. Ulcer of the gastric mucosa. Note how deeply the ulcer has penetrated into the stomach wall. (From Bockus: *Gastroenterology*, Vol. 1, 2nd Ed., W. B. Saunders Co., Philadelphia.)

such as over-indulgence in alcohol, highly seasoned foods, or an irregular pattern in mealtimes; and (3) an increased secretion of hydrochloric acid in the stomach.

Symptoms. The most common symptom of peptic ulcer is a burning and gnawing pain in the stomach region. This pain is more pronounced when the stomach is empty and is relieved by eating. The attacks of pain are seasonal; that is, they are more likely to occur during the spring and fall than at other times of the year. Other symptoms may include nausea, frequent belching, vomiting (vomitus may contain blood), and tarry stools.

An ulcer that becomes chronic may continue to erode into deeper tissue until it has finally penetrated the stomach wall. This complication is referred to as *perforation*. Other complications include *hemorrhage* and *obstruction*.

Medical Treatment and Nursing Care. Medical treatment of a peptic ulcer is aimed at relief of the patient's symp-

toms and removal of the causative factors.

REST. The patient is placed on bed rest. If hemorrhaging is present the patient is put on absolute bed rest. His environment must be controlled so that he may have relaxation and freedom from worry.

DIET. There are several dietary regimens useful in the medical management of peptic ulcer. They all are concerned with neutralizing gastric acid, preventing chemical or mechanical irritation of the gastric and intestinal mucosa and gradually progressing from small, frequent feedings to a more normal diet.

The Sippy diet and the Meulengracht diet, named after the physicians who devised them, are the two progressive diets most often used. The administration of milk and cream (90 ml. each), is an initial part of the Sippy diet and is frequently used with other diets. The purpose of giving milk and cream every hour can readily be understood when we realize the need for providing a continued supply of food or liquid in the stomach so that the gastric juices will digest the stomach contents rather than the stomach mucosa. Milk is given because it is a protein which will neutralize the acids of the stomach. Fat is given because it inhibits the flow of gastric juices and also slows down the passage of milk from the stomach.

The physician often orders milk and cream every hour on the hour and an antacid drug every hour on the half hour so that there is no time when the stomach acids are not being rendered neutral. Later on, small frequent feedings are given so that the stomach is not empty and there is no free hydrochloric acid present for long periods of time. The patient usually is not allowed raw fruits and vegetables or high residue foods that are capable of mechanically irritating the stomach or intestinal mucosa. Spices, meat broths, fried foods, coffee and alcoholic beverages usually are restricted because they stimulate the flow of gastric juices and increase the muscular action of the stomach.

MEDICATIONS. Specific drugs used in the treatment of a peptic ulcer are as follows:

1. *Antacids* which neutralize gastric acid. Examples: Amphogel, Gelusil and Maalox.

2. *Antispasmodics* which reduce muscle spasm and decrease gastric secretions. Examples: atropine, tincture of belladonna and Pro-Banthine.

3. *Sedatives* which reduce emotional tension. Examples: phenobarbital and the tranquilizers.

EDUCATION OF THE PATIENT. Before a peptic ulcer can be successfully controlled, the patient must understand how and why he probably developed an ulcer in the first place. Once he has understood the predisposing factors he must then be helped to avoid them as much as possible. Unless he can cooperate fully with the physician and nurses there is a strong possibility that he will continue to develop ulcers in spite of medical or even surgical treatment.

Below is a list of some of the important points to be emphasized in teaching a patient with a peptic ulcer.

1. He must learn to regulate the type of foods he eats and the manner in which he eats them. Mealtime should be unhurried, relaxed, and spaced at regular intervals.

2. His emotional health, ability to cope with distressing situations, and his occupation and home life are all important to his state of physical health. He must learn either to avoid situations of anxiety or to strive to develop a more placid and serene outlook on life.

3. Most patients who have peptic ulcers drink very little water. Since water dilutes the gastric juices and thereby makes them less corrosive, the patient should develop the habit of taking several swallows of water at least every hour during the day.

4. It is presumed that there is some relationship between the use of tobacco and aggravation of a peptic ulcer. If the patient is unable to discontinue smoking altogether he might at least use more moderation in his smoking habits.

5. The patient is encouraged to cooperate with his physician and remain under medical supervision for as long as the physician deems advisable. He must report regularly for periodic x-ray examinations of the stomach to determine his progress.

Surgical Treatment of a Peptic Ulcer.

INDICATIONS FOR SURGERY. Surgical treatment becomes necessary when a chronic ulcer fails to respond to medical treatment or when complications such as perforation, obstruction or hemorrhage occur.

TYPES OF SURGICAL PROCEDURES. *In plastic repair of a perforated ulcer,* the hole in the stomach is sutured and the area is reinforced with a graft from the peritoneal fold over the stomach.

Subtotal gastrectomy (gastric resection) is removal of a part of the stomach and then joining the remaining portion to the small intestine by *anastomosis.* Anastomosis is the joining of two hollow organs by suturing the open ends together so that they become one continuous tube.

Total gastrectomy is the surgical removal of all of the stomach. The esophagus is anastomosed to the small intestine.

The vagus (tenth cranial nerve) stimulates the stomach cells to secrete hydrochloric acid. A *vagotomy* is the cutting of the vagus nerve so that the stomach does not receive impulses from the brain and therefore does not secrete hydrochloric acid. A vagotomy is often done at the same time a gastric resection is performed.

PREOPERATIVE CARE. The patient who is to have gastric surgery will usually have an x-ray series and other diagnostic tests before the surgery is done. The exception to this rule is an emergency situation in which complications demand immediate surgery and there is not time for an extensive preoperative work-up.

A Levin tube is usually inserted the morning of the operation. This tube is left in place during and after surgery (see gastric decompression below).

The patient will receive routine preparations necessary for all major abdominal surgery. This includes enemas so that the colon is emptied of fecal material. In case the patient has had a barium enema, the practical nurse should look for and report returns which contain whitish material. This is barium and it will become hardened if left in the colon, thus presenting the possibility of a fecal impaction later on.

The diet of the patient is restricted to liquids only during the 24 hours before surgery. In case of obstruction a Levin tube is inserted and gastric suction begun to remove all stomach contents before surgery.

POSTOPERATIVE CARE. When the patient returns to his room and has fully recovered from the anesthesia, he is placed in semi-Fowler's position. This position is more comfortable and facilitates drainage from the stomach when a gastric tube is in place.

Gastric or intestinal decompression is used in almost all types of gastric or intestinal surgery. The type of tube used will depend on the area involved. The Levin tube is used to aspirate or convey liquids to the stomach (see Fig. 14-5). A Miller-Abbott tube and a Cantor tube are used to remove intestinal contents (see Fig. 14-6).

Gastrointestinal decompression is accomplished by connecting the nasogastric tube to a suction apparatus such as the Gomco electric suction machine. Common indications for gastrointestinal suction include (1) distention following surgery or accompanying intestinal obstruction, (2) withdrawal of specimens of stomach or intestinal contents, and (3) removal of stomach or gastrointestinal contents before surgery.

Figure 14-5. A Levin tube in place. The Levin tube is used to aspirate gastric contents or to convey liquids to the stomach.

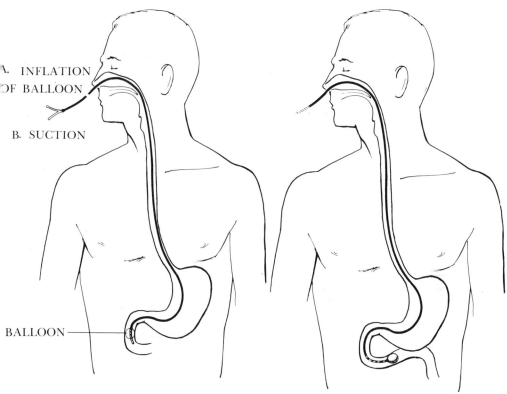

A. INFLATION OF BALLOON

B. SUCTION

BALLOON

Figure 14-6. *Left,* A Miller-Abbott tube in place. It is advanced through the intestines to the prescribed point. The Miller-Abbott tube has a double lumen. *A,* Portion of the metal tip leading to the balloon. *B,* Portion of the metal tip leading to the lumen that can be suctioned. *C,* Balloon inflated with air. *Right,* A Cantor tube in place. This intestinal tube ends in a bag that is filled with mercury to help it to pass along the gastrointestinal tract to the point prescribed by the physician. Intestinal tubes are not taped in place until they have advanced fully. The holes for suctioning are behind the balloon.

During continuous gastrointestinal decompression by electric suction the machine should be turned on "low." If the machine is left on "high" continuously it may cause damage to the gastric mucosa. It is important that the tube be kept open and draining freely. Irrigations, which can be helpful in removing mucus plugs and blood clots, are *not* routinely done; they require a physician's written order. The nurse should know what solution is to be used, how much to use and whether the procedure requires aseptic technique or clean technique.

All drainage obtained via the nasogastric tube should be measured accurately and the amount recorded on the patient's chart for every 24-hour period. Since fluids and electrolytes removed by suction must be replaced, the physician will use the nurse's notes

as a guide to fluid replacement. It is also important to record the color and consistency and any unusual odor or other characteristic noted in the fluid in the drainage bottle. Although some bloody drainage is to be expected after gastric surgery, an excessive amount of drainage or bright red blood coming through the tubing must be reported immediately.

The tubing connected to the nasal tube should be long enough to allow for adequate turning of the patient from side to side. The nostril into which the tube is inserted is very tender, and rough handling of the tubing will cause the patient much discomfort. A special clamp which attaches to the bedclothes should be used to prevent pulling and unnecessary motion of the tube.

After the tubing is removed the patient is given small amounts of liquids to determine if he can tolerate them. These liquids are gradually increased according to the patient's ability to take them without nausea, vomiting, or abdominal distress. If the liquids are well tolerated the patient then progresses to small, frequent feedings. Within six months most patients are able to take three regular meals a day as the remaining portion of the stomach stretches to accommodate more and more food. Patients who have had a *total* gastrectomy are usually restricted to small frequent feedings of easily digested semisolids for the rest of their lives. When the patient is to be dismissed from the hospital the hospital dietitian usually is called to help the patient and his family in the ways and means of planning and preparing his special diets after gastric surgery.

Some patients who have had gastric surgery experience a complication known as the "dumping syndrome." The patient feels weak and faint and may perspire profusely or experience palpitations of the heart. These sensations probably are due to the rapid passage of large amounts of food and liquid through the remaining portion of the stomach (if any) and into the jejunum. This occurs because part or all of the stomach and duodenum have been surgically removed and are no longer present to slow down the progress of the intestinal contents through the upper portion of the gastrointestinal tract. When a patient experiences the dumping syndrome he is instructed to avoid eating large meals and to drink a minimum of fluids during the meal. He may take the fluids in small amounts later, between meals. If sweet foods and liquids seem to aggravate the condition, and sometimes they do, the patient should try to avoid them. It also may be helpful for the patient to lie down flat in bed for 30 minutes after a meal.

CANCER OF THE STOMACH

Definition. Cancer of the stomach is a malignant growth within the stomach. It is frequently associated with chronic inflammation or ulceration of the stomach mucosa. It is often difficult to distinguish between gastric ulcer and gastric cancer without extensive diagnostic tests.

Symptoms. The symptoms of gastric cancer are very similar to those of a gastric ulcer. Frequently the symptoms are not severe until the malignancy has reached the advanced stages and spread to neighboring tissues.

Treatment and Nursing Care. When gastric cancer has been positively diagnosed the treatment is surgical removal of all or part of the stomach.

The nursing care of the patient having gastric surgery is discussed earlier in this chapter.

CANCER OF THE LARGE INTESTINE

Definition. Malignant growths within the large intestine occur most frequently in persons over 50 years of age and are among the most common diseases affecting this part of the digestive tract. The cause is unknown. Polyps or chronic ulcerations located in the large intestine tend to undergo malignant changes.

Symptoms. As in cancer of the stomach, cancer of the large intestine may present only mild symptoms until it has reached an advanced stage. Any change in an individual's bowel habits may be an early sign of cancer of the colon. Either constipation or diarrhea, or alternate attacks of each, are the most common signs. As the growth enlarges it obstructs the normal passage of fecal material through the colon and this results in changes in the shape of the stool and loss of blood rectally. If the growth completely obstructs the intestinal tract the patient experiences the symptoms of an intestinal obstruction.

Treatment and Nursing Care. Cancer of the colon is treated by surgical removal of the affected portion of intestine. There are several different operative procedures which may be carried out. The surgeon's choice will depend on the location of the growth and the extent of the area involved. The purpose of the surgery is to remove the diseased section of the intestine and at the same time provide a means of elimination of fecal material.

INTESTINAL OBSTRUCTION

Definition. Intestinal obstruction is a blocking of the intestinal tract, thereby preventing the normal passage of gastrointestinal contents through the intestine. The condition may occur suddenly or progress gradually over a period of time. Obstruction of the intestines may result from strangulated hernia, cancer, twisting of the bowel (*volvulus*), telescoping of one part of the bowel into another (*intussusception*), or interference with the passing of nerve impulses to the bowel.

Symptoms. In acute intestinal obstruction the onset is sudden with severe pain as a result of increased peristalsis above the point of obstruction. The abdomen becomes distended as the intestinal contents accumulate and fill the intestines. Increased pressure then may constrict blood vessels in the walls of the intestines, resulting in gangrene of the affected portion. Nausea and vomiting are common symptoms of intestinal obstruction. The vomiting is extremely forceful (*projectile*) and the emesis is often foul in odor because of the back flow of fecal material into the stomach.

In chronic intestinal obstruction the outstanding symptom is an increasing constipation as the bowel becomes occluded. Nausea and vomiting may be present and anemia is also frequently present as a result of loss of appetite.

Treatment and Nursing Care. The treatment of intestinal obstruction is immediate surgical correction of the condition. Any one of the surgical procedures listed below under "Types of Surgical Procedures" may be used in the treatment of intestinal obstruction.

The patient with acute intestinal obstruction is very seriously ill. He often has respiratory difficulty because of the pressure of the distended abdomen against the diaphragm. Placing the patient in Fowler's position will help relieve this pressure and also aids in the removal of gas and intestinal contents through the intestinal tube. This tube is inserted before the patient goes to surgery and offers some relief of the symptoms of intestinal obstruction until surgery can be performed.

The postoperative nursing care of the patient with surgery of the large intestine is discussed below.

NURSING CARE OF THE PATIENT WITH SURGERY OF THE LOWER INTESTINAL TRACT

Types of Surgical Procedures. COLECTOMY. This is simply the removal of the diseased portion of the colon.

COLOSTOMY. In this procedure an abdominal incision is made and the colon is brought to the outside for the purpose of providing a means of draining fecal material. A colostomy is usually done after a colectomy. The colostomy may be permanent or temporary. If it is a temporary colostomy the patient must return to surgery later for anastomosis of the open ends.

ABDOMINOPERINEAL RESECTION. This is a very extensive surgical procedure in which part of the colon and the entire rectum and anus are removed. Both an abdominal incision and perineal incision are necessary for this procedure. Because of the nature of the surgery a permanent colostomy is necessary.

Preoperative Care. Before surgery of the large intestine, efforts are made to remove as much fecal material from the colon as possible. To accomplish this the patient is usually placed on a low-residue diet as early as 7 to 10 days before surgery. The last 24 to 72 hours before surgery his diet is changed to liquids only. Vitamins and minerals may be given to supplement these restricted diets.

In addition to the dietary preparation, laxatives and enemas are administered to cleanse the lower bowel further. Contents of the stomach are removed by inserting a Levin tube and connecting it to a suction apparatus the morning of surgery. If it is necessary to remove the contents of the small intestine a specially designed tube which passes through the stomach and into the duodenum is inserted. This tube is called a Miller-Abbott tube. It is attached to the suction apparatus and given the same care as a gastric tube. The tube is usually left in place after surgery to remove accumulations of mucus and gas which may cause distention and strain on the sutures.

Postoperative Care. The immediate postoperative care is the same as for other patients having major abdominal surgery. Operations of the large intestine are usually of long duration. The prolonged period of anesthesia and exposure of the body, with loss of essential fluids, leaves the patient particularly susceptible to shock. Therefore, the patient must be watched more closely than usual for signs of shock during the immediate postoperative period.

Difficulty in voiding after surgery is a common problem with these patients. To avoid the retention of urine in the bladder during the postoperative period, a Foley catheter is usually inserted in the operating room. As soon as the patient returns to his room the catheter is connected to a sterile bedside bottle and an accurate record of his intake and output kept.

The gastric or intestinal tube is connected to an electric suction as soon as the patient is returned to his room. The physician usually does not want the patient to have anything by mouth for the first 48 hours after surgery. Peristalsis usually becomes active after this period of time and the patient will then be able to take liquids by mouth. The passing of gas, liquids, or solids through the rectum is an indication of active peristalsis. In any surgery of the intestine the surgeon is always concerned with the return of normal peristalsis. It is the nurse's responsibility to observe these patients carefully for evidence of the return of peristalsis and to report such evidence to the doctor.

Special Aspects in the Care of the Patient with a Colostomy

Preoperative Period. The prospect of having an artificial anus in an abdominal opening through which bowel movements will pass is a difficult situation for even the most stalwart of individuals to face. The first thoughts are those of repulsion and absolute despair that an adjustment can ever be made. The nursing staff must recognize the emotional shock for a patient having a colostomy and be prepared to offer adequate moral support. Preparation of the patient during the preoperative period will depend on the physician. He may or may not choose to explain a colostomy fully to the patient before surgery. He will have good reasons for his choice and the nursing staff must know and respect his wishes in this matter. It is not the responsibility of the nurse to inform the patient of the exact surgical procedure that will be done when he goes to surgery. Her responsibility lies in finding out how much the patient has been told so that she can exercise care in answering any questions he may ask. Some patients do not wish to be told, while others insist on a detailed explanation from the doctor. In other cases the surgeon does not know himself what procedure will be necessary until after he has opened the abdomen and evaluated the patient's condition.

If the surgeon does tell the patient that a colostomy will be done he will also explain what a colostomy is, how it works and methods which can be used to control the bowel movements so that the patient's activities are not restricted when he is discharged from the hospital.

There are times, however, when a patient will listen to every word the doctor says and apparently accept the situation calmly. Later, after the initial shock has worn off, he becomes extremely agitated or depressed and begins to display his true emotions. At this time the nurse must realize why the patient is behaving as he is and strive to help him by answering his questions with intelligence and encouragement.

There are thousands of individuals in every walk of life who have colostomies. They are able to continue their regular activities with few restrictions and most of their associates are not aware that they have a colostomy. It is important that a patient who must adjust to a colostomy knows and understands that such a surgical procedure does not mean invalidism and permanent withdrawal from society.

If there is a person available who has had a successful experience with his own colostomy, arrangements may be made for him to talk with the patient and tell him what he can expect immediately after surgery and during the convalescent period. Information should never be forced on the patient, however. Written material should be made available if he wishes to read about colostomies and how they are cared for, but if he is upset by thinking about his future life with a colostomy he may not want to discuss the subject with anyone. That is his choice and privilege.

Postoperative Period. Immediately after surgery the patient with a colostomy will receive the same general care necessary for any patient who has had surgery of the large intestine. Since the intestinal tract has been thoroughly cleansed before the operation there will be no fecal material passing through the colostomy for several days. The patient also has a gastric tube in place and this will remove secretions which might collect in the stomach. Later, as the intestinal tract resumes its normal functions and peristalsis begins, the stomach tube is removed and the patient is allowed liquids by mouth. If these are well tolerated the diet gradually progresses to a low-residue diet.

Most surgeons wish to have the patient get out of bed the first postoperative day. The gastric tube and retention catheter are clamped off while the patient sits up in a chair at the bedside.

On the third or fourth day after surgery the surgeon usually irrigates the colostomy for the first time. This is sometimes a difficult experience for the patient even though he has had some preparation and should have some idea of what to expect. His first glimpse of the colostomy is bound to produce some emotional shock and his eventual acceptance depends to a great extent on the reactions of those around him who must help him care for his colostomy. He must never be made to feel that the colostomy is an inconvenience to others or that they are repelled by the task of caring for him.

Gradually, the patient is taught to irrigate and care for his own colostomy. As long as there is some drainage through the colostomy the skin around the artificial anus must be kept clean and protected from irritation by applying ointments or salves as ordered. It may be necessary to change the dressings frequently at first and, if so, Montgomery straps should be used to hold the dressing in place (see Fig. 14-7). Soiled dressings must be wrapped in paper and removed from the patient's room immediately. It is encouraging to the patient if he understands that regular bowel movements

Figure 14-7. Dressing fastened with Montgomery tapes. (From Sutton: *Bedside Nursing Techniques*, 2nd Ed., W. B. Saunders Co., Philadelphia.)

will come in time and frequent changing of the dressings will no longer be necessary.

The restriction of the diet is a vital part of controlling the number and consistency of the stools. A low-residue diet is used until the patient learns to control the bowel movements with irrigations. As regularity is established and the patient gains self-confidence, the diet is changed to one that is less strict.

Establishing a regular pattern for evacuation of the bowel takes much time and patience on the part of the patient and the nurses who are teaching him to care for his colostomy. There are several important points to be considered.

1. The colostomy should be irrigated at the same time every day. Later on, the irrigations may be necessary only every two or three days. Some patients adjust very well and have spontaneous evacuations regularly without irrigations.

2. The length of time required for complete evacuation of the bowel varies from 15 minutes to one hour.

3. The amount of solution necessary may vary with individual patients from one pint to several quarts.

4. Irrigations and evacuation seem more normal to the patient if he is sitting on the toilet during the procedure.

5. If the patient is physically able he should begin irrigating his colostomy soon after surgery and gradually assume responsibility for its care.

6. Foods which are likely to cause

diarrhea or lead to the formation of gas should be avoided.

There are various kinds of appliances and colostomy bags available. These are used to collect the intestinal contents until the colostomy is under control. The patient may wish to use such equipment in the early stages of adjustment because it gives him a sense of security. Colostomy bags should not be used indefinitely, however, because they are a source of odor and do not allow the patient complete freedom. The ultimate goal is complete control of the bowel movements so that only a gauze square is needed over the opening to collect mucus that may leak from the colostomy.

ABDOMINAL HERNIA

Definition. The internal organs of the body are contained within their respective cavities by the outside walls of the cavity. In the abdomen the wall is muscular. If there is a defect in this muscular wall the contents of the abdominal cavity may protrude through the defect. This protrusion is called a *hernia.* The lay term for hernia is "rupture."

The most common locations for a hernia are in areas where the abdominal wall is normally weaker and more likely to allow protrusion of a segment of intestine. These areas include the center of the abdomen at the site of the umbilicus and the lower abdomen at the points where the inguinal ring and the femoral canal begin. Figure 14-8 shows the most common contributing factors in the development of a hernia.

Hernias are classified as *reducible,* which means the protruding organ can be replaced by pressing on the organ; and *irreducible,* which means that the protruding part of the organ is tightly wedged outside the cavity and cannot be pushed back through the opening. Another name for an irreducible hernia is *incarcerated* hernia. If the protruding part of the organ is not replaced and

1   STRAINING AT WORK

2   CHRONIC COUGH

3   STRAINING TO VOID

4   STRAINING AT STOOL

5   ASCITES

Figure 14-8.   The five major predisposing factors in hernia development. (From Le Maitre and Finnegan: *The Patient in Surgery*, W. B. Saunders Co., Philadelphia.)

its blood supply is cut off, the hernia is said to be *strangulated*.

Symptoms.   There is a "lump" or local swelling at the site of the hernia. The most common sites are the umbilicus, groin, or along a healed abdominal incision. When pressure on the abdominal wall is removed by lying down the swelling disappears. Lifting of heavy objects, coughing, or any activity which puts a strain on the abdominal muscles may force the organ back through the opening and the swelling reappears. Pain occurs when the peritoneum becomes irritated or when the hernia is incarcerated or strangulated. The flow of intestinal contents becomes blocked by an incarcerated hernia and the patient has the symptoms of an intestinal obstruction.

Treatment and Nursing Care.   Hernias are best treated by surgery. If surgery is not possible because of age or poor surgical risk then the patient may be fitted with an appliance called

a *truss*. The truss is put on each morning before the patient gets out of bed because the hernia is more likely to be reduced at that time. A truss simply reinforces the weakened cavity wall and prevents protrusion of the intestines. It is only a symptomatic measure and does not cure the hernia.

The surgical procedure used in the treatment of a hernia is called a *herniorrhaphy*, which means a surgical repair of a hernia. The defect is closed with sutures. If the area of weakness is very large a *hernioplasty* is done. In this procedure some type of strong synthetic material is sewn over the defect to reinforce the area.

During the postoperative period the patient must be protected from respiratory infections so that coughing does not place a strain on the abdominal wall.

The doctor instructs the patient in the activities he may perform during the convalescent period so that the surgical area will have time to heal completely before any strenuous activities are resumed.

DIVERTICULA

Definition. The term diverticula refers to small blind pouches resulting from a protrusion of the mucous membranes of a hollow organ through weakened areas of the organ's muscular wall. Diverticula occur most often in the intestinal tract, especially in the esophagus and colon. When they are present the patient is said to have *diverticulosis.* If the diverticula become inflamed or infected the condition is referred to as *diverticulitis.*

Symptoms. A person may have diverticulosis and remain unaware of his condition for quite a while because it often presents no symptoms. Eventually, however, the diverticula may fill with some material passing through the intestinal tract and become inflamed or infected, causing symptoms. If the diverticulitis is in the esophagus the patient may have difficulty in swallowing, foul breath and emesis of food that was eaten several days prior to the vomiting. Diverticulitis of the intestine produces symptoms of diarrhea or constipation, abdominal pain, fever and rectal bleeding. The condition may be complicated by intestinal obstruction or by peritonitis if the intestinal wall ruptures.

Treatment. The symptoms of the patient will govern to some extent the treatment necessary. Esophageal diverticulitis, if severe, usually is treated by surgical removal of the sacs and repair of the muscular wall. Intestinal diverticulitis often can be managed conservatively with low-residue diet and a lubricating, mild laxative such as mineral oil to control constipation. In some stubborn cases or those likely to be complicated by obstruction or rupture of the intestine wall, surgical removal of the affected portion of intestine may be necessary.

HEMORRHOIDS

Definition. Hemorrhoids are varicosities of the veins of the rectum. They may be *internal* (inside the sphincter muscles of the anus), or *external* (outside the sphincter muscles) (see Fig. 14-9).

Symptoms. Local pain and itching are the most common symptoms. Bleeding from the rectum at the time of defecation may also be present. External hemorrhoids are less likely to bleed but they are more evident to the examiner and appear as tumor-like projections around the rectum.

Constipation, prolonged standing or sitting, and pregnancy are predisposing causes of hemorrhoids. The habit of sitting on the toilet and straining at the stool for long periods of time is one of the primary factors responsible for many cases of hemorrhoids.

Treatment and Nursing Care. The symptoms of hemorrhoids may be relieved by elimination of constipation, local applications of heat or cold, sitz baths, and the use of ointments which contain a local anesthetic. The patient should also be instructed to wash the anal region with warm water and soap after each bowel movement.

The most effective treatment is surgical removal of the hemorrhoids. The procedure is called a *hemorrhoidectomy.*

Most patients experience a good bit of pain after a hemorrhoidectomy. This is relieved by cold applications or warm compresses to rectum as ordered, and the administration of pain-relieving drugs. Mild wet dressings which are commercially prepared may also be used on the operative area. These dressings have a glycerine base and contain a mild astringent which reduces swelling and relieves pain.

The patient may be more comfortable lying on a rubber ring so that pressure is removed from the rectal area. Sitz baths are also effective in the relief of

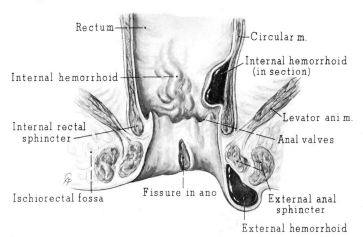

Figure 14-9. Common disorders of the anal canal. (From Jacob and Francone: *Structure and Function in Man*, W. B. Saunders Co., Philadelphia.)

pain. These are usually ordered twice a day.

After rectal surgery of any kind there is usually difficulty in voiding because the patient is afraid to completely relax the perineum and the sphincter muscles. Nursing measures to induce voiding should be tried first and if they are unsuccessful the patient must be catheterized.

Most patients dread the first bowel movement after a hemorrhoidectomy. There is no doubt that it will cause some pain and the usual procedure is the administration of mineral oil to soften the stool and thus make defecation less traumatic. A sitz bath after each bowel movement will offer relief and also cleanses the operative area, keeping it free from irritation. The practice of sitting in a tub of warm water may be continued after the patient goes home. During the convalescent period the patient should avoid roughage in his diet until the operative area has had time to heal completely.

PILONIDAL SINUS (PILONIDAL CYST)

Definition. The word pilonidal means "having a nest of hair." A pilonidal sinus is a lesion located in the cleft of the buttocks at the sacrococcygeal region. It is sometimes called a pilonidal cyst but it is believed to be a subcutaneous canal (sinus) with one or more openings into the skin, rather than a true cyst or fluid-filled sac. The condition occurs when the stiff hairs in the sacrococcygeal region irritate and eventually penetrate the soft skin in the cleft of the buttocks. Conditions which can lead to development of such a sinus include local injury, improper cleansing of the area, and obesity. Persons who have more than the usual amount of body hair are particularly susceptible.

Symptoms and Treatment. A pilonidal sinus may cause no trouble until it becomes infected, and then the patient experiences pain in the area with swelling and a purulent drainage. When this occurs the area must be incised surgically and the connecting canals opened and drained. Hairs and necrotic tissue must be removed so the area can heal.

Postoperative care includes changing of dressings and measures to avoid contamination of the wound. A lubricating laxative and oil enema usually are given before the first bowel movement to avoid strain on the sutures. Antibiotics may be given to control infection.

Part II—DISEASES OF THE ACCESSORY ORGANS OF DIGESTION

SPECIAL DIAGNOSTIC TESTS

X-ray Examinations. The gallbladder and ducts which carry bile to the small intestine may be visualized by x-ray if a contrast medium of radiopaque dye is used. The dye is given to the patient by mouth or directly into the vein. It is then carried to the liver where it is secreted with the bile. As the dye travels from the liver to the gallbladder and on through the bile ducts, the hollow structures may be outlined on the x-ray film. Obstructions within the ducts or failure of the gallbladder to fill are thus more easily diagnosed.

Cholecystogram, gallbladder studies, or *choleangiogram* are all terms which are used to describe x-ray examinations of the type described above. In the oral method the patient is given a fat-free meal the evening before the morning of the x-ray examination. After the meal is completed the dye is given orally in tablet form and then the patient receives nothing by mouth until after the x-rays are completed. Cleansing enemas and laxatives are usually given to prepare the patient for the test.

The *intravenous* method of administering the dye does not require the administration of laxatives and repeated enemas. This method of giving the

Table 20. *The Normal Hepatogram**

FUNCTION	TEST	NORMAL RANGE
Excretory	Bromsulphalein	With 2 mg./kg. dose, less than 4% retention at 30 min.
	Alkaline phosphatase	2-4 Bodansky units
	Bilirubin	Direct: 0.0-0.2 mg./100 ml.
		Total: 0.2-1.4 mg./100 ml.
	Icterus index	8 units or less
	Urobilinogen	Trace
	Cholesterol	Total: 135-260 mg./100 ml.
		Ester: 95-200 mg./100 ml.
	Cholinesterase	0.7-1.4 pH units/hr.
	Lactic dehydrogenase	Less than 300 units
	Transaminase (SGP-T)	5-35 units
	Serum proteins	Total: 6.5-8.0 Gm./100 ml.
		Albumin: 4.0-5.5 Gm./100 ml.
		Globulin: 2.0-3-0 Gm./100 ml.
		Fibrinogen: 0.2-0.3 Gm./100 ml.
	Prothrombin time	12-15 sec.
	Prothrombin production	Shortening of prothrombin time after dose of vitamin K
Metabolic	Galactose tolerance	Oral: less than 3 Gm. excreted in 4 hr.
		Intravenous: complete removal in 45-60 min.
Detoxication	Hippuric acid	Oral: at least 3 Gm. excreted in 4 hr.
		Intravenous: at least 1 Gm. excreted in 1 hr.
Miscellaneous	Cephalin flocculation	Negative to 2+
	Zinc turbidity	4-8 units
	Thymol turbidity	1-4 units

*From French: Nurses' Guide to Diagnostic Procedures, 2nd edition. Copyright McGraw-Hill, Inc., 1967. Reprinted with permission of McGraw-Hill Book Company.

dye is usually used for patients who cannot tolerate the dye orally. There is, however, some danger of a serious allergic reaction to the dye given by the intravenous route.

Specific orders for preparation of the patient for gallbladder studies may vary slightly according to the wishes of the radiologist in charge of the examination. The practical nurse is responsible for familiarizing herself with the routine used in the institution in which she works and for carrying out these directions conscientiously.

Bilirubin Test. Bilirubin is a pigment normally found in the blood as a result of the breakdown of hemoglobin and removed by the liver. The liver secretes the pigment in bile which enters the intestinal tract and gives the stools their characteristic brown color. When the liver is diseased bilirubin accumulates in the blood stream; thus a bilirubin test of the blood is a measurement of liver function.

Bromsulphalein Test. Bromsulphalein is a dye that is administered by injection. Under normal circumstances the liver will remove this dye from the blood stream. The Bromsulphalein test measures the rate at which the liver is able to remove the dye from the blood stream. If the liver is not functioning properly the dye will remain in the blood longer than it normally would.

Prothrombin Level. This test is sometimes used as a diagnostic test for liver disease because prothrombin is manufactured by the liver. For more details on the prothrombin test see page 43. Other liver function tests are included in Table 20.

JAUNDICE

Definition. Jaundice is actually a group of symptoms rather than a disease. It is only an indication of excessive amounts of bile pigment in the blood stream. When the bile pigment reaches a certain level it stains the skin a yellowish color and the patient is said to be jaundiced.

Types of Jaundice. Jaundice may be divided into three general types based on the underlying cause of the symptoms. The three types are:

1. *Obstructive jaundice:* caused by a plugging of the bile ducts which in turn causes a back flow of bile. The obstruction may be caused by gallstones or neoplasms in the ducts.

2. *Nonobstructive jaundice:* associated with damage to the cells of the liver. An inflammatory process within the tissues of the liver or nutritional deficiencies may cause this type of jaundice.

3. *Hemolytic jaundice:* Hemolysis means destruction of blood cells. When excessive amounts of red blood cells are destroyed their pigment is released into the blood stream and the patient becomes jaundiced. This condition is primarily a disease of the blood.

Nursing Care of a Patient with Jaundice. The other symptoms which accompany jaundice are not always so obvious as the yellowish cast to the skin but they nevertheless require attention and care from the nurse.

Itching of the skin frequently accompanies jaundice. The itching is of an intense nature and may be very disturbing to the patient. Baths of starch or sodium bicarbonate (baking soda) solutions offer some relief. Mild lotions and frequent changing of the patient's gown and bed linen are also helpful. If the itching is so severe that it disturbs the patient's rest the nurse should report the situation to the doctor. He may wish to order antihistamine drugs for relief of the itching.

Because the bile is not being secreted into the small intestine, fats eaten by the patient are not properly digested. This leads to *indigestion,* loss of appetite, flatulence, and constipation. The patient may be placed on a low-fat diet to avoid these distressing symptoms. A low-fat diet is sometimes difficult for the patient to accept, however, because the foods are not palatable. If the patient understands that fats are directly responsible for many of his digestive discomforts he may accept the restricted diet more readily. Some imagination in the use of other seasonings besides fat in the preparation of his meals will also help him remain within the limits of his restricted diet.

The stools of a patient with jaundice are lacking in the bile pigment and are therefore very light in color. The urine is very dark because the kidneys have removed some of the pigment from the blood stream and excreted it in the urine. The observations of the nurse in regard to the color of the stools and urine of the patient with jaundice are very important in helping the doctor determine the patient's progress.

Earlier in this chapter we mentioned the prothrombin level in the diagnosis of diseases of the liver. It was stated that prothrombin was manufactured by the liver; thus, a patient who has jaundice as a result of liver cell damage will also be expected to have a low prothrombin level. Prothrombin plays an important role in the clotting of blood and so we can expect a patient with a deficiency of prothrombin to hemorrhage easily. This condition demands intelligent observation on the part of the nurse so that she may protect her patient from massive hemorrhage or severe anemia from loss of blood. Any symptoms which might indicate the loss of blood internally as well as externally must be reported immediately so that treatment may be started.

VIRAL HEPATITIS

Definition. Viral hepatitis is an inflammation of the liver caused by a virus. Hepatitis may be caused by more than one virus. Consequently, a person who has had an attack of viral hepatitis is not immune to the disease if he is exposed to a different virus.

Types of Viral Hepatitis. Viral hepatitis is an infectious disease, which means that it can be transmitted from one individual to another. There are two general types of viral hepatitis according to the mode of transmission.

The first type is called *epidemic hepatitis* or *catarrhal jaundice.* This type is transmitted by the ingestion of foods or liquids contaminated by the virus. There is also a possibility that the virus may enter the body by way of the respiratory tract.

The second type of viral hepatitis is *serum hepatitis.* It gets its name from the serum of human blood which contains the virus. The source of infection may be whole blood or blood derivatives such as pooled plasma, or needles and syringes which contain the blood of individuals with the virus in their blood.

Symptoms. The early symptoms of viral hepatitis are very similar to those of an upper respiratory infection. The victim has a low-grade fever, malaise, indigestion, and loss of appetite. Later there is local tenderness in the region of the liver and some enlargement of the liver. As the inflamed liver cells cease to function, jaundice becomes evident and the stools become lighter and the urine darker than normal.

Treatment and Nursing Care. Bed rest is necessary until the patient is free of symptoms. After the symptoms subside the patient may have his physical activities restricted for as long as two or three months so as to avoid permanent damage to the liver. This limiting of activities may be difficult for the patient to understand because he usually feels well and quite able to resume his former activities. He must be encouraged to follow the doctor's orders because of the danger of possible cirrhosis of the liver and other complications if adequate rest is not provided during the long convalescent period.

The patient is isolated during the acute phase of the disease to prevent the spread of the infectious organism (see Chap. 8). Extreme care must be used with all needles and syringes used in treating the patient with hepatitis as these are dangerous sources of infection. Careless handling of contaminated needles may easily lead to a pricked finger and the entrance of the virus directly into the blood stream.

All articles and equipment containing bodily excretions from the patient also require special handling and disinfection.

The patient's diet is planned to provide an adequate intake of calories and protein. The diet is usually high in protein because protein helps in the repair and rebuilding of body tissues, and high in carbohydrates because these are thought to have a protective effect on the liver cells. Even though nausea is a common occurrence in hepatitis, the patient should eat everything on his tray. His refusal to eat all or part of his meals and extra feedings should be reported so that supplements may be given.

There are no specific drugs used in the treatment of infectious hepatitis other than antibiotics which may sometimes be given to prevent secondary bacterial infections.

CIRRHOSIS OF THE LIVER

Definition. Cirrhosis is a chronic disease characterized by degenerative changes within the structure of the liver cells. The cells are first loaded with fat and then they begin to degenerate and die. These necrotic cells are then replaced by scar tissue.

The specific cause of cirrhosis of the liver is not known. Although the incidence of cirrhosis is high among known alcoholics, this does not mean that all persons with cirrhosis have a history of excessive drinking. The underlying factor in cirrhosis is a nutritional deficiency and alcoholics are subject to cirrhosis because they prefer to drink alcohol rather than eat an adequate diet.

Symptoms. In the early stages of cirrhosis the patient has symptoms similar to those of acute hepatitis. As the disease progresses the liver cells begin to degenerate and the blood vessels within the liver also fail to function normally. This results in congestion of the blood vessels which drain the digestive organs and transport the blood to the liver. The next step in the process is an accumulation of fluids within the intestinal tract. The excess fluid produces symptoms of indigestion and diarrhea or constipation.

As the fluid in the intestines continues to accumulate it may eventually pass through the walls of the intestines and fill the abdominal cavity. This excess fluid within the abdominal cavity is called *ascites.* The patient's abdomen becomes extremely swollen and respiratory function may be affected. Ascites is relieved by tapping the abdominal cavity with a large needle and draining off the excess fluids. This procedure of withdrawing fluids from the abdominal cavity is called a *paracentesis.*

The backing up of venous blood may also lead to varicose veins of the esophagus. The varicosities tend to bleed easily and thus cause vomiting of blood. In some cases massive hemorrhage can occur in this way.

Other symptoms of cirrhosis include edema, jaundice, and small hemorrhages under the skin. These hemorrhages are very close to the surface of the skin and have a "spidery" appearance.

Treatment and Nursing Care. There is no known cure for cirrhosis of the liver and treatment is aimed at relief of the patient's symptoms.

Rest in bed becomes necessary as the disease progresses. The patient with ascites is usually more comfortable with his head and shoulders elevated. This position relieves some of the pressure of the abdomen against the diaphragm and thus facilitates breathing.

There is frequently generalized edema as well as the local collection of fluid within the abdomen. The patient's intake and output are carefully recorded. He is also usually weighed every day to determine the increase or decrease of fluids held in the body. A low-salt diet is given these patients.

Care of the skin is important, not only because of the edema, but also because the patient frequently has jaundice with severe itching.

Distended veins and a tendency to bleed are common and predispose the patient to hemorrhage. The nurse must be alert for early symptoms of hemorrhage and report them immediately. Loss of blood through the intestinal tract, no matter how slight it may appear, must be reported to the physician in charge.

The dietary treatment of cirrhosis consists of a high-protein, low-sodium, low-fat diet. Vitamins, especially the vitamin B group, are given in large amounts to supplement the diet.

In the last stages of cirrhosis some patients undergo mental and emotional changes. The edema may cause increased intracranial pressure and result in irritability and confusion. Depression and despair are also common because the patient realizes that very little can be done to help slow down the disease process and there is nothing which will cure him of the disease. Delirium and coma or convulsions must be watched for and all precautions taken to protect the patient from injury should these appear.

noticeable several hours after eating. There is usually a chronic pain in the upper part of the abdomen on the right side.

In an acute inflammation of the gallbladder the patient has severe pain in the gallbladder region, nausea and vomiting, and chills and fever. The gallbladder may become filled with pus and will eventually rupture, spilling its contents into the abdominal cavity and leading to a severe peritonitis.

Treatment and Nursing Care. Treatment may vary according to individual cases. The conservative medical treatment consists of measures to improve the general physical condition of the patient and relieve the symptoms until the inflammation has subsided.

Surgical treatment may be resorted to immediately during the acute stage to prevent complications, or the physician may choose to wait and perform surgery after the conservative treatment has had its effect. A *cholecystectomy*, or surgical removal of the gallbladder, is the surgical procedure performed. Nursing care of the patient having a cholecystectomy is presented on page 315. If the surgeon wishes to open and drain the contents of the gallbladder he performs a procedure called a *cholecystostomy*. The nursing care of the patient having this type of surgery is similar to that of the patient having a cholecystectomy.

CHOLECYSTITIS

Definition. Cholecystitis is an inflammation of the gallbladder. The cause of cholecystitis is not known but it is often associated with gallstones. It occurs most frequently in middle-aged women who are overweight.

Symptoms. The symptoms of cholecystitis may be mild or severe, depending on the degree of inflammation present in the gallbladder. In mild cases the symptoms are those of indigestion and abdominal distention, and are most

CHOLELITHIASIS

Definition. Cholelithiasis is the presence of gallstones within the gallbladder or bile ducts. The stones vary in size and may grow to be as large as an orange, but it is usually the smaller stones which cause the most trouble because they are passed into the bile ducts where they become lodged, causing an obstruction in the flow of bile (see Fig. 14-10).

Symptoms. The most outstanding symptom of cholelithiasis is a severe

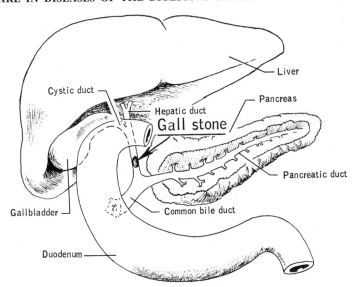

Figure 14-10. Bile is drained from the liver by the hepatic duct and from the gallbladder by the cystic duct. An obstruction due to a gallstone, as pictured above, prevents the flow of bile into the digestive tract. (Modified from Manner: *Elements of Anatomy and Physiology*, W. B. Saunders Co., Philadelphia.)

and almost intolerable pain in the region of the gallbladder. Nausea and vomiting are also present and the patient is frequently drenched in perspiration and near shock because of the pain. A history of intolerance to fatty foods over a period of time is a common complaint of patients with gallstones.

Treatment and Nursing Care. The treatment of gallstones is surgical correction of the condition. The specific type of surgical procedure will depend on the location of the stone and the condition of the gallbladder at the time of surgery.

The long names given to surgical procedures involving the gallbladder and ducts may seem very perplexing and difficult to understand but they are actually only various combinations of prefixes and suffixes.

CHOLECYSTECTOMY. *Chole* refers to gall, *cyst* means bladder, and *ectomy* is the surgical removal of. Thus cholecystectomy means the surgical removal of the gallbladder.

CHOLECYSTOSTOMY. The suffix *ostomy* means cutting into an organ for the purpose of providing drainage. Cholecystostomy is a surgical incision into the gallbladder and the insertion of a drain.

CHOLEDOCHOLITHOTOMY. *Lith* refers to stone, *docho* refers to duct. Thus a choledocholithotomy is a surgical incision into the bile duct for the purpose of removing a stone.

Nursing Care of the Patient Having Surgery of the Gallbladder. PREOPERATIVE CARE. Unless the surgery is performed for emergency relief of the condition, the patient will have extensive diagnostic tests before the operation is scheduled. These tests help the surgeon determine the location of the difficulty so that he may be prepared for the type of procedure he will need to perform. If jaundice is present the patient's prothrombin level may be checked to see if he may safely undergo surgery. Vitamin K is given to improve the clotting ability of the blood.

Patients who are having acute pain or abdominal distention often have Levin tubes inserted to remove the gastric and intestinal contents. This tube may be left in place during and after surgery.

POSTOPERATIVE CARE. Because the surgical incision is in the upper section of the abdomen the patient is placed in semi-Fowler's position after he recovers from anesthesia. Aside from the fact that he will be more comfortable and there will be less strain on the sutures, the patient will also be able to take deep breaths and cough more easily in this position.

One of the most confusing aspects of nursing a patient who has had gallbladder surgery is proper care of the drains or tubes which may be in place when the patient returns from the operating room.

In most cases the surgery has been performed to relieve an obstruction to the flow of bile through the bile ducts or to provide a means of draining purulent material to the outside. If the patient has had an infection of the gallbladder the drainage is absorbed by the dressings over the surgical wound. These must be changed often and should be checked quite frequently for signs of fresh bleeding. The drain is left in as long as necessary and is then removed by the surgeon.

When an obstruction of the common bile duct has occurred because of stones or tumors the surgeon may insert a small tube directly into the common bile duct. This tube is called a *T tube* because it is shaped like the letter T (see Fig. 14-11). This tube must be kept

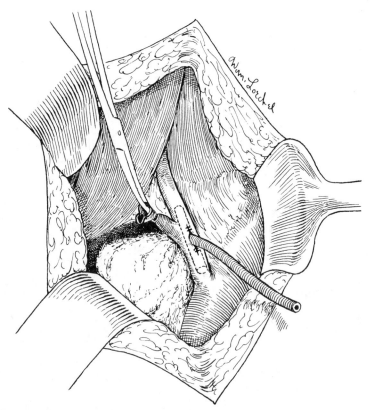

Figure 14-11. Diagrammatic drawing showing the T tube inserted into the common bile duct and sutured in place. The hemostat on the left holds the end of the cystic duct, which has been cut and tied. The gallbladder has been removed. The T tube is brought to the outside and attached to a drainage bottle. (From Ferguson and Sholtis: *Eliason's Surgical Nursing.* 11th Ed., J. B. Lippincott Co., Philadelphia.)

open at all times and is connected to a bedside bottle as soon as the patient returns to his room. The length of time the T tube is left in place depends on the condition of the patient. While the tube is in the common bile duct there will be no bile going to the duodenum as it normally would.

Precautions must be taken that no tension is put on tubes or drains which have been inserted in the surgical wound (see Fig. 14-12). T tubes are sutured in place and if they are accidentally pulled out the patient must be returned to the operating room and the incision reopened to replace the tube. Dressings must be changed with careful handling of the tube or drain. There is usually so much drainage that the dressings must be changed often and Montgomery straps are best for holding the dressings in place. The sight of so much greenish yellow discharge (bile) on the dressings may upset the patient unless he is told that this is to be expected.

Since the surgeon will be concerned with whether or not bile is beginning to flow through the duct and on into the duodenum as it normally should, the nurse must carefully observe the color of the patient's stools. A return

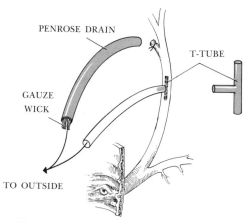

Figure 14-12. After cholecystectomy the Penrose drain helps to remove exudate from the area formerly occupied by the gallbladder. The T tube diverts bile to the outside.

of the characteristic brown color to the stools is an indication that bile is entering the small intestine. If the obstruction remains in the bile ducts the patient will show signs of jaundice. Light-colored stools, dark urine, and the early appearance of a yellowish cast to the skin must be reported as soon as any one of these is noticed by the nurse.

There is no specific diet recommended for the patient who has had surgery of the gallbladder, although he is usually warned to avoid excesses of fatty foods.

PANCREATITIS

Definition. Pancreatitis is an inflammation of the pancreas. It may be acute or chronic in nature, and frequently accompanies obstruction of the pancreatic duct due to gallstones or the back flow of bile into the pancreatic duct.

Symptoms. An attack of acute pancreatitis may be mistaken for an attack of acute indigestion. The patient experiences severe pain in the region of the stomach and nausea and vomiting are usually present. The pain radiates through to the back and may be so severe as to cause the patient to go into shock.

Treatment and Nursing Care. Pancreatitis is usually treated medically. Nitroglycerine under the tongue sometimes relieves the pain but morphine given intravenously may be necessary in extreme cases. The patient is allowed nothing by mouth during the acute phase so as to prevent stimulation of the pancreas and further aggravation of the inflammation. Fluids are given intravenously until the edema of the pancreas and the pancreatic duct has subsided and the digestive juices from the pancreas can once again flow into the duodenum. Most patients with acute pancreatitis recover with this type of treatment.

If the pancreatitis becomes chronic there is some destruction of the pancreas cells and the pancreatic duct becomes fibrotic. A diet low in fat and the administration of antispasmodic drugs are helpful in treating chronic pancreatitis. Alcohol is forbidden.

CLINICAL CASE PROBLEMS

1. Mr. Long, age 42, is admitted to the hospital with a diagnosis of bleeding gastric ulcer. He has had the ulcer for more than a year and even though he has been informed of the type of restricted diet he should follow, he does not always follow it.

Mr. Long is placed on milk and cream every hour on the hour and an antacid medication every hour on the half hour. While you are giving him P.M. care he becomes nauseated and begins to vomit bright red blood. He also complains of a sharp pain in his upper abdomen. His wife who is in the room at the time tells you that he has been vomiting blood at home and since milk and cream make him nauseated she thinks you should just omit them and he will be all right. Mr. Long seems resigned to letting his wife do all the talking.

> What problems do you see in this situation?
> Do you think it is necessary to report his episode of vomiting immediately?

2. Mrs. Knight is a 45-year-old mother of 5 children who has had a colostomy for treatment of an intestinal obstruction. On her fourth postoperative day she is assigned to your care. She has received instructions in the care of her colostomy from the nurse in charge but so far she has refused to take care of it herself.

Mrs. Knight has been told by the surgeon that he may be able to close the colostomy in several months if all goes well. When you enter her room to begin caring for Mrs. Knight she becomes very upset and tells you that she cannot face the future knowing that she may have to be inconvenienced by the colostomy. She feels that she will be a burden to her family and completely incapacitated by her illness.

> How can you help the patient accept her illness?
> What can you do to encourage her to take care of herself?
> What other problems can you see in this situation?

3. Mr. May is admitted to the hospital with a diagnosis of cirrhosis of the liver. He is 59 years of age and has been hospitalized several times for his condition. He suffers from shortness of breath due to a swollen and enlarged abdomen, is anemic because of minimal but constant esophageal bleeding, and appears jaundiced. He has several abrasions on his arms, legs and abdomen from repeatedly scratching to relieve his pruritus. Mr. May is very depressed and will not converse with you when you enter his room with his breakfast tray the first morning you are assigned to his care. He refuses to eat and indicates his attitude by pushing the tray away and turning on his side, face to the wall.

> What nursing measures might help relieve some of Mr. May's symptoms?
> Why do you think he is mentally depressed?
> How would you go about helping him emotionally?
> What special observations must you make while caring for Mr. May?
> How would you explain a paracentesis to Mr. May if one were ordered for him?

4. Mrs. Luke, age 46, is admitted to the hospital for a cholecystectomy. She is extremely obese and enjoys eating rich, fatty foods even though she knows this will add to her obesity and precipitate attacks of cholecystitis. You are assigned to care for Mrs. Luke when she returns from surgery.

> How will you position this patient postoperatively?
> If she has a large amount of drainage from the surgical incision how will you take care of this problem?
> When you get this patient out of bed the next day how are you going to manage the dressings and prevent strain on the sutures?
> What other problems might you anticipate?

REFERENCES

1. Brown, A. F.: *Medical Nursing*, 3rd edition. Philadelphia, W. B. Saunders Co., 1957.
2. Eichenwald, M. D.: "When Your Patient Has Hepatitis." RN, Sept. 1961, p. 71.
3. Glenn, F. A.: "Surgical Treatment of Biliary Tract Disease." Am. Journ. Nurs., May, 1964, p. 88.
4. Henderson, L. M.: "Nursing Care in Acute Cholecystitis." Am. Journ. Nurs., May, 1964, p. 93.
5. Howe, P.: *Nutrition for Practical Nurses*, 3rd edition. Philadelphia, W. B. Saunders Co., 1963.
6. Isler, C.: "Caring for Patients with Ulcerative Colitis." RN, Nov., 1962, p. 43.
7. Katona, E. A.: "Learning Colostomy Control." Am. Journ. Nurs., March, 1962, p. 43.
8. Palumbe, L. T.: "Present-day Treatment of Diseases of the Biliary Tract." Am. Journ. Nurs., Jan., 1960, p. 50.
9. Seide, D.: "Caring for Colostomy and Ileostomy Patients." RN, Sept., 1960, p. 37.
10. Shafer, K. N., Sawyer, J. R., et al.: *Medical-Surgical Nursing*, 4th edition. St. Louis, C. V. Mosby Co., 1967.
11. Smith, D. W., and Gips, C. D.: *Care of the Adult Patient*, 2nd edition. Philadelphia, J. B. Lippincott Co., 1966.
12. Usher, F., and Matthews, J.: "Surgery: Treatment of Choice for Hernias." Am. Journ. Nurs., Sept. 1964, p. 85.
13. Wolfman, E. F., and Flotte, C.: "Carcinoma of the Colon and Rectum." Am. Journ. Nurs., March, 1961, p. 60.

SUGGESTED STUDENT READING

1. American Cancer Society (pamphlets): "Care of Your Colostomy" and "The Patient with a Colostomy."
2. Courtney, L.: "Postoperative Cholecystectomy." Practical Nursing, May, 1962, p. 37.
3. DiPalma, J. R.: "Drugs in the Management of Peptic Ulcer." RN, April, 1963, p. 71.
4. Eichenwald, M. D.: "When Your Patient Has Hepatitis." RN, Sept., 1961, p. 71.
5. Fisk, J. E.: "Nursing Care of Patient with Surgery of the Biliary Tract." Am. Journ. Nurs., Jan., 1960, p. 53.
6. Hansen, D. E.: "Abdominal Hernia." Am. Journ. Nurs., March, 1961, p. 102.
7. Isler, C.: "Caring for the Patient with Ulcerative Colitis." RN, Nov., 1962, p. 43.
8. Jay, A. N.: "Colitis." Am. Journ. Nurs., Aug., 1959, p. 1133.
9. Katona, E. A.: "Learning Colostomy Control." Am. Journ. Nurs., March, 1967, p. 534.
10. Lamberty, K.: "Diet Therapy for Ulcers." Journ. Pract. Nurs., June, 1965, p. 25.
11. Seide, D.: "Caring for Colostomy and Ileostomy Patients." RN, Sept., 1960, p. 37.
12. Uhl, M., and Lyden, J.: "Viral Hepatitis:" Am. Journ. Nurs., March, 1961, p. 102.

OUTLINE FOR CHAPTER 14

I. Introduction

A. Digestive tract is concerned with digestion (physical and chemical changes which foods undergo) and absorption (passage of nutritive elements from the intestines to the blood).

B. Accessory organs of digestion: liver, gallbladder and pancreas.

Part I – Nursing Care of Patients with Diseases of the Digestive Tract

I. Diagnostic Tests

A. X-ray examinations—gastrointestinal series and barium enema.

B. Gastroscopy—direct visualization of the lining of the stomach.

C. Esophagoscopy—direct visualization of the esophageal lining.

D. Proctoscopy—direct visualization of the anus and rectum.

E. Sigmoidoscopy—direct visualization of the inner lining of the sigmoid colon.

F. Gastric analysis—examination and analysis of the contents of the stomach.

G. Stool examination—examination of fecal material for presence of blood, specific bacteria, cysts, ova or parasites.

II. Stomatitis (Inflammation of the Mucous Membranes of the Mouth)

A. May be caused by certain drugs, trauma, nutritional deficiencies, or pathogenic microorganisms.

B. Aphthous stomatitis, commonly called "canker sores," is probably a viral infection. No specific cure.

C. Vincent's angina ("trench mouth"). Caused by a combination of a bacillus and spirochete. Treated with sodium perborate mouthwashes and antibiotics.

III. Gastritis (Inflammation of the Mucous Membranes of the Stomach)

A. Main causes—overeating, excessive drinking, contaminated food or ingested poisons.

B. Symptoms—nausea, vomiting and tenderness in the gastric region.

C. Treatment—restriction of foods followed by a bland diet, medications that coat the gastric mucosa and antispasmodics.

IV. Ulcerative Colitis

A. Inflammation with formation of ulcers in the mucosa of the colon.

B. Symptoms—diarrhea, nausea and vomiting or loss of appetite. Dehydration and malnutrition may occur in chronic cases.

C. Treatment—rest, freedom from anxiety, and antidiarrheic drugs.

V. Peritonitis (Inflammation of the Peritoneum)

A. Common causes—ruptured appendix, perforated ulcer and ruptured ectopic pregnancy.

B. Symptoms—vomiting, severe abdominal pain, fever, tachycardia and symptoms of shock.

C. Treatment—massive doses of antibiotics, intravenous fluids and electrolytes, and gastrointestinal decompression.

D. Vital signs taken and recorded frequently, patient observed for signs of intestinal obstruction and protected from injury when delirium is present. Semi-Fowler's position helps localize purulent material in pelvis.

VI. Peptic Ulcer

A. Open lesion on the mucosa of the stomach (gastric ulcer) or small intestine (duodenal ulcer).

B. Exact cause unknown. Predisposing factors—anxiety, tension, poor eating habits and increased secretion of hydrochloric acid.

C. Symptoms—gnawing, burning pain in epigastrium (relieved by eating), frequent belching, vomiting and tarry stools.

D. Medical Treatment—rest and bland, non-irritating diet. Medications include antacids, antispasmodics and sedatives.

E. Surgical treatment for chronic ulcers that fail to respond to medical treatment or are complicated by perforation or hemorrhage.

VII. Nursing Care of Patient Having Gastric Surgery

A. Preoperative care—diagnostic tests, physical preparation of skin, enemas and insertion of Levin tube.

B. Postoperative care—semi-Fowler's position to facilitate drainage of stomach contents. Keep Levin tube open and draining freely. Irrigations if ordered. Mouth care while tube is in place. Observe drainage for color, consistency and amount.

C. "Dumping syndrome"—occurs in some patients who have had part or all of stomach removed. Occurs after eating when large amounts of food pass rapidly into small intestine. May be relieved by eating small meals, avoiding liquids during the meal and lying down after eating.

VIII. Cancer of the Stomach

A. Diagnosis difficult as symptoms may be quite similar to those of gastric ulcer.

B. Treatment—surgical removal of all or part of the stomach.

IX. Cancer of the Large Intestine

A. Symptoms—constipation or diarrhea (or alternate attacks of each) and rectal bleeding.

B. Treatment—surgical removal of the affected portion.

X. Intestinal Obstruction (Blocking of the Intestinal Tract)

A. Causes—strangulated hernia, twisting or telescoping of the bowel or interference with conduction of nerve impulses.

B. Symptoms—acute intestinal obstruction characterized by projectile vomiting, nausea and abdominal pain. Chronic type may have less abrupt onset. Symptoms include nausea, vomiting and constipation.

C. Treatment—surgical correction of obstruction and intestinal decompression.

XI. Nursing Care of the Patient with Surgery of the Lower Intestine

A. Types of surgical procedures: colectomy (removal of the diseased portion of colon), colostomy (creation of an artificial anus with bowel opening on the abdominal surface) and abdominoperineal resection (removal of the affected portion of colon, the entire rectum and the anus).

B. Preoperative care—low residue diet, cleansing of lower bowel and intestinal decompression.

C. Postoperative care—observation for signs of shock, care of retention catheter, care of gastrointestinal tube and observation of drainage. Watch for signs of returning peristalsis.

D. Special care of patient with colostomy
   1. Preoperative period should include adequate explanation of surgical procedure and plans for rehabilitation.
   2. Postoperative care includes instruction of patient in the care of his colostomy.

XII. Abdominal Hernia (a Protrusion of the Intestines through a Weakened Area in the Abdominal Wall

A. Most common sites are the umbilical area and beginning of inguinal canal and femoral canal.

B. Reducible hernia—protruding organ can be replaced by pressing on the organ. Incarcerated hernia—cannot be reduced. Strangulated hernia—blood supply to the organ has been obstructed.

C. Surgery most effective means for treating hernia (herniorrhaphy).

XIII. Diverticula

A. Small, blind pouches of mucous membrane that have protruded through a weakened wall of a hollow organ.

B. Symptoms not apparent until inflammation (diverticulitis) or infection occurs. Esophageal diverticulitis may produce difficulty in swallowing, foul breath and emesis. Intestinal diverticulitis produces abdominal pain, fever, diarrhea or constipation and rectal bleeding.

C. Treatment may be surgical removal of affected portion of organ or low-residue diet and lubricating laxatives.

XIV. Hemorrhoids (Varicose Veins of the Rectum)

A. Symptoms—local pain, itching and bleeding at time of defecation.

B. Treatment—hemorrhoidectomy. Postoperative care concerned with prevention of infection and relief of pain.

XV. Pilonidal sinus

A. Subcutaneous canal located in the cleft of the buttocks in the sacrococcygeal area. Produces pain and purulent drainage.

B. Treatment—surgical incision of canal, drainage of purulent material and removal of hairs and necrotic tissue. Antibiotics given to control infection.

Part II—Diseases of the Accessory Organs of Digestion

I. Special Diagnostic Tests

A. Cholecystogram and choleangiogram—x-rays of the biliary tract after injection of a radiopaque dye.

B. Bilirubin test—measurement of pigment normally removed from the blood by the liver.

C. Bromsulphalein test—done to determine the liver's ability to remove a dye from the blood stream.

D. Prothrombin level—the liver manufactures prothrombin.

II. Jaundice (Excessive Amounts of Bile Pigments in the Blood Stream)

A. Three types: (1) obstructive jaundice, (2) nonobstructive jaundice, and (3) hemolytic jaundice.

B. Nursing care—frequent bathing to relieve itching, low-fat diet, observation of stools and urine for bile pigments, observation for signs of bleeding.

III. Viral Hepatitis (Inflammation of the Liver)

A. Symptoms—low-grade fever, malaise, indigestion, local tenderness over liver and jaundice.

B. Treatment and nursing care—rest, isolation to prevent spread of infection, and high-protein, high-carbohydrate diet.

IV. Cirrhosis of the Liver

A. Specific cause unknown. Underlying factor seems to be prolonged. nutritional deficiency.

B. Symptoms—early symptoms similar to those of hepatitis. Later there is congestion of the portal circulation, edema, indigestion and diarrhea. Tendency to bleed. Jaundice and small hemorrhages under the skin.

C. Treatment and nursing care—rest, low-salt, high-protein diet and vitamin supplements. Paracentesis to relieve ascites. No cure.

V. Cholecystitis

A. Inflammation of the gallbladder. Often associated with gallstones.

B. Symptoms—indigestion, abdominal distention and chronic pain in the upper right abdomen. Severe, acute inflammation produces severe pain, chills, fever, nausea and vomiting.

C. Treatment—surgical removal of gallbladder (cholecystectomy) or incision and drainage of gallbladder (cholecystostomy).

VI. Cholelithiasis (Stones in Gallbladder or Biliary Ducts)

A. Symptoms—severe pain in gallbladder region, nausea, vomiting and history of intolerance to fatty foods.

B. Treatment—exact surgical procedure depends on location of stones.

VII. Nursing Care of the Patient Having Surgery of the Gallbladder.

A. Preoperative care—diagnostic tests, care of Levin tube and gastric suction and vitamin K to prevent bleeding.

B. Postoperative care—semi-Fowler's position. Care of tubes, frequent changing of dressings, careful observation of stools for indications of the return of bile to the intestine.

VIII. Pancreatitis (Acute or Chronic Inflammation of the Pancreas)

A. Symptoms—acute attack similar to acute indigestion. Patient has severe pain in the region.

B. Treatment and nursing care—medications to relieve pain, restriction of foods and fluids and intravenous feedings. Chronic pancreatitis treated with antispasmodic drugs and restriction of alcohol and fat.

Chapter 15

NURSING CARE OF PATIENTS WITH DISORDERS OF THE URINARY SYSTEM

VOCABULARY

Contour
Distention
Excreted
Hypercalcemia
Intracranial
Secreted

INTRODUCTION

The urinary system is composed of the kidneys, ureters, urinary bladder, and urethra. Their functions are secretion, storage, and excretion. The kidneys are two bean-shaped organs which lie on either side of the vertebral column at the level of the last thoracic and first lumbar vertebrae. They are richly supplied with blood from branches of the aorta and vena cava.

The need for an abundant supply of blood to the kidneys becomes apparent when one realizes that nearly one fourth of the body's blood is filtered by the kidneys at one time. Waste products are retained in the kidneys in urine to be excreted, while the remainder of the fluid is returned to the blood. During a 24-hour period the kidneys handle as much as 200 quarts of liquid, excreting only 1½ to 2 quarts as urine.

The *nephron* is the functioning unit of the kidney. Each kidney is composed of about one million nephrons and each nephron can form urine by itself. Thus, to understand the function of the nephron is to understand the function of the kidney. The basic function of the nephron is to filter a large portion of the blood plasma out of the blood stream and through the glomerular membrane. Unwanted substances such as urea, creatinine, uric acid and other wastes are retained in the tubules while water and many electrolytes are allowed to re-enter the blood stream. The water and wastes remaining in the tubules are excreted as urine.

The ureters, one from each kidney, convey the urine by *peristaltic* action from the kidney to the urinary bladder. The bladder serves as a reservoir and holds the urine until its normal distention of 300 cc. to 400 cc., when the urge to urinate compels emptying the bladder. The urine passes from the bladder through the urethra to the outside. The urethra is approximately 1½ inches long in the female and 8 inches in the male.

The kidneys and urinary tract are responsible for maintaining the proper balance of fluids, minerals, and organic

323

substances necessary for life. In view of this fact it is not surprising that a diseased condition of any one system of the body may have a direct effect on the kidneys and urinary tract. Generalized diseases such as arteriosclerosis, other circulatory lesions, infections, or disturbances in the metabolic processes may very seriously impair the proper functioning of the kidneys. Similarly, involvement of the heart, lungs or circulatory system can arise from kidney failure.

Diseases, like human beings, will not always conveniently fit into clearly defined categories. The body functions as a whole and the systems are interdependent. This chapter will be concerned primarily with diseases of the urinary system; however, it should be remembered that the nurse will frequently have need for a good working knowledge of the basic principles of urologic nursing in a wide variety of cases under her care.

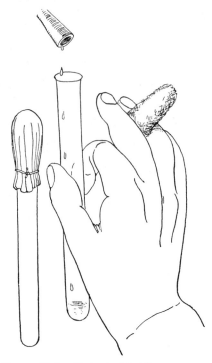

Figure 15-1.   Method of holding stopper and tube to collect urine for culture. At left is sterile tube with cotton stopper and paper wrapping. Newer tubes may have cork stoppers. (From Davis and Warren: *Urological Nursing,* 6th Ed., W. B. Saunders Co., Philadelphia.)

DIAGNOSTIC TESTS AND EXAMINATIONS

Urine Culture.   A sample of urine is taken by catheter under sterile technique and placed in a sterile culture tube (see Fig. 15-1). After the catheter has been inserted, a small amount of urine should flow through the catheter into the waste basin. This will flush out and partially cleanse the urethra. Approximately 10 cc. of urine should be allowed to drop into the tube, making sure not to let the catheter touch the inside of the tube. The culture tube must be maintained in an upright position so that the urine does not come in contact with the stopper. The tube is then carefully labeled and sent to the laboratory, where cultures are grown under controlled conditions to determine specific types of bacteria present in the urine.

P.S.P. Test.   These initials stand for phenolsulfonphthalein, which is a dye administered directly into the vein. The purpose of the test is to estimate the ability of the kidneys to excrete the dye in a given number of hours. Normally, the bright red color will become apparent in the urine within 30 minutes after injection and after 2 hours have elapsed more than half the dye should appear in the urine.

Fishberg Concentration Test.   This is a relatively simple method for determining the ability of the kidneys to concentrate urine. Normally the kidneys remove a large amount of water from the blood plasma as it passes through the nephron (this is called dilution). Waste products and some water are retained in the tubules while the remaining water and some minerals are reabsorbed into the plasma. If the renal tubules fail to allow for reabsorption of the water, it remains and is excreted as very dilute urine. If the nephron functions normally, the urine is more concentrated because it contains less water.

In the Fishberg concentration test the patient is allowed no food or water from after the evening meal the night before the test until after the test, which begins about 10:00 A.M. when the first specimen of urine is collected. An hour later a second specimen is obtained and both are properly labeled and sent to the laboratory where they are tested for specific gravity. A normal specific gravity is between 1.020 and 1.025. A lower specific gravity would mean more dilute urine and would indicate impairment of the kidney's ability to concentrate urine.

X-ray Examinations. Visualization of the urinary tract with x-ray may be achieved by the injection of a contrast medium (one that is opaque to x-ray). The medium used may be given in any one of three ways: (1) directly into the vein (for an *intravenous pyelogram*), (2) by way of a ureteral catheter (*retrograde pyelogram*), or (3) through a urethral catheter (*cystogram*).

The intravenous pyelogram is probably the one used most often, being the simplest and least dangerous method of examining the kidneys, ureters, or prostate. It is helpful in diagnosing impairment of kidney function, obstruction, foreign bodies, or tumors in the ureters or prostate. The urine should be concentrated in this test so as not to dilute the dye, thus preventing its effectiveness on x-ray film. For this reason fluids are restricted during preparation of the patient for this test.

The retrograde pyelogram must be done during *cystoscopy* (see below) because a catheter is inserted into the ureters and dye injected directly into the ureters.

The cystogram is done to visualize the bladder *contour*. X-ray films are taken before and after sodium iodide is injected into the bladder through a urethral catheter.

The success of an x-ray examination of the pelvic and abdominal area depends to a great extent on the thoroughness of the preparation. It cannot be stated too often or too strongly that the preparatory procedures done by the nurse must be carried out efficiently and well. Poor preparation leads to unnecessary expense of time and undue taxing of the patient's energy and pocketbook. Methods of cleansing the lower intestinal tract of gas and fecal matter for proper visualization of the urinary tract will vary according to the radiologist's and attending physician's wishes and the individual patient's needs. The nurse must understand the specific orders for catharsis and enemas, and carry them out effectively. She must personally supervise the procedures on all patients, male or female.

Blood Analysis. When the filtering plant of the kidney has been affected by disease there is a slowing down of absorption of wastes from the blood stream. These wastes then begin to accumulate in the blood, upsetting the normal balance in the body. The two most common laboratory tests for these waste products are *blood urea nitrogen* (B.U.N.) and *nonprotein nitrogen* (N.P.N.). Both of these must be a "fasting blood" specimen and are drawn in the morning before breakfast. The normal range for these two tests may be found in Chapter 4.

Following all tests requiring restriction of fluids there will be some dehydration; fluids should be forced during the day unless contraindicated.

Cystoscopy. This is a surgical procedure in which the physician inserts an instrument (the cystoscope) into the bladder through the urethra for the purpose of examining the interior of the bladder.

Patients who are not anesthetized for this procedure should be reassured and encouraged to relax as much as possible during the examination. This will decrease the pain and help the examining physician.

Following cystoscopy the patient may have a general reaction with chills and elevation of temperature. The patient may also have some low back pain and a full sensation with frequent desire to void because of irritation to the mucous membrane. Extensive bleeding or sharp abdominal pain should be reported.

MEASURING THE PATIENT'S LOSS OF FLUIDS

Because the functions of the urinary system are so closely related to the maintenance of the proper fluid balance in the entire body, the loss of fluids from the body is of primary importance in diseases of the urinary system. The physician must depend on the nursing staff for accurate and intelligent observation, measuring and reporting of the patient's output, or loss of fluids. If measurement of the *total urinary output* is required, the nurse must make sure that urine from all points of drainage is measured and the exact amount recorded. For example, urine from a ureterostomy tube and from a urethral catheter should both be included. When *total output* is to be measured this must include vomitus, watery stools, urine excreted, and an estimate of the amount of fluid lost through perspiration.

There are several terms used to describe abnormalities in the flow of urine. These include *retention, suppression,* and *residual urine.*

Retention of urine refers to a retaining or holding of urine in the bladder. It may be relieved by inserting a catheter and draining the urine from the bladder. If a catheter is not passed to relieve distention the bladder will not rupture but urine will begin to dribble out through the urethra. The retention of urine in the bladder and resulting stretching of the bladder cause severe discomfort to the patient. Nursing measures to induce voiding may be successful, but if they are not a catheter must be passed. Catheterizations may very easily lead to an infection of the urinary tract and should not be done without a written order from the doctor.

Suppression of urine indicates that the kidneys are unable to produce urine because of some serious malfunction of the kidney cells. There is simply little or no urine being filtered from the blood stream and if the condition cannot be relieved, uremia (and ultimately death) will follow.

Residual urine is urine retained in the bladder after voiding. When there is poor bladder tone or a partial obstruction of the urethra the patient may dribble or void only the "overflow," leaving the bladder still unemptied. Residual urine is measured by having the patient void as much urine as possible and then catheterizing him immediately after. Fifteen milliliters is considered a normal amount of residual urine. Any amount over this will become more and more concentrated over a period of time and may lead to an infection or the formation of stones in the bladder.

NURSING CARE OF THE PATIENT WITH A RETENTION CATHETER

A retention catheter is one which is inserted through the urethra into the bladder and left in place so that urine is constantly drained from the bladder. The catheter used most often for this purpose is the Foley catheter which is specially designed with an inflatable balloon at its tip. The balloon is inflated after the catheter is inserted into the bladder, thereby holding the catheter securely in place so that it is not easily pulled out (see Fig. 15-2).

A retention catheter should always be kept open and draining freely unless there are specific orders to clamp it off. Usually the urine drains by gravity flow, which means that the tube leading from the catheter must lead to a collection bottle which has been placed *below the level of the bladder* and there must be no looping of the tube below the level of the bottle. A closed container presents fewer possibilities for

Figure 15-2. Foley catheter with inflated balloon in place. The balloon may be deflated by releasing tie on small tube or by cutting the small tube if the catheter is the disposable type. The Foley catheter may be used for both male and female patients. The small tube to left of the Foley catheter is a ureteral catheter, which is passed through the bladder and into the ureter. (From Davis and Warren: *Urological Nursing*, 6th Ed., W. B. Saunders Co., Philadelphia.)

tubing and apparatus used in caring for the catheter must be sterile. One must use rigid asepsis when handling the connections for catheter, tubing and drainage bottle (see Fig. 15-3).

The amount, color, and content of the urine should be observed closely. Sometimes mucus shreds and bits of tissue or clots may be seen. Various antiseptics, such as pyridium, will cause the urine to be red. Other drugs, dyes, and some foods will sometimes change the color and odor of the urine. The presence of what appears to be bright red blood in the catheter should always be reported immediately, even though the practical nurse may suspect that the coloring is due to something other than blood.

While a catheter is in place the genitalia and surrounding skin will need extra care. The areas must be kept clean and dry and creams and powders avoided because they tend to cake and further irritate the skin. Soap and water gently and frequently applied, with thorough rinsing and drying, will do much to prevent odors, irritations, and general discomfort of the patient.

If there are clots, mucus plugs, or other material obstructing the flow of urine through the catheter the physician may order irrigations of the catheter. Sometimes it is possible to remove

introducing infectious agents into the urinary tract than does an open container. The amount of drainage in the bottle is measured at least every 8 hours and the amount recorded on the patient's chart. The nurse should report any sandy residue collecting in the tubing or catheter so that they may be changed before there is complete obstruction of the tubing. Sandy residue may be determined by rubbing the tube or catheter between the thumb and fingers. The urinary system is considered to be sterile. For this reason all

Figure 15-3. Sites at which contamination is most likely to occur.

obstructing material by alternately pinching and releasing the tubing as shown in Figure 15-4. The upper hand rapidly squeezes and releases the tube while the lower hand holds the catheter closed.

Constant or intermittent irrigation of the bladder may be necessary to cleanse the bladder and remove clots or other material which may obstruct the catheter. In order to accomplish this various types of apparatus may be used. The type of equipment will vary according to the wishes of the doctor and the equipment available (see Fig. 15-5). When caring for this type of irrigation the nurse must have a clear understanding of the type of fluid used for irrigation, any medications or antiseptics to be added to the fluid, and the rate of flow desired by the doctor. If measurement of the urinary output is ordered the amount used for irrigation must be subtracted from the total amount of fluid in the drainage bottle.

Figure 15-5. Simple apparatus for irrigating bladder through retention catheter. The upper jar is filled with irrigating fluid. Ordinarily clamp A is closed and clamp B is left open so that urine drains freely into bottle D. When irrigation is desired, clamp B is closed and clamp A is opened, thus allowing fluid to run into the bladder (Bl.). After desired amount runs into bladder, clamp A is closed and clamp B is opened. Bottle D rests in a metal frame hung from the bed rail. C is a glass coil used to keep air out of the drainage tube. (From Davis and Warren: *Urological Nursing,* 6th Ed., W. B. Saunders Co., Philadelphia.)

Figure 15-4. Method of "milking" a catheter for the purpose of removing a blood clot or mucus plug obstructing the catheter. (From Sutton: *Bedside Nursing Techniques,* W. B. Saunders Co., Philadelphia.)

Care must be taken to avoid contamination of fluids and equipment used for any irrigation because the irrigating fluid flows directly into the bladder and an infection can easily result.

When the doctor orders removal of the retention catheter the nurse accepts responsibility for removing the catheter and carefully observing the patient for signs of retention of urine. If a Foley catheter has been inserted, the balloon must, of course, be deflated before it is removed. The catheter is removed slowly while the patient takes a deep breath and lets it out slowly. This will relax the patient and reduce the discomfort. The genital area is washed thoroughly with soap and water and dried. The time of removal of the catheter is recorded and the patient is observed carefully for signs of difficulty in voiding. A patient with proper fluid intake ought to void within eight hours after removal of a retention catheter. The nurse should report any bleeding, incontinence, or dribbling of urine, the last of which may indicate an excessive amount of residual urine.

OTHER MEANS OF ESTABLISHING URINARY FLOW

Aside from the retention catheter mentioned above there are several other ways in which a urologist may provide for adequate drainage of urine. The term "retention catheter" or "indwelling catheter" usually refers to a catheter that has been inserted through the urethra. This is the most commonly used method of draining urine. Other means include the following:

Ureteral catheters are very small and of narrow gauge. They are inserted by the urologist directly into the ureters, usually by means of cystoscope. They may be attached to a urethral catheter (see Fig. 15-3).

A *ureterostomy* is a surgical incision into the ureter by way of the abdominal wall. A tube is left in the ureter and permits drainage to the outside.

Nephrostomy and *pyelostomy* tubes are placed directly into the kidney pelvis by way of a surgical wound over the kidney.

Care of these special tubes requires much skill and knowledge and is the responsibility of the physician or registered nurse. A practical nurse must have additional training in urological procedures before attempting to care for a patient who has any one of the above-mentioned tubes inserted.

NEPHRITIS

Definition. Nephritis, sometimes called Bright's disease, refers to a general inflammation and resulting degeneration of the cells of the kidney. The inflammation is not due to an invasion of bacteria and is therefore classified as a *noninfectious* disease. There are two specific diseases classified under the general heading of nephritis. These diseases are glomerulonephritis and nephrosclerosis. Glomerulonephritis may be acute or chronic.

Acute Glomerulonephritis

This condition occurs most frequently in the winter and spring months and is seen primarily in children and young adults. It affects males more often than females. There is no definite cause known; however, it is closely related to and believed to be a complication of an infection by some strains of streptococci. Usually the patient has a history of a recent attack of "strep throat," scarlet fever, or chickenpox.

Symptoms. The patient with acute glomerulonephritis usually becomes ill suddenly with widespread edema, puffiness about the eyes, visual disturbances, and marked hypertension. If treatment is not successful the disease will rapidly progress to uremia and death.

Treatment and Nursing Care. The nurse's first responsibility in the treatment of acute glomerulonephritis is to provide rest for the patient and for the kidney. Absolute bed rest is usually ordered. Though the patient may respond quickly to treatment and, feeling better, wish to become more active, the nurse must explain the need for continued rest and provide an atmosphere for rest. An attitude of willingness to do everything necessary for the patient cheerfully and efficiently will do much to assure the patient of the nurse's sincere interest in him. She should be especially aware of the need for special attention to the diet and fluid intake during the acute phase. The doctor will usually order a sodium restricted diet if edema is present, and a limiting of fluids if there is *oliguria* (diminished urine) or *anuria* (absence of urine). The nurse should be sure the patient understands the importance of these factors in the treatment of the disease and do all she can to encourage his cooperation.

Edema that is obvious from external signs may very well be present in the internal organs. For this reason the blood pressure and pulse must be checked frequently for indications of cerebral edema with increased *intracranial* pressure. Cardiac failure or pulmonary edema may also develop and the patient must be watched closely for extreme restlessness, increased respiratory difficulty, or cyanosis.

Prognosis for acute glomerulonephritis varies, depending upon the extent of permanent damage done to the kidneys or other vital organs.

Chronic Glomerulonephritis

Chronic glomerulonephritis may develop rapidly or progress slowly over a period of years.

Symptoms. There is insidious edema, headache associated with hypertension, and dyspnea. The prognosis for this disease is ultimately poor. However, the speed with which it progresses to renal failure and uremia varies with the individual. The exact reason for this is not known. Some patients who develop chronic glomerulonephritis may have acute exacerbations (flareups) which subside. Then they may live for several years before damage to the glomeruli of the kidney brings about the uremic state. Others will rapidly pass into uremia and succumb to the disease in a short period of time.

Treatment and Nursing Care. The treatment for chronic glomerulonephritis in the latent stage is primarily *symptomatic* with emphasis on avoiding fatigue and infections, particularly of the upper respiratory tract.

The patient with chronic glomerulonephritis requires much patience and understanding. Often he is aware of the eventual outcome of the disease and may appear stubborn and uncooperative with those who are trying to help him. The nursing care is essentially the same as for acute glomerulonephritis, but is more difficult because of the need for prolonged and constant care and attention to proper rest and diet, with prevention of an infection anywhere in the body. The patient will have periods of irritability and depression. Everything should be done to eliminate undue mental and physical strain on the patient. Obesity must be avoided and pregnancy is considered extremely dangerous because of the additional work placed on the kidneys during that time. The family will need help in understanding the severity of the disease and adjusting to the fact that the prognosis is poor and death is the eventual outcome.

NEPHROSCLEROSIS

Definition. The primary difficulty in this condition is the hardening and narrowing of the small arteries in the kidneys. As the blood supply decreases the kidney cells degenerate and lose their ability to function. Nephrosclerosis is frequently associated with hardening of the arteries elsewhere in the body.

Symptoms. The symptoms of nephrosclerosis are similar to those of the patient with chronic glomerulonephritis and the treatment and nursing care are also similar.

PYELONEPHRITIS

Definition. In contrast to the diseases which come under the heading of nephritis, pyelonephritis is an *infection* of the kidney. It is caused by bacterial invasion of the kidney and urinary tract.

Normally the glomeruli of the kidney not only filter the blood passing through them but also destroy the bacteria being carried by the blood. When something happens to interfere with this process the bacteria may enter and infect the kidney. There are three basic situations which may contribute to the development of a kidney infection: (1) an increase in the number and strength of the bacteria in the blood stream, (2) lowered resistance of the patient to the bacteria, and (3) back pressure of urine because of poor drainage from the kidney.

The terminology used in describing the various processes which take place in a kidney infection often confuses those who expect the various steps in the process to represent three distinct diseases. Actually the classification of infections of the kidney are three stages of the same disease process. *Pyelitis* is an infection of the pelvis of the kidney. *Pyelonephritis* is an inflammation of the kidney pelvis and the kidney cells. *Pyonephrosis* is a collection of pus in the kidney pelvis. So we can see that as the infection spreads and pus collects the diagnosis or name of the disease may change. For the sake of simplifying the discussion of these stages of an infection of the kidney, we will cover the symptoms, treatment, and nursing care of the patient with pyelonephritis.

Symptoms. In the acute stage of pyelonephritis the symptoms include fever, chills, nausea and vomiting, and pain in the flank radiating to the thigh and genitalia. The chronic phase is more often insidious with gradual scarring of the kidney tissues which results in loss of weight, low-grade fever, and weakness. Eventually the urine becomes loaded with bacteria and pus.

Treatment and Nursing Care. Since approximately 90 percent of the cases of pyelonephritis are associated with an obstruction in the urinary tract, treatment is aimed at removal of the obstruction as well as destruction of the bacteria causing the infection.

Bed rest and forcing fluids are important in the treatment of pyelone-phritis. In addition, the nursing care is basically the same as for any severe infection during the acute stage. The urine must be observed closely for amount, changes in color, and the presence of pus or a foul odor.

Special diagnostic tests may be done to determine the location of the obstruction if one is suspected.

Specific drugs to destroy the bacteria are usually chosen according to the sensitivity of the causative organism, so that the most effective antibiotic is given. Urinary antiseptics are useful because they are excreted and concentrated in the urine and are capable of inhibiting the growth of bacteria within the urinary system. The sulfonamides, Urotropin, and Mandelamine are examples of urinary antiseptics.

The prognosis of the patient depends on the success of the treatment of the active infection before destruction and scarring of the kidney cells can occur. If chronic pyelonephritis develops the patient may live for years without significant symptoms before renal damage leads to hypertension or uremia.

RENAL FAILURE

Definition. Renal failure or insufficiency means that the kidneys have ceased to function or are only partially functioning as filters. Some substances such as albumin, globulin, and red and white cells are not normally passed through the kidneys and into the urine. Their presence in the urine indicates kidney damage and disturbance of kidney function. When renal failure occurs, waste products such as urea salts remain in the blood and the patient is said to be in a state of *uremia.* Uremia may occur as an acute condition or develop slowly as a chronic condition.

Acute Uremia. In acute renal failure the damage is more sudden and rapid in its progress, with injury or total destruction of masses of kidney cells. The causes of acute uremia are usually poisoning from mercury, transfusion reaction, or prolonged shock or dehydration. The outlook for acute uremia is better than for chronic uremia; the prognosis depends on the successful restoration of kidney function before permanent damage has been done to the kidney cells.

Chronic Uremia. Chronic uremia is a much slower process, occurring over a period of time. It may present mild symptoms at first which increase in severity, or the symptoms may be severe at the outset. Prolonged inflammation or damage to the vesicles leads to scarring, and the glomeruli are permanently lost. Hypertension is usually present and *oliguria* and *anuria* are nearly always present.

Symptoms. Uremia is characterized by depression of consciousness, muscular twitching, impaired vision, convulsions, vomiting, acidosis, and dehydration. There is an elevation of nonprotein nitrogen in the blood. There is loss of appetite and there may or may not be edema.

Treatment and Nursing Care. Treatment is concerned with decreasing the work load of the kidney and establishing a normal fluid and electrolyte balance. Fluids may be restricted if there is edema and must be spaced at intervals over a 24-hour period.

Nursing care of the patient with uremia presents a real challenge to the nurse. Because the breath is foul and carries odors of urine, diligent mouth care is important. If vomiting is present there must be a careful measuring and recording of emesis. Fluids may be increased as edema subsides, but if nausea is present, fluids should be given in small amounts at intervals. The skin may itch and be very dry, increasing the irritability of the patient. Sponging the skin with a mild acid solution using two tablespoons of vinegar to one pint of warm water will help to relieve the *pruritus.* Constipation prevents elimination of wastes through the alimentary tract and must be avoided. Edematous extremities should be elevated on pil-

lows above the level of the heart. Pillows should be protected since there may be oozing of fluids through pores of the skin. Meticulous care is needed to prevent a breakdown of the skin and resulting pressure sores.

All precautions must be taken to prevent respiratory infections. The nurse must not allow the patient to become chilled, must prevent contact of the patient with others who may have an upper respiratory infection, and must turn the patient carefully at least every two hours, avoiding friction of the skin against the sheets.

Observe the patient at all times for twitching or impending convulsions as they may occur at any time if *intracranial* pressure increases. Keep equipment at the bedside for prevention of injury to the patient during convulsions (see Chap. 3). The patient may become extremely irritable and confused; all external stimuli such as noise, bright lights, and disturbing visitors should be kept at an absolute minimum.

The family will need help and sympathetic understanding from the nurse during the final stages of chronic uremia. The nurse should avoid assuming a morbid attitude, remembering that the patient may appear comatose, yet still be able to hear what is being said in the room. Attention should be given to the patient's spiritual needs as well as his physical needs. Whatever her personal beliefs may be, the nurse should do all that she can to cooperate with the patient's minister and offer any spiritual and moral support she may be able to give the patient and his family.

DIALYSIS WITH THE ARTIFICIAL KIDNEY

In recent years, medical science has made great strides in development of highly complicated machines and devices designed to assist the human body in its vital functions when trauma or disease have temporarily disrupted these functions. The artificial kidney is one such device that has been developed and is used in large medical centers. It has received much publicity, and since many patients have read or heard of the artificial kidney, the practical nurse should know something of its limitations and the principles on which it operates.

Essentially, the artificial kidney is used to remove from the blood waste products that ordinarily would be filtered by the normal kidney and excreted in the urine. The artificial kidney utilizes the principle of diffusion: solutes in a solution of higher concentration will pass through a semipermeable membrane into a solution of lower concentration. This natural movement of molecules will continue to take place until the two solutions are of equal concentration. In hemodialysis the blood of the patient represents the solution of higher concentration. As the blood is circulated through the tubing of the artificial kidney the impurities pass through the cellophane filter into a "bath" solution containing salt, sugar, sodium bicarbonate and other components of normal plasma. The waste products such as urea are thus removed from the patient's blood (see Fig. 15-6).

At the beginning of each treatment the artificial kidney is primed with blood that is of the same type as that of the patient. This insures a continuous flow of blood through the tubing. A small pump keeps the blood circulating through the artificial kidney during the treatment, which lasts from 10 to 16 hours depending on the patient's body size, the amount of renal function that remains and the amount of wastes to be removed.

Artificial kidneys have been used for treatment of patients with acute renal problems since the early 1900's, but it was not until 1960 that those with chronic renal failure could hope to benefit from the artificial kidney. It was at this time that a specialized type of cannula was devised (see Fig. 15-7). The cannula is left in the patient's arm at all times and is replaced only once or twice a year. It eliminates the need for a cutdown each time the patient receives hemodialysis and provides ready access to the patient's blood stream when hemodialysis is indicated.[5]

At the present time there are many patients whose lives depend on the artificial kidney. These people must return to a chronic dialysis unit in a hospital two or three times a week for

Figure 15-6. Schematic diagram of the artificial kidney. (From Jacob and Francone: *Structure and Function in Man,* W. B. Saunders Co., Philadelphia.)

A

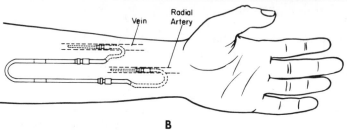

B

Figure 15-7. *A,* The cannula, the semipermanent appliance in a patient's arm. The Silastic material is shown coming out of the patient's skin; one side is long and the other side short. The Silastic is connected to the Teflon joint, and the metal rings hold the Teflon inside the Silastic so that the cannula does not come apart. *B,* Schematic drawing showing the two Teflon tips within the vein and artery. The diameter of the beveled tips that are inserted in the vessels ranges from size 13 ($\frac{1}{8}$ inch) to size 18 (less than $\frac{1}{16}$ inch). (From Fellows: *Nursing Clinics of North America,* December, 1966.)

an indefinite period. Since their kidneys are functioning very little or not at all, they must depend on the dialysis unit to remove urea and other waste from their blood. They must maintain strict adherence to a low-protein diet to help reduce the amount of waste products in the blood and they must limit their sodium intake so that edema and hypertension can be controlled.

One factor that limits the availability of hemodialysis to all patients who can benefit from it is the tremendous cost of the unit. Also, it is difficult or impossible for some individuals to make repeated visits to a clinic. At this writing there are more persons needing treatment than there are hemodialysis units available for their use. This means that someone must make the difficult decision as to who will receive the treatment and who will not. There has been some effort to establish a program whereby the hemodialysis unit is installed in the patient's home so that he can utilize the unit at night while he is sleeping. This program has many inherent problems for the patient and

his family and may not be feasible for a large number of patients, but it is less costly than a hospital unit and some patients feel that the advantages of a home unit outweigh its disadvantages.

PERITONEAL DIALYSIS

This procedure can be used as an alternative to the use of an artificial kidney. The semipermeable membrane in this case is the peritoneum and the "wash" solution is introduced into the space of the abdominal cavity. There are two phases in peritoneal dialysis — the infusion phase and the withdrawal phase.

In the infusion phase 2 liters of solution of glucose and electrolytes are introduced into the abdominal cavity via a catheter (see Fig. 15-8). The solution is left in the cavity about one hour, during which time the wastes in the patient's blood pass through the walls of the local blood vessels and into the solution in the abdominal cavity.

During the withdrawal phase the

Figure 15-8. Peritoneal dialysis. (From Watkins: American Journal of Nursing, July, 1966.)

fluid, which now contains the wastes, is removed by gravity flow. The cycle of infusion, dialysis and withdrawal is repeated until blood tests reveal a near normal level of chemicals in the blood.[14]

The chief disadvantage of peritoneal dialysis is the danger of peritonitis. One also should realize that peritoneal dialysis will not permanently relieve the symptoms of a patient with chronic renal failure. It can be used to remove wastes until a kidney transplant or other procedure is done or until an acute renal condition is corrected, but it is not a cure for renal failure.

CYSTITIS

Definition. Cystitis is an inflammation of the bladder and one of the most common disorders of the urinary tract. It is rarely a primary disease and is often a symptom of some other disturbance in either the urinary tract or the genital tract. Acute cystitis occurs more frequently in females because of the close proximity of the bladder to the genital area and the relative shortness of the female urethra in comparison to the male urethra.

Symptoms. The patient with cystitis is extremely uncomfortable with frequent and urgent desires to void. There is often a burning sensation at the completion of each act of voiding. Hematuria (blood in the urine) is sometimes present. A general reaction with fever and chills is not characteristic of cystitis and suggests an extension of the infection to the kidneys.

Treatment and Nursing Care. Treatment of cystitis is aimed at removal of the underlying cause and prevention of the spread of the infection beyond the bladder. Urinary antiseptics and, sometimes, antibiotics may be necessary to control the infection. The nursing care consists of simple measures to relieve the symptoms. Rest is important and heat in the form of sitz baths, vaginal douches, or suprapubic heat will do much to allay the discomfort.

URETHRITIS

Definition. Urethritis is an inflammation of the urethra. It can be caused by many different organisms. Urethritis is one of the most common symptoms of gonorrhea, however, and should be investigated when it is first noticed. In the female, trauma from childbirth and the proximity of the genital organs to the urethra predispose the urethra to infection.

Symptoms. The chief symptoms of urethritis are burning, itching, frequency in voiding, and painful urination. A discharge is present and becomes increasingly more purulent if gonorrhea is present. The urinary meatus is swollen and inflamed.

Treatment and Nursing Care. Treatment begins with determination of the causative organism and the administration of specific drugs to combat the infection. The nursing care is similar to that for the patient with cystitis. The nurse should be especially aware of the possibility of a gonorrheal infection until a definite diagnosis has been established and carry out the necessary precautions against spread of the infection to the eyes.

OBSTRUCTIONS OF THE URINARY TRACT

Hydronephrosis

Definition. Whenever the normal flow of urine is obstructed there follows a backward flow of fluid into the kidney pelvis. If this condition is not relieved by removal of the obstruction, the kidney becomes dilated and continues to fill with fluid. Soon the kidney cells will atrophy until all normal function ceases and the kidney becomes merely a thin, walled cyst. This condition is known as *hydronephrosis*. It can eventually result in complete destruction of the kidney. The condition may be *unilateral* or *bilateral* (one or both kidneys). If it occurs only on one side, the other kidney may enlarge and efficiently carry on the work of two kidneys. This is called *compensatory hypertrophy*.

Symptoms. Severe pain is present only if hydronephrosis develops rapidly. Otherwise there are no outstanding symptoms and the patient may develop signs of uremia only after serious damage has occurred.

Treatment and Nursing Care. The primary goal of the treatment is removal of the obstruction so the kidney may drain properly. The ideal situation is drainage of the kidney in the early stages. If the damage is irreparable the kidney is removed by surgery. The nursing care of the patient with hydronephrosis is concerned with close observation and accurate reporting of urinary output, and of early signs of impending uremia. If nephrectomy is necessary, the nursing care is the same as for any patient with nephrectomy.

Nephroptosis

Definition. The kidney usually lies with its flat surface against the posterior wall of the body and is well padded with fat. If the pad of fat is absent or the *pedicle* of the kidney is longer than usual, the kidney may move backward and forward freely or sag below its normal position when the patient stands. This condition is known as nephroptosis or "floating kidney." It occurs most commonly in middle-aged women who are thin and long waisted.

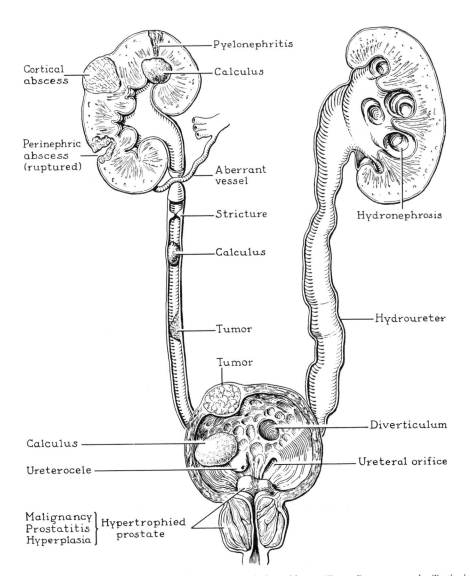

Figure 15-9. Commonly encountered male urogenital problems. (From Brunner et al.: *Textbook of Medical-Surgical Nursing*, J. B. Lippincott Co., Philadelphia.)

Symptoms. Nephroptosis may cause no symptoms or disability; however, it has the potential of causing a twisting or kinking of the ureters with resulting hydronephrosis. In some patients there is pain in the kidney region aggravated by standing and relieved by lying down and elevating the hips.

Treatment and Nursing Care. Palliative treatment is directed at relief of symptoms by bed rest, weight-gaining techniques, and abdominal support with belts or braces. The patient wearing supporting belts or braces should be instructed to apply them on arising in the morning when the kidney is nearest to its normal position after a night's rest. Surgical fixation of the kidney by suturing it in its normal position *(nephropexy)* is sometimes done when other measures fail. The nursing care after nephropexy is the same as for nephrectomy though there is less danger of hemorrhage and the patient should have a more rapid recovery. The foot of the bed is sometimes elevated postoperatively to help the kidney maintain a normal position and to avoid strain on the sutures.

Renal Calculi

Definition. For reasons not yet fully determined, some people have a tendency to manufacture stones in the kidney from deposits of crystalline substances normally excreted in the urine. These stones may vary in size from "sand or gravel" to large stones the size of an orange. Some are star-shaped and are called "renal stars." They may be found anywhere in the urinary tract and, if small enough, are flushed out by the urine without any noticeable symptoms. Otherwise they may obstruct the flow of urine at any point from the kidney to the bladder. These stones are closely associated with urinary tract infections, hyperparathyroidism and its accompanying *hypercalcemia*, or bone lesions. Men are more often affected than women.

Symptoms. Usually there is a dull aching in the lower back with increased production of urine. Blood and pus are found to be present in the urine. If the stone is small and attempts to pass through the ureter it will often scrape the lining of the ureter and present the dramatic symptoms of *renal colic*. The pain of renal colic is a sudden agonizing pain starting in the flank of the affected side and radiating from there down the ureter to the genitalia and along the inner side of the thigh. These symptoms are frequently accompanied by nausea and vomiting and extreme *diaphoresis*.

Treatment and Nursing Care. The simplest method of treating stones would be by dissolving them or causing them to pass spontaneously; however, though much research is being done, at present there is no way known to accomplish this. When a patient is admitted for kidney stones most urologists choose to wait a reasonable length of time for the stone to pass spontaneously, as a large percentage do. During this period the nurse should encourage fluids, unless otherwise ordered and strain all urine through cheesecloth or gauze in order to catch the stone should it pass with the urine. If the stone is not passed, a surgical procedure is necessary to remove it. The type of surgery will depend upon the location of the stone.

TUMORS OF THE KIDNEY

Definition. *Neoplasms* of the kidney are fairly uncommon, actually constituting less than 1 percent of all malignant tumors of the body. They are, however, nearly always cancerous and are extremely difficult to treat in the later stages. Except for Wilms's tumors (see below) they occur mostly in middle life.

Symptoms. The principal symptom of malignant tumors of the kidney is *hematuria* (blood in the urine), which is usually not accompanied by pain in the early stages. There may be an enlargement of the affected kidney. Diagnosis can be made fairly easily by a retrograde pyelogram.

Treatment and Nursing Care. The only treatment that has met with any degree of success is surgical removal of the affected kidney before *metastasis* has occurred. Unfortunately this is difficult to achieve because the patient usually does not have symptoms severe enough to send him to the doctor until it is too late. Postoperative radiation is sometimes used to deter further involvement after nephrectomy. The nursing care of the patient is that for patients receiving radiation therapy and postoperative care following nephrectomy.

Wilms's Tumors

Definition. Wilms's tumors of the kidney are thought to be congenital in origin. The average age of onset is three years. Since these tumors are highly malignant and metastasize quickly, the death rate is very high.

Treatment and Nursing Care. Treatment of Wilms's tumor is by nephrectomy. If the tumor is caught early and the kidney removed during the first year of life the chances of cure are much better.

CARE OF THE PATIENT WHO HAS HAD SURGERY OF THE KIDNEY

Types of Surgery. The two main types of surgical procedures which may be performed on the kidney are *nephrectomy* and *nephrostomy.*

Nephrectomy is the surgical removal of the kidney. Although this is always a serious operation, a person may live with only one kidney. The remaining kidney enlarges and is usually able to carry on the work formerly done by two kidneys.

Nephrostomy is a surgical incision into a kidney for the purpose of providing an artificial means of draining the kidney. This procedure may be done in the treatment of obstructions from large stones or strictures of the ureter, or to drain purulent material from an infected kidney.

Nursing Care. In either a nephrectomy or nephrostomy the surgical incision may be lumbar, transabdominal, or thoracic. When the patient returns from surgery the nurse must check carefully for the location of the surgical wound and the presence of any drains or tubes that may have been inserted during the operation. Attachment of these tubes to drainage bottles or other bedside equipment is the responsibility of the nurse in charge.

Dressings over the surgical wound may be reinforced but they should not be changed by the nurse unless there are specific written orders to do so. The drainage on these dressings will be blood-tinged at first, but it should gradually become clearer. If bright red blood appears or there is a sudden change in the amount of drainage, the doctor should be notified. Sometimes the drains will have a sterile safety pin attached to the end. This pin must be kept closed at all times and must never be attached to the dressings, the patient's gown or the bedclothes. Extreme care must be taken during the changing of dressings that the drains or tubes are not dislodged or pulled from the surgical incision.

Positioning of the patient depends on the wishes of the surgeon. He may prefer to have the patient lie only on the operative side. The nurse must determine his wishes and follow his orders explicitly in this matter. Turning the patient may be difficult at first because it is usually quite painful for him to move about. The nurse should explain the need for frequent turning and deep breathing so that complications may be prevented.

Hemorrhage is always a danger after surgery of the kidney. It will be remembered that the kidneys have a very rich supply of blood directly from the aorta and vena cava. The vital signs are carefully checked and any indication of shock or hemorrhage reported immediately.

Adequate drainage from the opposite kidney after surgery is of great concern to the physician. Urinary output must be very carefully measured and recorded. Fluids are usually restricted immediately after surgery and then are gradually increased as the remaining kidney compensates for the loss of its partner. If a nephrostomy has been done, fluids are restricted until the affected kidney can recover sufficiently and resume its functions.

TUMORS OF THE BLADDER

Definition. Most tumors of the bladder are malignant and the prognosis for cure is generally not good. However, superficial tumors, if detected in the early stages, have a more favorable prognosis.

Symptoms. Frequency of urination, *dysuria* (painful or difficult urination) and hematuria are the most common symptoms of bladder tumor. In the later stages, as the tumor becomes larger, there may be an obstruction of the flow of urine.

Treatment and Nursing Care. The treatment for bladder tumor is complete or partial removal of the bladder with transplantation of the ureters to the outside or to the intestinal tract. During the preoperative period, extra care must be taken to observe the patient for hemorrhage from the bladder. Clots or obstruction of the urinary flow or the tumor itself may cause severe bladder spasms and pain. If the patient has a retention catheter in place, care must be taken to maintain open drainage.

CARE OF THE PATIENT HAVING SURGERY OF THE BLADDER AND URETERS

Types of Surgery. *Cystectomy* is the surgical removal of the bladder. *Ureterostomy* is a surgical incision into the ureter for the purpose of diverting the flow of urine. If the bladder is removed, there obviously must be some means of diverting the flow of urine that normally would pass through the ureters and into the bladder. One procedure is a *cutaneous ureterostomy* in which the ureters are transplanted to the skin on the abdomen (see Fig. 15-10). This is a relatively safe procedure but it frequently is complicated by stricture of the ureter at the point where it joins the skin or fascia.

Another surgical procedure necessitated by cystectomy is ureterosigmoidostomy in which the ureters are attached to the sigmoid colon which then acts as a reservoir for the urine (see Fig. 15-11A).

A third procedure involves suturing the ureters to an isolated section of ileum that is connected to an opening in the skin (see Fig. 15-11B). The open ends of intestines where the section of ileum was removed are rejoined by anastomosis.

Figure 15-10. Cystectomy and cutaneous ureterostomies. (From *Essentials of Cancer Nursing,* American Cancer Society, Inc.)

Figure 15-11. *A*, Ureterosigmoidostomy. This is performed for congenital malformations of the bladder and carcinoma of the bladder and pelvic organs. Problems: chronic infection of the urinary tract, reabsorption of urinary electrolytes, and malignancy at the site of ureter implantation. *B*, Ileal conduit. Performed when the bladder (and often the rectum also) has been removed. Problems: patient must wear ileostomy appliance and stricture may develop at the implant site. (From Bloom and Merrill: G. P. *23*:91, 1961.)

Nursing Care. Nursing care following cystectomy is always difficult because of the danger of hemorrhage and infection. There are also problems involved in devising a satisfactory arrangement for the collection of urine. If ureterostomy tubes have been inserted and brought to the outside, the drainage will keep the dressings wet because urine is constantly dribbling through the ureters from the kidney. The dressings must be changed quite frequently and some waterproof material used to protect the patient's gown and bed linens. The skin around the tubes must also receive special attention to prevent irritation.

There are special cups and appliances available for the collection of urine after a cutaneous ureterostomy or ileal conduit (see Fig. 15-12). These are similar in principle to the colostomy bag, but must be worn constantly because there is no way to control the flow of urine from the kidneys. The patient must have adequate instruction in the daily care of his ureterostomy cup. It is possible for many patients to wear these appliances, resuming their former activities without embarrassment or restriction.

Practical nurses wishing to know

Figure 15-12. A rubber leg urinal draining urine from a ureter implanted into the skin. The end of the bag can be unplugged periodically during the day to allow the urine that has collected to flow out.

more about cutaneous ureterostomies are referred to references at the end of this chapter.

TRAUMATIC INJURIES TO THE KIDNEY AND URETERS

Definition. Accidental injury to the kidneys, ureters, bladder, or urethra occurs frequently and should always be considered a possibility whenever there has been trauma to the abdominal cavity or thoracic cage.

Symptoms. The chief symptoms indicating trauma to the kidney are: gross hematuria, pain and tenderness in the renal area, and an enlarged mass in the flank.

Treatment and Nursing Care. Since bleeding in the kidney is often self-limiting, most urologists advocate a period of watchful waiting before doing surgery. This is done with the hope that the kidney may be saved. During this time of observation the nurse must be constantly alert for the early signs of shock and hemorrhage in the patient. Strict bed rest must be enforced and precautions taken against infections. Nephrectomy may be necessary if there is persistent hemorrhage or an infection developing. Nursing care of the patient with a nephrectomy is discussed above.

TRAUMATIC INJURIES TO THE BLADDER

Definition. Any violent blow or crushing injury to the lower abdomen may result in rupture or perforation of the bladder wall with resulting leakage of the urine into the pelvic tissues or peritoneal cavity. This brings about a severe inflammation in these areas.

Symptoms. Early symptoms of bladder injury are painful hematuria, or inability to void, marked tenderness and spasm in the suprapubic area, or

the development of a large mass in that area.

Treatment and Nursing Care. If the bladder has ruptured or is perforated, treatment consists of a suprapubic cystostomy for the purpose of providing drainage of blood and urine. Care of the patient demands meticulous care and attention to drains and dressings to avoid infection and maintain good drainage. Cold applications may be ordered to the swollen area before surgery and to the operative area following surgery. The nurse should observe the patient carefully for postoperative shock and massive hemorrhage. Any formation of a mass in the suprapubic area before or after surgery, or any change in the vital signs, should be reported immediately.

In addition to physical distress, the patient with bladder injuries is likely to have emotional difficulties in dealing with the problems arising from the sudden loss of his control over the urinary flow and the intimate procedures and treatments necessary. The nurse must be prepared for this and do all she can to encourage and help the patient through this difficult period of adjustment.

Regardless of the diagnosis, patients with urological problems must be approached with an attitude of dignity and composure. Depending on his age, personality, place in the family and community, and severity of his illness the male patient's attitude toward these problems will vary. Whatever his reaction to necessary treatments and nursing care, the nurse must remain in control of the situation. By her professional bearing and dignity she can alleviate much embarrassment, indicating that her primary concern is for the welfare of the patient.

CLINICAL CASE PROBLEMS

1. Mrs. Spence, age 45, is admitted to the medical service with a diagnosis of chronic glomerulonephritis. Her blood

pressure is 190/80, pulse 88 and irregular. She has generalized edema and shortness of breath. Her skin is very dry and shows marked excoriation where she has scratched herself to relieve itching. She has very long, heavily polished fingernails in which she takes great pride.

Mrs. Spence's two children, aged 25 and 23 years, have heard about the artificial kidney, and are very anxious to have Mrs. Spence sent to the city 80 miles away for treatment. They ask you if you think they should change doctors and have her transferred.

Mr. Spence travels and on his visits to his wife he displays an attitude of indifference and impatience toward her illness. In an effort to show some interest, he usually brings her a box of chocolate candy and salted nuts.

What nursing problems do you find in this situation?

How would you, as a practical nurse, be able to help in the solution of some of these problems?

What special nursing care would you expect this situation to require?

2. Mrs. Downs is a 35-year-old patient who has had a nephrostomy for treatment of hydronephrosis. She returns from surgery with a urethral catheter, a ureteral catheter, and a rubber Penrose drain in place.

Explain the purpose of a ureteral catheter.

What special care must be taken with the urethral catheter and the drainage apparatus?

What information should you have before irrigating the urethral catheter?

What special care will be required by the drain that has been inserted in the operative area?

3. A friend of yours tells you that she has been very uncomfortable during the past week because of frequency of urination and burning when she voids. Last night she had a severe chill and some elevation of temperature. She has been told that she probably has a very common ailment in women and that if she will drink a lot of fluids it will probably go away.

What would be your advice to this person?

How would you explain the need for her to follow your advice?

REFERENCES

1. Brand, L., and Komorita, N. I.: "Adapting to Long-term Hemodialysis." Am. Journ. Nurs., Aug., 1966, p. 1778.
2. Brunner, L. S., et al.: *Medical-Surgical Nursing.* Philadelphia, J. B. Lippincott Co., 1964.
3. Davis, J. E.: "Drugs and Urologic Disorders." Am. Journ. Nurs., Aug., 1965, p. 107.
4. Downing, S.: "The Patient Who Has Peritoneal Dialysis." Am. Journ. Nurs., July, 1966, p. 1572.
5. Fellows, B. J.: "The Role of the Nurse in a Chronic Dialysis Unit." *Nursing Clinics of North America.* Philadelphia, W.B. Saunders Co., Dec., 1966.
6. Fellows, G.: "Hemodialysis at Home." Am. Journ. Nurs., Aug., 1966, p. 1775.
7. Hand, J. R.: "Infections of the Urinary Tract." Am. Journ. Nurs., Aug., 1957, p. 1008.
8. Isler, C.: "G. U. Nursing Updated." RN, Nov., 1960, p. 37.
9. Jacob, S. W., and Francone, C. A.: *Structure and Function in Man.* Philadelphia, W. B. Saunders Co., 1966.
10. Rodman, M. J.: "Diuretics to Fight Edema." RN, June, 1959, p. 22.
11. Shafer, K. N., Sawyer, J. R., et al.: *Medical-Surgical Nursing,* 4th edition. St. Louis, C. V. Mosby Co., 1967.
12. Smith, D. W., and Gips, C. D.: *Care of the Adult Patient,* 2nd edition. Philadelphia, J. B. Lippincott Co., 1966.
13. Trusk, C. W.: "Hemodialysis for Acute Renal Failure." Am. Journ. Nurs., Feb., 1965, p. 80.
14. Watkins, F. I.: "The Patient Who Has Peritoneal Dialysis." Am. Journ. Nurs., July, 1966, p. 1575.

SUGGESTED STUDENT READING

1. Ansell, J. S., and Tauffie, M. R.: "Nephrectomy and Nephrostomy" and "Nursing the Patient after Nephrectomy." Am. Journ. Nurs., Oct., 1958, p. 1394.
2. Brand, L., and Komorita, N. I.: "Adapting to Long-term Hemodialysis." Am. Journ. Nurs., Aug., 1966, p. 1779.
3. "Charting Intake and Output." RN, Nov., 1958, p. 33.
4. Davis, J. F.: "Drugs for Urologic Disorders." Am. Journ. Nurs., Aug., 1965, p. 107.
5. Santora, D.: "Preventing Hospital-acquired Urinary Infection." Am. Journ. Nurs., April, 1966, p. 790.

6. Spellman, R. M., and Swanwick, M. H.: "The Management of Cutaneous Ureterostomies." Am. Journ. Nurs., July, 1955, p. 800.
7. Winter, C. C., Reehm, M. M., and Watson, H. G.: "Urinary Calculi" and "Nursing Care." Am. Journ. Nurs., July, 1963, p. 72.
8. Zielinski, J.: "Terminal Uremia." Journ. Pract. Nurs., Feb., 1965, p. 33.

OUTLINE FOR CHAPTER 15

I. Introduction

A. Urinary system composed of kidneys, ureters, urinary bladder and urethra.

B. Urinary system maintains proper balance of fluids, minerals and organic substances necessary for life.

C. Generalized diseases such as circulatory disorders and metabolic disturbances can affect function of the kidneys.

II. Diagnostic Tests and Examinations

A. Urine culture determines specific microorganisms causing infection.

B. P.S.P. test estimates ability of kidneys to excrete dye.

C. Fishberg concentration test determines kidney's ability to concentrate urine.

D. X-ray examinations visualize the urinary tract through the use of a radiopaque material, which can be given directly into the vein (intravenous pyelogram), by way of a ureteral catheter (retrograde pyelogram) through a urethral catheter (cystogram).

E. Blood analysis determines the kidney's ability to remove wastes such as urea nitrogen and nonprotein nitrogen from the blood.

F. Cystoscopy is insertion of a cystoscope into the bladder for the purpose of examining the interior surface.

III. Measuring the Patient's Loss of Fluids

A. Nursing staff responsible for accurate measuring and recording of output.

B. Total urinary output measures all urine obtained from all catheters.

C. Total output must include vomitus, watery stools, urine excreted and an estimate of fluid lost through perspiration.

D. Retention of urine means urine is held in the bladder, patient is unable to void.

E. Suppression of urine means kidneys are unable to produce urine.

F. Residual urine remains in the bladder after the patient has voided.

IV. Nursing Care of Patient with Retention Catheter

A. Catheter must be kept open and draining freely.

B. Drainage bottle must be kept lower than bladder.

C. Tubing and container must be handled with care to avoid introducing infection into the bladder. Tubing is changed when sandy residue builds up.

D. Urine amount is measured at intervals. Urine is observed for color, content, peculiar odor or other noticeable characteristics.

E. Genitalia and surrounding skin must receive extra care.

F. Irrigations should be done according to the physician's orders. Nurse must be sure to use correct solution and amount.

G. After removal of retention catheter patient is watched for ability to void, bleeding, incontinence, and dribbling of urine.

V. Other Means of Establishing Urinary Flow

A. Ureteral catheter—inserted directly into the ureter.

B. Ureterostomy—a surgical incision into the ureter to insert catheter or drain.

C. Nephrostomy—surgical incision into kidney for the purpose of drainage.

VI. Nephritis (General Inflammation and Resulting Degeneration of the Renal Cells)

A. Acute glomerulonephritis—closely related to streptococcal infections.
   1. Symptoms—widespread edema, visual disturbances and marked hypertension.
   2. Treatment—rest, low-sodium diet and observation for signs of increased intracranial pressure, cardiac failure or pulmonary edema.

B. Chronic glomerulonephritis— may develop rapidly or over a period of years.
   1. Symptoms—insidious edema, headache associated with hypertension and dyspnea.
   2. Treatment and nursing care— primarily symptomatic with emphasis on avoiding fatigue and infections. No cure.

C. Nephrosclerosis—hardening and narrowing of the small arteries in the kidneys leading to degeneration of renal cells.
   1. Symptoms and treatment similar to those of chronic glomerulonephritis.

VII. Pyelonephritis (Infection of the Kidneys Due to Bacterial Invasion)

A. May develop from (1) increase in strength and number of bacteria in the blood stream, (2) lowered resistance of the patient or (3) back pressure of urine because of poor drainage from kidney.

B. Symptoms—fever, chills, nausea and vomiting and pain in the flank radiating to the thigh and genitalia. Later symptoms—weight loss, weakness, and bacteria and pus cells in the urine.

C. Treatment and nursing care—bed rest, fluids, careful observation of urine for amount, color and odor, urinary antiseptics and antibiotics.

VIII. Renal Failure (Renal Insufficiency)

A. Kidneys fail to function as filters. Indicated by the presence in the urine of albumin, globulin and red and white blood cells.

B. Uremia—the accumulation in the blood stream of waste products such as urea and urea salts.

1. Acute uremia—sudden and rapid injury or destruction of masses of renal cells. Caused by poisoning from mercury or other heavy metals, transfusion reaction, prolonged shock or dehydration.

2. Chronic uremia. Caused by prolonged inflammation or damage to renal cells.

   a. Symptoms—depression of consciousness, muscular twitching or convulsions, impaired vision, vomiting, acidosis and dehydration. Elevation of nonprotein nitrogen in the blood.

   b. Treatment and nursing care—concerned with decreasing workload of kidneys and establishing normal fluid and electrolyte balance. Mouth care, skin care, prevention of respiratory infections, observation of patient for convulsions, delirium and disorientation and provision of nonstimulating environment.

IX. Artificial Kidney

A. Utilizes the principle of dialysis for removal of waste products.

B. Patient's blood is circulated through tubes of cellophane that filter out waste products. Cleansed blood is returned to the patient's body.

C. Development of a specialized type of cannula has made hemodialysis with artificial kidney feasible for patients with chronic renal failure.

X. Peritoneal Dialysis

A. Similar to the artificial kidney, but using the peritoneum as semipermeable membrane. Fluid is injected into the abdominal cavity. Waste products leave blood stream and enter fluid, which is then removed by gravity flow.

B. Chief disadvantage is danger of peritonitis.

XI. Cystitis (Inflammation of the Bladder)

A. Often a symptom of some other disturbance in the urinary tract.

B. Occurs most often in females.

C. Symptoms—frequent urge to urinate, burning sensation during voiding and hematuria; fever and chills in more extensive involvement of urinary tract.

D. Treatment—urinary antiseptics, antibiotics, sitz baths and rest.

XII. Urethritis (Inflammation of the Urethra)

A. Can be caused by many different organisms but often is a symptom of gonorrhea.

B. Symptoms are burning, itching, frequent voiding and painful urination. Purulent discharge may indicate gonorrhea.

C. Treatment involves determination of causative organisms and specific antibiotic to control infection.

XIII. Obstructions of the Urinary Tract

A. Hydronephrosis—flow of urine from the kidney obstructed. Kidney becomes dilated and fills with fluid.

1. Symptoms—severe pain occurs only if condition develops rapidly. Otherwise symptoms are mild and patient may not be aware of condition until uremia develops.

2. Treatment—aimed at removal of obstruction. Patient observed closely for signs of impending uremia and urinary output noted and recorded.

Nephrectomy may be necessary if damage is extensive.

B. Nephroptosis—a sagging of the kidney below its normal position. Condition can lead to kinking of ureter, causing hydronephrosis.

1. Symptoms—sometimes pain in the kidney region that is aggravated by standing.

2. Treatment—bed rest, weight gain, abdominal support with belt or brace and possibly surgical fixation of the kidney by suturing it in its normal position (nephropexy).

XIV. Renal Calculi (Kidney Stones)

1. Exact cause unknown but closely associated with urinary tract infections, hyperparathyroidism and bone lesions.

2. Symptoms—dull aching pain in lower back with increased urine production. Attempt to pass stone down ureter may cause patient renal colic.

3. Treatment—stone may pass spontaneously, so fluids are encouraged and urine is strained. Surgical removal necessary for stones which cannot be passed in the urine.

XV. Tumors of the Kidney

A. Neoplasms fairly uncommon but nearly always malignant.

1. Symptoms—hematuria and enlargement of affected kidney.

2. Treatment—surgical removal of affected kidney before mestastasis has occurred.

B. Wilms's tumor—a tumor of the kidney thought to be congenital.

1. Average age of onset—three years. Highly malignant and metastasizes rapidly.

2. Treatment—surgical removal as soon as possible.

XVI. Care of the Patient Who Has Had Surgery of the Kidney

A. Two main types of surgery—nephrectomy and nephrostomy.

B. Nursing care.

1. Patient must be checked carefully for catheters and drains and turned carefully to avoid tension on them.

2. Dressings may be reinforced but usually are changed by the surgeon.

Some blood-tinged drainage is expected but bright red drainage must be reported. Most common complication is hemorrhage.

3. Urinary output is measured carefully. Fluids may be restricted.

XVII. Tumors of the Bladder

A. Usually malignant. Prognosis generally not good.

B. Symptoms—frequency of urination, dysuria and hematuria. Possibility of later obstruction to the flow of urine from the bladder.

C. Treatment—surgical removal of part or all of bladder.

XVIII. Care of the Patient Having Surgery of the Bladder and Ureters

A. Cystectomy—surgical removal of the bladder.

B. Ureterostomy—surgical incision into ureter for purpose of providing drainage.

C. Surgical procedures to provide for diversion of flow of urine: (1) cutaneous ureterostomy (ureters are transplanted to the skin), (2) ureterosigmoidostomy (ureters are attached to the sigmoid colon), and (3) ileal conduit (a section of ileum connects ureters to abdominal opening).

D. Patient must wear some type of bag or cup for collection of urine. Will require instruction similar to that given a colostomy patient.

XIX. Traumatic Injuries to the Kidney and Ureters

A. Always a possibility when there has been trauma to the abdominal cavity or thoracic cage.

B. Symptoms—gross hematuria, pain and tenderness in renal area and an enlarged mass in the flank.

C. Treatment—watch for signs of shock and hemorrhage. Strict bed rest. Surgery, possibly nephrectomy.

XX. Traumatic Injuries to Bladder

A. Caused by violent or crushing blow to lower abdomen.

B. Symptoms—painful hematuria, inability to void and marked tenderness, spasm or large mass in suprapubic area.

C. Treatment—meticulous care of drains and dressings to avoid infection and to maintain good drainage of urine.

Chapter 16

NURSING CARE OF PATIENTS WITH DISORDERS OF THE ENDOCRINE SYSTEM

VOCABULARY

Atrophy
Coma
Hypothalamus
Lethargy
Idiopathic
Pruritus

INTRODUCTION

The endocrine system is composed of glands which have no ducts; that is, they pour their secretions directly into the blood stream. These secretions are of great importance to the health of an individual because they affect the activities of the body tissues; in fact, the nervous system and the endocrine system share the responsibility for controlling *all* activities of every cell in the human body.

The secretions from the endocrine glands are called *hormones*. Hormones are chemical substances capable of stimulating or inhibiting the activities of the cells. They do this by acting as catalysts, which means that they speed up or slow down the chemical changes which take place within the cells and tissues.

The glands of the endocrine system do not always function independently of one another. In some instances the hormones from one endocrine gland may directly affect the function of other endocrine glands, thus making the study of these glands and their functions very complex and somewhat difficult to understand. There is still much research and scientific investigation to be done before the endocrine glands and the part they play in our health and well-being can be completely understood.

Diseases resulting from an abnormal functioning of the endocrine glands may result from overactivity and increase in secretions from the gland, or underactivity and a decrease in production of hormones. The prefixes *hyper-* and *hypo-* are often used to designate the condition present. For example, hyperthyroidism means overactivity of the thyroid gland and an increase in the secretion of its hormone, *thyroxine*. Hypothyroidism is just the opposite; that is, underactivity of the gland and deficiency in the secretion of thyroxine.

DISEASES OF THE THYROID GLAND

Introduction. The thyroid gland is located below the pharynx in front of and on either side of the trachea. It secretes *thyroxine* and several other closely related hormones that regulate the rate at which the tissues of the body work. Since thyroxine acts to increase the metabolic activities in most cells of the body it can, by increasing the nutritive demands of the tissues, affect the heart rate, blood flow, respiration, secretion of gastric juices and muscular functions.

In order to maintain a normal basal metabolic rate there must be precisely the right amount of thyroxine secreted at all times. The control of the rate of thyroid secretion is a function of the adenohypophysis (anterior lobe of the pituitary gland), which is often called the master gland. The adenohypophysis secretes a hormone called thyrotropin or thyroid-stimulating hormone (TSH). As is obvious from its name, TSH stimulates the thyroid gland to secrete *its* hormone thyroxine. This process of one hormone's regulating the secretion of another hormone is just one example of the many ways in which the endocrine glands affect one another.

Special Diagnostic Tests. Basal Metabolic Rate. Because thyroxine is so closely related to metabolism, a measurement of the metabolic rate when the body is completely at rest will give important information on the functioning of the thyroid gland. The reader is referred to page 52 of this text for more detailed information on the testing of the basal metabolic rate of an individual.

Radioactive Iodine Uptake. The thyroid gland readily absorbs and utilizes the mineral *iodine* in the process of manufacturing thyroxine. To test the activity of the thyroid gland, radioactive iodine is given to the patient by mouth, and after 24 hours the amount of iodine taken up by the thyroid is measured with a Geiger counter. The overactive thyroid gland will accumulate more iodine than one that is normal or underactive.

Protein-bound Iodine. This test is another way of measuring iodine content, except that the iodine measured is that which is found in the plasma of the patient's blood. It is called protein-bound iodine because the iodine is chemically bound to proteins in the plasma. Normally there are 4 to 8 μg. (micrograms) of such iodine in the plasma. In hyperthyroid individuals the iodine content is above normal.

Cholesterol Level. Cholesterol is the principal animal sterol and it is found in many tissues of the body. The concentration of cholesterol in the serum is high when the thyroid is underactive and low when the thyroid is overactive. Although a change in the cholesterol level does not necessarily indicate a disorder of the thyroid gland, determination of the cholesterol level can be used with other diagnostic tests to confirm or rule out thyroid disease.

Simple Goiter

Definition. There is often some confusion as to the proper classification of diseases of the thyroid, especially those concerned with enlargement of the gland. A *simple goiter* is only an enlargement of the thyroid and there is no oversecretion of thyroxine in this condition. The cause of simple goiter has been proven to be a deficiency of iodine in water or food.

Symptoms. As stated before, there are no constitutional symptoms or changes in the metabolic rate of individuals with simple goiter. The first sign to be noticed is enlargement of the neck. Later as the goiter continues to grow it presses against the esophagus and causes *dysphagia* (difficulty in swallowing). The goiter may also press against the trachea and produce dyspnea.

Table 21.   *Functions of Endocrine Glands*

GLAND	HORMONE	ACTION OF HORMONE
PITUITARY **Anterior lobe**	Thyrotropic hormone Somatotropic hormone Gonadotropic hormones (LH, FSH, LTH)	Stimulates thyroid gland. Stimulates growth. Affect growth, maturity, and functioning of primary and secondary sex organs.
	Adrenocorticotropic hormone (ACTH)	Stimulates cortex of adrenal glands.
Posterior lobe	Antidiuretic hormone	Decreases production of urine.
	Oxytocic principle	Stimulates uterine contractions.
THYROID	Thyroxin	Stimulates metabolism (catabolic phase).
PARATHYROID	Parathormone	Regulates blood calcium level.
ADRENAL **Cortex**	Hormones divided into three main groups: Glucocorticoids	Tend to increase amount of sugar in blood.
	Mineralocorticoids	Tend to increase amount of blood sodium and decrease amount of potassium in blood.
	Androgens (male hormones)	Govern certain secondary sex characteristics. All corticoids important for defense against stress or injury to body tissues.
Medulla	Epinephrine (adrenalin); "fight or flight" hormone	Elevates blood pressure. Converts glycogen to glucose when needed by muscles for energy. Increases heartbeat rate. Dilates bronchioles.
OVARIES	Estrone and progesterone	Stimulate development of seconddary sex characteristics. Affect repair of endometrium after menstruation
TESTES	Testosterone	Essential for normal functioning of male reproductive organs. Stimulates development of male secondary sex characteristics.
ISLANDS OF LANGERHANS ON PANCREAS	Insulin	Promotes metabolism of carbohydrates.

Treatment and Nursing Care. If goiter is treated early with medications containing iodine, the growth of the gland may be halted and the enlargement may even disappear eventually. These medications must be given well diluted and administered through a straw because they may stain the teeth. Examples of iodine preparations are *Lugol's solution* and a saturated solution of *potassium iodide* (S.S.K.I.).

A very large goiter which continues to grow and produce local symptoms of pressure, or presents the possibility of the development of malignancy in the gland, may be removed surgically.

Hyperthyroidism

Definition. Hyperthyroidism is a systemic condition resulting from overactivity of the thyroid gland and overproduction of the hormone thyroxine. This disorder is also known as *Graves' disease, toxic goiter,* and *thyrotoxicosis.*

The reason for this increased activity of the gland is not known. In some cases there has been a history of severe emotional distress or physical strain just before development of the symptoms.

Symptoms. The symptoms produced by the disease are all a result of an increase in metabolism in the body tissues. The patient is extremely nervous, tense and overactive. He seems compelled to indulge in physical activities even though he has an increasing sense of fatigue. He is very sensitive and may laugh or cry at the slightest provocation. His appetite is enormous and he eats great quantities of food but does not gain weight. The thyroid gland may or may not be greatly enlarged.

Another symptom found in about one third of all patients with hyperthyroidism is protrusion of the eyeballs (exophthalmos) (see Fig. 16-1). The exact cause of this condition is not fully understood but it may be quite severe. It can lead to blindness through stretching of the optic nerve or through ulcera-

Figure 16-1. Patient with exophthalmic hyperthyroidism. Note protrusion of the eyes and retraction of the superior eyelids. The basal metabolic rate was +40. (Courtesy of Dr. Leonard Posey. From Guyton: *Textbook of Medical Physiology,* W. B. Saunders Co., Philadelphia.)

tion of the cornea due to incomplete closure of the eyes while the patient is sleeping, which lets the epithelial surfaces of the eyes become dry, irritated and eventually infected.

Treatment and Nursing Care. Hyperthyroidism may be treated by conservative medical methods or it may be treated surgically, depending on the individual case and the response of the disease to conservative measures.

Physical and mental rest are of extreme importance because of the relationship between physical stress or emotional upset and increased activity of the thyroid gland. Rest also helps to conserve the strength of the patient.

The diet of the hyperthyroid individual is based on his metabolic needs. If his metabolic rate is very high he must eat enough to compensate for this so that he will have sufficient energy to carry on his daily activities. The diet is high in carbohydrates, which we know are good sources of quick energy, high in vitamins, and high in calories. The patient will need to receive instruction in the particular foods which will meet his dietary requirements, and should be encouraged to substitute those foods for others less beneficial to him.

There are several drugs available which temporarily inhibit the release of thyroxine. These drugs greatly reduce the symptoms of hyperthyroidism and in many instances eliminate the need for hospitalization and surgical treatment.

Lugol's solution and potassium iodide are both examples of iodine preparations which temporarily inhibit the release of thyroxine. Another drug called *propylthiouracil* also blocks the release of thyroxine.

In recent years *radioactive iodine* has been given to reduce the size and activity of the thyroid gland. Those on the nursing staff who must constantly handle the drug need to take radium precautions, but the patient is not exposed to enough radiation to cause concern. Radioactive iodine is excreted in the urine and the patient must be instructed to dispose of the urine promptly if he is receiving this drug as an out-patient. In the hospital, the nursing staff should use caution in handling the bedpans and urinals and quickly dispose of the urine of all patients receiving radioactive iodine.

The surgical removal of the thyroid gland is called a *thyroidectomy*. If a malignancy of the gland is diagnosed the entire gland is removed. In other cases, such as unsightly simple goiter, or highly toxic goiters, only a portion of the gland is removed and the remaining portion continues to secrete thyroxine. Thyroidectomies are not as common as they formerly were because the newer antithyroid drugs have made medical control of hyperthyroidism more successful.

PREOPERATIVE NURSING CARE. The preoperative nursing care of the patient having a thyroidectomy is much less difficult than it was before the antithyroid drugs became available. Most patients who enter the hospital for this type of surgery are much calmer emotionally and less active physically than formerly because they have received medications to stabilize the activity of the gland.

Whereas the practice of "stealing a thyroid" used to be a common occurrence so that the patient would not be unduly upset by surgery, the patients today usually know the exact day and hour of surgery and the type of surgery to be done. The responsibility of the nurse for preparation of the patient who is to have a thyroidectomy is essentially the same as for other types of major surgery. If the patient does appear nervous, tense and apprehensive, his condition should be reported to the physician. These symptoms may indicate improper control of the activities of the thyroid gland and may predispose the patient to the postoperative complication of "thyroid crisis" (see below).

POSTOPERATIVE NURSING CARE. As soon as the patient returns from the operating room he is placed in *high Fowler's* position to facilitate breathing and reduce swelling of the operative area. The head may be supported with sandbags on either side to relieve tension on the sutures.

Close observation of the patient is an essential part of postoperative care. The vital signs are checked at frequent intervals and the patient is watched closely for signs of bleeding and swelling of the operative area. Any rise in the temperature, pulse, or respiration rate should be reported when first noticed since they may indicate a high level of thyroxine in the blood stream. External swelling may cause constriction of the bandage around the neck. Difficulty in swallowing or breathing should also be reported immediately as they may indicate internal edema and pressure on the esophagus and trachea. In many hospitals a tracheostomy set is kept at the bedside of the postoperative thyroidectomy patient in case severe respiratory embarrassment develops. Persistent hoarseness or loss of the voice are other symptoms to be reported as they may indicate damage to the vocal cords.

Tetany and *thyroid crisis* are other complications of a thyroidectomy which may occur. These complications are rare, but when they do occur the surgeon expects the nurse to be alert for the beginning signs and report her observations immediately.

Tetany is actually a symptom and results from injury to, or accidental removal of, the parathyroid glands. These small glands are located on the posterior surface of the thyroid gland. *Parathormone* is secreted by the parathyroid glands and is important in the regulation of the calcium and phosphorus level in the body tissues. A deficiency of this hormone produces muscle cramps, twitching of the muscles, and in some cases severe convulsions.

This complication is treated by the administration of calcium intravenously during the emergency stage, and subsequent maintenance doses of parathyroid hormone to maintain the proper calcium and phosphorus balance in the body.

Thyroid crisis, sometimes called *thyroid storm*, is another complication to be considered following a thyroidectomy. The condition is caused by a sudden increase in the output of thyroxine due to manipulation of the thyroid as it is being removed. Another cause may be improper reduction of thyroid secretions before surgery (see Preoperative Nursing Care).

The symptoms of thyroid crisis are produced by a sudden and extreme elevation of all the body processes. The temperature may rise to 106° or more, the pulse increases to as much as 200 beats per minute, respirations become rapid, and the patient exhibits marked apprehension and restlessness. Unless the condition is relieved, the patient quickly passes from delirium to coma to death from heart failure.

Treatment of thyroid crisis must be begun immediately after the first symptoms are noticed. Measures are employed to reduce the temperature,

cardiac drugs are given to slow the heart beat, and sedatives, such as one of the barbiturates, are given to reduce restlessness and anxiety.

Hypothyroidism

Definition. Underactivity of the thyroid gland with a deficiency in the production of the hormone thyroxine is called hypothyroidism. The symptoms vary according to the age at which the disease presents itself. In young children the condition is called *cretinism*, whereas if the disease develops in adulthood the condition is called *myxedema*.

Symptoms. The child who has a deficiency in thyroxine has retarded physical and mental growth and development. Adults who have myxedema have a decrease in appetite but an increase in weight gain. In both children and adults there is a tendency to sleep for long periods of time, the speech is slurred, and the individual is very sluggish in his mental and physical activities. The skin is dry and scaly and the patient often complains of increased sensitivity to cold.

Treatment. Hypothyroidism is successfully treated with the administration of thyroid extract. The dosage is gradually increased until a proper level has been reached and then a delicate balance must be maintained so that the patient does not suffer from either hypothyroidism or hyperthyroidism.

The results of treatment of hypothyroidism are very striking and most patients show a remarkable abatement of their symptoms. The practical nurse may not see many cases of hypothyroidism in the hospital because treatment usually does not require hospitalization. If the patient is admitted for some other condition of illness and is also being treated for hypothyroidism, some special considerations must be made. As stated above, these patients have very rough and dry skin and they will need massage with lotions and creams to prevent cracking and peeling of the skin. Provisions for extra warmth must also be made for those patients who have an increased sensitivity to cold as a result of their hypothyroidism.

The nurse must also bear in mind the psychological aspects of hypothyroidism. She must avoid rushing these patients or giving them the impression that she is annoyed and inconvenienced by their sluggishness. Forgetfulness, inability to express themselves vocally, and physical inertia are mannerisms which are a direct result of the deficiency in thyroxine and the nurse must recognize them as unavoidable and embarrassing to the patient as he struggles to overcome his handicap.

DISORDERS OF THE PARATHYROIDS

Introduction. The parathyroid glands, usually four in number, are located on the posterior aspect of the thyroid gland. The parathyroid hormone exerts an important regulating effect on the calcium and phosphorus concentration of body fluids. In general, the parathyroid hormone depresses the concentration of phosphorus, and increases the concentration of calcium in the blood by removing the calcium from the bones so that it circulates in the blood stream.

In order to understand the disorders produced by malfunctioning parathyroid glands one must be familiar with the metabolism of calcium and phosphorus. Calcium is important to four main functions of the body: bone formation, blood clotting, maintenance of normal cell permeability so that nutrients may enter and waste products may leave and proper conduction of nerve impulses to and from the muscles. Phosphorus also is essential to bone formation and to the metabolism of carbohydrates and proteins.

Hypoparathyroidism (Tetany)

Definition. Hypoparathyroidism is a deficiency of the parathyroid hormone. It sometimes is seen following thyroidectomy when too much of the parathyroid tissue is accidentally removed. It also can occur with idiopathic atrophy of the parathyroid glands.

Symptoms. A deficiency of the parathyroid hormone is accompanied by a drop in the level of calcium in the blood and an increase in the phosphorus level. The chief symptom occurring as a result of the lowered calcium level is *tetany*. Muscular twitching and spasms occur due to extreme irritability of the muscular tissue. If the calcium level continues to fall the patient will suffer from severe convulsions and spasms of the larynx.

Treatment. Acute hypoparathyroidism is treated by oral or parenteral administration of calcium salts. In chronic hypoparathyroidism treatment is aimed at restoring and maintaining normal calcium levels in the blood. This can be accomplished by injections of parathyroid extract, vitamin D in massive doses to enhance the absorption of calcium by the small intestine, and oral administration of calcium salts.

Hyperparathyroidism (von Recklinghausen's Disease)

Definition. Excessive secretion of the parathyroid hormone is due to an overgrowth of the parathyroid glands. It also can occur in a patient with chronic nephritis. High levels of parathyroid hormone in the blood leads to removal of calcium from the bones (*decalcification*) and accumulation of this mineral in the blood (*hypercalcemia*). The calcium is then precipitated in the kidney where it brings about the formation of kidney stones.

Symptoms. Hyperparathyroidism is characterized by fatigue, muscular weakness, formation of kidney stones and changes in the skeletal system. The bones become tender and painful and are easily fractured or deformed.

Treatment. The condition is treated

by surgical removal of the excess glandular tissue so that sufficient parathyroid tissue is left to maintain a normal calcium and phosphorus level.

DISEASES OF CARBOHYDRATE METABOLISM

Introduction. When carbohydrates are taken into the body they are converted into simple sugars which can readily be absorbed into the blood stream. Some of the sugar remains in the blood stream as glucose so that it is available when needed for energy. The excess sugar is carried to the liver where it is stored as glycogen. When a demand for more energy arises, the liver reconverts the glycogen into glucose and releases it into the blood stream so that it can be carried to the muscles and other body tissues. In order for this process to take place the hormone *insulin* is necessary. Insulin is secreted by the *islets of Langerhans*, which are located on the surface of the pancreas.

An excess of insulin leads to a condition called *hypoglycemia* (low blood sugar). A deficiency in the supply of insulin or interference with the normal physiologic action of insulin results in a condition known as *diabetes mellitus.*

Special Diagnostic Tests and Examinations. URINALYSIS. Sugar is not present in the urine of a normal individual. When it is found in the urine this is an indication of a high level of sugar in the blood because excess blood sugar is spilled over into the urine.

Many unsuspected cases of diabetes mellitus have been discovered when a routine urinalysis was done as a part of a physical examination.

The testing of urine for sugar is now a relatively simple matter and most diabetics check their own urine at home after they have been discharged from the hospital.

BLOOD SUGAR. There is always a certain amount of sugar in the blood of a normal person (80 to 120 mg. of sugar per 100 ml. of blood). This sugar is constantly being used for the production of energy to carry on the daily activities of the body. However, an increase in the blood sugar level indicates a disorder of glucose metabolism. A high level of blood sugar is found in diabetes, in chronic liver disease, and in overactivity of some of the endocrine glands.

GLUCOSE TOLERANCE. All starches and sugars taken into the body must be eventually reduced to glucose before they can be absorbed into the blood stream and utilized by the body tissues for food and energy. When diabetes is suspected the physician orders a glucose tolerance test to determine the patient's ability to utilize glucose.

In this test a "fasting blood sugar" and urinalysis are done first and then the patient is given a solution of glucose to drink. Samples of urine and blood are taken later at regular intervals to determine their level of glucose. A normal individual's blood sugar will drop back to normal levels within 2 hours. A diabetic's blood sugar will remain high.

Diabetes Mellitus

Definition. Diabetes is a disease which results from an inability of the body to use and store carbohydrates in a normal manner. Even though insulin is necessary for the proper usage of carbohydrates, recent investigations have shown that other endocrine glands and their hormones may play some part in the development of the symptoms of diabetes.

The exact cause of diabetes is not known. However, there are at least four factors which may contribute to the development of this disease. These are:

1. There may be an inability to produce

enough insulin because the pancreas is diseased or absent.

2. There may be an increase in the rate at which the body uses up insulin. This may be caused by overeating or by overactivity of the thyroid gland. Where this creates an insulin shortage, diabetes results.

3. There may be an increase in the rate at which insulin is destroyed in the body. It has been shown that the liver and other tissues contain an enzyme *insulinase* which can inactivate insulin.

4. There may be a drop in the efficiency of insulin due to liver disease or the introduction into the system of certain chemicals which impede insulin activity.[5]

Statistics indicate that from 20 to 50 percent of all diabetic individuals have a positive history of diabetes in the family. Authorities classify the trait as mendelian recessive. When a diabetic marries a nondiabetic who is not a carrier of the trait, none of their children will have diabetes but all will be carriers. If two diabetics marry, all of their children will become diabetic eventually.

In older persons heredity may be a predisposing factor rather than a direct cause of diabetes. In these persons there seems to be a condition resulting from "using up" all the insulin the islets of Langerhans can produce and the cells seem no longer capable of secreting sufficient insulin. Elderly diabetics usually have a less severe form of the disease than do younger persons and they are less likely to develop keto-acidosis (diabetic coma). The vascular problems due to atherosclerosis are a common problem in the older diabetic.

Until the discovery of insulin many diabetics who developed the disease in early childhood did not live to reach child-bearing age. Now that the disease can be controlled, and diabetics are able to marry and have children, we can expect the incidence of diabetes to increase. At present it is believed that there are more than one and a half million people in the United States who are known to have diabetes and probably as many more who have not yet been diagnosed as having the disease.[16]

There are four groups of people who are most susceptible to diabetes: those who are over 40 years of age, those who are overweight, women, and those who have had diabetes in their family. Anyone fitting into any of these four categories should be tested for early signs of diabetes at least once a year.

Symptoms. The elevation of the blood sugar level and the presence of sugar in the urine are the two most outstanding symptoms of diabetes. These are found only by special laboratory work, however, and are not apparent to the individual who has not yet sought medical attention. Other warning signals which a person may recognize as symptoms of illness are also present in diabetes. These symptoms are known as the three "polys": *polyuria* (increased urinary output), *polydipsia* (excessive thirst), and *polyphagia* (an increase in appetite).

Fatigue and muscular weakness, pruritus, and numbness and tingling of the hands and feet are also symptoms of diabetes.

Treatment and Nursing Care. The treatment of diabetes must continue as long as the patient lives, and demands his complete cooperation with the physician. For this reason, education of the patient is a very important aspect of the treatment.

Diabetes is never *cured* in the true sense of the word, but it may be controlled by diet and the administration of insulin according to the needs of each individual patient. There are also several systemic complications which may result from an excessive amount of sugar in the blood and these must be diligently guarded against throughout the life of the patient.

According to the American Diabetes Association a person's diabetes is well controlled when:

1. The person feels well.

2. He maintains normal weight on a well-balanced diet.

3. His urine tests are usually negative.

4. His blood sugar tests are usually normal.

As long as a diabetic can meet these four requirements and follows his doctor's orders faithfully he need not worry about the progress of his disease or the development of complications.

DIET. The diet of the diabetic must be calculated on an individual basis. The amount of physical activity performed, the usual amount of food the individual eats, and the severity of his disease are some of the factors to be considered. Some physicians require accurate weighing and measuring of each gram of food on the diet, while others prefer to give the diabetic an exchange list of foods and allow the patient to restrict his diet accordingly.

Although the calculation of a diabetic diet seems to be confusing and extremely difficult at first, it should be remembered that such a diet is actually only a modification of a normal diet. *If the principles of basic nutrition are thoroughly understood,* the exchange of certain foods for others less rich in carbohydrates becomes a relatively simple matter.

The American Diabetes Association and the American Dietetic Association have worked together to devise a simplified method of calculating a diabetic diet and planning a diabetic's meals. The booklet in which this information is published is entitled "Meal Planning with Exchange Lists." The principal foods are divided into six groups: milk, vegetables, fruits, breads, meats and fat. Each group contains foods that are similar in kind and have equal nutritional value in regard to carbohydrate, protein and fat. For example, more than 20 fruits from which the diabetic can choose are listed, each providing 10 Gm. of carbohydrate, a negligible amount of protein and fat, and 40 calories per serving. Other lists contain similar information for a great variety of foods. With this simple method of choosing a menu from the exchange lists a diabetic or a member of his family can calculate the caloric value and nutritional value with ease.

The nurse as well as the patient must not develop a defeatist and negative attitude toward the diabetic diet. The word "restriction" should be avoided because it implies a great inconvenience and limiting of the patient's choice. This is not actually the case. There are, after all, only three food constituents which supply calories: carbohydrates, proteins, and fats. Of these three, carbohydrates are most likely to create problems for the diabetic. Thus, foods such as sugar, which contains only carbohydrate, and starches, which are very high in carbohydrate content, must be replaced by foods which contain many food constituents and a low percentage of carbohydrate.

In his choice of foods the diabetic must simply be a bit snobbish; "just anything to eat" won't do. He must have the best of foods to eat. This, of course, is an attitude even the nondiabetic would do well to develop.

In order to help the diabetic and his family learn which foods he should eat and those he should avoid, the physician, the dietitian, and the nurse must all participate in the instruction. Fortunately, there are available many well-written and clearly illustrated booklets and pamphlets which are most helpful to the diabetic and his family. Such organizations as the American Diabetes Association* and the American Medical Association† will send instructive material on request. This material not only covers diets, but also warns the diabetic against misleading or fraudulent information in regard to quick "cures" or special diets which will cure diabetes.

---

*Address: 18 E. 48 St., New York 10017.
†Address: 535 North Dearborn Street, Chicago, Ill. 60611.

ADMINISTRATION OF INSULIN. There are some individuals who cannot control their diabetes with diet alone. This is especially true of children who have developed diabetes at an early age, and older diabetics with a moderate or severe case of diabetes. In these cases exogenous insulin prepared by a pharmaceutical firm must be administered parenterally at regular intervals so that the body's metabolic processes can function normally. Exogenous insulin is a liquid hormonal preparation obtained from the pancreas of animals. Insulin was first discovered in 1921 by Sir Frederick G. Banting and Dr. Charles H. Best. This was plain insulin and is known today as *regular insulin.* This type of insulin will last in the body only 6 to 8 hours (see Table 22).

In 1936 a Danish physician, Dr. Hagedorn, discovered that by adding a protein *(protamine)* to insulin its action could be prolonged to a period of 12 hours. It was later found that by adding *zinc* to the protamine, insulin blood sugar levels could be controlled for as long as 24 hours with a single injection. This combination of protamine, zinc and insulin is known as *protamine zinc insulin* or *PZI.*

The discovery of this long-acting insulin eliminated the need for several daily injections of regular insulin, but it did not prove to be ideal for those who had moderately severe or severe diabetes. In these cases it was still necessary for the patient to take regular insulin in order to augment the action of the PZI.

The development of an intermediate-acting insulin which would strike a happy medium and reach its peak of action at some time between that of the fast-acting regular insulin and the long-acting PZI came only after much research and study. The first to be used was *globin* insulin and later NPH insulin and *lente* insulin were finally developed.

PZI, NPH and lente insulin are all cloudy and milky in appearance and must be thoroughly mixed before they are administered, so that the proper proportions of the crystals are given. This is done by *gently rolling* the bottle between the palms of the hands. The bottle is *not shaken* because this produces air bubbles in the solution which may alter the dosage being given.

Insulin is always measured in units. U-40 means that there are 40 units of insulin per milliliter, U-80 means that there are 80 units per milliliter. A specially marked insulin syringe must be used when administering insulin so that there will be no error in the calculation of the dosage.

The diagnosis of diabetes is usually definitely established by laboratory tests requiring admission to the hospital. Thus, an individual learns he is a diabetic while he is a patient in the hospital. When the physician feels that the patient is ready to accept the fact that he is a diabetic he may ask the nurse in

Table 22. *Types of Insulin*

TYPE OF INSULIN	APPEARANCE	ACTION BEGINS	PEAK OF ACTION	ACTION LASTS
Regular	Clear	30 minutes to 1 hour	2 to 3 hours	6 to 8 hours
Globin Zinc	Amber	2 hours	8 hours	24 hours
Protamine Zinc	Cloudy	4 to 6 hours	12 to 24 hours	48 hours
N P H	Cloudy	4 hours	8 to 12 hours	28 to 30 hours
Lente	Cloudy	1 to 2 hours	8 to 12 hours	28 to 30 hours

charge to instruct the patient in self-administration of insulin. It is natural that there will be some resistance from the patient at first and some individuals never can bring themselves to the point of actually sticking a needle in their own skin. The practical nurse and all other members of the nursing staff must appreciate the patient's feeling in this matter and offer sympathetic encouragement and understanding. If the patient flatly refuses to learn to give his own insulin, or is physically unable to do so, a member of the family is taught to give the injections under supervision before the patient is discharged from the hospital. Rotation of sites for insulin injections is necessary to avoid irritation and assure absorption (see Fig. 16-2).

The diabetic or a member of his family must also learn to test the urine for sugar and acetone, and to give insulin according to the amount of sugar present.

SYNTHETIC HYPOGLYCEMIC AGENTS. All types of insulin must be given by injection. There are, to date, no insulin pills, capsules or liquids that can be taken by mouth. In recent years at least three new drugs have been developed which act to lower the blood sugar. These drugs are rather limited in their usefulness because they do not take the place of insulin in the body and are effective only in older patients who have a relatively stable, nonketotic type of diabetes. They are of no value in a patient with ketosis or in diabetic acidosis.

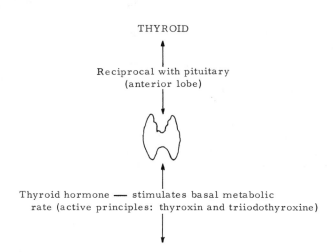

THYROID

Reciprocal with pituitary
(anterior lobe)

Thyroid hormone — stimulates basal metabolic
rate (active principles: thyroxin and triiodothyroxine)

Drug therapy: Used to stimulate basal metabolic
activity and to treat many conditions

For stimulation or substitution:
Thyroid extract, U.S.P.
Refined thyroid, U.S.P
Thyroxin, U.S.P.
Sodium liothyronine, U.S.P. (Cytomel)
Sodium levothyroxine, U.S.P. (Synthroid

To depress activity of gland:

Strong iodine sol., U.S.P.
Sodium iodide, U.S.P.
Potassium iodide, U.S.P.
Sodium radioiodide sol., U.S.P.
    tracer — 1-100 microcuries
    therapy — 1-100 millicuries
Thiouracil
Propylthiouracil
Methylthiouracil (Methiacil,
    Muracil, Thimecil)
Iothiouracil sodium (Itrumil)
Methimazole, U.S.P. (Tapazole)
Carbimazole

Figure 16-2. Endocrine system in relation to drug therapy. (From Falconer, Norman, Patterson and Gustafson: *The Drug, The Nurse, The Patient,* 3rd Ed., W. B. Saunders Co., Philadelphia.)

Tolbutamide (Orinase) is a sulfonamide derivative. It reaches its peak in 5 to 8 hours and is very rapidly excreted. *Chlorpropamide* (Diabinese) reaches its peak in about four hours and is less rapidly excreted. Both of these drugs require that the diabetic have at least a small amount of insulin production. *Phenformin* (DBI) is another hypoglycemic agent that sometimes is used in the treatment of juvenile diabetes but it does not take the place of insulin.

All hypoglycemic agents are capable of producing gastric irritation with nausea, vomiting and diarrhea. There also may be liver damage with jaundice, bone marrow depression, or an allergic reaction. All patients taking one of these drugs should be informed of the early symptoms of hypoglycemia (drowsiness, nausea and deep breathing) because these drugs can produce hypoglycemic shock very rapidly.

PREVENTION OF COMPLICATIONS. The diabetic is subject to a variety of complications. These may be the result of an extreme elevation in blood sugar, too much insulin, or gradual changes within the blood vessels and other tissues.

The proper balance of glucose and insulin in the body may be compared to a scale. As long as there are equal parts on either side of the scale there will be an even balance. In normal individuals this balance is maintained, but in a diabetic the balance may be easily upset by failing to follow his diet, administering himself too much insulin, or an infection or other illness which may increase the need for insulin in the body.

Too much glucose may produce a condition known as *diabetic coma*, and too much insulin may produce *insulin shock*. Both of these conditions may be found as complications of diabetes.

Table 23 describes the symptoms of diabetic coma as opposed to insulin reaction. In studying these symptoms the reader must remember that each person reacts differently in a given situation and not all of the symptoms

Table 23.   *Symptoms of Diabetic Coma and Insulin Reaction*

DIABETIC COMA	INSULIN REACTION
Gradual onset, may be more rapid in active children	Sudden onset, begins abruptly
Skin hot and dry, face may be flushed.	Perspiration, skin pale, cold and clammy
Deep, labored breathing	Shallow breathing
Nausea	Hunger
Drowsiness and lethargy	Mental confusion, strange behavior, nervousness
Fruity odor to breath	Double vision
Loss of consciousness	Loss of consciousness, convulsions (rarely)
Urine contains much sugar	There may be sugar in the urine, depending on the type of insulin and when it was taken
Blood sugar high	Blood sugar low

will be present in every case. Some of the symptoms may be entirely absent and some may not be as obvious as others.

The patient with diabetic acidosis must have immediate treatment or the condition can be fatal. He is given insulin, glucose and water intravenously in doses calculated according to his current blood sugar level and urinalysis. The urinalysis is done on an hourly basis until the diabetic acidosis is brought under control.

A mild insulin reaction may be relieved by a glass of orange juice or some other source of simple sugars. Severe insulin shock requires intensive treatment to prevent circulatory collapse. Glucose is often administered intravenously. The amount of glucose given is also calculated according to the patient's current urinalysis for sugar and his blood sugar level.

Diabetic coma, also called ketoacidosis or diabetic acidosis, is the result of a complicated chemical derangement in the body due to metabolic disturbances. When the body is unable to utilize carbohydrate for energy it resorts to the metabolism of fat for its energy source. In diabetes, the amount of insulin is insufficient for proper carbohydrate metabolism, and so large amounts of fatty acids are removed from the body's adipose tissue to supply energy. The liver then breaks down these fatty acids into acetoacetic acid which accumulates in the blood and body tissues because the cells cannot handle it as rapidly as the liver produces it. This acid and two other chemicals into which it is converted are called *ketone bodies*. One of these chemicals is acetone, a highly volatile substance that causes a sweet, fruit-like odor to the breath in patients with metabolic acidosis. As the ketone bodies (two of which are acid) collect in the body fluids they upset the normal acid-base balance and the patient is said to be in *acidosis*. The ketoacids are excreted by the kidneys, and that is why a diabetic's urine is tested for

acetone when ketoacidosis is suspected or likely to develop.

The person who has diabetes cannot always control his mealtime or emotional crises in his life any more than anyone else. He may be delayed by traffic or miss his train home after work and wait an hour or two for the next one. Or a death or sudden financial loss may cause him to become emotionally upset. Missing a meal can easily result in insulin reaction if the diabetic is taking an intermediate or long-acting insulin, and a sudden emotional upset may use up all available glucose and result in a drastic lowering of the blood sugar.

If the diabetic is alone and away from home at the time he suffers from insulin reaction or diabetic acidosis his condition may be mistaken for drunkenness or mental derangement. To avoid confusion and delay in obtaining medical attention all diabetics should carry an identification card (see Fig. 16-3), or wear an identification bracelet stating that he is a diabetic. Several drug companies as well as the American Diabetes Association have these cards available and will mail them upon request.

Other complications of diabetes arise from the fact that diabetics have a tendency to develop *arteriosclerosis*. The arteries which may be affected are the peripheral blood vessels, the vessels serving the kidney, and those serving the heart. In view of this, it is obvious that such complications may easily lead to serious illnesses and even death.

The lower extremities of the diabetic are particularly susceptible to disturbances arising from poor circulation. That is why amputations of the lower limbs are a relatively common occurrence in many diabetics, especially those who have difficulty keeping the diabetes under control and their blood sugar level low.

Exercises and special care of the feet and legs as discussed previously under diseases of the peripheral vessels (p. 249)

Figure 16-3. Front and back of identification card. This type of identification is recommended for all persons who have diabetes or some other type of chronic disease, or a serious allergy to certain drugs.

are essential in the prevention of complications arising from poor circulation of the lower limbs of the diabetic (see Fig. 16-4).

In addition to poor circulation, the diabetic also has an impaired resistance to infection. This situation demands meticulous care of the skin and careful attention to breaks in the skin through which bacteria may enter and cause an infection. It is believed that the high level of sugar in the blood provides an excellent breeding ground for bacteria and they multiply much more rapidly in a diabetic than in a normal individual.

A slight cold or minor infection will also increase the need for insulin as the body speeds up its metabolism to fight the infection. The diabetic should know and understand this so that he will be prepared for an elevation of blood sugar and an increased need for insulin while he has an infection. He should be advised to notify his physician at once should an infection develop so that plans can be made for increasing the dosage of insulin when necessary.

Every nurse should appreciate the value of good habits of personal hygiene and recognize them as essential to the health of everyone. High standards of personal hygiene are even more important to the diabetic because they may mean the difference between life and death for him. He cannot afford to be careless in matters of cleanliness or fail to avoid extremes in eating, physical activities and exposure to infections. Every person who takes insulin must establish a regular pattern for meals, rest, work, and play so that the amount of insulin available in the body at a given time will be in balance with the amount of sugar present. Physical exhaustion, emotional upsets, or worry and anxiety can use up the supply of glucose in the blood and decrease the need for insulin.

Changes in vision are often associated with diabetes. These changes may be caused by a *retinitis* or by the formation of cataracts. Regular visits to an eye specialist are necessary so that early changes in vision may be discovered and treatment begun before there is a serious loss of sight. Many visual disturbances are relieved when the diabetes is brought under control and the blood sugar lowered.

HYPOGLYCEMIA

Introduction. The term hypoglycemia refers to an abnormally low level of glucose in the circulating blood. The patient with this condition utilizes the available glucose in his blood at a very rapid rate causing his blood sugar to drop to a seriously low level within a few hours after he has eaten a meal or after exercise.

In most cases of chronic hypoglycemia there is no known cause. In others the condition can be traced to a tumor

CARE OF FEET IN DIABETES
1. Keep feet clean
   Dry thoroughly after washing.

2. Cut toenails frequently
   They should be cut
   straight across.

3. Wear properly fitting shoes.

Corns grow from pressure
by shoes that are too tight.
Relieve the pressure.

4. Avoid constricting
   the circulation.

5. Avoid burning or freezing, bruising or cutting the feet.
6. Report any sore anywhere, but especially one on the
   foot that fails to heal.

Figure 16-4. The care of the feet in diabetes. (From Dowling and Jones: *That the Patient May Know,* W. B. Saunders Co., Philadelphia.)

of the pancreas, liver disease or a disorder of the pituitary gland or the adrenal glands.

Symptoms. The patient with hypoglycemia has a limited supply of glucose available for energy, so he feels weak and faint, appears pale and may have slight tremors. These symptoms are familiar to all of us who have, for some reason, gone too long without an adequate intake of food. If hypoglycemia becomes severe there may be excessive perspiration, convulsions and coma. Many times the symptoms can be relieved temporarily by eating a carbohydrate food such as candy or by drinking a sweetened fruit juice.

Treatment. There is no cure for hypoglycemia when the basic cause is unknown. It can be controlled by diet and limiting of strenuous physical exercise to periods when glucose is readily available. The patient should eat regularly spaced meals that are high in protein. The body converts carbohydrates to glucose quite readily but proteins are utilized more gradually and a high protein diet is more likely to supply a more constant source of energy. Most physicians instruct hypoglycemic patients to carry candy or sugar with them at all times so that they can have a source of quick energy available in case they experience weakness and faintness.

DISORDERS OF THE ADRENAL GLANDS

Introduction. The adrenal glands are composed of two distinct parts, neither of which apparently has any direct functional relationship with the other. The *adrenal medulla* (middle portion) secretes two hormones, *epinephrine* and *norepinephrine.* These substances are secreted in response to stimulation from the sympathetic nervous system and their effects are, in turn, almost the same as direct stimulation of the sympathetic nerves. Epinephrine prepares

the body to meet stress or emergency situations and prevents hypoglycemia. Norepinephrine functions as a pressor hormone to maintain blood pressure.

The *adrenal cortex* (outer covering) secretes two major types of hormones, the *mineralocorticoids* and the *glucocorticoids.* It also secretes small amounts of *androgenic hormones,* which have effects similar to the male and female sex hormones. Normally the androgenic hormones have very little effect in comparison to the sex hormones secreted by the gonads, but in some abnormalities of the adrenal cortex such large amounts of androgenic hormones are poured into the blood stream that they can present symptoms of sexual changes in the patient.

The mineralocorticoids and glucocorticoids are so named because of the effects they have on the body. The mineralocorticoids affect the electrolytes, particularly sodium, potassium and chloride. Without the mineralocorticoids an individual would die within three to seven days, because these hormones directly control fluid balance, blood volume, cardiac output, exchange of nutrients and wastes in each cell, and in effect, all chemical processes and glandular functions within the body. Little wonder that they are said to be "life-saving hormones." The glucocorticoids are almost equally important because they are essential to the metabolic systems for proper utilization of carbohydrates, proteins and fats.

Addison's Disease (Hypoadrenalism)

Definition. This disease is a result of *underactivity* of the adrenal cortex. It can be caused by an inflammation, infection, or tumor of the adrenal gland which interferes with the production of secretions from the gland.

Symptoms. The symptoms in the early stages of Addison's disease are so vague they often are considered to be annoying, but not serious enough to consult a physician. These symptoms include malaise, chronic fatigue, irritability, and loss of weight. Pigmentation of the skin and mucous membranes develops later and gives the skin a brownish, "tanned" appearance. Nausea and vomiting appear and become increasingly persistent and the patient may eventually collapse with dehydration and circulatory failure.

Treatment and Nursing Care. Treatment of Addison's disease consists of replacement of the adrenal hormones lacking in the body. *Cortisone* is given in regular doses to maintain a proper level. Cortisone may be given as often as two to three times daily. Hydrocortisone, prednisone or prednisolone also may be used.

Infections are likely to increase the need for adrenal hormones just as they increase the need for insulin in a diabetic. Moderation in all activities and habits of good personal hygiene are as essential for the person with Addison's disease as they are for those suffering from diabetes.

Those who have Addison's disease should carry an identification card or wear an identification bracelet in the event they become ill from an acute episode while away from home. Such acute flare-ups may occur from failure to take the hormones regularly as ordered, or from some physical or mental stress. During this acute stage the patient may die from circulatory collapse and shock if treatment is not begun immediately.

Cushing's Syndrome (Hyperadrenalism)

Definition. This disease is a result of an *increased* production of hormones from the adrenal cortex. It may be caused by a tumor or other disease of the adrenal gland or it may result from overstimulation of the adrenal glands by the pituitary gland.

Symptoms. The person with Cushing's syndrome has a wide variety of symptoms too numerous to mention here. Briefly it may be stated that the condition is characterized by a typical "moon" face, muscular weakness, abnormal sexual development, and some mental disturbances.

Treatment and Nursing Care. Treatment is usually based on the primary condition causing the increase in production of the hormones. But this is not always a simple matter and in some cases the cause cannot be found. Supportive treatment consists of administration of potassium chloride by mouth and measures which will improve the patient's general physical health and mental stability.

While potassium is being given the nurse must keep an accurate record of the patient's intake and output. A low-sodium, high-potassium diet may be ordered as a means of maintaining the proper balance of these salts in the body.

Severe mental depression is often present and the nursing staff must be alert for indications that the patient is contemplating suicide.

Surgical removal of the adrenal gland (adrenalectomy) may be carried out if other measures fail to relieve the symptoms of the disease. The surgeon leaves only an appropriate amount of adrenal cortical tissue so that normal function can be maintained.

PHEOCHROMOCYTOMA

Definition. This is a relatively rare tumor that usually is located in the adrenal medulla but occasionally occurs in other chromaffin tissues of the sympathoadrenal system. It causes an increased secretion of epinephrine and norepinephrine which in turn produces hypertension, severe headache, visual disturbances and tachycardia.

There is a test, called the Regitine test, that is specifically used for diagnosis of pheochromocytoma. The drug Regitine neutralizes the effect of epinephrine. If the blood pressure drops when the drug is administered, the presence of the tumor is strongly suspected.

Treatment of pheochromocytoma involves surgical removal of the tumor. During the postoperative period the patient must be watched closely for extreme fluctuations in blood pressure. Although pheochromocytoma can be fatal, surgical treatment is usually successful and the patient can be cured if there has been no damage to the cardiovascular system.

DISORDERS OF THE PITUITARY GLAND

Introduction. The pituitary gland (*hypophysis*) lies at the base of the brain and is connected with the hypothalamus by the hypophyseal stalk. It is only 1 cm. in diameter but is a key organ because it influences all systems and organs of the body. The hypophysis is divided into two distinct portions: the anterior pituitary, known as the *adenohypophysis,* and the posterior pituitary gland, known as the *neurohypophysis.* The adenohyseal hormones and their functions are presented in Table 21. One can readily see that hypofunction or hyperfunction of the gland can produce a variety of symptoms, depending on the particular organs involved.

Adenohypophysis

Gigantism. This condition results when hyperplasia or tumors of the adenohypophysis occur during the rapid growth before adolescence. Because there is overproduction of the growth hormone (somatropin) at a time when the epiphyses of the long bones have not become fused with the shafts, the bones lengthen very rapidly and gigantism develops. The patient also may have diabetes mellitus as a result of overstimulation and eventual degeneration of the islets of Langerhans on the pancreas. Treatment involves irradiation of the hypophysis to reduce hormonal secretion. This is accomplished by insertion of a radioactive needle directly into the tumor or excessive glandular tissue.

Acromegaly. When there is an excessive secretion of the growth hormone after adolescence, the soft tissues continue to grow and the bones grow thicker but not longer. In this situation the disorder is called acromegaly. Enlargement is especially marked in the bones of the cranium, lower jaw, hands and feet. It also involves soft tissue such as that of the tongue and liver, which become greatly enlarged. Treatment usually is irradiation of the hypophysis in a manner similar to that used for gigantism. This reduces the secretion of hormones, but nothing can be done about the enlargement that has already taken place in the bones and soft tissues.

Dwarfism. Some types of dwarfism occur when there is undersecretion of the adenohypophyseal hormones. In one type, called the Lorain type, the condition is present at birth and, though the features of the body develop in proportion to one another, the rate of growth is much slower than normal. There is no mental retardation in the Lorain type of dwarfism. In other types there may be thyroid deficiency and poor sexual development as well as retarded physical growth.

Panhypopituitarism in the Adult. This condition, also called Simmonds' disease, is very rare. It occurs as a result of tumors, surgical trauma, or thrombosis of the hypophyseal blood vessels. There are three general effects of panhypopituitarism: thyroid deficiency, depressed secretion of adrenal glucocorticoids, and loss of sexual function, due to decreased production of hormones from the gonads which depend on the pituitary gland for stimulation. The patient becomes emaciated, ages prematurely, and loses sexual function. Treatment is by administration of hormones of the glands that depended on the adenohypophysis for stimulation.

Neurohypophysis

Diabetes Insipidus. This condition is characterized by the production of copious amounts of dilute urine, often as much as 15 to 20 liters in every 24-hour period. Diabetes insipidus occurs as a result of decreased production of the antidiuretic hormone (ADH). This hormone regulates reabsorption of water in the kidney tubules. When it is not present in sufficient amounts the water remains in the tubules and is excreted as urine. Restriction of fluid intake does not control the excessive flow of urine and the only satisfactory treatment is administration of posterior pituitary extract (pituitrin) on a regular basis for the rest of the patient's life.

CLINICAL CASE PROBLEMS

1. You are assigned to the evening care of Mrs. Tate, age 33, who had a thyroidectomy early that morning. Mrs. Tate has completely recovered from the anesthesia and has made a good recovery so far.

What precautions must you take in turning and positioning Mrs. Tate? What special observations would you be expected to make while caring for this patient?

2. Mrs. Loomis is 62 years of age and has been a known diabetic for 20 years. She was admitted to the hospital with an infection of the great toe, resulting from improper care of an ingrown toenail. Before admission to the hospital, Mrs. Loomis had been taking Orinase and staying within the limits of her diet. With the development of the infection she began have a 3+ and 4+ sugar with each urinalysis and finally informed her physician of her difficulties only after the infection was well under way.

What complications may develop from Mrs. Loomis' infection? Why are these complications likely to develop and how could Mrs. Loomis have avoided them?

What type of insulin would you expect her to receive while in the hospital?

REFERENCES

1. Beland, I.: *Clinical Nursing.* New York, The Macmillan Co., 1965.
2. Brown, A. F.: *Medical Nursing,* 3rd edition. Philadelphia, W. B. Saunders Co., 1957.
3. Brunner, L. S., et al.: *Medical-Surgical Nursing.* Philadelphia, J. B. Lippincott Co., 1964.
4. DiPalma, J. R.: "Drugs for Diabetes." RN, Oct., 1967, p. 71.
5. Delger, H., and Seeman, B.: *How to Live with Diabetes.* New York, W. W. Norton Co., 1960.
6. French, R. M.: *Nurse's Guide to Diagnostic Procedures,* 2nd edition. New York, McGraw-Hill Book Co., 1967.
7. Guyton, A. C.: *Textbook of Medical Physiology,* 3rd edition. Philadelphia, W. B. Saunders Co., 1966.
8. Jacob, S. W., and Francone, C. A.: *Structure and Function in Man.* Philadelphia, W. B. Saunders Co., 1965.
9. King, B. G., and Showers, M. J.: *Anatomy and Physiology,* 5th edition. Philadelphia, W. B. Saunders Co., 1963.
10. Krensnick, A.: "Diabetic Neuropathy." Am. Journ. Nurs., July, 1964, p. 106.
11. Krysan, M.: "How Do We Teach Four Million Diabetics?" Am. Journ. Nurs., Nov., 1965, p. 510.
12. Martin, M. M.: "Diabetes Mellitus: Current Concepts." Am. Journ. Nurs., Nov., 1965, p. 105.
13. Martin, M. M.: "Insulin Reaction." Am. Journ. Nurs., Jan., 1967, p. 328.
14. Moore, M. L.: "Diabetes in Children." Am. Journ. Nurs., Jan., 1967, p. 104.
15. Nordyke, R. A.: "The Overactive and the Underactive Thyroid." Am. Journ. Nurs., May, 1963, p. 66.
16. Rosenthal, H. and Rosenthal, J.: *Diabetic Care in Pictures,* 3rd edition. Philadelphia, J. B. Lippincott Co., 1967.
17. Shafer, K. N., Sawyer, J. R., et al.: *Medical-Surgical Nursing,* 4th edition. St. Louis, C. V. Mosby Co., 1967.
18. Shea, K. M., et al.: "Teaching a Patient to Live with Adrenal Insufficiency." Am. Journ. Nurs., Dec., 1965, p. 80.
19. Smith, D. W., and Gips, C. D.: *Care of the Adult Patient,* 2nd edition. Philadelphia, J. B. Lippincott Co., 1966.
20. Weller, C.: "Oral Hypoglycemic Agents." Am. Journ. Nurs., March, 1964, p. 90.

SUGGESTED STUDENT READING

1. Caso, E. K., and Youland, D. M.: "An Apple for an Orange." Am. Journ. Nurs., Aug., 1955, p. 942.

2. Cooley, D. G.: "Hormones: Your Body's Chemical Rousers." Today's Health, Nov., 1962, p. 28; December 1962, p. 28.
3. Crosby, A. V.: "Diabetes Mellitus." Practical Nursing, April, 1962, p. 25.
4. DiPalma, J. R.: "Drugs for Diabetes." RN, Oct., 1967, p. 71.
5. Horgan, P. D.: "The Changing Care of Patients with Thyroid Disease." RN, Feb., 1962, p. 50.
6. Hubay, C. A., and Evans, R. D.: "Hyperthyroidism." Am. Journ. Nurs., Oct., 1955, p. 1206.
7. Martin, M. M.: "Detection Is Your Protection." Am. Journ. Nurs., Nov., 1960, p. 1608.
8. Martin, M. M.: "The Unconscious Diabetic Patient." Am. Journ. Nurs., Nov., 1961, p. 92.
9. Martin, M. M.: "Insulin Reaction." Am. Journ. Nurs., Jan., 1967, p. 328.
10. Martin, M. M.: "Foot Disorders in Diabetes." Journ. Pract. Nurs., April, 1967, p. 32.
11. Martin, M. M.: "Insulin, the Life-giving Hormone," Part I, Part II. Journ. Pract. Nurs., March-April, 1968, p. 42.
12. Moss, J. A., and Delawter, D.: "Oral Agents in the Management of Diabetes Mellitus." Am. Journ. Nurs., Nov., 1961, p. 1610.
13. Rodman, M. J.: "Drugs Used in Thyroid Disease." RN, March, 1962, p. 61.
14. Root, H. F., Roehrig, C. B., and Pond, M. R.: "Diabetic Coma: Medical Aspects, Nursing Care." Am. Journ. Nurs., Oct., 1955, p. 1196.

OUTLINE FOR CHAPTER 16

I. Introduction

A. Endocrine system is composed of ductless glands that pour their secretions (hormones) directly into blood stream.

B. Hormones are chemical substances that speed up or slow down activities of the cells of the body.

C. Overactivity or underactivity of a gland may cause disease.

II. Diseases of the Thyroid Gland

A. Special diagnostic tests—basal metabolic rate, radioactive iodine uptake, protein-bound iodine, and cholesterol level.

B. Simple goiter—thyroid enlarged but not oversecreting thyroxine. Caused by deficiency of iodine in the diet.

  1. Symptoms—enlargement of the neck, dysphagia and dyspnea.

  2. Treatment and nursing care—Medications with iodine. Surgical removal of the goiter may be necessary if it is greatly enlarged.

C. Hyperthyroidism—a systemic condition resulting from overactivity of the thyroid gland and overproduction of thyroxine. Also called Graves' disease, toxic goiter or thyrotoxicosis.

  1. Symptoms—result of increased metabolic rate. Patient extremely nervous, tense and overactive increasingly fatigued and very hungry. May be very unstable emotionally.

  2. Treatment—rest and diet high in carbohydrates, calories and vitamins. Drugs—iodine preparations, thyroid blocking agents such as propylthiouracil and radioactive iodine.

    a. Surgical treatment—thyroidectomy.

      (1) Preoperative care—observation of the patient for signs of overactivity or other indications that his metabolic rate may be too high for safety during surgery.

      (2) Postoperative care—patient placed in high Fowler's position. Vital signs checked frequently and patient watched for signs of bleeding or swelling in the operative area. Two most dangerous complications are thyroid crisis and tetany.

D. Hypothyroidism—underactivity of the thyroid gland with a deficiency in the production of thyroxine.

  1. Symptoms vary. In children the symptoms of *cretinism* are retarded physical and mental growth. In adults the condition (*myxedema*) is characterized by slurred speech, reduced mental activity, sluggishness, dry and scaly skin and increased sensitivity to cold.

  2. Treatment with thyroid extract usually successful.

III. Disorders of the Parathyroids

A. Parathyroids are located on the posterior aspect of the thyroid. Parathyroid hormone regulates calcium and phosphorus concentration in body fluids.

B. Hypoparathyroidism (tetany) is due to a deficiency of parathyroid hormone.

  1. Can occur following thyroidectomy in which parathyroid tissue has been removed accidentally or with idiopathic atrophy of the parathyroid glands.

  2. Chief symptom is extreme irrita-

bility of muscle tissue resulting from calcium deficiency.

3. Acute condition treated by administration of calcium salts. Chronic condition treated by injections of parathyroid extract, vitamin D in massive doses and calcium salts.

C. Hyperparathyroidism (von Recklinghausen's disease) is due to excessive secretion of parathyroid hormone.

1. Symptoms brought about by removal of calcium from bones and its accumulation in the blood include fatigue, kidney stones and changes in the skeletal system.

2. Treatment is surgical removal of the excess glandular tissue.

IV. Disorders of Carbohydrate Metabolism

A. The hormone insulin that is secreted by the islets of Langerhans on the pancreas is necessary for proper utilization of carbohydrates. An excess of insulin leads to hypoglycemia; a deficiency in insulin leads to diabetes mellitus.

B. Diagnostic tests include (1) urinalysis for sugar, (2) blood sugar level (a high level is found in diabetes mellitus, chronic liver disease, and overactivity of some of the endocrine glands), and (3) glucose tolerance (measures the body's ability to utilize glucose).

C. Diabetes mellitus is a chronic disease resulting from inability of the body to use and store carbohydrates normally.

1. Exact cause not known. Contributing factors may include inability to produce enough insulin, increase in the rate at which the body uses up insulin, increase in the rate at which insulin is destroyed in the body and drop in the efficiency of insulin.

2. Symptoms are polyuria, polydipsia, polyphagia, fatigue, muscular weakness, pruritus and numbness and tingling of hands and feet.

3. Treatment. No cure, but it can be controlled by diet, proper exercise and administration of insulin or a hypolycemic drug.

   a. Diet is generally low in carbohydrate, high in protein, and moderate in fat. The patient is given an exchange list from which his menus are planned.

   b. Insulin is administered by hypo-

dermic. Hypoglycemic agents may be used for some diabetics who develop the disease in adult life.

4. A serious deficiency of insulin can lead to diabetic acidosis, which can be fatal. Too much insulin can cause an insulin reaction.

5. The uncontrolled diabetic is more likely to develop arteriosclerosis with accompanying circulatory disturbances, especially in the lower extremities, and is prone to infections and visual disturbances.

D. Hypoglycemia is an abnormally low level of glucose in the blood.

1. Condition can be due to a tumor of the pancreas, liver disease or a disorder of the pituitary or adrenal glands.

2. Symptoms are weakness, pallor, excessive perspiration, convulsions, and coma.

3. Treatment of the primary disorder (if one can be found) is first step. Patient should eat high-protein, regularly spaced meals, and should carry candy or sugar as a quick source of energy.

V. Disorders of the Adrenal Glands

A. The adrenal medulla secretes epinephrine and norepinephrine; the adrenal cortex secretes the mineralocorticoids, the glucocorticoids and the androgenic hormones.

B. Addison's disease (hypoadrenalism).

1. Result of underactivity of the adrenal cortex.

2. Symptoms — malaise, chronic fatigue, pigmentation of skin, dehydration and circulatory collapse.

3. Treatment — replacement of the adrenal hormones lacking in the body.

C. Cushing's syndrome (hyperadrenalism).

1. Result of increased activity of adrenal cortex.

2. Presents a wide variety of symptoms including muscular weakness, abnormal sexual development and some mental disturbances.

3. Treatment of primary condition when it is known. Also supportive measures, administration of potas-

sium chloride and a low-sodium, high-potassium diet. Surgical treatment is removal of most of the adrenal gland, leaving enough to provide necessary hormones.

D. Pheochromocytoma—a tumor located in the adrenal medulla or in other chromaffin tissues of the sympathoadrenal system.
1. Causes an increased secretion of epinephrine and norepinephrine.
2. Symptoms—hypertension, severe headache, visual disturbances and tachycardia.
3. Treatment—surgical removal of the tumor.

VI. Disorders of the Pituitary Gland

A. Introduction. The hypophysis influences all systems and organs of the body.

B. Gigantism. The growth hormone is overproduced during childhood causing rapid growth and lengthening of the long bones. Patient also may have diabetes mel-litus. Treatment involves irradiation of the tumor or excessive glandular tissue.

C. Acromegaly. Overproduction of the growth hormones after adolescence affecting growth of the soft tissues and the bones of the cranium, hands, feet and lower jaw. Treated by irradiation of the hypophysis.

D. Dwarfism. Some types may be due to undersecretion of the adenohypophyseal hormones. May be some thyroid deficiency and poor sexual development as well as retarded physical growth.

E. Panhypopituitarism in the adult (Simmond's disease). A very rare disorder of the pituitary gland causing thyroid deficiency, loss of sexual function, and depressed secretion of the adrenal glucocorticoids. Treated by administration of deficient hormones.

F. Diabetes insipidus. Result of decreased production of the antidiuretic hormone (ADH). Characterized by production of copious amounts of dilute urine. Treated by administration of posterior pituitary extract (pituitrin).

Chapter 17

NURSING CARE OF PATIENTS WITH DISORDERS OF THE REPRODUCTIVE SYSTEM

INTRODUCTION

The male and female reproductive systems have one basic function in common: *procreation* or *reproduction of the species*. Aside from this similarity in function there are some basic similarities in the structure of the male and female organs of reproduction. Generally these organs may be divided into glands, tubes or ducts, and reservoirs.

The glands of the female reproductive system are the ovaries, which lie on either side of the pelvis and are attached to the uterus. The ovaries are both *endocrine* and *exocrine glands* because they secrete hormones directly into the blood stream (estrogen and progesterone) and they also have external secretions which contain an ovum or egg.

The glands of the male reproductive system are called the testes and they too have internal secretions of a hormone (testosterone) and external secretions which contain the spermatozoa. The testes, like the ovaries, are oval; however, they are located outside the abdominal cavity in the scrotal sac. The prostate gland, which is located just below the bladder and completely surrounds the urethra, is one of several auxiliary glands which secrete a lubricant for the urethra.

The second group of organs are the tubes. In the female these tubes are the uterine tubes, which conduct the egg from the ovary to the uterus, and the vagina, or birth canal, which serves as a passageway for either the menstrual flow or the products of conception, depending on whether or not the ovum has been fertilized.

In the male the system of tubes is much more complex. These tubes include the epididymis, the ductus deferens, the ejaculatory duct, and the urethra, and they are all responsible for transporting the spermatozoa from the testes to the outside.

The third group of organs consists of the reservoirs. In the female the ovary contains and allows for maturation of the egg, or ovum; the uterus serves as a reservoir for the fertilized egg and assists in its maturation and development until the birth of the infant.

In the male the epididymis stores the spermatozoa until ejaculation, at which time the sperm are transported in the seminal fluid through the ducts to the outside.

The normal development and proper functioning of the reproductive organs in both the male and female depend to a great extent on the proper functioning of hormones from the pituitary gland.

In spite of the basic similarities mentioned above, there are many and diverse pathological conditions affecting the male or female reproductive system. This chapter is divided into Part I, which covers the female reproductive system, and Part II, which is concerned with the male reproductive system.

Part I – DISEASES OF THE FEMALE REPRODUCTIVE SYSTEM

SPECIAL DIAGNOSTIC TESTS AND EXAMINATIONS

Pelvic Examination. The examination of the genital organs by palpation and visualization is one of the most commonly used methods of diagnosing diseases of these organs. There are several duties and responsibilities of the nurse in assisting with this examination.

Physical and mental preparation of the patient is of utmost importance. The success of the examination will depend to a great extent on the ability of the patient to relax and cooperate with the examining physician. Proper draping of the patient and providing privacy for such an examination are considered to be an essential part of the nursing procedure and every practical nurse is expected to know this procedure and carry it out efficiently and quickly without giving the patient the impression of being rushed into the procedure. The necessary equipment, such as a vaginal speculum, gloves, and lubricant, must be assembled and conveniently arranged before the physician is summoned to begin the examination. The nurse should remain with the patient during the examination and assist her in dressing after the

examination is completed. She should avoid all signs of haste or lack of interest in the patient's feelings and attitudes toward the examination. A few moments should be taken to explain the procedure if the patient does not know what to expect, and to relieve her anxieties and fears by answering her questions simply and honestly. We repeat, *the success of the examination depends to a great extent on the patient's ability to relax and cooperate.*

While preparing her patient for a gynecological examination the nurse must be sure to have the patient empty her bladder completely. Otherwise the distended bladder will interfere with the examination.

The best time for a pelvic examination is between menstrual periods. This is sometimes taken to mean that a pelvic examination is dangerous and undesirable if the patient is bleeding. Actually, the presence of persistent vaginal bleeding for several weeks or months may indicate a serious disease which should be investigated *immediately*, rather than delaying the examination in the hope that the bleeding will stop. Thus there is no reason that a pelvic examination should not be done when the patient is bleeding.

Sometimes patients who have an abnormal amount of vaginal discharge will administer a vaginal douche to themselves before going to the doctor's office, unaware that this procedure washes away secretions which may help the physician in diagnosing the cause of the discharge. The nurse may need to explain this to her patients so that they will understand why douching is not advisable immediately before a gynecological examination.

Smears and Cultures. In both of these tests samplings of material from the reproductive tract are taken and examined in the laboratory. As is true for all other smears and cultures, these tests are useful in determining specific diseases present or the microorganisms causing the disease.

A Papanicolaou smear is used specifically for diagnosing cancer of the cervix. For further details on this particular type of smear and also for a cervical biopsy the reader is referred to pages 144 and 145.

Dilatation and Curettage. This is actually a minor surgical procedure done under general anesthesia, and may be used to treat certain diseases of the reproductive system. However, the endometrial tissue removed during the operation is often sent to the laboratory for microscopic examination to aid in the diagnosis of the patient's condition. For this reason we consider dilatation of the cervix and curettage (scraping of the uterus) as both a diagnostic and therapeutic procedure.

Mammography. This is an x-ray examination of the soft tissues of the breast without the injection of a contrast medium. It can be used in diagnosing lesions of the breast such as tumors and abscesses, but requires a skilled and experienced radiologist to read the films properly. One of the most difficult tasks is distinguishing between benign and malignant lesions, and so mammography cannot take the place of biopsy, palpation and other examinations of the breast. It should be accepted as one more means of detecting breast disorders rather than as a specific examination that eliminates the need for further study. It has been suggested that mammography could be useful in screening the general population for breast lesions that require further examination.

DISORDERS OF MENSTRUATION

Amenorrhea

Definition. The word "amenorrhea" means absence of menstruation, and this term is used to cover the absence of regular monthly periods at any time between the onset of puberty and the menopause. Amenorrhea is usually classified as *primary amenorrhea*, in which the menses have never occurred, and *secondary amenorrhea*, in which there is an absence of menstrual periods in individuals who have formerly had normal menstrual cycles. (See Table 24 for explanation of normal menstrual cycle.)

Symptoms. The symptoms of amenorrhea are obvious—there is simply no evidence of the monthly menstrual flow. The causes of amenorrhea are many and complex, and are most often associated with disturbances in the hormonal activities of one of the glands, such as the ovaries, thyroid, or pituitary gland. Other causes include malformations of the vagina or uterus, acute or chronic disease, or some emotional disturbance. Sometimes the cessation of menstruation indicates pregnancy.

Treatment. The treatment of amenorrhea must be directed toward the cause of the condition. Most physicians advise a thorough check-up by a gynecologist if a girl has not menstruated by her fifteenth birthday. All mature women who have an unexplained cessation of menstruation should consult a gynecologist, since absence of the menstrual flow may be symptomatic of many different diseases of the genital tract.

Table 24. *Periods of the Menstrual Cycle**

FIRST TO FIFTH DAY	SIXTH TO FOURTEENTH DAY	FIFTEENTH TO TWENTY-EIGHTH DAY
Menstrual Period	Period of Growth and Repair	Secretory Period
1. Endometrium sloughs away as menstrual flow begins.	1. Follicle grows and egg matures.	1. Progesterone and estrogen are secreted.
2. Progesterone and estrogen are no longer secreted.	2. Endometrium returns to normal state and then begins to thicken because of action of estrogen.	2. Endometrium continues to thicken and becomes filled with blood in preparation for receiving the fertilized egg.
3. New follicle starts to mature.	3. Ovulation occurs about fourteenth day when follicle ruptures and releases the egg.	

*NOTE: In order for menstruation to occur, two organs are essential: (1) the uterus, because menstruation is the sloughing away of the lining of the uterus; and (2) at least part of one ovary, because the ovary secretes the hormones which cause the endometrium to thicken.

Dysmenorrhea

Definition. Dysmenorrhea refers to the association of pain with the menstrual flow. It is estimated that at least 50 percent of all menstruating women experience some degree of discomfort during their menstrual periods at some time or other. However, this percentage cannot be considered an accurate statistic because individuals react differently to pain and discomfort and most women do not have difficulty with every menstrual period.

Symptoms. It should be emphasized that menstruation is a normal function and should not be accompanied by severe cramps or a steady aching type of pain. Dysmenorrhea refers to an *abnormal amount* of pain and discomfort. Therefore, severe or persistent dysmenorrhea should be reported to a gynecologist.

Treatment and Nursing Care. Dysmenorrhea is treated according to its cause. Surgery is rarely indicated and usually when congenital malformations or tumors are the direct cause of the condition. Endocrine disorders causing dysmenorrhea may be treated by the administration of hormones in some cases.

An individual's general physical condition and mental attitude toward menstruation may have a direct effect on the success of treatment for dysmenorrhea. The nurse may be of great help to young girls first learning about and adjusting to monthly periods if she will help them understand that menstruation should not restrict most of their usual activities. The person who is busy and happily engaged in her normal activities is less likely to be bothered by the minor discomforts of menstruation than one who considers the monthly cycle as a great inconvenience and an excellent opportunity to lie in bed and receive attention. Adequate rest, warm, soothing baths, removal of tight clothing, and a well-balanced, nonconstipating diet should be all that is necessary for relief of the minor discomforts of menstruation.

Menorrhagia

Definition. Menorrhagia is an excessive loss of blood in the menstrual flow during the regular monthly period. It is frequently due to a disturbance in the function of the endocrine glands, in which case it is called *functional bleeding.* Other causes may include uterine tumors, pelvic inflammatory disease, and an abnormal condition of pregnancy.

Curettage of the uterine cavity is sometimes done for treatment of the condition as well as for diagnosis of the cause of the excessive bleeding.

Metrorrhagia

Definition. Metrorrhagia is uterine bleeding or spotting which occurs at times other than the regular menstrual cycle. Even a slight spotting should be reported to a gynecologist since it may be the only symptom of a serious pelvic disease, as for example, malignant diseases of the genital tract.

INFECTIONS OF THE GENITAL TRACT

Gonorrhea

Definition. Gonorrhea is a venereal disease caused by a specific organism called the *gonococcus.* Venereal diseases are infections usually spread by sexual contact.

Of the many venereal diseases, gonorrhea is the most common and, in spite of intensive efforts to eradicate the disease, it is still a menace to public health.

Symptoms. The symptoms of gonorrhea usually appear within 48 hours after exposure and include burning on urination and itching in the vaginal region. Within a few days a profuse and purulent vaginal discharge appears. The disease spreads upward from the vagina, involving the endometrium (lining of the uterus) and then spreading to the uterine tubes. The symptoms of the acute stage may then subside somewhat and the disease becomes chronic if left untreated. A definite diagnosis may be made by discovering the *gonococcus* in a specimen of the vaginal discharge.

Treatment and Nursing Care. In caring for these patients the nurse must remember that gonorrhea is a highly infectious disease that may easily be spread to the eyes (gonorrheal conjunctivitis). In procedures such as douches or assisting with a pelvic examination the nurse's hands must be thoroughly washed and kept away from the face. It is best if the nurse wears rubber gloves while administering any treatment which involves contact with the genital area or discharge from the vagina.

The antibiotics such as penicillin or streptomycin are used in the treatment of gonorrhea. Early treatment may prevent spreading the disease to others, or complications such as sterility.

Syphilis

Definition. Syphilis is also a venereal disease, but it is a more generalized disease affecting the entire body and not limited to the genital organs only. It is caused by a spirochete, *Treponema pallidum.* The causative organism of syphilis cannot survive without moisture and it can be destroyed with plain soap. Since the spirochete must be wet and warm to survive, syphilis is nearly always transmitted by direct bodily contact; it is extremely rare for the disease to be transmitted by inanimate objects such as toilet seats or eating utensils.

It is possible for an infant to be born with an active case of syphilis because the spirochete can pass the placental barrier once the fetus has reached the fourth month of development. About one half of the expectant mothers who have an active case of syphilis that is not treated will bear an infant with congenital syphilis. The disease can be fatal to the infant or it can lead to physical deformities and mental disorders.

Diagnosis. A positive diagnosis of syphilis is established by finding the treponema in a smear made from exudate taken from a chancre. Blood tests such as the Wasserman, Mazzini, Kahn and Kolmer also can detect syphilis once it has been established in the body. This is usually within three weeks of the initial infection. A serologic test for syphilis (S.T.S.) can be falsely positive however, and newer tests such as the TPI (*Treponema pallidum* immobilization) test are considered more accurate.

Symptoms. Unfortunately, the symptoms of syphilis are not very severe in the earlier stage of the disease. Some have a way of subsiding and then reappearing, and the infected person may not be aware of the serious and permanent damage being done to vital organs of his body until it is too late. This is doubly tragic because the disease can be cured and serious complications avoided if it is treated in its earliest stages.

There are three stages of syphilis: *primary, secondary,* and *tertiary.* In the primary stage a chancre or hard sore appears on the mucous membrane of the mouth or genitalia. The chancre is teeming with spirochetes and so the individual is highly infectious at this stage. Within three days after infection the spirochetes enter the blood stream, where they begin to multiply rapidly. Other symptoms of the first stage may include headache and some enlargement of the lymph glands near the chancre, but generally, the infected person does not feel very sick. The chancre and other symptoms disappear within three to eight weeks, and if the patient has used some salve or patent medicine with the mistaken idea that the chancre was a minor infection he may falsely conclude that the medicine had cured him. Nothing could be further from the truth, because the disease has now entered the second stage and spirochetes have invaded his blood stream.

Symptoms of the secondary stage of syphilis vary in individuals. Some may feel fairly well with only slight malaise or headache. Others may develop a skin rash or sore throat or they may lose patches of hair from the scalp. There also may be some arthritis, neuritis, or retinitis. Eventually these symptoms subside (though they may reappear) and the disease enters a latent period.

The tertiary stage of syphilis can begin one year after infection but more often it is four or five years before the serious effects of the infection are first noticed. In some individuals the disease may lie dormant for 20 years before symptoms of the third stage appear. Since the spirochetes have had free access to all tissues of the body, the damage they have caused can present a wide variety of symptoms. The nervous system, blood vessels, and eyes are most often affected.

Treatment and Nursing Care. Penicillin is the drug of choice in treating syphilis in its primary stage. Other drugs that can be used as alternatives in case of sensitivity to penicillin include tetracycline and erythromycin. Usually the patient receives a single, massive dose of long-lasting penicillin which destroys the spirochetes in his body. He is instructed to return for periodic checkups to be sure he is rid of the disease. There is no immunity conferred by an attack of the disease and an individual can become infected with syphilis again and again.

One of the most important aspects of treating and controlling syphilis and other venereal diseases is proper education of the public so that their cooperation can be gained. One promiscuous individual can be responsible for infecting several others who in turn become sources of infection for still others and the chain reaction can be almost endless. Locating those who have been in contact with an infected individual can be a time-consuming and often thankless job because it necessarily involves asking personal questions and requires convincing the contacts that a simple treatment can prevent very serious complications in later life. The nurse should realize that many infected persons are teenagers who fear being found out by their families and friends and who do not fully understand the disease or appreciate its seriousness. She must use tact and understanding with these patients, avoid treating them with disgust or censuring them, and encourage them to cooperate with Public Health Officials and other members of the health team who are striving to locate and treat infected individuals.

Pelvic Inflammatory Disease

Definition. This is a general term used to include any inflammation in the pelvis *outside the uterus.* If the inflammation is located in the uterine tubes it is called a *salpingitis*, if the ovaries are affected the term used is *oophoritis*, and involvement of the pelvic peritoneum is called *pelvic peritonitis.*

The organisms causing the infection are usually introduced from the outside and then spread upward through the uterus without affecting the endometrium. Sometimes, however, in an infection following delivery the inflammatory process may extend outward from the uterus and involve adjoining connective tissues of the pelvis. When this happens the patient has a *pelvic cellulitis.*

Many people are under the impression that pelvic inflammatory disease is caused only by the gonococcus, probably because it was once the most common causative organism before the discovery of penicillin and the sulfonamides. Now that gonorrhea may be cured in its early stages before it spreads upward through the genital tract it is less common as a cause of pelvic inflammatory disease. Any organism capable of producing an infection can cause pelvic inflammatory disease.

Symptoms. The patient with acute pelvic inflammatory disease is very ill and appears to be in acute distress. She experiences severe abdominal and pelvic pain, elevated temperature, nausea and vomiting, and frequently has a purulent, foul-smelling vaginal discharge.

If the disease progresses to the chronic stage there are usually disturbances of menstruation, backache, and a feeling of heaviness in the pelvis.

Treatment and Nursing Care. Ideally the condition should be treated in its earliest stages so that further spread of the infection and complications from scarring of the tissues may be avoided. Antibiotics are administered for control of the infection and hygienic measures to improve the general health of the patient are also employed.

The patient is usually placed on bed rest and positioned in a semi-Fowler's position so that any abscess which may form will be low in the pelvis where drainage is most easily established. Heat is usually applied to the lower abdomen and hot vaginal douches are ordered to facilitate drainage of the exudate from the site of the inflammation. Any change in the amount, color, or odor of the vaginal discharge should be reported immediately.

The most common complication of pelvic inflammatory disease is *sterility.* This is a result of the narrowing or complete closure of the uterine tubes which prevents passage of the sperm through the tube. Sometimes, even if the sperm can pass through and fertilize the egg, there is not room for the enlarged fertilized egg to pass back through the tube into the uterus and it becomes lodged in the tube, thus leading to a *tubal* or *ectopic* pregnancy.

Trichomonas Vaginitis

Definition. This is an inflammation of the vaginal mucosa. It is a very common condition and is caused by the protazoon *Trichomonas vaginalis*, a parasite which thrives in the vaginal canal. Since these organisms are found in the vaginal secretions of women who do not have any symptoms at all, it is believed that other factors such as changes in the physiologic condition of the vagina contribute to the growth of the parasite and the development of an infection.

Symptoms. The symptoms of a trichomonal infection of the vagina include a persistent *leukorrhea* (white vaginal discharge) which causes irritation of the vaginal mucosa, and a swelling and inflammation of the vulva and perineum.

Treatment and Nursing Care. Trichomonal infections are very difficult to control and in many cases the condition may persist for years in spite of treatment. There are several suppositories and powders which may be prescribed for local application, but their success depends on the individual case. Vinegar douches which change the chemical environment of the vagina are often beneficial. Scrupulous cleansing of the perineum with soap and water after each voiding or defecation may help in the control of the primary infection and prevent a secondary infection from other bacteria.

Monilial Vaginitis

Definition. This is an inflammation of the vagina caused by *Candida albicans*, a member of the yeast family that thrives in warm, moist places. The condition is often seen in uncontrolled diabetics because the sugar provides an excellent medium for the growth of the yeast.

Symptoms. The most outstanding symptom is a watery vaginal discharge, often containing white, cheeselike flakes, and producing severe itching and inflammation of the vulva.

Treatment and Nursing Care. If the condition can be traced to uncontrolled diabetes, it is obvious that lowering the blood sugar will greatly facilitate elimination of the infection. In other cases local treatment is used. This consists of frequent applications of gentian violet or one of the other drugs used specifically for treating yeast infections.

Douches are not advisable as long as the local medication is being applied.

TUMORS OF THE UTERUS

Definition. Tumors within the uterus are very common in women between the ages of 25 and 40. Those tumors which are benign are commonly called *fibroids*, and involve the uterine wall. Malignant tumors most often affect the cervix; in fact, 66 percent of the malignancies involving the genital tract in the female are located in the cervix.

Symptoms. Bleeding is the most common symptom of all uterine tumors in their early stages. Later as the tumor becomes larger it causes symptoms of pressure within the abdominopelvic cavity.

Treatment and Nursing Care. The treatment of a nonmalignant tumor of the uterus is entirely different from that of a malignant tumor. It is well known that a malignancy requires immediate surgical removal of the affected part, and possibly additional radiation therapy to destroy any remaining malignant cells. A benign uterine tumor, however, may subside spontaneously, especially at the time of menopause because it is at this time that ovarian hormones which stimulate the growth of these tumors are no longer secreted.

The choice of treatment of a benign tumor of the uterus depends on the age of the patient and the symptoms brought about by the tumor. In younger women the tumor is removed surgically and an effort made to preserve the functions of the ovaries. Patients near the age of menopause or older may be treated conservatively unless severe bleeding or pressure symptoms require radium therapy or surgery.

UTERINE DISPLACEMENTS

Definition. The uterus is normally suspended in the abdominopelvic cavity by ligaments and is attached to the floor of the pelvis. It is not in a *fixed position*, however, and can be moved about to some degree. An extreme tilting of the uterus away from its normal position is considered to be abnormal and does create some difficulty. This condition is referred to as a uterine displacement.

Types of Displacement. The uterus may be bent forward or tilted backward. It may also slip downward out of its normal position. Figure 17-1 shows the major displacements of the uterus in comparison to its normal position.

Anteflexion is a bending forward of the uterus.

Retroflexion is a bending backward of the uterus.

Retroversion is a tilting backward of the uterus without bending.

Retrocession is a backward displacement of the uterus without bending.

Prolapse of the uterus is a falling or lowering of the uterus into the vagina.

Symptoms. Not all uterine displacements produce symptoms. Those that are severe cause symptoms of backache, feeling of heaviness or "drag" in the pelvis, white vaginal discharge, and fatigue.

Treatment and Nursing Care. Treatment is considered necessary only when symptoms are annoying or cause discomfort. In minor displacements the uterus may be replaced manually during a pelvic examination and a *pessary* inserted to hold the uterus in place. This is considered to be a temporary measure and is used to find out whether displacement is the cause of the patient's difficulties. In young women, if the pessary does prove to relieve the symptoms, the physician may correct the displacement by surgery. In this procedure the ligaments are shortened so that they hold the uterus more securely.

In older women who are poor surgical risks, the pessary may be used perma-

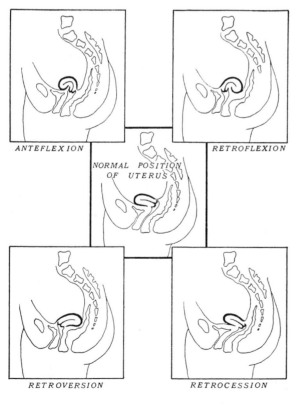

Figure 17-1. Types of forward and backward uterine displacements. (From Miller and Avery: *Gynecology and Gynecologic Nursing,* 4th Ed., W. B. Saunders Co., Philadelphia.)

nently. Vaginal douches daily and frequent visits to the physician are necessary because this device is a foreign body in the vagina and is therefore likely to be irritating to the vaginal mucosa.

NURSING CARE OF THE PATIENT HAVING VAGINAL SURGERY

Introduction. Surgery of the female genital organs may be done by way of the abdomen or by way of the vagina. Surgical procedures such as those involving repair of the vaginal canal or pelvic floor, with restoration of these tissues and organs to their normal structure and function, will obviously involve vaginal surgery. Removal of part or all of the uterus, tubes, and ovaries may be done by way of an abdominal incision or by way of the vagina. Table 25 gives a brief description of some of

the more common types of gynecological surgery.

Preoperative Nursing Care. The physical preparation of the patient involves shaving of the pubic and perineal hair and a thorough cleansing of the area with a surgical detergent or pHiso-Hex. Care must be taken to clean between the folds of the labia and around the clitoris so that all secretions are removed. Vaginal douches may be ordered the evening and morning before surgery. Other physical aspects of the preoperative care are the same as for any patient having major surgery.

Postoperative Nursing Care. When the patient returns from surgery she must be watched closely for signs of hemorrhage because bleeding is a common complication of vaginal surgery. Some physicians do not allow patients with perineal stitches to wear perineal pads during the immediate postoperative period because they consider them

Table 25. *Types of Gynecological Surgery*

NAME OF SURGICAL PROCEDURE	EXPLANATION
Dilatation and curettage	Widening the cervix and scraping away the inner lining of the uterus (endometrium).
Conization, or conical excision	Removal of a cone of inflamed tissues of the cervix. Conization is done with an electric cutting wire. Conical excision is done with a surgical knife.
Total hysterectomy	Removal of the entire uterus.
Radical panhysterectomy	Removal of the entire uterus, tubes, and ovaries.
Partial hysterectomy or surgical hysterectomy	Removal of part of the uterus, leaving a portion of the body of the uterus and endometrium.
Anterior and posterior colporrhaphy	Repair of the anterior and posterior wall of the vagina.
Salpingectomy	Removal of a uterine tube.
Oophorectomy	Removal of an ovary.

to be a source of infection. The practical nurse should not apply any pads or dressings to the perineal area unless specifically ordered to do so.

Some drainage containing blood may be expected following vaginal surgery, but any change in the amount or color of vaginal discharge should be reported immediately. A foul odor may indicate the presence of an infection. When caring for the patient with vaginal surgery the nurse must always bear in mind the proximity of the rectum and recognize it as a source of infection. When cleansing the area or removing perineal pads, care must be taken to wipe from front to back and to avoid dragging the pad across the perineum from the rectum. Special irrigations of normal saline or a mild antiseptic may be ordered to keep the operative area clean, especially when there has been plastic surgery of the vagina or perineum. Heat lamps may be ordered once or twice daily to keep the area dry and to promote healing of the surgical wound. Aerosol sprays containing local anesthetics may be soothing and comforting when applied to the suture line.

Defecation may become a problem for the patient who has had a repair of the anterior and posterior walls of the vagina. To prevent straining at the stool, and subsequent stress on the sutures, mineral oil is usually given each night at bedtime.

An indwelling catheter is usually inserted before or during surgery to insure proper drainage of the bladder. This catheter must be kept open so that distention of the bladder does not place an undue strain on the sutures of the repaired tissues. When the cather is removed on the third or fourth postoperative day the patient must be checked frequently for voiding so that the bladder is not allowed to become distended. If the patient cannot void, an order for catheterization must be obtained. The physician will also usually order that the patient's *residual urine* be checked.

Early ambulation and nursing measures to prevent pulmonary and circulatory complications are necessary as for any patient having major surgery.

Mental depression and anxiety are commonly associated with surgical procedures involving removal of the female genital organs. The nurse must use much patience and tact in dealing with the patient who seems unreasonable or unduly worried about the changes brought about by the surgery. We cannot ignore the fact that such surgery may have altered the parts of her body which are closely associated with sexual activities and womanliness. In spite of a full explanation by the physician the patient may continue to wonder about the effect the surgery may have on her femininity, her ability to have children, or her fulfillment of her role as a wife. Even though such fears and anxieties are, in many cases, unfounded, the nurse must realize that the patient needs sympathetic care and understanding while she is going through this difficult period of adjustment.

ENDOMETRIOSIS

Definition. Endometriosis is a rather common disorder in which endometrial tissue (that of the inner lining of the uterus) is found outside the uterus, especially in the ovaries, recto-vaginal septum and other areas of the pelvis and abdomen. The misplaced tissue usually undergoes changes during the menstrual cycle in the same way normal endometrium does and there may be some bleeding at the time of menstruation.

Symptoms. Because the aberrant endometrial tissue can cause bleeding into spaces that have no outlet and are likely to be irritated by the blood, the patient experiences pain and often has adhesions in the area of bleeding Other symptoms may include excessive menstrual flow, bleeding between menstrual periods, and pain on defecation or during sexual intercourse. Some patients have dysmenorrhea that is so severe as to be almost incapacitating.

Treatment. The most efficient method for eradicating the symptoms of endometriosis is the removal of the ovaries, which are necessary for continued growth of endometrial tissue. This is not always a simple matter, however, because endometriosis is a disease of young women in their child-bearing years. If the patient is young and anxious for future pregnancies, the gynecologist usually tries more conservative treatment. This usually involves surgical removal of only one ovary or resection of an endometrial cyst of an ovary and fulguration of other areas of endometrial tissue in the pelvic or abdominal cavity. If the conservative treatment does not relieve the severe symptoms of endometriosis there may be no choice but to return the patient to surgery and remove both ovaries.

Although ectopic endometrial growths rarely become malignant, they can and often do lead to sterility. Most physicians advise their young patients with endometriosis to complete their families as quickly as possible before they become sterile.

OVARIAN TUMORS

Definition and Types. Tumors of the ovary are generally classified as benign or malignant. These new growths can arise from misplaced endometrial tissue (see above) or they can develop from tissues of the ovary itself. Some tumors are cystic, that is, sac-like structures, while others are solid. Dermoid cysts are neoplasms of the ovary that are believed to be the result of spontaneous growth of an unfertilized ovum.

Symptoms. Ovarian tumors do not, as a rule, present specific symptoms until they are fairly well advanced. For this reason many malignant ovarian tumors are not detected until other organs have become involved. Some ovar-

ian tumors such as the fibroma can become very large, weighing as much as fifteen pounds and interfering with normal motion of adjacent organs. Most ovarian tumors cause irregular bleeding, or there may be a palpable mass or a vague feeling of fullness in the abdomen. When an ovarian tumor is found in its very early stages it is usually discovered during a routine examination.

Treatment and Nursing Care. If the tumor is benign, involves only one ovary and the patient is relatively young, the surgeon may treat it conservatively with surgical removal of the ovary and a section of the uterine tube, leaving the other tube and ovary intact. Patients with malignant tumors are treated more radically, usually with a panhysterectomy in which both ovaries, both uterine tubes and the uterus are removed. Radiation therapy is sometimes used to destroy the tumor and stop ovarian function when the patient is considered a poor surgical risk.

DISORDERS OF THE BREAST

Introduction. The most common disorder of the breast is cystic disease (dysplasia); the most serious is carcinoma or cancer of the breast. Cystic disease is not an inflammatory disease even though it is sometimes called cystic mastitis. The condition usually presents only mild symptoms and requires no extensive treatment. If, however, there are multiple cysts and more severe symptoms of pain and tenderness, a simple mastectomy may be performed as treatment.

Carcinoma of the breast is the most common type of malignancy in females in the United States. It occurs most often during and after menopause and is more common in women who have a relative who has had the disease. For reasons not fully understood the incidence of breast cancer is lower in women who have nursed babies. The cause of carcinoma of the breast is unknown. The belief that a blow to the breast can lead to cancer is unfounded and probably has arisen from the fact that a lump has been found following a blow that produced some tenderness and led the individual to examine her breast and thus discover the lump.

Signs and Symptoms of Breast Tumors. A lump in the breast is one of the prime symptoms of a breast tumor (see Fig. 17-2). Pain is symptomatic of cystic disease but is not usually associated with a malignant growth until it is in an advanced stage. Abnormal discharge from the nipple can be symptomatic of almost any breast disorder but it should be considered significant and have prompt medical attention. Dimpling of the breast tissue and overlying skin and retraction of the nipple can occur when a tumor near the surface adheres to underlying structures. Other symptoms include swelling or enlargement of one breast, a change in firmness, or the appearance of a reddened area.

Treatment. The safest, most effective treatment for cancer of the breast is radical mastectomy in which the entire breast, the pectoral muscles, the lymph nodes under the arm and all adjacent tissues are removed. A simple mastectomy may be performed for cystic mastitis, a well defined benign tumor, or an advanced malignancy in which an ulcerated and draining carcinoma demands removal of the breast but cannot offer hope of a cure.

NURSING CARE OF THE PATIENT HAVING A MASTECTOMY

Preoperative Nursing Care. The physical preparation of the patient having a mastectomy differs very little from the routine preoperative care of any patient having major surgery. The emotional preparation, however, demands additional explanation of the type of surgery to be done and the formulation of plans for rehabilitation and pros-

thesis after surgery. These are the responsibility of the surgeon, but the nurse must be aware of the emotional upheaval that some patients experience when they realize that the breast must be removed. The same fears and anxieties associated with surgery of the genital organs are frequently seen in the mastectomy patient. Since the breasts are secondary sex organs, and as such are closely related to femininity and motherhood, it is only natural that removal of a breast will cause some emotional reaction. The nurse must try to understand her patient's problems in adjusting to this type of surgery and give her all the moral support and comfort she needs preoperatively as well as postoperatively.

Postoperative Nursing Care. A mastectomy is an extensive surgical procedure, one that may take 4 to 6 hours, and may involve the loss of more than a pint of blood. Transfusions are usually started during surgery and may be continued until several pints of blood have been given.

Since there is a loss of so much blood, the surgeon usually applies a pressure dressing over the wound to prevent further bleeding after surgery. This dressing must be watched carefully for signs of hemorrhage during the first few days postoperatively. In observing for bleeding the nurse must remember to turn her patient and check the back of the chest as well as the front because the blood may have seeped downward by gravity flow and collected on the bottom sheet. The pressure dressing may be reinforced but is never changed without specific orders to do so.

During the first 24 hours after surgery there may be some swelling under the dressing, causing it to become tighter and constrict the blood vessels leading to the arm. When this happens the patient will complain of numbness of the lower arm, inability to move the fingers, or swelling of the lower arm. Such symptoms should be reported immediately.

Deep breathing and coughing should

1. Careful examination of the breasts before a mirror for symmetry in size and shape, noting any puckering or dimpling of the skin or retraction of the nipple.

2. Arms raised over head, again studying the breasts in the mirror for the same signs.

3. Reclining on bed with flat pillow or folded bath towel under the shoulder on the same side as breast to be examined.

4. To examine the inner half of the breast the arm is raised over the head. Beginning at the breastbone and, in a series of steps, the inner half of the breast is palpated.

5. The area over the nipple is carefully palpated with flats of the fingers.

6. Examination of the lower inner half of the breast is completed.

7. With arm down at side self examination of breasts continues by carefully feeling the tissues which extend to the armpit.

8. The upper outer quadrant of the breast is examined with the flat part of the fingers.

9. The lower outer quadrant of the breast is examined in successive stages with flat part of the fingers.

Figure 17-2. Self-examination of the breast. (From the American Cancer Society booklet, "The Nurse and Breast Self Examination," 1952.)

Figure 17-3. Arm exercise #1. Stand with feet 8″ apart. Bend forward from the waist allowing arms to hang toward the floor by gravity. Swing both arms together describing an arc from one shoulder to the other. Do not bend elbows. Stand and allow arms to fall to side. Arm exercise #2. Stand facing the wall at arm's length with feet 8″ apart. Place hands against the wall at shoulder level parallel to each other. Slowly flex the elbow bending the trunk forward until forehead touches wall. Straighten elbows slowly until body is upright. Repeat. Note: Keep head, trunk, and legs in straight line. Arm exercise #3. Stand with feet 8″ apart. Extend arms sideways to shoulder level. In rhythm: Flex elbows clasping fingers at nape of neck. Rotate elbows forward until they touch. Rotate elbows sideways. Unclasp fingers and extend arms sideways at shoulder level. Repeat. Arm exercise #4. Lie on back with arms against the side of the body (use firm surface as floor with rug, pad or blanket, or firm mattress without a pillow). In rhythm: Raise arms to shoulder level (do not flex elbow). Extend arms above head. Return arms to shoulder level. Lower arms to side. Repeat. (From Wolf: *Nursing Clinics of North America*, December, 1967.)

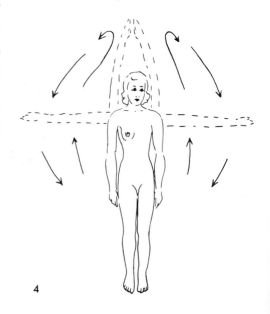

be encouraged even though they will most certainly cause some discomfort in the operative area. The patient is usually allowed out of bed the first postoperative day. When getting the patient up the nurse should be aware that the patient will have some difficulty in balancing herself as long as she cannot use one arm, and will therefore be very likely to fall if she does not have adequate support from those helping her out of bed.

Special exercises of the arm and shoulder on the affected side are begun as soon as the physician feels the patient may safely do them. Most patients are very cooperative and anxious to do these exercises regularly if they understand how these exercises will prevent deformities and disabilities. The most commonly used exercises are hand wall climbing, hair brushing exercises, elbow pull-in and paddle swinging. These exercises are fully described and illustrated in the booklet, "Help Yourself to Recovery," published by the American Cancer Society and available at any local Cancer Society office. This booklet also contains some excellent information on the selection and fitting of breast forms and specially designed brassieres for the patient who has had a mastectomy. Other post-mastectomy exercises are shown in Figure 17-3.

Part II — THE MALE REPRODUCTIVE SYSTEM

INFECTIONS OF THE MALE GENITAL TRACT

Introduction. A variety of pathogenic organisms may cause an infection anywhere within the male genital tract. The terminology used for each infection depends on the location of the infection. *Urethritis*, for example, is an inflammation of the urethra, *prostatitis* an inflammation of the prostate, *epididymitis* an inflammation of the epididymis, and *balanitis* an inflammation of the glans penis.

Urethritis

Definition. This is simply an inflammation of the urethra. It may be caused by the staphylococcus, streptococcus, *Escherichia coli* (from the colon) or the gonococcus.

Symptoms. The patient with urethritis has symptoms of frequency and urgency, and burning on urination. The urinary meatus is swollen and inflamed and a discharge from the urethra may be present.

Treatment and Nursing Care. Medications used in the treatment of urethritis include the antibiotics and the local application of a mild antiseptic to control the infection. Hot sitz baths may relieve some of the discomfort associated with this condition. Fluids are forced to increase the flow of urine and aid in prevention of urinary complications.

Prostatitis

Definition. This is an inflammation of the prostate gland. It also may be caused by any pathogenic organism which has found its way into the male genital tract.

Symptoms. Because the prostate encircles the urethra just below the neck of the bladder, an inflammation of the prostate produces symptoms of urinary obstruction to some degree. There may be painful urination or difficulty in voiding. The patient also has tenderness and pain in the perineal area.

Treatment and Nursing Care. Prostatitis is treated by antibiotics and local applications of heat in the form of hot sitz baths or low rectal irrigations. Fluids are forced and the patient is encouraged to rest in bed until the infection is under control.

Epididymitis

Definition. Inflammation of the epididymis may be caused by any pathogenic organism and is one of the most common infections of the male genital tract. It is a common complication of gonorrhea.

Symptoms. In epididymitis there is local pain and tenderness in the scrotal area. Walking may cause pain and in order to protect the scrotum the patient assumes an unnatural, stiff-legged gait. A high fever and extreme fatigue usually accompany epididymitis.

Treatment and Nursing Care. In the treatment of epididymitis cold applications are applied rather than hot because extremely high temperatures may destroy the sperm cells. The scrotum should be elevated and an ice bag placed under it. Later when the patient is allowed out of bed an athletic support must be worn.

Balanitis

Definition. This is an inflammation of the glans penis. It is most often the result of *phimosis*, a condition in which the foreskin of the penis cannot be pulled back over the glans penis, thus preventing proper cleansing of the area.

Symptoms. The symptoms of balanitis are swelling of the penis with visible signs of a local inflammation.

Treatment. The first step in the treatment of balanitis is removal of the cause. The surgical procedure for correction of phimosis is *circumcision*. Antibiotics may be given for control of the infection.

Orchitis

Definition. This is an inflammation of the testicle. It is frequently found to be a complication of mumps in adult males. In many cases this condition leads to sterility.

Symptoms. The symptoms of orchitis are very similar to those of epididymitis. The patient experiences local pain and tenderness in the scrotal area and frequently has an elevated temperature.

Treatment. Because orchitis is a common complication of mumps in adult males, gamma globulin should be given routinely to all individuals past puberty who have been exposed to the disease and have not had mumps before. The orchitis is treated in the same manner as epididymitis.

TUMORS OF THE PROSTATE GLAND

Definition. Neoplasms, or the growth of new cells, within the prostate gland commonly occur in men over the age of 55. These tumors may be benign *(benign prostatic hypertrophy)*, or malignant *(cancer of the prostate)*.

Symptoms. Benign prostatic hypertrophy produces no symptoms until the growth becomes large enough to press against the urethra. Then the patient begins to experience difficulty in urinating and in the later stages there is complete obstruction of the urinary flow.

Carcinoma of the prostate is usually not discovered until the later stages of development when it begins to cause symptoms of obstruction of the urinary flow. This is unfortunately true of most malignancies and is all the more reason why individuals past the age of 40 should have a complete physical check-up every 6 months even though they may feel perfectly well.

Treatment and Nursing Care. Surgical removal of all or part of the prostate gland is the choice of treatment for tumors of the prostate. Whenever a biopsy shows the tumor to be malignant the entire prostate and its capsule must be removed.

The location of the incision and the amount of tissue to be removed will depend on the individual patient, his general physical condition, and the type of tumor present.

Radical prostatectomy is the removal of the entire prostate gland and its capsule. The incision is made through the perineum.

Suprapubic prostatectomy is surgical removal of the prostate through an incision directly over the bladder. The bladder is opened and the urethral mucosa is incised. The tumorous tissue is removed through this incision.

Retropubic prostatectomy involves a low abdominal incision but the bladder is not opened.

Transurethral prostatic resection is removal of part of the prostate gland by way of the urethra. There is no surgical incision in this procedure and the postoperative period is much shorter.

Preoperative Nursing Care. The patient who is admitted to the hospital for a prostatectomy will inevitably have some difficulty in voiding. The retention of urine may be so severe that an indwelling catheter is necessary to drain the bladder. In less severe cases the patient may be able to void but probably cannot completely empty his bladder. In either case the physician usually wishes to have an accurate record of the patient's intake and urinary output during the preoperative period.

Since most of the patients requiring a prostatectomy are older men beyond the age of 60, the nurse may need to give these patients the special attention required by all geriatric patients. Side rails should be applied to the bed, especially if a sedative has been given. Adequate explanation of the purpose of the indwelling catheter may help the patient accept this inconvenience more readily.

Preoperative medications are given according to the age and general physical condition of the patient since elderly people cannot tolerate heavy sedation.

Postoperative Nursing Care. The postoperative nursing care of the patient will vary according to the type of surgery used in removing the prostate gland (see types of surgery above). The general principles of postoperative nursing care which apply to all patients having major surgery are necessary for the patient having a prostatectomy. In addition, the nurse must pay special attention to drainage through the catheter leading from the bladder. This is of primary importance because occlusion of the catheter may lead to more bleeding, cystitis, or an upper urinary tract infection.

The patient who has had a transurethral resection will not have a surgical incision; however, this is still a major surgical procedure and postoperative hemorrhage is always a possibility to be considered. In order to check the amount of drainage and loss of blood through the urethral catheter, the drainage bottle may be marked with adhesive tape. An excessive increase of bright red drainage in a given period of time should be reported.

The catheter and tubing should be checked frequently to make sure that they are not obstructed in any way. Clots or bits of tissue within the catheter may lead to severe spasms of the bladder which are extremely painful. Before administering any analgesic medication the nurse should first note whether or not the catheter is draining properly. If the catheter is obstructed irrigations may be ordered by the surgeon. These irrigations should not be done without a written order and then only under sterile conditions because infection is a very real danger after prostatectomy. If the patient continues to complain of severe pain even though the bladder is empty the physician should be notified at once because unusually severe pain and abdominal rigidity may indicate a perforated bladder.

When a suprapubic prostatectomy has been done the surgical incision will lie directly over the bladder. The cavity left by the removal of the prostate may be packed with gauze or Gelfoam to prevent hemorrhage; or a large Foley catheter may be inserted into the cavity and traction applied so that the balloon of the catheter presses against the blood vessels. This traction is usually applied for as long as 6 to 8 hours and must not be disturbed while administering care to the patient.

Dressings over the wound must be changed frequently because they collect urinary drainage from the bladder. The skin around the surgical wound must be washed frequently to remove urine, which is very irritating to the skin.

The patient with a perineal incision usually returns from surgery with a small cigarette drain extending through the incision. There may be urinary drainage through this drain as well as through the urethral catheter in the bladder. The principles of cleanliness recommended for the patient having vaginal surgery are equally important in the care of the male patient with a perineal incision. Dressings over the incision must be changed as often as necessary to keep the patient dry and comfortable.

CLINICAL CASE PROBLEMS

1. Your brother, whose wife is dead, has asked you to explain menstruation to his daughter, who is reaching the age of puberty. You know that the child has some idea of what to expect but most of her information has come from her friends who are no better informed than she. Her mother has been dead for two years and even though you have tried, you have never been able to gain the child's confidence completely.

How would you go about explaining menstruation to her?

2. Miss Lawrence is a 40-year-old school-teacher who has just had a radical mastectomy for treatment of cancer of the breast. She is a very well-adjusted individual and does not seem to be seriously disturbed by her operation. She wishes to have some information on procuring a prosthesis and the exercises she should take to regain use of her arm and shoulder.

How can you help this person?

3. Mr. Williams, age 67, has been admitted to the hospital for a transurethral resection of the prostate. He is assigned to your care his second postoperative day. Mr. Williams seems disoriented and restless and when you begin to give him his bath he tells you that his bladder is full and he needs to urinate. You check the catheter and find that it apparently is not draining as it should.

What would you tell Mr. Williams about his need to void?
What would you do about the catheter that seems obstructed?
What observations should you make while caring for this patient?
What special precautions should be taken for his safety?

REFERENCES

1. Alford, D. A.: "Nursing Care of the Patient with Endometriosis." *Nursing Clinics of North America*, vol. 3, no. 2. June, 1968, p. 229.
2. Brown, A. F.: *Medical and Surgical Nursing II.* Philadelphia, W. B. Saunders Co., 1959.
3. Crossen, R. J., and Campbell, A. J.: *Gynecologic Nursing*, 5th edition. St. Louis, Mo., C. V. Mosby Co., 1956.
4. Davis, D. M., and Warren, K. C.: *Urological Nursing*, 6th edition. Philadelphia, W. B. Saunders Co., 1959.
5. Egan, R. L.: "Mammography." Am. Journ. Nurs., Jan., 1966, p. 108.
6. Ferguson, L. K., and Sholtis, L. A.: *Eliason's Surgical Nursing*, 11th edition. Philadelphia, J. B. Lippincott Co., 1959.
7. Funnell, J. W., and Roof, B.: "Before and after Vaginal Hysterectomy." Am. Journ. Nurs., Oct., 1964, p. 120.
8. Kasselman, M. J.: "Nursing Care of the Patient with Benign Prostatic Hypertrophy." Am. Journ. Nurs., May, 1966, p. 1026.
9. Larsen, G. I.: "What Every Nurse Should Know about Congenital Syphilis." Nurs. Outlook, March, 1965, p. 52.
10. Mayo, P., and Wilkey, N. L.: "Prevention of Cancer of the Breast and Cervix." *Nursing*

Clinics of North America, vol. 3, no. 2. June, 1968, p. 229.

11. McGowan, L.: "Before and after Vaginal Surgery." Am. Journ. Nurs., Feb., 1964, p. 73.
12. Miller, N. F., and Avery, H.: *Gynecology and Gynecologic Nursing*, 4th edition. Philadelphia, W. B. Saunders Co., 1959.
13. Noval, E. R.: "Benign Ovarian Tumors." Am. Journ. Nurs., Nov., 1964, p. 104.
14. Shafer, K. N., Sawyer, J. R., et al.: *Medical-Surgical Nursing*, 4th edition. St. Louis, Mo., C. V. Mosby Co., 1967.
15. Smith, D. W., and Gips, C. D.: *Care of the Adult Patient*, 2nd edition. Philadelphia, J. B. Lippincott Co., 1966.
16. Wolf, E. S.: "Nursing Care of Patients with Breast Cancer." *Nursing Clinics of North America*, vol. 2, no. 4. Dec., 1967, p. 587.

SUGGESTED STUDENT READING

1. American Cancer Society (pamphlet): "Help Yourself to Recovery after Mastectomy."
2. Bolton, W.: "Why Girls Menstruate." Today's Health, April, 1962, p. 12.
3. Felton, C.: "The Long Road Home." Journ. Pract. Nurs., July-Aug., 1965, p. 34.
4. Funnell, J. W., and Roof, B.: "Before and after Hysterectomy." Am. Journ. Nurs., Oct., 1964, p. 120.
5. Lewison, E. F.: "The Treatment of Advanced Breast Cancer." Am. Journ. Nurs., Oct., 1962, p. 107.
6. McGowan, L.: "Before and after Vaginal Surgery." Am. Journ. Nurs., Feb., 1964, p. 73.
7. Schussman, M.: "What It Means to Have a Mastectomy." RN, May, 1961, p. 33.
8. Suiter, J. A.: "Clinical Picture of Advanced Carcinoma of the Breast." Practical Nursing, Oct., 1962, p. 14.

OUTLINE FOR CHAPTER 17

I. Introduction

A. Reproductive system handles procreation or reproduction of the species.

B. Male and female organs of reproduction are glands, tubes or ducts and reservoirs.

1. Female glands (ovaries) secrete estrogen and progesterone and excrete ova. Male glands (testes) secrete testosterone and excrete spermatozoa.
2. Uterine tubes of female conduct ova from ovary to uterus. Vagina conducts menstrual flow or baby. Complex system of tubes in male serves as passageway for spermatozoa.
3. Reservoirs in female are the ovary

and the uterus. In the male the epididymis stores spermatozoa until ejaculation.

Part I – Diseases of the Female Reproductive System

I. Special Diagnostic Tests and Examinations

A. Pelvic examination.

B. Smears and cultures – sampling of material from the reproductive tract is taken and examined in the laboratory.

C. Dilatation and curettage – dilation of the cervix and curettage (scraping) of the endometrial lining of the uterus.

D. Mammography – x-ray examination of the soft tissues of the breast without injection of a contrast medium.

II. Disorders of Menstruation

A. Amenorrhea – absence of menstruation.

1. Causes – hormonal imbalance, malformation of the reproductive tract, chronic disease or emotional disturbance.
2. Treatment directed toward primary cause.

B. Dysmenorrhea – painful menstruation.

1. Severe pain, but not minor discomfort that usually accompanies menstruation, should be reported to gynecologist.
2. Treatment concerned with primary cause.

C. Menorrhagia – an excessive loss of blood during menstruation.

1. Frequently due to an endocrine disturbance, uterine tumors or an abnormal condition of pregnancy.
2. Curettage of the uterine cavity sometimes done to relieve bleeding and to aid in diagnosis.

D. Metrorrhagia – bleeding at times other than menstrual cycle.

1. May be a symptom of serious pelvic disease and should be investigated.

III. Infections of the Genital Tract

A. Gonorrhea – a venereal disease caused by the gonococcus and spread by sexual contact.

1. Symptoms – purulent vaginal discharge, dysuria and itching. Can cause sterility.

2. Treatment—penicillin and streptomycin.

B. Syphilis—a venereal disease caused by a spirochete called *Treponema pallidum.*

1. Spread by direct bodily contact. Can be transmitted by a mother to her unborn child.
2. Diagnosis—presence of treponema in smear taken from chancre or by blood test.
3. Symptoms.
   a. Primary stage—chancre, headache and enlarged lymph glands.
   b. Secondary stage — no symptoms, or patient may have rash, loss of hair in patches, sore throat or arthritis and neuritis.
   c. Tertiary stage—symptoms depend on organs affected; do not appear until damage has been done. Organs most often affected are the blood vessels and heart, nerves and eyes.
4. Treatment — penicillin or some other antibiotic in primary stage will cure and prevent complications. Disease in the tertiary stage beyond treatment.

C. Pelvic inflammatory disease—any inflammation in the pelvis outside the uterus.

1. Caused by microorganisms that spread upward through the uterus and uterine tubes.
2. Symptoms—severe abdominal and pelvic pain, nausea and vomiting, foul-smelling, purulent vaginal discharge.
3. Treatment—antibiotics and measures to localize infection and prevent complications.

IV. Vaginal Infections

A. Trichomonas vaginitis—inflammation of the vaginal mucosa, caused by *Trichomonas vaginalis.*

1. Symptoms—persistent white vaginal discharge that irritates the vaginal mucosa and swelling and inflammation of the vulva and perineum.
2. Treatment—various suppositories, powders or other local applications may be used but infection difficult to control.

B. Monilial vaginitis—inflammation of the vagina caused by *Candida albicans.*

1. Symptoms—watery vaginal discharge containing cheese-like flakes and intense itching and inflammation of the vulva.

2. Treatment—local applications of drugs.

V. Tumors of the Uterus

A. Most common benign tumors (fibroids) involve the uterine wall. Malignant tumors most often affect the cervix.

B. Abnormal bleeding first symptom. If tumor grows it can cause symptoms of pressure.

C. Treatment. Benign tumors may subside at menopause or may require a simple hysterectomy. Malignant tumors demand prompt removal and possibly irradiation to eliminate the danger of metastasis.

VI. Uterine Displacements

A. An extreme tilting of the uterus away from its normal position in the pelvis.

B. Symptoms (may be none)—backache, feeling of heaviness in the pelvis, vaginal discharge and fatigue.

C. Treatment—insertion of pessary for milder cases; surgical fixation for more severe ones.

VII. Nursing Care of the Patient Having Vaginal Surgery

A. Preoperative preparation varies. Usually the patient is given a vaginal douche, the vulva and perineal area are shaved and cleansed with a surgical detergent and the intestines are emptied.

B. After surgery patient is watched closely for signs of unusual bleeding. If there is no catheter the patient must be checked for ability to void. Early ambulation or sitting up help prevent circulatory complications, such as thrombophlebitis, and pulmonary complications.

VIII. Endometriosis (Endometrial Tissue Outside the Uterus)

A. Symptoms—severe pain in lower abdomen or pelvis, excessive menstrual flow, metrorrhagia and pain on defecation or during sexual intercourse.

B. Treatment—varies with location of misplaced tissue, age of patient and her desire to have children and severity of symptoms. Surgical removal of one or both ovaries or a panhysterectomy most often done.

IX. Ovarian Tumors

A. Symptoms very slow to develop. Irregular bleeding, palpable mass in abdomen and vague feeling of fullness in abdomen.

B. Treatment depending on type and size of tumor, age of patient and severity of symptoms. Surgery or radiation therapy common.

X. Disorders of the Breast

A. Cystic disease, also called dysplasia or cystic mastitis, is most common disorder of breast. Symptoms are mild and treatment (simple mastectomy) necessary for very few cases.

B. Carcinoma of the breast.
    1. Cause unknown.
    2. Symptoms are a lump in the breast, dimpling, retraction of nipple, abnormal discharge from nipple, swelling, change in firmness or appearance of redness.
    3. Treatment is radical mastectomy.

XI. Nursing Care of the Patient Having a Mastectomy

A. Simple mastectomy—removal of a breast. Radical mastectomy—removal of entire breast, underlying pectoral muscles and axillary lymph nodes.

B. Preoperative care—shaving and cleaning operative area and emotional support.

C. Postoperative care—pressure dressing watched closely for sign of hemorrhage, checked for being too tight and reinforced as necessary (changed only on specific orders). Deep breathing and coughing encouraged. Special exercises of arm and shoulder necessary to prevent deformities and disabilities.

Part II—The Male Reproductive System

I. Infections of the Male Genital Tract

A. Urethritis—an inflammation of the urethra.
    1. Symptoms—frequent urge to void and burning on urination.
    2. Treatment—antibiotics and local applications of a mild antiseptic.

B. Prostatitis—an inflammation of the prostate gland.
    1. Symptoms—painful urination, dif-

ficulty in voiding and pain and tenderness in perineal area.
    2. Treatment—antibiotics, local applications of heat and bed rest.

C. Epididymitis—inflammation of the epididymis. A common complication of gonorrhea.
    1. Symptoms—local pain and tenderness in scrotal region, high fever and severe fatigue.
    2. Treatment—cold applications to scrotum, antibiotics and wearing an athletic support.

D. Balanitis—an inflammation of the glans penis often caused by phimosis.
    1. Symptoms—swelling and signs of local inflammation.
    2. Treatment—circumcision and antibiotics.

E. Orchitis—an inflammation of the testes. Can be a complication of mumps.
    1. Symptoms—pain and local tenderness in scrotal area and fever.
    2. Treatment—bed rest, elevation of scrotum and applications of ice bags.

II. Tumors of the Prostate Gland

A. Classified as benign or malignant. Occur most often in men over 55 years of age.

B. Symptoms—tumors usually cause no symptoms until they have grown large enough to obstruct the flow of urine from the bladder.

C. Treatment is surgical removal of all or part of the prostate gland.
    1. Radical prostatectomy—entire prostate gland and its capsule removed.
    2. Suprapubic prostatectomy—removed by incision into the bladder.
    3. Retropubic prostatectomy—removed by low abdominal incision.
    4. Transurethral prostatic resection—removed by way of the urethra.
    5. Preoperative care—maintenance of urinary flow, protection of the patient from self-injury and adequate explanation of necessary procedures.
    6. Postoperative care—postoperative hemorrhage guarded against, urinary flow maintained and dressing changed to keep patient dry and comfortable.

Chapter 18

NURSING CARE OF PATIENTS WITH DISORDERS OF THE NERVOUS SYSTEM

Aneurysm
Cerebrospinal
Hematoma
Occiput
Palliative

INTRODUCTION

The nervous system is the communication system of our bodies. It acts as coordinator for all sensory and motor activities, receiving, interpreting, and relaying messages which are vital to the proper performance of all the body's activities. The nervous system is composed of nerve cells and their branches which interlace with one another to form a dense network of nerve tissue. There are a number of different types of nerve cells, but they all have two physiological properties in common, *excitability* and *conductivity*.

Nerve cells are excited, or spurred into action, by a stimulus. This stimulus sets up an impulse which is conducted along the nerve pathways until it reaches the tissues of the organ which are controlled by the nerve cells. Should anything happen to impair the ability of certain nerve cells to receive and conduct impulses, the tissues which these cells control cease to function normally. An example of this would be trauma to the spinal cord. All parts of the body below the point of injury would be paralyzed and have no sensation of heat, cold, pressure, or pain if the spinal cord had been severed and the flow of impulses interrupted.

Neurology is the branch of medicine concerned with the study of the nervous system and its diseases. It is a highly specialized branch of medical practice. Neurological nursing also requires special training and scientific knowledge above the level of basic nursing. The practical nurse should become familiar with some of the more common neurological terms and basic principles of neurological nursing, but she should realize that most patients with serious neurological disorders should be cared for by nurses who have had formal training as well as additional experience in the field of neurological nursing.

COMMON NEUROLOGICAL TERMS

Paraplegia: paralysis of the lower extremities or lower part of the body. Commonly associated with spinal injury.

Hemiplegia: paralysis of one side of the body. Commonly associated with cerebral damage.

Quadriplegia: paralysis of all four extremities.

Flaccid paralysis: paralysis in which the muscles are limp and flabby.

Spastic paralysis: paralysis in which the muscles are tense and rigid.

Amnesia: loss of memory.

Aphasia: loss of the ability to speak. In total aphasia the individual cannot comprehend language in any form, written or spoken.

SPECIAL EXAMINATIONS AND DIAGNOSTIC TESTS

Neurological Examination. The complete neurological examination measures the ability of the body to perform certain motor and sensory functions. It is a very intensive and prolonged procedure, sometimes requiring several days to complete if the examination is done in its entirety. It is not within the scope of this text to cover the neurological examination in detail, but some general aspects of the examination may help the practical nurse understand the purpose of the examination.

The *cranial nerves* control both sensory and motor activities within various parts of the body. The patient will be tested for his sense of taste, smell, sight, and hearing. His facial expressions, gag reflex, and ability to move his eyes are also included in the testing of the cranial nerves.

Groups of large muscles are tested for strength and coordination during a neurological examination. The physician will evaluate the patient's gait while walking and running, his posture while standing, and the strength of his hand grip.

Involuntary muscular contractions in response to a stimulus are called reflexes. These reflexes are impaired or entirely absent in some types of neurological disorders. The knee jerk in response to tapping below the kneecap with a percussion hammer is a well known example of a reflex.

When the physician suspects an inflammation or traumatic injury to the protective coverings of the brain and spinal cord, he will perform certain tests for signs and symptoms of meningeal irritation. Stiffness of the neck, unusual sensitivity of the skin, and an involuntary flexion of the hip and knee joints when the head is flexed are all indications of an irritation of the meninges.

Lumbar Puncture. The meninges covering the brain and spinal cord are composed of three layers; the second, or middle layer is called the *arachnoid* because it resembles a cobweb. The spaces within the arachnoid layer are filled with cerebrospinal fluid which bathes and protects the spinal cord and brain. To obtain a sampling of this fluid for examination in the laboratory, the physician inserts a hollow needle into the arachnoid space between the third and fourth lumbar vertebrae. The spinal cord does not extend this far down the vertebral column so there is no danger of puncturing the cord with the needle. The specimen of spinal fluid obtained through a lumbar puncture is collected in a sterile test tube and sent to the laboratory for microscopic examination and chemical analysis.

The lumbar puncture (or spinal tap as it is sometimes called) may also be done for any of the following reasons:

1. To measure the pressure within the cerebrospinal cavities.

2. To determine whether there is a blockage of the flow of spinal fluid.

3. To remove blood or pus from the arachnoid space.

4. To reduce intracranial pressure.

5. For spinal anesthesia.

6. To inject air for x-ray examination of the skull (pneumoencephalogram).

The patient is usually kept flat in bed for at least 8 hours after a lumbar puncture to reduce headache.

Cisternal Puncture. In this type of spinal tap the needle is inserted just below the occipital bone into the cisterna magna (see Fig. 18-1). Some authorities feel that this procedure is less likely to cause headache than a lumbar puncture. Cisternal puncture is often done in out-patient clinics and on children and other patients who are unable to cooperate during a lumbar puncture. Complications seldom occur but the patient should be observed immediately after the procedure for signs of respiratory difficulty or the appearance of cyanosis.

Electroencephalogram. This test records the activity of the brain tissues and is similar in principle to the electrocardiogram (see p. 53).

X-ray Contrast Studies. There are three types of x-ray examinations commonly done in the diagnosis of intracranial disorders. These tests help determine the presence or absence of "space-taking" lesions such as tumors and other conditions such as atrophy of cerebral tissue and vascular disorders and malformations.[12]

Angiography involves injection of a radiopaque liquid into the common carotid or vertebral arteries and taking a series of x-ray films as the solution fills the cerebral vessels. If a tumor is present in the brain the blood vessels will appear dislocated or pushed aside at the tumor site. Other abnormalities such as aneurysms, thromboses, or hematomas also can be diagnosed by angiography.

Pneumoencephalography utilizes a gas, usually air or oxygen, as a contrast medium. The gas is injected during a lumbar puncture and then routine x-rays from varied angles are taken of the patient's head. Abnormalities of the brain structure will show up on the x-ray film. This procedure is not done if the patient shows signs of increased intracranial pressure because the injected gas may serve to increase the pressure and damage the brain tissue.

Ventriculography involves the boring of two holes in the skull for the purpose of injecting air into the ventricles of the brain. This procedure must be done in an operating room. After air is injected, the wounds are closed and x-rays are taken of the skull. This type of test is most helpful in diagnosing and locating brain tumors.

Radioisotopes. Because some brain tumors accumulate more than a normal amount of radioactive isotopes,

Figure 18-1. The position of the needle when a cisternal puncture is done. Note the needle length and the short bevel. (From Shafer et al.: *Medical-Surgical Nursing,* 4th Ed., The C. V. Mosby Co., St. Louis.)

A

B

Figure 18-2. *A,* Normal brain scan. Note normal increased uptake in areas such as venous sinuses, nasopharyngeal mucosa, and scalp. *B,* Abnormal brain scan. Note large density seen in the left temporal area resulting from increased uptake by abnormal tissue. *C,* Normal liver scan. The reticuloendothelial portions of the liver are seen, as well as small portions of the pulmonary area. Uptake in the left upper quadrant is the spleen. Note that normal tissue concentrates the isotope. (All three scans courtesy of the Department of Nuclear Medicine, St. Mary's Hospital, St. Louis, Mo. From French: *Nurse's Guide to Diagnostic Procedures,* 2nd Ed., McGraw-Hill Book Co., New York.)

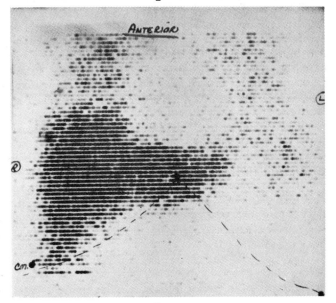

C

a substance such as radioactive iodine combined with serum albumin can be injected intravenously and then traced to the brain. Figure 18-2A shows the distribution of radioactive iodine in a normal brain scan. Figure 18-2B shows a dense area of radioactivity in the temporal area suggesting a tumor that has accumulated the radioactive iodine.

GENERAL NURSING CARE OF THE PATIENT WITH A NEUROLOGICAL DISORDER

The patient with a neurological disorder has some *organic* disease of the nervous system. His condition should not be confused with mental derangements or emotional illness which are psychiatric problems resulting from difficulties in adjusting to one's environment. Even though neurological diseases do affect an individual mentally and emotionally, these effects are a direct result of physical changes and loss of function, or degeneration of nerve tissues.

There are many diseases that can cause disturbances in the functions of the nervous system. These include infectious diseases, tumors, trauma, disorders of the cerebral blood vessels, and congenital malformations. The symptoms produced by these diseases are many and complex, and the nursing care required by each patient will depend on the type and location of the lesion and the effect the pathological changes have on his ability to help himself. In serious neurological disorders the patient may have complete loss of function and control of many of his bodily activities. He will then be totally dependent upon those who care for him. In less serious neurological diseases there may be varying degrees of helplessness and dependency on others.

Hygiene. Proper care of the skin to prevent pressure sores and breaks in

the skin are especially important in neurological nursing. We must remember that with a loss of motion of the various parts of the body there is also a loss of feeling. The patient does not complain of discomfort from pressure or lying in one position too long because he does not *feel* any discomfort. He has been robbed of one of nature's ways of warning that something is wrong. This places an added responsibility on the nursing staff, since they cannot depend on the patient to remind them when he needs his position changed.

A regularly scheduled routine must be established for skin care, turning the patient and proper positioning so that the body is in good alignment.

Providing for Self-care. The nurse should not assume that all patients with neurological disorders are totally helpless. She should take every opportunity to help the patient *help himself* as long as there are no contraindications for his doing so. If the physician grants permission for the patient to move about as much as he is physically able, the nurse may feel free to encourage her patient and provide him with the means to care for himself as much as possible. Doing too much for the patient may be as harmful to him as not doing enough.

The furniture in the patient's room should be arranged so that he can conveniently reach his bedside table and drawer if he wishes to get something for himself. Side rails should be applied to prevent falling out of bed and also to provide the patient with something to grasp so he can assist the nurses in turning him. A trapeze bar may be installed over the bed and the patient instructed in the way he might use this to lift himself up in bed or onto a bedpan.

Feeding himself may be slow or clumsy for the patient, but it is best if he manages this for himself as much as he is able. There are many things we do in the process of eating that require the use of both hands. For hemiplegics such maneuvers as cutting up food, spreading butter or jelly on bread, and opening milk cartons are extremely difficult if not impossible.

The patient should not be rushed through a meal, nor made to feel that it would be best if he did not feed himself because he is so awkward. Accidental spilling of food or liquids should be treated as a matter of course and no comment made on the mess such accidents may make.

While encouraging the patient to help himself the nurse should avoid pushing him into activities beyond his physical limitations. If the patient seems easily discouraged and unwilling to try to help himself, the practical nurse should consult the physician or nurse in charge and determine how much activity can be expected from the patient.

Prevention of Complications. Proper positioning of the patient and passive exercises to prevent contractures, foot drop and wrist drop, and fixation of the joints are especially important in the care of the paralyzed and bedridden patient. The general principles and specific practices discussed in Chapter 11 in regard to orthopedic patients are equally important in neurological nursing.

Emotional Aspects. In view of the fact that impairment of motion and sensory perception are so often the result of neurological disorders, it is not surprising that emotional disturbances and personality changes should accompany these disorders. It is never easy for a formerly active individual to adjust to a loss of his physical independence. Such a situation is extremely frustrating and the patient may express his resentment in a number of ways. Emotional outbursts of anger or depression are not uncommon and in some cases the individual may show a loss of the will to live. The nurses who care for patients with neurological disorders must be prepared for such emotional storms and crises and do their best to help these patients adjust to their illness and their handicaps and the problems they bring.

Perhaps the following quotation from a person whose muscles have been rendered all but useless by *myasthenia gravis* will help the reader gain some insight into the problems these individuals must face.

If nurses and others would look past the body which is weak, and the face which probably looks expressionless, with its drooping lids or mouth half open because the patient is unable to close it, they would find a perfectly sane, reasonable human being. These patients are like a competent driver sitting in a faulty vehicle. No matter how hard he tries, he cannot make the car behave as he knows he could with a perfect machine which would respond to his control. However, it is not pity alone which is needed; in fact, that is usually not wanted. There are, however, some small things which mean much and can be done. The myasthenic is always a frustrated person because he usually has a strong will, and the greater his will, the greater the frustration when his muscles will not obey.*

Rehabilitation. The success of rehabilitation and preparation of the patient for his return to home, family, and community will depend on the type of disorder affecting the nervous system. In some degenerative diseases such as multiple sclerosis, Parkinson's disease, or myasthenia gravis there is a gradual deterioration of the nerve cells and progressive loss of function. In these cases rehabilitation is limited to keeping the patient happily occupied, if not gainfully employed, as the disease progresses.

When traumatic injury, cerebrovascular accidents (strokes) or tumors have brought about loss of function in specific areas of the body rather than a generalized paralysis, rehabilitation must be planned so that the individual is eventually able to function as an active member of the family and com-

---

*Quoted from *Medical and Surgical Nursing II* by Amy Frances Brown. Philadelphia, W. B. Saunders Co., 1959, p. 568.

munity in spite of his handicap. For further information on rehabilitation the reader is referred to page 110.

INFECTIOUS DISEASES OF THE BRAIN AND SPINAL CORD

Meningitis

Definition. Meningitis is an inflammation of the membranous linings of the brain and spinal cord. The infection may be carried to the meninges by way of the blood stream, or by direct extension from neighboring tissues, such as from a severe infection of the sinuses. Many different bacteria and viruses can cause meningitis, but when the disease occurs in epidemic form it is usually caused by a specific organism called *meningococcus.* The disease is then spread by healthy meningococcal carriers.

Symptoms. The most outstanding symptom of meningitis is a severe and persistent headache that is greatly aggravated by shaking the head. There are also other signs of meningeal irritation; for example, pain and stiffness of the neck, irritability, photophobia, and hypersensitivity of the skin. Nausea and vomiting and signs of an upper respiratory infection are usually present.

When meningitis is suspected, a spinal tap is done and the cerebrospinal fluid examined for the number and types of cells and organisms in it. In meningitis the spinal fluid will often appear milky due to the increase of white cells suspended in the fluid.

In the late stages of severe meningitis the back may be bowed so that the head is extended back toward the heels and the trunk and legs are rigid.

Treatment and Nursing Care. Successful treatment of meningitis and prevention of permanent disability depend on early recognition and diagnosis of the disease. Once the causative

organism has been determined specific antibiotics are given in large doses. The drugs may be administered by mouth or intramuscularly, and penicillin is sometimes given directly into the spinal fluid circulation *(intrathecally).* Anticonvulsive drugs are given to control seizures. As long as the disease is in the acute stage, the patient is placed in strict isolation to prevent contamination of others. Meningococcal infection is spread by droplet infection, which means that all secretions from the respiratory tract are sources of infection.

Nursing care is primarily concerned with supportive measures to conserve the strength of the patient, and close observation of the patient for signs of chills, elevation of body temperature, and convulsions.

The patient's room should be quiet and dimly lighted. Sudden noises or a bright flash of light, such as occurs when an overhead light is switched on, may easily precipitate a convulsion. Every detail of the patient's environment must be considered and all stimuli which may excite the patient removed. It is obvious from his outward appearance that the patient with meningitis is acutely ill. He resents any disturbance because motion of the head or extremities increases pain and adds to his discomfort. He must be turned very gently and disturbed as little as possible for necessary treatments. Meningitis often produces mental confusion and delirium as well as the possibility of convulsions. Padded side rails and other safety measures should be used to prevent self-injury. Cool compresses on the forehead or an ice bag on the head often help relieve delirium.

Herpes simplex (fever blisters) frequently accompany meningitis. The presence of these sores, plus drying of the lips and mouth due to high temperatures and dehydration, demand special mouth care. The lips and mouth should be cleansed and lubricated at least every two hours during the acute stage of the disease.

Dehydration is often a problem and most physicians wish to have a record kept of the patient's intake and output. Excessive vomiting or outward signs of early dehydration should be reported so that fluids may be given intravenously when necessary.

A decrease in peristaltic action of the intestines often occurs in meningitis and thus leads to an accumulation of flatus and fecal material with severe abdominal distention. Rectal tubes, suppositories or *small low* enemas may be ordered for relief of this condition. Large amounts of water should not be given rectally because they may increase intracranial pressure and lead to convulsions or severe headache.

Once the acute stage of the disease is over the patient is allowed to gradually resume his former activities. Residual effects of the disease, such as paralysis, deafness, or visual defects, sometimes occur but these *sequelae* of meningitis do not usually occur if the disease is diagnosed and treated in the early stages before permanent damage is done.

Encephalitis

Definition. Encephalitis is an inflammation of the brain tissues. The disease is most often caused by a virus, or from toxins produced by the organisms which cause chickenpox, measles, or mumps. Some chemicals such as lead and arsenic can also cause encephalitis.

Symptoms. The onset of encephalitis may be sudden or insidious and is characterized by headache, fever, extreme restlessness, or lethargy and muscular weakness. The lethargy may progress to coma. Mental confusion, visual disturbances, and disorientation may also be present.

Treatment and Nursing Care. The treatment of encephalitis is mainly symptomatic with general supportive measures to maintain the strength of the patient. Isolation of the patient may be necessary if the encephalitis is of the infectious type.

Side rails and constant attendance to prevent the patient from injuring himself are necessary during the period of disorientation. Mechanical restraints should be used only when absolutely necessary, for example, when the patient is receiving intravenous fluids and may dislodge the needle. The head of the bed and the side rails are padded and a tongue blade wrapped with gauze is kept at the bedside in case the patient has convulsions.

The vital signs are carefully checked at frequent intervals so that any change may be reported immediately. If the body temperature becomes excessively high, measures are taken to bring it down to within normal limits. The environment of the patient is kept quiet and restful and sedatives are sometimes given to control restlessness and induce sleep. Should the patient become extremely restless or display any signs of respiratory difficulty his condition should be reported immediately.

The convalescent period for the patient with encephalitis is essentially the same as that for a patient with meningitis.

Poliomyelitis

Definition. Poliomyelitis is an acute inflammation of the anterior horn of the spinal cord. The disease may be caused by three different strains of viruses, all of which have a special affinity for nerve tissue. Since the discovery of the exact cause of poliomyelitis, it is now possible to immunize individuals against this disease. The Salk vaccine and Sabin vaccine are used and have greatly reduced the incidence of poliomyelitis in this country.

Symptoms. Poliomyelitis may present such mild symptoms that the disease often goes unrecognized and leaves no residual paralysis. In fact, some authorities state that as high as 80 percent of the people in this country have had poliomyelitis at some time without realizing they had the disease.[1]

The symptoms of severe poliomyelitis are very similar to those of other neurologic infections. Signs of an upper respiratory infection, fever, severe headache and soreness and stiffness of the neck, back and hamstring muscles are usually present. As the disease progresses paralysis may occur.

Treatment and Nursing Care. There is no cure for poliomyelitis and no specific treatment. It is a tragic disease in its more serious form, and the adage, "an ounce of prevention is worth a pound of cure," could not be more aptly applied than in this instance. In spite of the fact that immunization is possible, recent statistics show that almost half the schoolchildren in this country still have not been immunized against poliomyelitis. The practical nurse should take every opportunity to encourage parents to have their children protected against this crippling disease.

During the acute febrile stage of the disease the patient is kept on complete rest. No specific positioning is necessary beyond maintenance of good posture and frequent turning. All muscular strain and rough handling should be avoided in moving the patient. The nurse should place the palms of her hands under the *joints* rather than on the muscular part of the extremities because the skeletal muscles are subject to painful spasms when stimulated by pressure (see Fig. 18-3).

Urinary retention and fecal impaction are common problems, especially in patients with paralysis of the lower extremities. The urinary output is measured and recorded and a careful checking of bowel movements is necessary. The nurse should not mistake a "dribbling" of overflow from a distended bladder as emptying of the bladder. She can determine bladder distention by gently pressing her hand over the bladder region. If the bladder is full it is plainly felt under the palm of the hand.

Figure 18-3. Proper method of handling a limb when muscle spasm is likely to result from stimulation. Note that the palms of the hands are used and the joints above and below the affected muscles are supported. (From Wiebe: *Orthopedics in Nursing*, W. B. Saunders Co., Philadelphia.)

The application of heat to the muscles for the relief of painful contractions has been found to be very helpful. The form of heat to be applied will depend on the wishes of the physician. Most patients with poliomyelitis are under the care of a physiotherapist who supervises the administration of hot packs and passive exercise of the extremities.

Patients with poliomyelitis frequently have difficulty swallowing and may also have respiratory problems requiring the use of an artificial respirator. These patients require expert nursing care from persons trained and experienced in this specialized area of nursing.

HEAD INJURIES

Definition and Types. A blow to the head may cause *open* injuries, with lacerations of the skin and scalp, and fracture of the skull; or *closed* injuries in which the scalp and skull remain intact but the underlying brain tissue is damaged. The term "*concussion*" is used to describe a closed head injury in which the brain is compressed by a portion of the skull at the time of the blow and temporary anemia of the brain tissue results. In a *contusion* the brain tissue is bruised and swelling occurs, pressing the brain tissues against the skull.

Symptoms. The severity of brain damage from a head injury is best judged by the symptoms presented by the patient, the history of the type of blow received, and whether or not the victim lost consciousness. No head injury should be considered completely harmless. They are all potentially dangerous because there may be a delayed reaction in which there is hemorrhage into the brain tissues or the formation of a blood clot (hematoma). These conditions build up over a period of time and result from weakening and rupture of the small blood vessels in the brain. Sometimes the bleeding is so slow that it takes weeks or even months for the symptoms of pressure within the skull to appear.

Aside from the obvious lacerations of the scalp, or fractures of the skull which may be seen on x-ray, intracranial hemorrhage or the formation of a blood clot must always be considered a possibility in a head injury. The observations of the nurse in regard to the patient's behavior and the symptoms he manifests may be of great help to the physician in determining the extent of damage to the brain.

Treatment and Nursing Care. The patient with a head injury is treated conservatively at first unless a compound fracture of the skull demands surgical debridement of the wound and removal of splintered bone from the brain tissues. Other surgical procedures to relieve pressure from intracranial bleeding may be necessary if the pressure in the skull builds up to a dangerous level. (See page 402 for nursing care of the patient having brain surgery.)

As we have stated above, the nurse's observations are extremely important in the diagnosis and treatment of head injuries. Any one of the symptoms listed below should be reported immediately should they occur.

1. Changes in the patient's blood pressure, pulse or respiration.

2. Extreme restlessness or excitability following a period of apparent calm.

3. Deepening stupor or loss of consciousness.

4. Headache which increases in intensity.

5. Vomiting, especially persistent, projectile vomiting.

6. Unequal size of pupils.

7. Leakage of cerebrospinal fluid (clear yellow or tinged with pink) from the nose or ear.

8. Inability to move one or more extremity.

These observations are continued until the physician feels that the patient has passed the critical stage of his illness.

Most patients with head injuries are placed on bed rest and kept absolutely quiet until the doctor orders otherwise. Narcotics and other pain-relieving drugs may be prohibited by the physician if he thinks these will mask any of the symptoms the patient may exhibit. Positioning of the patient will also depend on the wishes of the physician. In some cases he may order the patient flat in bed without a pillow, or, if there are signs of increased intracranial pressure and cerebral compression, he may order the head of the bed slightly elevated.

Patients who are unconscious must be watched closely for respiratory difficulties or inability to swallow. If the patient cannot swallow, his head must be turned to the side and his mouth and trachea suctioned as necessary to prevent aspiration of mucus into the lungs. A tracheostomy set and/or respirator may be required in severe head injuries in which there is severe respiratory embarrassment.

When delirium or disorientation is present and convulsions are anticipated, the patient must be protected from self-injury.

Sometimes the patient remains unconscious for weeks or months and a stomach tube must be passed and tube feedings given regularly to maintain adequate nutrition. Intake and output records are kept and the patient is observed for signs of urinary retention, incontinence, abdominal distention or bowel complications.

BRAIN TUMORS

Definition. Tumors of the brain are abnormal growths of cells within the brain tissue or the coverings of the brain. As with other tumors, the cause is not known.

Symptoms. There may be as many symptoms of brain tumors as there are functions of the brain. Symptoms may be produced by actual destruction of portions of brain tissue or they may result from increased pressure within the skull and compression of the brain as the tumor grows inward.

The symptoms may appear gradually, or, if the tumor is a highly malignant, fast-growing type, they may appear suddenly. In a slow-growing type of tumor the individual first shows personality changes, disturbances in judgment and memory, loss of strength, or difficulties in speaking clearly. Headache and vomiting usually do not appear early in the disease because they are a result of increased intracranial pressure which occurs only after the tumor has grown to considerable size.

Treatment and Nursing Care. Brain tumors are treated by surgical removal of the tumorous mass and removal of adjacent tissues which may contain cancer cells. Radiation therapy may also be used in some types of tumors. Localization of the tumor is sometimes very difficult and is determined by observation of the patient's symptoms and by x-ray studies. If the tumor is located in the *cerebrum,* an operation called a *craniotomy* is done. In this procedure a flap of scalp and bone is cut and pulled down, the dura (first meningeal layer) is opened, and the tumor is removed.

Tumors in or near the *cerebellum* are removed through an incision under the occipital bone. This is called a *suboccipital craniectomy* and part of the skull is permanently removed, leaving a defect in the skull.

If the tumor cannot be removed, a portion of the skull (usually in the temporal region) may be removed to relieve compression of the brain against the skull. The tumorous mass then bulges through the opening. This procedure is only a temporary measure to relieve the patient's symptoms.

NURSING CARE OF THE PATIENT HAVING BRAIN SURGERY

Preoperative Care. During the preoperative period in which diagnostic tests and x-ray examinations will be done to determine the location of the tumor, the nurse should familiarize herself with the patient's symptoms. She later uses these observations as a basis for comparison of the patient's condition postoperatively.

Physical preparation of the patient includes shaving of the scalp, which is a painful procedure physically, as well as an emotional shock for the patient. In most hospitals the shaving of the scalp is done in the operating room after the patient has been anesthetized. The hair removed from female patients is saved so that a wig or other type of hairpiece may be made to cover parts of the head while the hair is growing back.

Postoperative Care. The patient's unit is prepared as soon as he is taken to the operating room. This includes the making of a postoperative bed as for other surgical patients, except that the linen is arranged so that the patient's head will be at the foot of the bed. This arrangement makes changing of the dressings and observation of the drainage from the surgical wound easier for the nurses and doctors and less disturbing to the patient. Side rails are applied to the bed.

Equipment assembled at the bedside should include: (1) a suction machine and two rubber catheters, (2) blood pressure apparatus, pencil, and pad to record vital signs, (3) an emergency medicine tray containing stimulants and sedatives, (4) a tourniquet, needles and syringes, (5) a padded tongue blade, (6) a rubber airway, (7) a tracheostomy set (usually necessary only when surgery is done in the area of the cerebellum).

As soon as the patient returns from the operating room he is placed on his side to facilitate drainage of mucus from the mouth and pharynx. Whether or not the head is elevated will depend on the wishes of the surgeon. The vital signs are taken and recorded at frequent intervals and any change is to be reported without delay.

The dressings must be checked often for signs of drainage. If the dressings become soaked with drainage they must be covered with a *sterile* towel to prevent contamination of the wound and possible meningitis.

A thin, watery, yellowish or pink-tinged discharge from the nose or ear may indicate a leakage of cerebrospinal fluid. This drainage is collected in a sterile gauze square loosely applied to the orifice from which the fluid is leaking. No attempt should be made to plug the orifice and stop the flow of fluid.

All of the observations listed on page 401 for patients with head injuries will apply to the patient having brain surgery.

Elevation of the body temperature may occur as a result of a disturbance of the temperature control center in the brain. Most surgeons wish to have the patient's temperature taken rectally every 2 hours for 24 hours after cranial surgery. Nursing measures to reduce the body temperature are used in the event that the temperature becomes excessively high.

As the patient recovers from the surgical procedure his nursing care is planned according to his individual needs. Adequate nutrition and a normal fluid and electrolyte balance must be maintained, either through oral feedings or intravenous therapy, depending on the patient's ability to chew and swallow. Records of intake and output are kept and the patient is observed for urinary retention or incontinence.

Plans for rehabilitation are made according to the residual effects of the surgery. Every attempt is made to salvage the patient's remaining abilities and use them to the greatest advantage. The prevention of complications by proper positioning, frequent turning and passive exercises during the postoperative period is one of the most important aspects of rehabilitation.

INJURIES OF THE SPINAL CORD

Definition. An individual may suffer from injury to the spinal cord in a number of ways. When we speak of injury our first thought is a violent traumatic type of injury in which the spinal cord is severed or partially severed by a direct blow. Automobile accidents, gunshot wounds and other forms of violence do often inflict severe damage to the spinal cord, but tumors, degenerative diseases, and infections can also impair the functions of the spinal cord and its branches.

Generally speaking, spinal cord injuries are classified according to their anatomical location; that is, *cervical, thoracic,* or *lumbosacral.*

Symptoms. Whatever the cause of the damage to the spinal cord, the symptoms of the patient are essentially the same. A complete severance of the cord results in a total loss of function and control in the parts of the body below the point of injury. If the cord is severed in the cervical region the paralysis and loss of sensory perception will include both arms and both legs. Severe injury to the cord above the level of the fifth cervical vertebra is often fatal because the *phrenic* nerves have their origin in the third, fourth and fifth cervical segments. Branches of these nerves play a major role in the control of respiration.

Injury to the spinal cord that does not involve complete severance of the cord may result in a temporary paralysis which will subside as the spinal cord recovers from the initial shock of the injury.

Treatment and Nursing Care. There are four main objectives in the treatment and nursing care of the patient with an injury of the spinal cord: (1) to save the victim's life, (2) to repair as much of the damage to the cord as possible, (3) to prevent further injury to the cord by careful handling of the patient, and (4) to establish a routine of care which will maintain and improve the patient's physical condition, prevent complications, and make his eventual physical, mental, and social rehabilitation possible.

IMMEDIATE CARE. As soon as an individual suffers a sudden injury to the spinal cord he must be handled with extreme care. Even though the nurse or doctor may not be at the scene of the accident to supervise the moving of the victim, they can teach others the proper emergency care of such injuries. If the injured person complains of neck pain, cannot move his legs, and has no feeling in them he should be treated as though he had a spinal cord injury.

Transfer of the patient to the hospital should be done only by trained ambulance attendants or other persons qualified to administer first aid. The victim is moved on a stretcher or board and taken directly to the hospital. His back is kept straight. *No pillow should be placed under the head;* however, rolled towels may be placed under the neck and small of the back so as to maintain the normal curvature of the spine.

In the emergency room of the hospital the patient is treated for shock and an examination is made to determine the extent of his injuries. His hospital room is fully prepared *before* he leaves the emergency room.

The type of bed to be used will be decided by the physician. In many cases a Stryker frame or Foster frame is preferred. In other cases a regular bed with cotton mattress and bed boards may be used and the bed is made up so that the head of the patient is at the foot of the bed.

The physician may also apply traction to the neck through the use of a head halter or Crutchfield tongs (see Fig. 18-4).

Once the patient is in bed or on the orthopedic frame the true test of nursing care begins. All the principles and practices of urologic, orthopedic, and neurologic nursing must be used. The nursing staff must wage a continuous battle with three formidable enemies: *decubitus ulcers, urinary complications,* and *orthopedic deformities.*

SKIN CARE. Frequent turning of the patient is made easier when the patient is on a frame, but it should be remembered that simple changing of position does not guarantee protection against decubiti. All points of pressure, especially the shoulder blades and sacral region, must be checked frequently, cleansed and dried often, and gently massaged to increase circulation to the area.

One factor that contributes to the formation of decubitus ulcers is the poor circulation of blood to any part of the body which has been deprived of its nerve supply. This is because limited muscular activity makes the flow of blood sluggish and inadequate. In view of this, one must also realize that intramuscular injections *should not be given* in the areas of the body which have no "feeling," even though this may appear to be an advantage since the patient cannot feel the injection. The tissues at the site of the injection tend to become inflamed and an abscess may develop because the medication is

Figure 18-4. *A*, Crutchfield tongs. They are inserted through two holes drilled half way into the inner plate of the patient's skull. *B*, Direct alignment of patient's head with his cervical spine is always maintained; three persons are required to turn him on his side. (From Hunkele and Lozier: American Journal of Nursing, September, 1965.)

not properly absorbed into the blood stream.

ELIMINATION. Kidney disorders are likely to develop because bladder function is partly controlled by the autonomic nervous system. A Foley catheter is usually inserted and irrigations of the bladder begun. In some cases there is a return of bladder control after the initial "spinal shock" has subsided.

Liquids by mouth are pushed to 3000 ml. daily to insure adequate flow of urine and elimination of wastes. The juices of citrus fruits are not allowed because these tend to make the urine alkaline. It has been definitely established that an alkaline urine supports the growth of bacteria and the formation of renal stones. Apple, cranberry, grape and cherry juices are excellent substitutes for citrus juices.

Bowel function is also partially controlled by the autonomic nervous system. When injury to the spinal cord impairs the flow of nerve impulses there is a decrease in peristalsis. Thus, gas-forming foods and those that are high in residue are eliminated from the diet.

During the period immediately following injury to the spinal cord the patient may be incontinent of feces because he does not feel the impulse to defecate. To avoid embarrassment and inconvenience he should be offered the bedpan at frequent intervals. Later, a routine may be set up by the physician and nursing staff. This includes the use of suppositories, mild cathartics or low enemas to stimulate defecation at a given time each day until the patient is able to establish his own schedule for regularity of bowel movements. Establishing this routine takes some time and much patience, and the patient should understand that only with determination and a willingness to try again and again can this obstacle to his return to society be overcome.

MUSCLE SPASMS. Immediately after a cord injury the patient will usually have a flaccid type of paralysis. Later, as the cord adjusts to the injury, the paralysis will become *spastic* and there will be strong, involuntary contractions of the skeletal muscles.

These muscle spasms may be violent enough to throw the patient from his bed or wheelchair and must be anticipated so that such accidents can be avoided. If the patient is on a frame a protective strap is placed across the thighs (see Fig. 18-5A). If the upper extremities are involved he is likely to tip over glasses, water pitchers or anything within reach of his arms when he is seized with uncontrollable muscle spasms.

The patient and his family may interpret these spasms as a return of voluntary function of the limbs and will thus have false hopes of complete recovery. It is best if the nurse in charge or the physician explains to them that such is not the case.

POSITIONING OF THE PATIENT. Every practical nurse should be fully aware of the complications resulting from poor posture, in or out of bed. The principles and practices of good positioning of the patient who is bedridden have been described in detail in Chapter 11 of this text, and in Chapter 12 under nursing care of a patient who has had a stroke. The only point to be emphasized here is a reminder that these principles and practices are of extreme importance in the care of a patient with an injury of the spinal cord. The success of his rehabilitation will depend to a great extent on the preservation of the remaining functions of his body. Through the use of footboards, hand rolls, trochanter rolls, sandbags, and other devices, the joints and muscles of the unaffected parts of his body can be kept intact (see Fig. 18-5B). To allow the loss of these remaining assets through negligence on the part of the nursing staff is unforgivable. The partially paralyzed patient has so little to work with in his efforts to adjust to a new way of life, it seems incredible that anyone would willingly or knowingly deny him the little he has.

Rupture of Intervertebral Disc

Definition. The bodies of the vertebrae lie flat upon one another like a stack of coins. Between each of the vertebral bodies there is a disc of fibrous cartilage which acts as a cushion to absorb shocks to the spinal column (see Fig. 18-6). This disc may be ruptured by some type of injury such as lifting a heavy object or wrenching or falling on the back. When the disc ruptures, part of it squeezes out from between the vertebrae and pinches the

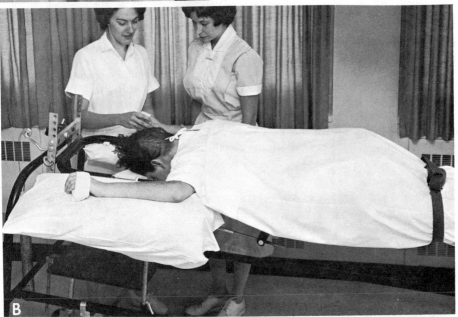

Figure 18-5. *A,* The patient's heels should be suspended above the frame, with the feet at a 90° angle against the foot support. Elastic bandages have been applied to improve circulation. Drainage tubing from the Foley catheter rests between the patient's legs and feet. *B,* This patient, being cared for on a frame and with Crutchfield tongs used for traction, illustrates several important points in care: arm pillows placed at shoulder height, hand rolls used to prevent contractures, and a protective strap at midthigh to prevent injury or a fall from bed during a muscle spasm. (From Martin: American Journal of Nursing, March, 1963.)

Figure 18-6. The articular disc, made of fibrous cartilage, is pictured here showing the manner in which it separates the body of each vertebra. When back strain or injury causes a slipping of the disc from between the vertebrae, there is a pinching of the spinal nerves located in that area. (From King and Showers: *Human Anatomy and Physiology,* 5th Ed., W. B. Saunders Co., Philadelphia.)

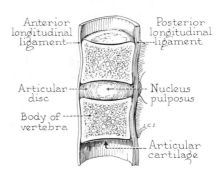

adjacent nerve root by pressing it against the bone. Thus, the individual suffers from what is sometimes called a "slipped disc." Another name for this condition is *hernia of the nucleus pulposus*.

Symptoms.   Most ruptured or slipped discs occur in the lower lumbar and lumbosacral region. The patient experiences pain in the lower back radiating down the back of one leg to the foot. Walking is extremely painful and the discomfort is aggravated by coughing, sneezing, or straining.

Treatment and Nursing Care.   In most instances the physician will treat the condition with conservative measures in the hope that surgical correction will not be necessary.

The patient is placed on a firm cotton mattress with bed boards under it. The bed is kept flat and the patient is placed on bed rest. When he is turned off his back he is "log-rolled"; that is, he is turned without bending his back. In order to accomplish this the patient folds his arms over his chest, flexes the knee opposite the side on which he is to turn, and then is rolled over, just as a log would be rolled.

Hydrocollator packs or some other form of local heat is applied to reduce muscle spasm in the back. Pelvic traction may be applied and mild exercises ordered by the physician (see Fig. 18-7). These treatments are usually done under the guidance of a physiotherapist. Specially designed corsets or back braces are sometimes used to maintain proper alignment of the spine when the patient is allowed up out of bed.

If these measures do not eventually relieve the symptoms, surgery is performed to relieve the damaged disc. The surgical procedure is called a *laminectomy*. The affected vertebrae may be fused together (spinal fusion).

The postoperative care is very much the same as for any patient with major surgery. The positioning of the patient following laminectomy is the same as before surgery: flat in bed and log-rolled to prevent bending the spinal column (see Fig. 18-8).

Figure 18-7.   Patient in pelvic traction for relief of muscle spasm due to ruptured intervertebral disc. Note that knee rest is slightly elevated and pillow is used to support leg and prevent pressure against heels. (From Pasternak: American Journal of Nursing, February, 1962.)

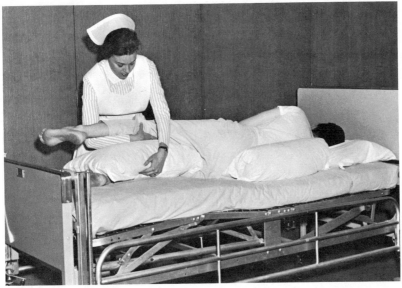

Figure 18-8. Proper alignment of back and support with pillows when patient is "log-rolled" following surgery. This method of turning and support is used for patient who has had laminectomy or a spinal fusion. (From Pasternak: American Journal of Nursing, February, 1962.)

MYASTHENIA GRAVIS

Definition. The words "myasthenia gravis" literally mean *grave muscle weakness.* This disease is fairly uncommon, occurring most frequently in females in their early twenties and thirties.

Symptoms. Severe muscle weakness is the outstanding symptom. Any of the skeletal muscles may be involved, while the muscles of the intestine, bladder and heart are not affected.

The onset is gradual, usually beginning with double vision, ptosis (drooping) of the eyelids, and progressive weakness in the arms and legs. The fatigue is relieved by rest but soon returns and is more severe than is to be expected from the amount of activity the person performs.

Diagnosis is established by administering an injection of *neostigmine.* If there is a dramatic return of strength within 15 to 20 minutes after the infection the diagnosis of myasthenia gravis is confirmed. Another test using edrophonium (Tensilon) produces similar results and the marked increase in muscular strength occurs within one minute of injection.

Treatment and Nursing Care. *Neostigmine* (Prostigmin) and *pyridostigmine* (Mestinon) are the two drugs most commonly used in treating myasthenia gravis. The dosage depends on the individual patient. Whereas some require two to four tablets a day, others who are severe myasthenics need as many as 20 or 30 a day. These medicines are classified as anticholinesterase drugs. They are used because they inactivate acetylcholinesterase, a substance that prevents accumulation of acetylcholine at the neuromuscular junction (point at which nerve impulses are transmitted to the muscle) (see Fig. 18-9). Since acetylcholine improves muscle strength in persons with myasthenia gravis (but not in normal persons) those drugs which remove the barrier to its accumulation indirectly prevent muscle weakness.

The physician usually gives the myasthenic patient a thorough explanation of his disease and encourages him to learn all he can about his illness. The

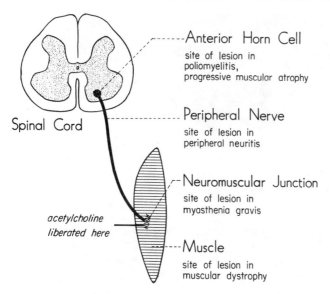

Spinal Cord

-----Anterior Horn Cell
site of lesion in
poliomyelitis,
progressive muscular atrophy

-------- Peripheral Nerve
site of lesion in
peripheral neuritis

*acetylcholine
liberated here*

--Neuromuscular Junction
site of lesion in
myasthenia gravis

----Muscle
site of lesion in
muscular dystrophy

Figure 18-9. A cross section of the spinal cord showing sites of lesions in four nervous system disorders. Special attention is directed to the neuromuscular junction, site of the chemical abnormality present in myasthenia gravis. This lesion is the basis for present forms of treating the disease. (From Magee: Journal of Practical Nursing, November, 1965.)

Myasthenia Gravis Foundation with headquarters at the New York Academy of Medicine, 2 East 103rd St., New York City, 10029, promotes research for discovery of the cause and cure for the disease and disseminates information about the disease through its local chapters.

There are some myasthenic patients who become rapidly worse despite treatment by rest and medication. This severe weakness is called "myasthenic crisis," and may result in death from weakness of the throat muscles and respiratory failure. The patient with this condition is admitted to the hospital and a tracheostomy and artificial respirator may be necessary to maintain life.

During the myasthenic crisis, a nurse should be in constant attendance, assisting the patient in maintaining a clear airway by suctioning the mouth and throat to remove mucus which cannot be swallowed, and reassuring the patient by her calm and competent manner.

It is understandable that these patients are extremely apprehensive when left alone because they are too weak to summon help when needed. Emotional excitement uses up their limited amount of energy just as physical activity does. A quiet atmosphere and anticipation of the patient's every need will do much to conserve the patient's energy until he has recovered from the crisis. In some cases there will be a spontaneous remission of symptoms in which the severe weakness subsides almost as rapidly as it appeared. The reason for this abatement of symptoms is not known.

PARKINSON'S DISEASE

Definition. Parkinson's disease is a degenerative disease of the nerve cells in the brain. The cause of the disease is not known but it sometimes follows encephalitis or carbon monoxide poisoning. The disease is most common in persons over 55 years of age.

Symptoms. There are two symptoms which are characteristic of parkinsonism. One is a *tremor* which is most marked in the fingers, causing the individual constantly to perform an involuntary "pill-rolling" movement; the second is *rigidity* of the skeletal muscles. This rigidity affects the individual's posture and gait so that walking becomes increasingly difficult. There may also be personality changes and intellectual deterioration as the disease progresses.

Treatment and Nursing Care. Treatment for Parkinson's disease is palliative and symptomatic. Medications used are those drugs which produce mild sedation and muscular relaxation. The patient is encouraged to continue his usual activities as much as possible within the physical limitations of the disease and to avoid emotional upsets or physical exhaustion.

In recent years some patients with Parkinson's disease have been successfully treated with neurosurgical procedures which destroy certain areas of nerve cells and thereby eliminate the tremor and muscular rigidity. This type of treatment offers encouragement and hope for recovery for certain selected patients but is not a cure for every person with parkinsonism. (See Reference 16 for details on neurosurgical procedures in the treatment of Parkinsonism.)

MULTIPLE SCLEROSIS

Definition. Multiple sclerosis is a chronic and progressive disease of the central nervous system. It is characterized by a sclerosing (scarring) of the *myelin sheath* which covers the nerve fibers, and may occur anywhere along the nerve pathways. In a normal individual the myelin sheath functions in the same way as insulation on an electric wire. If the protective covering is worn away and replaced by scar tissue, nerve impulses cannot travel along the nerve pathways. Thus, the muscles do not receive these impulses and cease to perform in a well coordinated and useful manner.

The cause of multiple sclerosis is not known. It tends to run in families and most often affects persons between the ages of 20 and 40.

Symptoms. Multiple sclerosis has a very slow and insidious onset with disturbances in vision, muscular weakness and gradual loss of coordination in muscular activities. The symptoms may completely subside for a while and then return with greater severity than before.

Treatment and Nursing Care. There is no cure for multiple sclerosis. Treatment is aimed at relief of symptoms and avoidance of infection, fatigue, poor nutrition or emotional upsets, all of which may precipitate an attack and increase the severity of the symptoms.

EPILEPSY

Definition. Epilepsy is a term used to describe sudden and uncontrollable seizures or "fits" in which the individual has muscular twitching and a temporary loss of consciousness. Epilepsy may be either a symptom or a disease in itself. When the seizures are due to a tumor, infection, or injury to the brain, it is considered to be a symptom. When the cause is not known and there is no demonstrable pathology found the condition is called *idiopathic epilepsy.*

Although epilepsy has sometimes been considered to be an inherited disease, it does not follow the laws of inheritance and there are no dependable statistical studies to justify the importance some authorities have attached to heredity as a cause of the disease.

Symptoms. The signs and symptoms of epilepsy may vary from minor (*petit mal*) to major (*grand mal*). In a minor seizure the attack may pass unnoticed by a casual observer because it often consists of only a very brief loss of consciousness and a "vacant stare" which lasts for a second or two.

The grand mal seizure is often preceded by an *aura.* This is a specific warning (varying in individual patients) which enables the epileptic to sense that an attack is coming on and prepare himself by lying down so that he will not be injured during the seizure. An epileptic may describe the aura as a flash of light, a dimming of vision, a peculiar odor, or any number of sensory changes of which he is aware just before the attack.

Treatment and Nursing Care. The care of an individual during a seizure is the same as for any person who is in convulsion (see p. 34).

The most useful and effective drugs for control of epileptic seizures are the barbiturates, diphenlyhydantoin sodium (Dilantin Sodium) and trimethadione (Tridione). There are quite a few other anticonvulsant drugs that can be used when a patient cannot tolerate one of those listed above, or when one specific drug loses its effectiveness for a patient. Toxic effects of anticonvulsants include drowsiness, rash, fatigue and sometimes blood disturbances. Patients taking these drugs regularly should remain under close medical supervision.

Through the efforts of the Epilepsy Association of America (111 W. 57 St., New York, 10019), the general public has become increasingly aware of the true nature of epilepsy. Research continues in an effort to find the cause and successful cure for this disease. In the meantime we all have a responsibility to help these people gain steady employment and lead useful, active lives. Most epileptics are perfectly normal between seizures; they are not mentally retarded, and are quite capable of becoming contributing members of our society if only they are given the chance to prove their worth.

CEREBRAL PALSY

Introduction. Cerebral palsy is a type of paralysis with lack of muscle coordination that is due to cerebral damage generally thought to occur at or near the time of birth. The exact cause is not known, but the condition is believed to be associated with oxygen lack, premature birth, blood type incompatibility, trauma during birth or infection involving the brain or meninges.

Symptoms. Although there may be a wide variety of muscular disorders and some disturbances of sensory perception, most cerebral palsy victims have one of three types: *Spastic paralysis,* in which there are exaggerated reflexes, increased deep tendon reflexes and muscle spasms; *athetoid type,* in which there are random and purposeless movements and a high degree of muscle tension; and *ataxic type,* in which there is a disturbance of coordination with poor balance and a staggering gait. The patient also may suffer from defects of hearing, vision or speech.

Treatment. There is no cure for cerebral palsy, but early muscle training and special exercises can be of benefit if they are started before a child develops faulty habits of movement and incorrect muscle patterns. In some cases orthopedic surgery and the use of devices such as braces and casts can be used to correct orthopedic deformities and disabilities.

Attitude of the Nurse. Most victims of cerebral palsy, be they men, women or children, long to be treated as normal, sane individuals. For some reason many people conclude that the speech difficulties and uncoordinated movements characteristic of cerebral palsy indicate mental retardation or total disability. Although the cerebral palsy victim may be somewhat slower and clumsier in accomplishing relatively simple tasks or more difficult to understand when he is talking, he can be fairly independent if one is patient with him and willing to make the effort to communicate with him. What can happen to a person with this disorder when he enters a general hospital for a physical illness? We have presented below the memories of one cerebral palsy victim who was hospitalized for appendicitis. It is hoped that those who read her story will strive to have a better understanding of the problems such a person may encounter and avoid the common misconceptions about a cerebral palsy victim.

* * *

A PATIENT'S HUMILIATION*

To the palsied patient, who cannot communicate clearly, any kind of operation can be terrifying. Terrified is how I felt when I entered a hospital for an appendectomy, recently. No member of my family could stay with me to interpret my needs, as I attended a boarding school 250 miles from home. Although the school is for the handicapped, I couldn't expect any of the nurses to be released from their regular duties at the school to stay at my side.

My first problem in the hospital arose when several nurses' aides came in to take a specimen of my urine. One of the problems of a cerebral palsy victim is that the harder he tries to do something, the tenser his muscles become, making the simplest commands almost impossible to obey. The aides tried everything to make me cooperate, but my tense muscles refused, no matter how hard I kept trying.

As they stood around my bed watching me, they began discussing my handicap. They discussed what a tragedy it was that I was so disabled and how sorry they felt for my parents. They must have thought me retarded, which frequently happens, as they ignored my presence. Several times, they spoke to me in language meant only for children. "Please try to go potty," was an example.

To anyone with normal intelligence, this would be very humiliating. In all my 19 years, I had detested self-pity, but now I wanted to turn my face to the wall and cry. However, I knew crying wouldn't solve anything and would even make me seen more retarded. After about an hour the aides gave up and left. I knew they were exasperated.

*Kay Stoll, in the American Journal of Nursing, October, 1965, p. 95. Reproduced by permission.

In a little while, a familiar face appeared at my door. She was one of the student nurses who had been affiliated with our school for two weeks. As she was accustomed to cerebral palsied speech, we were able to begin a friendly conversation. I mentioned my problem with the aides and told her that if she would leave me alone for a few minutes I knew I would have success. Later, when she returned, my specimen was ready for the laboratory.

The pain in my side increased through the night robbing me of sleep. Two or three times I put on my signal light, but the nurse who came couldn't understand me either. She thought I was just restless. Finally, streaks of dawn appeared and I could hear breakfast trays rattling. I could hear the aides discussing me outside my door. "Do I have to feed her?" one asked. "Yes, I did it last night and it's a slow and tedious job. She can't swallow too well and her head moves so much that she spills most of it."

"Well I guess I have to do it, but I dread it."

Knowing the nurses' aide dreaded feeding me made me all the more unsteady. I wanted to tell her that when I was in my wheelchair sitting at a table, I wasn't shaky at all; but I knew that to try talking to her was useless. It would not help.

The morning passed slowly. My pain subsided and I felt rather chipper by noon. As the afternoon wore on, my pain became worse again, and blood tests revealed that my white blood count was up and other symptoms of appendicitis were appearing.

The only thing I remember about my operation is being wheeled into the operating room and given an injection. When I came out of the anesthetic, I was terribly nauseated. Two of the school nurses and the principal were beside me when I awoke, but I was too sick to care. Later, after they left, I longed for their return because a tube had been placed in my nose, and the foot of my bed was raised on blocks. I knew no one would understand if I asked why these things were needed, so I didn't even try. Finally, after about three hours of misery, the tube was removed from my nose and I was able to drift into a peaceful sleep.

Shortly after I awoke in the morning, mom came. Words cannot express my happiness in seeing her. I was alone no longer; someone was there who could understand what I said and needed. For the next five days mom was beside me doing most of my personal nursing herself. On the following Sunday, I was released from the hospital and driven back to school. There were many depressing moments during my hospital stay. Some could not have been avoided; others might have been if personnel had known that what I needed most was to be treated as any patient would be—and as the 19-year-old adult I am.

* * *

CLINICAL CASE PROBLEMS

1. John Powers, age 16, is admitted to the hospital with a diagnosis of meningitis. He had been ill several days before admission and complained of having a head cold and aching all over. The morning of admission he began to experience severe headache and stiffness of the neck and was taken to the doctor's office by his parents.

Two days after his admission to the hospital John is assigned to your care. He is beginning to feel better but has still not completely recovered from the acute stage of his illness. John is a very popular teenager and his friends and classmates are anxious to visit him and keep him company and they cannot understand the doctor's order restricting visitors.

What special precautions should you take while caring for this patient?
How can you keep him quiet yet help pass the time for him?
What special observations should you make while caring for John?
How can you help his friends understand his need for rest?

2. Mrs. Lewis has been in the hospital for five days following an automobile accident in which she received a severe blow to the head, but there was no open wound and no fracture of the skull. She regained consciousness the day after the accident but is still somewhat disoriented and confused. You are assigned to the care of Mrs. Lewis the fifth day after the accident.

What special observations must you make in caring for this patient?
What equipment would you need at the bedside?
What problems in nursing care would you expect this patient to present and how would you go about solving them?

3. Mr. Connors is admitted to the hospital with a diagnosis of rupture of an intervertebral disc. The physician has chosen to treat the condition conservatively and orders the patient placed on a cotton mattress with bed boards under it.

How would you give the patient a bed bath and back care?
What special treatment would you anticipate his receiving which might require alteration in the scheduling of his A.M. care?
How would you serve his meals if his head cannot be elevated?
Will he need any help with his tray?

REFERENCES

1. Brown, A. F.: *Medical-Surgical Nursing II.* Philadelphia, W. B. Saunders Co., 1959.
2. Carini, E., et al.: "Head Injuries." Am. Journ. Nurs., Jan., 1956, p. 54.
3. Creighton, H.: "Brain Injuries and Care of the Patient." RN, April, 1961, p. 57.
4. DeGutierrez-Mahoney, C. G., and Carini, E.: *Neurological and Neurosurgical Nursing,* 3rd edition. St. Louis, Mo., C. V. Mosby Co., 1960.
5. Ferguson, L. K., and Sholtis, L. A.: *Eliason's Surgical Nursing,* 11th edition. Philadelphia, J. B. Lippincott Co., 1961.
6. Golub, S.: "Parkinson's Disease Today." RN, Oct., 1967, p. 59.
7. Haber, M. E.: "Operative Procedures in Brain Surgery." Practical Nursing. April, 1962, p. 16.
8. Hilkemyer, R., Fleming, E. B., and Kincaid, M.: "Nursing Care of Patients with Brain Tumors." Am. Journ. Nurs., March, 1964, p. 81.
9. Hunkele, E., and Lozier, R.: "A Patient with Fractured Cervical Vertebrae." Am. Journ. Nurs., Sept., 1965, p. 82.
10. Iverson, S. M.: "Helping a Quadriplegic Patient Adjust." Am. Journ. Nurs., Jan., 1964, p. 128.
11. King, B. G., and Showers, M. J.: *Human Anatomy and Physiology,* 5th edition. Philadelphia, W. B. Saunders Co., 1963.
12. Leavens, M. E.: "Brain Tumors." Am. Journ. Nurs., March, 1964, p. 78.
13. Magee, K. R.: "Myasthenia Gravis." Am. Journ. Nurs., March, 1960, p. 336.
14. Martin, A. M.: "Nursing Care in Cervical Cord Injury." Am. Journ. Nurs., March, 1963, p. 60.
15. Moser, D.: "Nursing Care of the Myasthenic Patient." Am. Journ. Nurs., March, 1960, p. 340.
16. Olson, C. K.: "Chemosurgery of Parkin-

sonism." Am. Journ. Nurs., Oct., 1959, p. 1400.

17. Shafer, K. N., Sawyer, J. R., et al.: *Medical-Surgical Nursing*, 4th edition. St. Louis, Mo., C. V. Mosby Co., 1967.

18. Smith, D. W., and Gips, C. D.: *Care of the Adult Patient*, 2nd edition. Philadelphia, J. B. Lippincott Co., 1966.

19. Stoll, Kay: "A Patient's Humiliation." Am. Journ. Nurs., Oct., 1965, p. 95.

SUGGESTED STUDENT READING

1. "Epilepsy—Today's Outlook." Journ. Pract. Nurs., Nov., 1966, p. 37.

2. Creighton, H.: "Brain Injuries and Care of the Patient." RN, April, 1961, p. 57.

3. Golub, S.: "Parkinson's Disease Today." RN, Oct., 1967, p. 59.

4. Haber, M. E.: "Operative Procedures in Brain Surgery." Practical Nursing, April, 1962, p. 16.

5. Magee, K. R.: "Myasthenia Gravis." Journ. Pract. Nurs., Nov., 1965, p. 23.

6. Magee, K. R., and Elliott, A.: "Parkinson's Disease—Neurological Management, Nursing Care." Am. Journ. Nurs., July, 1955, p. 814.

7. Pasternak, S.: "The Patient with a Ruptured Disk." Am. Journ. Nurs., Feb., 1962, p. 77.

OUTLINE FOR CHAPTER 18

I. Introduction

A. Nervous system is body's communication system.

B. All nerve cells are excitable and conductive.

C. Impairment of nerve cells' ability to receive and conduct impulses affects normal function of tissues controlled by those nerves.

II. Special Examinations and Diagnostic Tests

A. Complete neurological examination is a very intensive and prolonged procedure in which physician may test normal functioning of cranial nerves, strength and coordination of groups of large muscles and involuntary muscular contractions.

B. Tests done for signs of irritation of the meninges.

C. Lumbar puncture—needle inserted into spinal cavity to measure pressure or to obtain specimen of spinal fluid.

D. Cisternal puncture—spinal tap needle is inserted just below occipital bone into cisterna magna.

E. Electroencephalogram records the activity of brain tissues.

F. X-ray studies of the skull are done after injection of a contrast medium.

1. Angiography involves injection of a radiopaque solution.

2. Pneumoencephalography utilizes a gas as contrast medium.

3. Ventriculography uses air injected via two holes bored in the skull.

G. Radioisotopes used to locate tumors of the brain.

III. General Nursing Care of the Patient with a Neurological Disorder

A. Patient suffers from some organic disease of the nervous system rather than from mental illness or personality disorder.

B. Patient may not be able to move or to recognize dangers of immobility.

C. Nurse should guide patient to help himself.

D. A neurological disorder can cause severe emotional upset. Patient will need help in adjusting to his illness.

E. Patient is rehabilitated to live a full life within the physical limitations imposed by his illness.

IV. Infectious Diseases

A. Meningitis is an inflammation of the membranous linings of the brain and spinal cord.

1. May be caused by a variety of organisms (meningococcus causes epidemics).

2. Symptoms are severe headache, stiff neck, nausea, vomiting and signs of an upper respiratory infection. Spinal fluid contains increased number of white cells and causative organisms.

3. Treatment and nursing care. Specific antibiotics and anticonvulsants may be given. Provide rest and fluids.

a. Patient may be isolated as all secretions from nose and mouth are highly infectious.

b. Protect patient from injury during delirium and convulsions.

c. Small, low enemas prevent abdominal distention.

B. Encephalitis is an inflammation of the brain tissues.

1. Caused by a virus or toxins from organisms and some chemicals.

2. Symptoms are fever, headache and extreme restlessness or lethargy and muscular weakness.

3. Treatment and nursing care is like that of the meningitis patient. Check vital signs frequently.

C. Poliomyelitis is an acute inflammation of the anterior horn of the spinal cord caused by three different strains of viruses. Vaccine is now available.

1. Symptoms may be so slight as to cause no great discomfort. Severe infection produces signs of upper respiratory infection, fever, severe headache, stiff neck and sore back and hamstring muscles. Paralysis may occur as disease progresses.

2. Treatment and nursing care. There is no cure. Give patient complete bed rest and apply heat to muscles. Watch for urinary retention and fecal impaction, respiratory failure and difficulty in swallowing.

V. Head Injuries

A. Concussion is a closed injury in which a portion of the brain tissue suffers from a temporary anemia. Contusion is bruising and swelling of brain tissues.

B. There may be a delayed reaction to any head injury.

C. Extent of damage to the brain is determined by patient's behavior and symptoms.

D. Treatment is conservative unless fracture or increased intracranial pressure is present. Patient placed on bed rest and kept quiet until physician decides danger has passed. May need help in swallowing or breathing.

VI. Brain Tumors (Abnormal Growths of Cells Within the Brain or Its Coverings)

1. Symptoms are quite varied. There may be personality changes, disturbances in judgment and memory, loss of strength, speech and visual disturbances, headache and vomiting.

2. Treatment: tumors must be removed surgically or destroyed by radiation.

VII. Nursing Care of a Patient Having Brain Surgery

1. Preoperative observations are used as a basis for comparison after surgery.

2. Postoperative care. Vital signs are taken frequently. Dressings are checked and reinforced when necessary.

VIII. Injuries of the Spinal Cord

A. Are classified as cervical, thoracic, or lumbosacral.

B. Symptoms depend on location of nerve damage and severity of damage.

C. Treatment: repair damage to cord, prevent further injury to spinal cord by careful handling and immobilization, improve patient's physical condition, prevent complications (decubitus ulcers, urinary complications and orthopedic deformities) and make rehabilitation possible.

D. Nursing care is concerned with proper care of skin, attention to proper elimination, prevention of muscle spasms and proper positioning of patient.

IX. Rupture of Intervertebral Disc

A. Symptom is pain in lower back and one leg.

B. Treatment and nursing care. Patient given bed rest with firm spinal support and heat to relieve muscle spasm. Pelvic traction sometimes used. Surgical treatment (laminectomy and spinal fusion) fuses the affected vertebrae together.

X. Myasthenia Gravis (Grave Muscular Weakness)

A. Symptoms—severe muscle weakness and fatigue.

B. Treatment—drugs (usually neostigmine and pyridostigmine).

XI. Parkinson's Disease

A. A degenerative disease of the nerve cells in the brain. Cause unknown.

B. Symptoms—tremor and rigidity of the skeletal muscles.

C. Treatment—drugs to produce mild relaxation and sedation. Surgical treatment successful in some cases.

XII. Multiple Sclerosis

A. A chronic and progressive disease of the central nervous system. Cause unknown.

B. Symptoms—slow onset with disturbance in vision, muscular weakness and gradual loss of coordination. There may be remissions of symptoms after which they are more severe.

C. Treatment—symptomatic. No cure.

XIII. Epilepsy (Sudden and Uncontrollable Seizures)

A. May be symptom of a disorder of the brain or idiopathic (in which there is no pathology).

B. Symptoms. Grand mal—severe convulsive movements and loss of consciousness. Often preceded by some sensory change. Petit mal—seizure very mild with only momentary loss of consciousness.

C. Treatment—protection from injury during convulsion and anticonvulsants.

XIV. Cerebral Palsy

A. A type of paralysis with lack of muscle coordination. Due to cerebral damage possibly stemming from oxygen lack at birth, traumatic birth, premature delivery or infection.

B. Symptoms—exaggerated reflexes, poor coordination of voluntary muscles, high muscle tension and sometimes a defect of hearing, speech or vision.

C. Treatment—early muscle training and special exercises. Orthopedic surgery, braces or casts can correct some orthopedic deformities and disabilities. Patient as independent as possible.

Chapter 19

NURSING CARE OF PATIENTS WITH DISORDERS OF THE EYES, EARS, AND THROAT

Part I—DISORDERS OF THE EYES

Introduction. According to statistics, there are two million persons in the United States who have inadequate vision even with glasses, and another million who are blind. In fact, probably a little over half the people in this country have defective vision to some degree. The emotional, physical, and financial burdens brought about by such visual defects would be impossible to estimate.

The sense of sight is such a priceless possession it would seem that everyone would exercise extreme care in taking care of his eyes, yet many of the persons included in the above statistics could have prevented their loss of vision if they had known and applied the fundamental principles of good eye care. Some of them may have been ignorant of these principles, others may have deliberately neglected their eyes, and still others may have been hopelessly confused by misinformation and super-stitious beliefs. Whatever the reason for improper eye care, all members of the health team have the responsibility of health education in prevention of injuries and diseases of the eyes.

In her work or at home among friends and relatives, the practical nurse will have many opportunities to correct mistaken ideas and give factual information about the eyes and their care. Some of the basic facts of eye care are listed below.

1. The term "eyestrain" has been greatly abused and overused. It has often been a catchall to explain various and sundry visual defects and diseases of the eye. It is actually very difficult to strain the eye. Inadequate light or excessive use of the eyes for close work can cause the eye muscles to become overly tired just as any other muscle of our bodies becomes tired from overuse, but such use will not damage the eyes any more than straining to hear a dis-

418

tant sound can damage the ears. The eye muscles should be rested periodically while the person watches television, reads, sews or performs other activities which require constant use of the eyes. If the eyes seem to tire easily, or if there is headache, burning, itching, and redness of the eyes, this is not eyestrain. These are symptoms of a visual defect and are an indication that the individual's eyes should be examined by a physician.

2. Adequate diet and good nutrition play an important role in the conservation of sight, but eating large amounts of carrots and other yellow vegetables will *not improve eyesight.* A lack of vitamin A in the diet often results in an inflammation of the lids and conjunctiva and an increased sensitivity to light. A deficiency of vitamin B in the diet can cause irreparable damage to the retina and permanent visual defects.

3. Normal eyes do not require irrigations or periodic "washing out" with boric acid solutions or other commercial preparations. The normal secretions of the conjunctiva and tear glands are sufficient to lubricate the eye and remove small particles of dust which may collect in the eye. Accumulation of purulent material, or itching and burning of the eyelids may indicate diseases and should be reported to a physician.

4. Children do not outgrow crossed eyes. Until a baby reaches the age of 6 or 9 months he may have some difficulty focusing his eyes but this condition should not persist past that age. Neglect of crossed eyes (*strabismus*) can cause a serious loss of vision. It is generally agreed by ophthalmologists that the sooner treatment is begun the better the chance of correcting the condition and preserving the child's eyesight. A child who has only one crossed eye will not use the affected eye and will eventually become blind in that eye if the condition is not corrected.

5. Every person over the age of 40 should have a periodic examination of the eyes. It is particularly important that a test for glaucoma be made at the time of the examination since this disease usually does not present symptoms of pain or discomfort until it reaches the advanced stages. It is also believed that this disease runs in families and any person who has a relative with glaucoma should be especially alert for the development of the disease in himself.

6. Every year there are at least 100,000 schoolchildren who suffer from some serious accidental injury to the eye. Many of these accidents could be avoided if parents, teachers, and the children themselves were made aware of the danger of sharp pencils, paper wads, small stones, or other objects children may be tempted to hurl at one another while playing.

7. Visual defects cannot always be corrected by the purchase of a pair of glasses or the changing of the lenses in glasses. Many people who otherwise demand the best of medical care for their physical ailments will not hesitate to purchase "reading glasses" from a dime store counter in an effort to improve their vision, or consult an optometrist for treatment of a serious eye disease. Both practices are foolish. The dime store clerk is only trained to collect the price of the glasses and make the correct change. A reputable optometrist will usually refer the individual to a physician when he recognizes the need for medical treatment of the eyes, but he is not qualified to diagnose diseases of the eyes and much precious time may be lost while he futilely attempts to correct the condition by changing the lenses of the patient's glasses.

8. One of the reasons for improper care of the eyes stems from the layman's confusion about the terminology used to designate the various persons concerned with the prescribing and fitting of eye glasses. The practical nurse should know and understand the various functions and qualifications of such persons so that she can offer intelligent advice to those who seek her help on disorders of the eye.

An *ophthalmologist* or *oculist* is a medical doctor who specializes in the diagnosis and treatment of visual defects and diseases of the eye.

An *optometrist* is one who is trained only in scientific examination of the eyes for the purpose of prescribing glasses. He is not a physician and cannot treat diseases of the eye.

An *optician* is one who is trained to make glasses and optical instruments. He grinds the lenses and fits glasses according to a prescription from the ophthalmologist or optometrist.

DIAGNOSTIC TESTS AND EXAMINATIONS

Snellen Chart. This chart is quite familiar to most of us even though we may not have known it by name. The chart is usually designed so that there is one large letter at the top and subsequent rows of letters under it, each row in smaller print than the one above it. The Snellen chart is read from a distance of exactly 20 feet and the letters are scaled according to normal vision. A person with normal visual acuity can read the top letter from a distance of 100 feet, the second row of letters from 70 feet, the third at 50 feet, and so on down to 10 feet for the last row of letters.

The visual acuity of the person being tested is expressed as a fraction. The *numerator* indicates the distance between the patient and the chart (20 feet), and the *denominator* indicates the distance at which a person with normal vision can read the letters. For example, 20/50 vision means that the person being tested can only read the letters of the third row at a distance of 20 feet while a person with normal visual acuity could easily read these letters from a distance of 50 feet. If the vision is 20/20 it is considered to be normal distance vision. A vision of 20/200 is used in defining blindness.

Near Vision. In order to test an individual's ability to see objects close at hand, the physician uses a test known as *Jaeger's Test Types.* The patient is given a card which is printed with different sizes of ordinary printer's types. The smallest and finest type is used for line one and each successive line is printed with larger types. A piece of cardboard is placed over one eye and each eye is tested separately.

Refraction. When light rays enter the eye they are "refracted" or bent so that they focus on the retina. The lens, aqueous humor and vitreous humor are responsible for bending these light rays. Disorders of the lens which prevent the proper focusing of light rays upon the retina are diagnosed by a *refraction.* This eye examination makes use of various glass lenses of different shapes through which the patient reads the Snellen chart. When he chooses the lens through which he can best read the chart the ophthalmologist prescribes the same kind of lenses to be ground by the optician and fitted as glasses for the patient.

Intraocular Pressure. The chambers of the eyeballs in front of the lenses are filled with a watery substance called the *aqueous humor.* This fluid is constantly being produced and drained off in equal proportions so that there is a normal amount of pressure within the chambers. An increase or decrease in the amount of pressure being exerted by the aqueous humor within the chambers of the eye can be measured with an instrument called a *tonometer.* The testing of intraocular pressure is extremely important in the diagnosis of glaucoma in which intraocular pressure is increased.

COMMON VISUAL DEFECTS

The most common visual defects are those of *refraction.* This means that light rays entering the eye are not "refracted," or bent, at the correct angle and therefore do not focus on the retina. Errors of refraction may be caused by a number of structural defects within the eyeball itself. For ex-

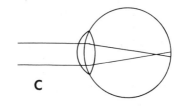

Figure 19-1. *A,* Normal vision. Lens bends light rays so that they focus directly on the retina. *B,* Hyperopia. Lens is too close to retina. Thus light rays converge at point beyond the retina. *C,* Myopia. Lens is too far away from retina, causing light rays to converge before they reach the retina. (Modified from Sackheim: *Practical Physics for Nurses,* 2nd Ed., W. B. Saunders Co., Philadelphia.)

ample, if the eyeball is constructed so that the distance between the lens and retina is too short, the light rays focus behind the retina. This causes difficulty in seeing objects close at hand and is called farsightedness *(hyperopia)* (see Fig. 19-1).

If the opposite is true, and the lens is situated too far from the retina, the light rays will converge and focus in front of the retina. The individual then has difficulty in seeing objects at a dis-

tance and is referred to as nearsighted. Nearsightedness is called *myopia.*

Light rays from distant objects do not enter the eye at the same angle as light rays from near objects. When we look off into the distance and then quickly look down at a book in our hands our eyes must make an adjustment to the difference in the light rays entering the eye. This adjustment is called *accommodation* and is accomplished by ciliary muscles and ligaments

Ligaments tight—lens flattened

Ligaments relaxed—lens more rounded

Rays from a distant object are focused on the retina by a flattened lens

Rays from a nearby object are properly focused on the retina by a more rounded lens

Figure 19-2. Defects of the eye. (From Sackheim: *Practical Physics for Nurses,* 2nd Ed., W. B. Saunders Co., Philadelphia.)

which change the shape of the lens, making it more rounded or flatter (see Fig. 19-2).

As we grow older our ciliary muscles become less elastic and cannot readily accommodate to the needs of distant and near vision. This hardening of the ciliary muscles occurs in many persons over 40 years of age and is known as *presbyopia*. Bifocal glasses are usually prescribed for this condition because they allow for two sets of lenses in one pair of glasses, one set for viewing distant objects and one for seeing close objects.

Astigmatism is a visual defect resulting from a warped lens or irregular curvature of the cornea, either of which will prevent the horizontal and vertical rays from focusing at the same point on the retina. Actually there are very few people who have perfectly shaped eyeballs and so there are very few who do not have some degree of astigmatism. If the astigmatism is very slight the eye can accommodate for its imperfection by changing the shape of the lens. If there is a serious error of refraction the eyes will tire very easily or the individual will have defective vision because the eyes cannot change the shape of the lens enough to compensate for the abnormality. The treatment for serious errors of refraction is the prescription of artificial lenses and the fitting of glasses so that the light rays are brought into proper focus on the retina.

INJURIES AND INFECTIONS OF THE EYE

Foreign Bodies

The human eye is situated within the eye socket of the skull so that it is partially protected from direct blows. The quick-acting lids, the eyelashes, and the eyebrows also serve to protect the eye from injury. But in spite of nature's attempts to protect the eye, there are still many instances in which foreign bodies become lodged in the eye (see Fig. 19-3).

If the foreign body is not deeply embedded in the tissues of the eye, it can easily be removed by touching it with the corner of a clean handkerchief. Should the object remain lodged in spite of this effort to remove it, a physician should be consulted at once. Many eyes have been damaged and vision permanently impaired by a layman's well-meaning attempts to remove foreign objects from the eyes.

Conjunctivitis

Definition. The term "conjunctivitis" is used to describe any inflammation of the mucous membrane lining the upper and lower lids and covering the front part of the eyeball. This condition may be caused by a number of organisms including the staphylococcus, streptococcus, and gonococcus.

"Pinkeye" is a conjunctivitis caused by a specific organism called the Koch-Weeks bacillus.

Symptoms. Objective symptoms of conjunctivitis include redness and swelling of the conjunctiva and the production of a watery secretion in the eyes. Later this secretion may become purulent and, if not properly treated, the eyes may be partially closed and covered with crusts of dried exudate. In addition to these outward signs, the patient may also complain of local itching and burning.

Treatment and Nursing Care. Conjunctivitis should be treated as quickly as possible and all precautions taken to prevent its spread to other persons. "Pinkeye" is highly infectious and is quite common in schoolchildren.

The treatment of conjunctivitis will depend on the organism causing the infection. Some types of conjunctivitis may resist local treatment of antibiotic ointments and eye drops and require the administration of antibiotics systemically. Gonorrheal conjunctivitis demands immediate attention because of

Figure 19-3. *A*, Foreign body often can be seen only if the upper lid is everted. *B*, Acute meibomitis (internal sty) may require surgical treatment. (From Gordon: American Journal of Nursing, November, 1964.)

the danger of blindness as a result of the infection. In this type of conjunctivitis the exudate from the eyes must be handled with extreme care and isolation precautions taken to prevent spread of the disease to the eyes of others.

In addition to the administration of ointments or eyedrops ordered by the physician, nursing care is also concerned with hot or cold moist compresses and irrigations of the eye to remove the exudate and relieve the local itching and burning.

Sty (Hordeolum)

Definition. The sty is one of the most common infections of the eye. It is usually a staphylococcus infection of a follicle of an eyelash.

Symptoms. Redness, burning, and itching of the eyelids are usually the first symptoms of a sty. Very soon after these symptoms develop a small pustule forms on the lid and the lid becomes red and swollen. Even though a sty is not especially painful it may be very annoying and uncomfortable. A general state of poor health or a need for glasses may predispose an individual to repeated development of stys.

Treatment and Nursing Care. Most stys will rupture and drain without incision if warm, moist compresses are applied regularly to the affected eye. Those which do not respond to this treatment must be surgically incised by a physician.

Infections of the meibomian glands (small lubricating glands around the edge of the eyelids) often are mistaken for sties. These infections cause considerably more pain than the more common sty and usually do not respond to hot wet compresses alone. If antibiotic ointments do not eliminate the infection, surgical treatment is necessary. Frequent infections of the eyelids can be symptomatic of diabetes mellitus.

Cataract

Definition. The word "cataract" literally means a waterfall. The term is used to designate an opacity of the lens of the eye because the vision of the person with this condition is impaired as if he were trying to see through falling water. His vision is blurred because the lens of the eye is cloudy and opaque, thus preventing proper entrance and focusing of light rays on the retina.

Cataracts are sometimes present at birth *(congenital cataracts)*. But they most often occur as a result of the aging process and are found in persons in their seventies or eighties *(senile cataracts)*.

Treatment. The only effective method of treating cataracts is surgical removal of the affected lens. This procedure is called a *cataract extraction.* It should be understood that while this procedure does *improve* vision, it does not restore the eye to a perfectly normal condition. The patient must have glasses prescribed and they must be worn at all times. The reason this is necessary is that the process of accommodation (see p. 421) is no longer possible once the lens has been removed. The glasses prescribed are usually bifocals. The practice of waiting until a cataract has grown to full maturity (ripened) is no longer practiced and the present trend is toward removal of the lens as soon as the cataract is noticed.

Nursing Care of the Patient Having a Cataract Extraction. PREOPERATIVE. Since the great majority of these patients are elderly and therefore most likely to be suffering from some additional chronic disease, the nurse must remember the need for applying the principles of geriatric nursing in administering nursing care to a patient with a cataract. Fear, anxiety over the surgery, and confusion about the expected results of the surgery are all factors to be considered in the preparation of the patient for the operation.

When the patient is admitted to the hospital he should be given adequate instruction in the physical layout of his room and the ways in which he can call for the nurse should he need her. Side rails are usually necessary to prevent falls and the patient should be cautioned against getting out of bed without assistance.

Preoperative medications include the local application of an antibiotic ointment to reduce the chances of a postoperative infection, and the administration of *mydriatic* eyedrops to dilate the pupil. The drugs must be given with extreme care and accuracy, especially if only one eye is affected. If the symbols "o.d." and "o.s." are used to designate the right eye and the left eye, the nurse must be sure that the medication is applied to the correct eye.

POSTOPERATIVE CARE. The patient may receive a general anesthetic for this surgical procedure or the physician may prefer to use a local anesthetic. There are several advantages to a local anesthetic but his choice will depend on the general health of the patient and his ability to cooperate with the surgeon.

In either case the nurse must help the patient understand the importance of avoiding stress on the suture line within the eye. Coughing, sneezing, squeezing the eyelids, or sudden movements of the head should be avoided. Policies regarding the amount of bodily activity allowed the patient vary in different institutions and some doctors permit their patients more freedom than others. In recent years there has been a trend toward allowing the patient more activity and many patients begin ambulation the day after surgery. The surgeon is usually very clear and explicit in his instructions to the patient and the nursing staff so there should be no excuse for failure to follow his orders precisely.

As long as the patient has dressings and eyeshields over both eyes he will need the same considerations as one who is blind. If he is allowed out of bed, he must have assistance (see Fig. 19-4).

Compresses and saline irrigations of the eye are usually ordered to remove drainage and exudate from the eyes. It should be remembered that the eyeball itself is never touched during this procedure. Only the lids are cleansed, using gentle vertical strokes, and working from the inner corner of the eye outward. If some bits of exudate cannot be removed with this gentle cleansing, they should be left for the surgeon to remove.

Occupational therapy and some diversional activities should be planned to prevent boredom and help the patient pass the long hours of waiting. Before the patient goes home he will receive instructions from the physician about the amount of activity he may be allowed. Usually he is told that lifting, bending, or otherwise straining his muscles should be avoided. He will also be told when he must return to the doctor's office for checkups and the prescribing of glasses.

Adjusting to cataract glasses can be very frustrating and even frightening for the patient and will require much patience and understanding from those trying to help him during this difficult period. The lenses of cataract glasses are very thick and the edges tend to curve straight lines. This produces a kind of rounded tunnel vision in which everything in the peripheral vision curves around the center and depth perception becomes greatly distorted, and the patient has great difficulty judging distances. If he turns his head suddenly the curved lines are set in motion and his only clear vision is directly through the center of the glasses. Another problem is a blind area, between 11 and 20 feet away, in which the patient cannot see objects. Thus, he has the unnerving experience of seeing someone approach him, disappear from his sight and then reappear much closer to him. In time the patient will adjust to this and he will barely notice the blind spot, but at first such a difficulty can be very frightening and discouraging.

Figure 19-4. When a patient is allowed up to walk after eye surgery, the nurse must realize that attempting to walk with both eyes covered is a frightening experience. The nurse who assists the patient must give adequate guidance and a feeling of safety, yet not make the patient feel that he is being pushed forward. This is accomplished by having the patient hold the guide's arm and by giving precise verbal directions, including an estimate of the distance to be covered. (Courtesy of Cora L. Shaw, Institute of Ophthalmology; and the American Journal of Nursing.)

The nurse can help the patient in his adjustment by reassuring him that such difficulties are to be expected at first and that eventually he can become accustomed to his glasses. He should be instructed to move slowly at first, feeling his way through doorways and other close quarters through which he feels unable to move about. He should make a special effort to get into the habit of moving his head from side to side rather than shifting his eyes, and he must always try to look directly through the center of his glasses. The adjustment can be more rapid if the patient is able to use his hands and eyes for fine work such as knitting, carving, whittling or sewing. This type of precision work trains the eyes to focus through the cataract glasses properly and also serves as a form of occupational therapy that can do wonders for the morale of a person who could barely distinguish between light and dark shadows before surgery.

Glaucoma

Introduction. The aqueous humor (watery fluid) which flows within the eyeball in front of the lens normally is constant in volume and exerts a well-balanced pressure within the chambers of the eye. When there is an increase in production of the aqueous humor, or when there is a hindrance to its outflow, the pressure within the eyeball increases. This increase of intraocular pressure can damage the optic nerve and produce varying degrees of visual impairment. Glaucoma is the condition in which increased intraocular pressure is present. It usually results from an obstruction to the outflow of the aqueous humor in the anterior chamber of the eye.

Symptoms. "Glaucoma must be considered a very serious condition because (1) it is frequently not diagnosed, (2) it often leads to irreversible loss of vision, and (3) the disease process may be extremely difficult to slow down."[2]

The disease is particularly treacherous because symptoms during the early stages are very mild and many patients are not aware that anything is wrong until vision has been completely lost in one eye, or until headache and pain in the eye during an acute attack bring about a visit to the physician.

The National Society for the Prevention of Blindness lists the following symptoms as danger signals of glaucoma:

1. Glasses, even new ones, don't seem to help
2. Blurred or hazy vision which clears up after a while
3. Trouble in getting used to darkened rooms, such as at the movies
4. Seeing rainbow-colored rings around lights
5. Narrowing of vision at the sides of one or both eyes

The society also recommends regular eye examination at least every two years after the age of 40.

Treatment and Nursing Care. Glaucoma is primarily treated medically. If the medications are not effective, and the disease continues to progress, a surgical procedure involving removal of a section of the iris *(iridectomy)* may be performed so that outflow of the aqueous humor is established.

The first drugs used in the treatment of glaucoma are usually those which constrict the pupil *(myotics)*. *Pilocarpine,* which acts on the sphincter muscle of the pupil, and *eserine* and *neostigmine,* which inhibit the nerve impulses to the pupil and prevent dilatation, are the drugs most often used. Other drugs, such as Diamox and other carbonic anhydrase inhibitors, which decrease the production of aqueous humor, are often used in conjunction with the myotic drugs.

Glaucoma is essentially a chronic disease. It develops slowly and if left untreated will relentlessly progress to total blindness in the affected eye. Both eyes are usually involved, although one may show evidence of the disease before the other will. This disease is the main cause of blindness in adults in this country and as such must be considered of primary importance in education of the public about the disease.

The patient with glaucoma is usually not hospitalized unless he suffers an acute glaucomatous attack. In this instance he will experience a severe pain which may be localized in the eye or may involve the entire head. The pain is so excruciating that nausea and vomiting will often occur. During this episode the patient should be kept very quiet and disturbed as little as possible, and sedatives, and analgesics for relief of pain are given until the attack subsides. If the condition is not treated the attack may persist for several days or weeks and complete blindness will result.

There is evidence that emotional upsets, worry, or poor general health further aggravate glaucoma and precipitate attacks of acute symptoms. The patient and his family will need help in understanding the disease and avoiding situations which increase intraocular pressure. These include family arguments, quarrels, and other situations which produce mental anxiety and tension. Physical exertion, heavy lifting, or tight-fitting clothing may also increase the pressure. Use of the eyes should be limited and watching television, sewing or reading should be interspersed with periods of rest for the eyes.

Detached Retina

Introduction. The retina is the innermost layer of the eye. It is composed of two layers: a pigmented layer that is in close contact with the choroid (vascular wall) of the eye and which supplies nutrients for both layers; and a sensory layer that receives visual stimuli and therefore is essential to normal vision. In detached retina there is a hole or tear in the two layers and vitreous fluid leaks under the retina, separating it from the vascular wall and depriving it of its blood supply. Once the retina is detached from the wall of the eye it no longer receives a clear image and vision is greatly impaired.

There are many possible causes of detached retina. The condition can result from a sudden blow or a penetrating injury to the eye or following surgery of the eye. Predisposing factors include myopia and diabetic changes in the retina.

Symptoms. There may be a gradual or sudden onset depending on the cause and size and location of the area involved. The patient may see flashes of light and then days or weeks later notice cloudy vision or loss of central vision. Another common symptom is the sensation of spots or moving particles in the field of vision. In severe cases there may be complete loss of vision.

Diagnosis of detached retina can be done with a direct ophthalmoscope but it is greatly simplified by a newer instrument called a stereoscopic indirect ophthalmoscope. This instrument permits visualization of the entire retina and produces an image of the retina with less magnification and distortion.

Treatment and Nursing Care. The only treatment for retinal detachment is surgery. During the preoperative period the patient usually is extremely apprehensive because of his fear of blindness and will need reassurance that newer techniques of surgery promise success in more than 85 per cent of all cases of retinal detachment. Physical preparation of the patient includes instillation of eye drops that dilate the pupil. These eye drops are extremely important and must be given precisely as ordered by the surgeon. Prior to surgery the upper and lower eyelashes of the affected eye are clipped close to the lid margin using scissors whose blades are covered with petroleum jelly so that the eyelashes adhere to the blades and do not fall into the eye. The patient's face usually is washed several times with a surgical soap. Male patients must be clean-shaven so that adhesive dressings can be applied without difficulty.

There are several new surgical procedures used for the repair of detached retina. Almost all of them utilize diathermy to seal the retinal break firmly so that vitreous fluid cannot leak between the retina and the choroid and thereby produce recurrence of retinal detachment. Another aim of surgery is to drain off fluid that has accumulated so that the retina can be returned to its normal position.

The amount of activity allowed during the postoperative period will depend on the type of surgery done and the specific directions of the surgeon. Patients having the newer types of surgery usually are allowed out of bed the day after surgery though they must use care not to move their heads too vigorously. Others who have had sutures applied to hold the retina in place may be confined to bed for two weeks postoperatively and they must keep their heads as still as possible during that time.

NURSING CARE OF THE PATIENT HAVING EYE SURGERY

Preoperative Care. During the preoperative period the individual needs of each patient anticipating surgery of the eye must be determined and his nursing care planned accordingly. Some patients will have nearly normal vision while others may be almost totally blind. At the time of admission the nurse should make a special effort to orient the patient to his environment. This is true for every patient having eye surgery, for even though he may be able to see fairly well before surgery, he may have his eyes bandaged after the operation. The physician or nurse should explain the reason for postoperative bandaging of both eyes, if this is expected, so that the patient will not be upset by the bandages when he recovers from anesthesia. In most instances, especially following cataract extraction, the unaffected eye is covered so that the patient will not be tempted to move his eyes during the immediate postoperative period.

Preoperative medications such as ophthalmic ointments and eye drops must be given exactly on time because they are important to the success of the surgery. When these medications are instilled, the eye is held open by resting the fingers on the bones of the face. Never press against the eyeball. The hand administering the drops should be firmly pressed against the patient's forehead so that any sudden movement of the head will not cause the container to injure the eye. After the eyelids are separated the patient is asked to look up and the medication is administered along the lower lid. The patient is then instructed to close his eye slowly so that the medication will not be squeezed out of the eye.

Physical preparation for surgery may include an enema or suppository to evacuate the lower bowel. This is done to prevent straining at stool during the immediate postoperative period. If the eyelashes are to be clipped, they should be cut with small curved scissors with blunt points. Petroleum jelly is applied to the blades of the scissors so that the eyelashes will adhere to the blade and will not fall into the eye. Some physicians direct the patient to wash his face with surgical soap several times during the evening before surgery and a sterile eye pad may be placed over the eye.

If the nurse notices any symptoms of a respiratory infection or allergy that will bring about coughing and sneezing during the postoperative period she should notify the surgeon. Since such violent motions can bring about hemorrhage within the eye or rupture the surgical incision the physician may postpone surgery until a later date.

Postoperative Care. In all types of eye surgery the key word is gentleness. The patient's head must be firmly supported when he is transferred from the operating table or stretcher to his bed and all movements by those moving him should be slow, deliberate and gentle. While he is confined to his bed small pillows may be used on either side of his head to help support it in the proper position. Remember that you should always speak softly before touching a patient who is blind or wearing bandages over his eyes. If he did not hear you enter the room or was napping at the time you entered he may be frightened and move suddenly and violently when he feels someone touch him. Children or older patients who are unable to cooperate may need someone in constant attendance to prevent their pulling at the bandages. Nausea and subsequent vomiting can wreak havoc with delicate suture lines in the eye. If the patient becomes nauseated, all food and liquids should be withheld and the physician notified so that an anti-emetic drug can be ordered. A sudden pain in the eye may indicate hemorrhage and should be brought to the attention of the physician immediately.

Irrigations of the eye and wet compresses sometimes are ordered to remove exudate and reduce swelling of the eyelids and surrounding tissues. These procedures must be done with the utmost care, cleansing only the lids and avoiding any contact with the eyeball.

Because there can be such a wide difference in the amount and type of activity allowed a patient and the positioning preferred by the surgeon, the practical nurse must be thoroughly familiar with the individual care of each patient who has had surgery of the eye. She should know whether or not the patient can be turned on one or both sides or whether he must remain flat on his back, whether pillows are allowed under the head and how high the head of the bed may be raised. At meal times she must know whether the patient can feed himself and whether there are restrictions on food or fluid intake. If the patient is allowed out of bed he must take care not to jar his head or move too suddenly; all straining and lifting must be avoided. The patient and his family should be encouraged to follow the physician's directions faithfully during the convalescent period at home so that nothing will be done to jeopardize the success of the surgery.

GENERAL PRINCIPLES IN THE CARE OF THE BLIND

Emotional Aspects of Blindness. Those of us who are fortunate enough to have adequate vision cannot fully realize the tremendous adjustments to be made by those who are deprived of their sight. If we were to put on a blindfold and stumble through one day of our usual activities, we might have some slight comprehension of the obstacles to be overcome, but we still would not experience the same sense of hopelessness and despair which besets those who have lost their sight. We would have the satisfaction of knowing that we could regain our sight by simply removing the blindfold. The permanently blind person has no such promise in the future.

These feelings of depression and despair in the person who has lost his sight are to be expected, and are considered by some psychologists to be a necessary step in the direction of adjustment to blindness. The following quotation from an article in the January 1956 edition of the American Journal of Nursing[6] may emphasize and clarify this very important point in the care of those who have lost their sight.

The important lesson for all who work with the blind—friends, nurses, and ophthalmologists—is to realize that the various stages through which the newly blinded person passes are fundamental to his rehabilitation. Unfortunately, we are told there seems to be a "concerted effort of society to prevent the patient from accepting his blindness." Everyone—frequently even the doctor who is treating the patient— tries to "cheer him up," to prevent him from grieving; many even offer hope that his sight may yet return. Rarely is any hope offered that the patient may yet have a full life as a blind man, and that it is only a *different kind of life* he must learn to live.

The patient must, in fact, "die as a sighted person in order to be reborn as a blind man," and he usually experiences a very welcome relief from struggle once he accepts his condition. Once he realizes that he is a new person, he can begin to investigate both his limitations and his capacities, and actually learn a new way of life.

SPECIAL RULES TO FOLLOW IN HELPING A BLIND PERSON

1. Remember that the individual is *blind*, not deaf. There is no reason to shout at him or address him as though he were either deaf or a child. Speak normally and do not try to avoid using the words "I see." Blind people use this phrase themselves without hesitation.

2. Speak to the blind person as you enter the room and do not touch him until after you have spoken to him. This prevents startling or frightening the blind patient who may not have heard you enter the room.

3. The prevention of accidents is an important part of the care of the blind. Aside from the physical effects of bumping into objects or falling over them, the blind person also suffers from a loss of self-confidence and security if he cannot move about safely and independently. Doors should be kept closed or completely open. They must never be left ajar. If it is necessary to move a piece of furniture in the patient's room, tell him about its new location.

4. When you leave the room tell the blind person that you are going. He will not then resume the conversation later and find that he is talking to someone who is not there.

5. Pity is neither expected nor appreciated by the blind. They only want to be treated as normal people, and would prefer to ask for your help when they need it rather than have you do everything for them. It is also important to remember that there are no such things as "extra senses of blindness" which many people mistakenly believe blind people are given to compensate for their loss of sight. Whatever the blind person has learned about living with his blindness he has accomplished through hard work and determination.

6. If you are assigned to the care of a blind person admitted to a general hospital, determine the amount of assistance the patient desires and needs. Do not embarrass him by assuming that he is helpless but avoid neglecting him when he needs your help. When serving a meal to the blind patient tell him what foods are on his plate and their location (see Fig. 19-5). Do not use a straw or drinking tube unless requested by the patient because it may be awkward for him to use. If you must feed him all of the meal work slowly and calmly. Inform him of hot and cold foods and alternate dishes rather than feed him all of one thing and then another. Avoid talking too much and forcing the patient either to stop eating or to answer you with a mouth full of food. Whenever possible allow the patient to feed himself finger foods such as bread and raw vegetables or fruit. Bear in mind that your goal is to help the patient maintain his dignity and self-respect while meeting his personal needs.

Figure 19-5. Telling the patient that his meat is at 6 o'clock, potato at 2 o'clock, and vegetable at 10 o'clock helps him to locate them on his plate.

Part II – DISORDERS OF THE EARS

INTRODUCTION

It is estimated that one out of every ten persons in this country suffers from hearing loss to some degree. Deafness, like blindness, burdens its victims with emotional problems as well as physical, financial, and social handicaps. Communication with others is of primary importance in daily living; to be deprived of the essentials of social intercourse leaves most individuals completely out of the group. Because this is true, the person who hears only distorted sounds or no sounds at all tends to withdraw from others and live within a world of his own.

Children who have hearing difficulties may be considered disobedient, stupid, or even seriously mentally retarded. A baby who is deaf at birth has great difficulty learning to speak because he cannot hear the words of the language and therefore is unable to repeat them. The adult who has a hearing deficiency may lose his job and alienate his friends because of his handicap in communicating with others.

Normal hearing depends on the conduction of sound waves through the ear to the auditory nerve, and the transmission of impulses along this nerve to the brain. Sound is described as occurring in waves because the vibrations of sound are similar to the ripples in a pond produced by throwing a pebble into the water. The length of the waves determines its *frequency*, the height of the waves determines the sound's *intensity*. Both of these are important in the detection of sound by the human ear.

A loss of hearing may be *sensorineural* or *conductive*. A sensorineural loss of hearing is brought about by a disorder of the eighth cranial nerve (the auditory nerve) and is sometimes called nerve deafness. Conductive loss of hearing occurs when there is a barrier in the canal, drum, or middle ear which prevents the progress of sound waves from the environment to the auditory nerve. Obstruction of the movement of the tiny ossicles within the middle ear will also produce a conductive loss of hearing.

SPECIAL DIAGNOSTIC TESTS AND EXAMINATIONS

Tuning Fork Tests. The tuning fork is a simple, inexpensive instrument which may be used to test hearing. The fork is struck with a rubber reflex hammer and its vibrations produce sound waves which can be heard by a person with normal hearing.

The *Weber test* is done by striking the tuning fork and then placing the handle of the tuning fork on the patient's forehead. If the patient has normal hearing or is equally hard of hearing in both ears he will hear the sound in the middle of his head. A comparison of hearing acumen in both ears can be made with this test.

The *Rinne test* is done by striking the tuning fork and then placing the handle against the mastoid bone. The fork is removed and struck again; this time it is held beside the ear. The patient is then asked in which position he heard the sound better or longer. The Rinne test is used to determine whether a hearing loss is sensorineural or conductive.

Audiometry. The audiometer is a special machine used in the measurement of sound perception. It is especially useful in the testing of speech perception because it is in this area that loss of hearing creates the most problems. The administration of tests using the audiometer requires special training and experience and must be done by an audiologist. A list of all the hearing centers where these tests are available may be obtained by writing to the American Hearing Society, 919 Eighteenth Street, N.W., Washington, D.C., 20006.

INFECTIONS OF THE EAR

Otitis Media, Tympanitis

Definition. Otitis media is an abscess or inflammation of the middle ear (tympanum). It is the most common of all ear infections and usually is a complication of an acute infection of the throat or sinuses. Otitis media may also occur as a result of the collection of fluid within the middle ear due to an allergy.

Symptoms. Pain in the ear, fever, and drainage from the ear are the common symptoms of this condition. In some cases of chronic otitis media these symptoms may be controlled by the administration of antibiotics, and the only indication of an inflammation will be a loss of hearing.

Treatment and Nursing Care. General treatment of otitis media is rest and the relief of pain through the use of analgesics and the application of heat to the ear. Antibiotics are given to inhibit the growth and development of the causative organisms. Because of the danger of eliminating the symptoms without curing the disease, most physicians also administer hearing tests during and after treatment to be sure that the infection has completely subsided and there is no remaining fluid left containing pathogenic organisms.

Incision and drainage of the eardrum to allow for removal of the inflammatory exudate from the middle ear is called a *myringotomy*. This procedure may also be done as a diagnostic test to determine the presence of specific types of pathogenic organisms in the fluid.

Nosedrops may be given at regular intervals during the day so that the eustachian tube is kept open and drainage encouraged. These drops are given

Figure 19-6. Recommended position for administering nose drops to patient who has otitis media and needs to have the eustachian tube kept open and draining. (From Boies: *Fundamentals of Otolaryngology*, 4th Ed., W. B. Saunders Co., Philadelphia.)

with the head inclined toward the affected ear (see Fig. 19-6).

Mastoiditis

Definition. Mastoiditis is a bacterial infection of the cells of the mastoid bone. The infection is usually streptococcal and spreads to the mastoid from the middle ear.

Symptoms. Earache with tenderness in the area of the mastoid bone, and elevation of the body temperature are the outstanding symptoms of mastoiditis. Upon visual examination the eardrum appears congested and is bulging. Incision of the eardrum brings about the flow of a large amount of purulent, foul-smelling drainage. The drum may rupture spontaneously if the pressure behind it becomes too great.

Treatment and Nursing Care. When antibiotics were first used in the treatment of middle ear infections it was hoped that the spread of infection to the mastoid cells would be prevented, thereby eliminating mastoiditis as a complication of otitis media. Unfortunately, this has not happened. Instead, the antibiotics often mask the symptoms, giving the impression that complete recovery has taken place, when in reality the infection smolders and spreads from the middle ear to the mastoid cells.

When mastoiditis is diagnosed it is treated surgically and with medication. The first step is usually myringotomy to drain off the purulent matter, and the administration of antibiotics and sulfonamides to destroy the causative organism. If x-ray examinations of the mastoid bone show that there is necrosis of the bone cells, the surgical removal of the cells becomes necessary. The operation is called a *mastoidectomy* and may be simple or radical, depending on the amount of dead bone tissue which must be removed.

Nursing Care of the Patient Having a Mastoidectomy.

PREOPERATIVE CARE. Physical preparation of the patient is basically the same as for other types of major surgery. The hair should be washed before the day of surgery and the area around the affected ear shaved (see Fig. 19-7).

Many of these patients are children and the nurse must recognize the need for eliminating safety hazards and providing emotional support for the child during the preoperative period. If possible, the same nurses should be assigned to the care of the child during the preoperative and immediate postoperative periods. This gives the child a sense of security and reduces the anxiety produced by unfamiliar surroundings and the child's natural fear of pain and discomfort.

POSTOPERATIVE CARE. When the patient returns from the recovery room he must be watched closely until fully conscious so that he will not disturb the surgical dressings or any drains which may have been inserted during the operation. Very small children may require tongue-blade restraints on their arms to keep their hands away from the operative site. Bleeding, elevation of temperature, or changes in the vital signs should be reported immediately.

The patient is usually placed on a semisoft diet of foods which require a minimum of chewing until the soreness in the operative area has subsided.

A   **B**

Figure 19-7. Area to be shaved for mastoid operation *(A)* on female patient and *(B)* on male patient. Note that hair of male patient has been parted very low on side of head where surgery is to be performed. (From Manhattan Eye, Ear and Throat Hospital: *Nursing in Diseases of the Eye, Ear, Nose and Throat,* 10th Ed.)

DISORDERS OF THE INNER EAR

Introduction. The inner ear is a very complex structure located deep in the temporal bone. It consists of bony and membranous labyrinths filled with fluid and its functions are hearing and maintaining equilibrium. Because of the location and complexity of structure of the inner ear, its disorders are difficult to treat and tend to become chronic, producing loss of hearing that can be permanent.

Labyrinthitis. This is an inflammation involving the labyrinths of the inner ear and usually occurs as a complication of chronic otitis media. The symptoms of labyrinthitis include loss of hearing in the affected ear, dizziness with nausea and vomiting and abnormal jerking movements of the eyes (*nystagmus*).

Treatment is aimed at removal of the source of infection and relief of symptoms. Antibiotics may be given in massive doses to control the infection, which often is quite persistent and difficult to clear up completely. The patient is kept in bed to minimize vertigo and to avoid injury from falls. Side rails must be applied to the bed and the patient should be told the reason for this and why he should not try to get out of bed without assistance. Dimenhydrinate (Dramamine) or other drugs to control motion sickness may be given. If the source of infection is a chronic mastoiditis that does not respond to medical treatment, a mastoidectomy may be done.

Meniere's Syndrome. This is a group of symptoms in which there is an increase in fluid within the spaces of the labyrinths with swelling and congestion of the mucous membranes of the cochlea. The symptoms include attacks of dizziness, ringing in the ear (tinnitus), headache, poor coordination that makes walking difficult or impossible and loss of hearing. Any sudden movement of the head or eyes during an attack usually produces severe nausea and vomiting. The condition occurs most often in persons who have had chronic ear disorders and allergic symptoms involving the upper respiratory tract. The exact cause is unknown.

Diagnosis of Meniere's syndrome usually is not difficult, but since these symptoms could indicate a tumor of the auditory mechanism, a special test may be done to confirm the diagnosis. This test, called the *caloric test,* involves instilling very warm or cold fluid into the auditory canal. A patient with Meniere's syndrome will experience a severe attack while a normal person will complain of only slight dizziness. A person with a tumor of the auditory mechanism will have no reaction at all.

Treatment of Meniere's syndrome is primarily concerned with relief of symptoms; there is no cure for the condition although it does disappear spontaneously in some cases. In order to control edema and reduce pressure in the inner ear, the patient may be placed on a low-sodium diet, his fluid intake restricted, and his urinary output increased by means of a diuretic drug. Drugs such as Dramamine and Bonamine may be given to control nausea and vomiting. The patient is kept quiet in bed to avoid aggravating his symptoms. He may be very irritable and withdrawn and refuse to eat or drink because of fear of vomiting. One should be very careful to avoid increasing his irritation by jarring his bed, turning on bright overhead lights or making loud noises.

These measures help control the severe symptoms during an attack but the patient's hearing is not improved. If the attacks continue and are very severe in spite of medical treatment, surgical destruction of the eighth nerve may be necessary. Although this produces permanent deafness in the affected ear, the severe attacks are eliminated and in most persistent cases of Meniere's syndrome the patient will have experienced a serious or even total loss of hearing eventually no matter what treatment was used.

OTOSCLEROSIS

Definition. Much of our hearing depends on the proper vibration of the small bones of the inner ear. The *stapes,* or stirrup, is particularly important because it transmits the sound waves to the fluid in the semicircular canals. In *otosclerosis* the stapes becomes fixed and cannot move because of destruction of normal bone and the laying down of sclerotic bone cells. When the stapes is locked in a fixed position it cannot vibrate and therefore is no longer able to transmit sound waves.

Symptoms. The patient who has otosclerosis has a peculiar type of hearing disability. He has difficulty hearing the voices of others, yet his own voice sounds unusually loud to him. In response to this he lowers his voice to the point that he can scarcely be understood by others. His reaction is characteristically one of criticism in which he complains that everyone is mumbling and they do not pronounce their words distinctly. His attitude can be understood when we realize that because of cranial bone conduction of sound waves he does not have an overall loss of hearing and can hear fairly well over a telephone or in a noisy atmosphere in which other people are speaking loudly above the surrounding noise.

Treatment and Nursing Care. Otosclerosis may be treated by a properly fitted hearing aid or by surgical means. Newer methods of surgery, using a microscope because the ossicles of the middle ear are so small, have greatly increased the success of surgical treatment of this condition.

The operative procedure is called a *stapedectomy,* in which the stapes is removed and is replaced with a prosthetic device. This device may be a steel wire and fat implant, a wire and a segment of vein, or a vein graft with polyethylene tubing. In any case, the prosthesis is attached to one end of the incus (anvil of the middle ear) so that sound can be transmitted to the inner ear.

The surgical procedure is extremely delicate and would not be possible without the fairly recently developed dissecting binocular microscope and other modern surgical instruments that allow visualization and manipulation of the very small structures of the middle ear.

Postoperative nursing care is concerned with keeping the patient quiet and flat in bed for forty-eight hours. The head is turned so that the operative ear is uppermost. When the patient is allowed to move about he must be warned that dizziness is likely to occur, especially if he turns his head suddenly. Side rails are applied to the bed and the patient must have assistance when getting out of bed and walking. Coughing, sneezing, and other violent movement of the head should be avoided, and the patient must be warned not to blow his nose, as this may introduce organisms into the middle ear via the eustachian tube. The physician will instruct the patient in which activities are allowed and which are to be avoided during his convalescence at home.

NURSING CARE OF THE PATIENT HAVING SURGERY OF THE EAR

Preoperative Care. The nursing care of the patient during the preoperative period usually is rather routine except for administration of ear drops or other special medications and treatments. The physical preparation may or may not involve removal of some of the hair from the scalp. Most patients having a mastoidectomy do have some hair removed on the affected side. Male patients should be clean-shaven the morning of surgery. The external ear and surrounding skin should be thoroughly cleaned, preferably with a surgical soap. Female patients with long hair should have it braided or pinned back securely so that it will not become soiled by drainage from the ear or serve as a source of infection at the operative site.

Postoperative Care. Positioning of the patient after surgery will depend on specific instructions from the physician. Usually the patient is placed flat in bed and his head is supported so that he does not turn it from side to side. In addition to noting the vital signs, the nurse should watch for signs of injury to the facial nerve. These would include inability of the patient to close his eyes, wrinkle his forehead or pucker his lips. Such symptoms should be reported to the surgeon. If they appear later than 12 hours after surgery they may be due to edema and the physician may order a loosening of the dressings.

Precautions such as side rails to the bed should be taken to avoid injury due to dizziness and loss of balance which can occur temporarily as a result of disturbance to the equilibrium mechanism. When the patient is allowed up and about he should have someone in attendance to prevent falls.

Because the ear is so near the brain, a special effort must be made to avoid contamination of the operative area. Dressings may be reinforced to keep them dry but excessive drainage must be reported to the surgeon. The patient must keep his hands away from the bandages and if he is unable to do so he should be restrained.

Sneezing, coughing and nose-blowing are all ways in which the operative site may be disturbed to the detriment of the patient's welfare. If sneezing cannot be controlled, the patient should be told to keep his mouth open while sneezing so that the force of the sneeze will exit through the mouth rather than the eustachian tube. Sneezing and blowing the nose also may force bacteria and other infectious material into the operative area.

The nurse should know beforehand exactly what outcome is to be expected from the surgery. If the patient's hearing is slightly impaired immediately after surgery because of edema or bandages but is expected to improve in time, she should know this so that she can sincerely reassure the patient that it will improve. She should be able to give encouragement to her patient but must avoid giving false hopes or telling him that he has nothing to worry about when he will indeed have to make an adjustment to a disability.

GENERAL PRINCIPLES IN THE CARE OF THE DEAF

Terminology. The terms "deaf" and "hard of hearing" are sometimes taken to mean the same thing, when, actually, they represent two separate conditions.

The *deaf* are those in whom the sense of hearing is entirely absent. The *congenitally deaf* are those who are born without the sense of hearing, the *adventitiously deaf* are those who are born with the sense of hearing but, by illness or accident, have lost their hearing.[5]

The *hard of hearing* are those in whom hearing is defective but not totally absent.

Signs of Hearing Loss. Many cases of deafness could have been prevented if the condition had been detected in the early stages and treatment begun. The value of public health education in the early signs of hearing loss cannot be estimated. Nurses must be familiar with these signs and accept some of the responsibility for educating parents and teachers in the health of the ears and preservation of the sense of hearing.

SIGNS OF HEARING LOSS*
1. A listless or weary expression.
2. Frequent requests for repetition.
3. Mispronunciation of words.
4. Habitually turning one ear toward the speaker.

---

*Quoted from "Hearing and Deafness." Am. Journ. Nurs., May, 1950, p. 305.

5. Inattention or failure to respond when questioned.

6. Voice or speech peculiarities.

7. Continued failure in school.

8. Earache, head noises, discharging ears.

9. Tendency to avoid people.

THE NURSE AND THE DEAF AND HARD OF HEARING

We have discussed earlier the emotional aspects of hearing loss (see introduction to Part II of this chapter). When a person who is deaf or hard of hearing enters a hospital he brings with him some of the emotional scars resulting from his struggle to live with his handicap. Like the blind patient, he does not want pity. He *does* appreciate understanding and consideration from those who must care for him while he is ill. The following rules are given in the hope that they will help the practical nurse when she is assigned to the care of patients who suffer from a loss of hearing.

1. Do not shout at the person who is hard of hearing. Speaking slowly and distinctly is more help than raising the voice.

2. Face the person when you speak to him. Your facial expressions are helpful in understanding what you are saying even if the person cannot read your lips.

3. Keep questions to a minimum, but when you must ask a question, phrase it so that his answer will require more than a yes or no. For example, "What is your name?" is better than "Are you Mr. Lowe?" In this way you avoid getting an incorrect answer from the patient who does not wish to ask you to repeat the question and will just say "Yes" because he thought you had asked if he was Mr. Long.

4. Because the patient either cannot hear, or often misinterprets the sounds he does hear in the unfamiliar surroundings of the hospital, he is more likely to be upset and frightened his first few days in the hospital. He will appreciate frequent visits from the nurse to reassure him that she is genuinely interested and close at hand should he need her.

The Hearing Aid. Many hearing aids are bought, worn for a few days, and then relegated to the depths of a dresser drawer. This unfortunate situation is often the result of improper fitting of the hearing aid and inadequate instruction in its use.

The hearing aid should do more than amplify sound. Less expensive aids do make sounds louder but they often distort the sounds. The patient who has a conductive hearing loss but normal sensory function is usually satisfied with amplification alone because he has no problem with sound perception. The patient who has sensorineural hearing loss may actually have poorer hearing with the hearing aid than without it if the appliance distorts sounds as it amplifies them.

It is obvious, then, that the choice of a hearing aid and the preparation and instruction of the patient are very important factors in the successful use of such an appliance. Just as the proper fitting of glasses for correction of visual defects demands more than a trip to the local dime store for a pair of reading glasses, the fitting of a hearing aid requires more than purchasing an amplifier and applying it to the ear. The individual who wishes to improve his hearing through the use of a hearing aid must have persistence, determination, and adaptability. He must be willing to cooperate with the audiologist who prescribes the aid, learn to use the aid intelligently, and care for it properly.

Part III — DISORDERS OF THE THROAT

PHARYNGITIS

Definition. The throat has been described as the "crossroads of the human body." It has openings leading from the nose and ears and also serves as a passageway for food and air. It is little wonder then that inflammation of the throat (pharyngitis) is such a common condition. Considering the exposure of the throat to the hordes of bacteria present in our environment, it is remarkable that more infections do not occur there.

Symptoms. Most of us are quite familiar with the symptoms of pharyngitis—the dry, "scratchy" feeling in the back of the throat, slight fever, chills, and malaise. These symptoms are usually accompanied by a sinusitis or an inflammation of the nasal mucosa.

Treatment and Nursing Care. Local treatment consists of hot saline throat irrigations and, if the discomfort is severe, the application of an ice collar to the throat. Aspirin gargles (5 grains of aspirin and ½ tsp. of baking soda dissolved in a glass of warm water) are also helpful in the relief of local symptoms. Antibiotics or sulfonamides are sometimes given to prevent secondary infection if the patient has a chronic illness or is physically weak and debilitated.

TONSILLITIS

Definition. An inflammation of the tonsils is usually caused by streptococci or staphylococci and is completely different from pharyngitis even though the symptoms may be somewhat alike. Acute tonsillitis may occur repeatedly, especially in those who have a low resistance to infection. Chronic tonsillitis usually produces enlargement of tonsillar tissue and adjacent adenoidal tissue as well.

Symptoms. *Acute tonsillitis* occurs most often in young children. There is an elevation of the temperature, sore throat, general malaise, and chills. Inspection of the throat reveals redness and swelling of the tonsils and surrounding tissues.

Chronic infection of the tonsils produces symptoms which may not be as dramatic but most certainly are capable of making the individual uncomfortable. The child with chronic tonsillitis and enlarged adenoids has frequent colds and appears to be in poor health. He gives the impression of being dull or mentally retarded because he constantly holds his mouth open to breathe and he often has difficulty in hearing. These children also are mouth breathers when they sleep and are very likely to snore.

Treatment and Nursing Care. Acute tonsillitis is treated with hot saline throat irrigations and the administration of specific antibiotics for the destruction of the causative organism. Bed rest, nursing measures to reduce the fever, and liquid diet to minimize trauma to the tonsils are also included in the treatment.

Chronic tonsillitis is treated surgically when accompanied by enlargement of the tonsils and adenoids. The practice of indiscriminately removing tonsils "just in case tonsillitis may develop" has been discontinued. Most physicians usually will not remove the tonsils unless the child fails to respond to medical treatment and has symptoms of enlarged tonsils and adenoids.

Nursing Care of the Patient Having a Tonsillectomy and Adenoidectomy. Pre-operative Care. Most tonsillectomies are performed on young children who have had no previous admissions to a hospital and are not yet old enough to fully understand the need for the surgical procedure. Every nurse who expects to care for a child in a hospital should have a thorough understanding of the essentials of child psychology. Even those nurses who have had training and experience in pediatric nursing are sometimes surprised to find that they are not able to gain the confidence and cooperation of a child and allay his fears and anxieties while he is in the hospital. It is to be expected, then, that those who do not understand children are even less likely to have any success in this area of nursing. The reader is referred to texts on pediatric nursing and child psychology for the essential principles of child care.

Physical preparation of the patient having a tonsillectomy involves administration of preoperative medications as ordered and restriction of the patient's diet for 6 to 8 hours prior to surgery. It is especially important that the child's temperature is taken for signs of fever, so that an elevation of temperature or any signs of an upper respiratory infection may be reported. Surgery is usually postponed if these signs are present.

POSTOPERATIVE CARE. Following tonsillectomy or adenoidectomy the nurse's chief concern is observation for hemorrhage. Even though about one million tonsillectomies are performed in the United States each year, and nurses may tend to become somewhat complacent about the routine care of these patients, it must be remembered that *a tonsillectomy or adenoidectomy should never be considered a minor operation.*

Since hemorrhage is always a possibility following a tonsillectomy the vital signs are checked quite frequently. If the patient appears to be swallowing often, seems unusually restless, or has a change in pulse rate and blood pressure, excessive bleeding should be suspected even though there are no outward signs of bleeding. An ice collar may be placed around the neck to reduce swelling and prevent the oozing of blood from the operative site.

Even though it is difficult to keep a child in one position for very long he should be kept on his side or abdomen as long as there is drainage from the surgical wound. If the child is thrashing about in the bed when recovering from the anesthesia it is best to collect secretions from the mouth in a large towel rather than use a metal emesis basin which may injure him. Older children may sit up in semi-Fowler's position after they have recovered from the anesthesia and are often more comfortable this way. Younger children usually can be kept calm and quiet if someone holds them and rocks them. This is not spoiling the child; he needs to keep as quiet as possible to prevent hemorrhage from the operative site and he needs love and affection to reassure him at a time when he is frightened and uncomfortable. It should be emphasized that every child is an individual. He has his own likes and dislikes, his own preferences. The nurse who bears this in mind is more likely to keep her patient calm and cooperative than the one who insists on following the rules to the letter.

The postoperative diet usually consists of ice-cold liquids, ice cream, jello, custards, and other semisolid foods for the first 24 hours. Citrus fruits, hot fluids, and rough foods should be avoided until the throat has completely healed.

CANCER OF THE LARYNX

Introduction. Cancer of the larynx occurs most often in men of middle age or older, but it can strike anyone, especially those over the age of 18. It is one of the most easily cured of all malignancies because of its location and adjacent tissues, and about 80 per cent of all cases treated by early surgery are cured. The cause of cancer of the larynx is not known but there is some evidence that predisposing factors are cigarette smoking, chronic laryngitis, abuse of the vocal cords, and a familial tendency toward cancer.

Symptoms and Diagnosis. Since the larynx, sometimes called the voice box, is directly concerned with the production of vocal sounds, a tumor of the larynx will quickly produce persistent hoarseness that does not respond to usual methods of treatment. After the cancer has spread beyond the vocal cords (and is much more difficult to treat) the symptoms may include difficulty in swallowing or breathing, a sensation of having a lump in the throat, cough, enlarged lymph nodes in the neck, and pain in the region of the Adam's apple.

Diagnosis is established by visualization of the larynx via a laryngoscope and microscopic examination of the sample of tissues taken from the tumor.

Treatment. There are two types of surgical procedures that may be done for treatment of a laryngeal malignancy. If the tumor is restricted to the vocal cords the surgeon may perform a partial laryngectomy in which the thryroid cartilage is split and only the tumor and involved portion of the vocal cords are removed. In more advanced cases metastasis may demand a total laryngectomy, in which the surgeon excises the entire larynx, epiglottis, thyroid cartilage, hyoid bone, cricoid cartilage and two or more rings of the trachea.

A partial laryngectomy does not permanently eliminate voice sounds. A tracheostomy may be done for temporary facilitation of breathing, but this eventually is closed and the patient may resume talking after the operative area is healed completely.

In a total laryngectomy the trachea is diverted to a surgically constructed opening (stoma) in the neck. The patient then has a permanent tracheostomy with no connection between the nose and mouth and the lower respiratory system and must depend on the stoma for breathing. The laryngectomy tube is inserted in the stoma and resembles a tracheostomy tube except that it is somewhat shorter and wider. Usually the laryngectomy tube can be removed within six weeks after surgery.

Nursing Care. The patient who has had a laryngectomy will require adequate instruction in the care of his stoma and laryngectomy tube. He will need help and guidance in facing a future in which he will not be able to speak until he learns esophageal speech or uses an artificial "voice box." He also may have difficulty eating and swallowing until he gets accustomed to the sensations of choking and gagging that frequently occur with a laryngectomy.

Feedings through a nasogastric tube may be prescribed by the physician if the patient has great difficulty swallowing or if the surgeon feels that there is danger of contaminating the operative area. Tube feeding is then given at regular intervals and the nasogastric tube is inserted before each feeding and removed when the feeding is completed. Some patients can be taught to pass their own tubes and give their own feedings because this gives them a feeling of independence. Others will refuse to take any active part in the procedure.

Protection of the tracheal opening from dust and lint can be accomplished by a simple gauze covering or high-necked clothing. The patient also should be told to avoid swimming and to use care when taking a shower or tub bath so that water is not aspirated through the opening. In order to protect the patient from inhalation of extremely cold air (he no longer breathes through his nose and mouth, which normally warm inspired air) the patient may wear a small scarf over the opening during winter weather.

Proper rehabilitation of the patient plays a very important part in his acceptance of surgery and its consequences. Many persons are able to learn esophageal speech in which they first master the art of swallowing air and then moving it forcibly back up through the esophagus. They then learn to coordinate lip and tongue movements with the sound produced by the air passing over vibrating folds of the esophagus. The sounds may be somewhat hoarse but they can be understood as speech and are more natural than the sounds produced by an artificial larynx.

In various parts of the United States there are several groups organized for laryngectomy patients who wish to get together for social and rehabilitation purposes. These clubs have names like Lost Cord, New Speech, New Voice and Esophageal Speech. Information regarding these clubs and other aspects of post-laryngectomy rehabilitation can be obtained by writing to the American Speech and Hearing Association, 1001 Connecticut Ave., Washington, D.C. 20036.

CLINICAL CASE PROBLEMS

1. Mr. Wilson, aged 72, is admitted to the hospital for surgical treatment of cataracts of both eyes. His poor eyesight has prevented his earning a living for quite a few years and he has been totally dependent on his son. He did not consult a doctor until recently because he has always heard that cataracts had to be "ripe" before they could be treated and he felt that he could not afford frequent trips to the doctor when nothing could be done for his eyes.

When you take Mr. Wilson to his room after admission to the hospital he tells you that he is used to being "almost blind" and can take care of himself. He does not want side rails on his bed and insists he can get up to the bathroom without any help. From your observations of the patient you can see that Mr. Wilson does need help but is apparently too proud to ask for it.

The day after his operation Mr. Wilson is again assigned to your care. He seems more cooperative and somewhat frightened by his experience in the hospital. He is very anxious to walk down the hall and the doctor has stated that he can be ambulatory for a very brief period of time.

What nursing problems are presented by Mr. Wilson's attitude of independence when he is admitted to the hospital?
What precautions must be taken for his safety?
What special nursing care will he require postoperatively?

How will you accompany Mr. Wilson as he takes a walk down the hall?

2. A neighbor tells you that her 4-year-old son seems to have more than his share of colds and sore throats. She feels that these could be eliminated by having the child's tonsils removed but her physician advises against surgery. The neighbor asks your advice about changing doctors because she is convinced that a tonsillectomy is the only solution to the frequent colds and sore throats.

How would you advise this person?

3. Janice is a 7-year-old who has been admitted to the hospital for a tonsillectomy and adenoidectomy. She has been emotionally prepared for the stay in the hospital and seems happy and satisfied before surgery.

Following the surgical procedure Janice is taken to the recovery room and then is brought to her room after she has recovered sufficiently from the anesthesia. When she is placed in the crib bed she begins to thrash about, screaming for her mother. All this activity causes an attack of vomiting and increases the flow of blood from the operative site. The mother of the child becomes very upset and cannot stay with her. The nurse in charge gives Janice a sedative and then asks you to stay with her and keep her quiet.

How will you handle the secretions from the operative site?
How would you keep the child quiet?

REFERENCES

1. Bender, R. E.: "Communicating with Deaf Adults." Am. Journ. Nurs., April, 1966, p. 757.
2. Blodi, F. C.: "Glaucoma." Am. Journ. Nurs., March, 1963, p. 78.
3. Bosanko, L.: "Nursing Care of a Patient with a Cataract Extraction." Am. Journ. Nurs., Oct., 1960, p. 1435.
4. Brockhurst, R. J., and O'Donnell, C. T.: "Detachment of the Retina." Am. Journ. Nurs., April, 1964, p. 96.
5. Brown, A. F.: *Medical-Surgical Nursing II.* Philadelphia, W. B. Saunders Co., 1959.
6. Cholden, L.: "Problems in Adjusting to Blindness. Am. Journ. Nurs., Jan., 1956, p. 74.
7. Cooper, S.: "Giving Eye, Ear, and Nose Drops." RN, March, 1960, p. 69.
8. Covey, J. K., and Balanka, C.: "Myths and

Facts about Eye Care." Today's Health, June, 1962, p. 8.

9. Gordon, D. M.: "The Inflamed Eye." Am. Journ., Nurs., Nov., 1964, p. 113.

10. Haddad, H. M.: "Drugs for Ophthalmologic Use." Am. Journ. Nurs., Feb., 1968, p. 325.

11. Hoehnig, L.: "A Hearing Program for School Children." Am. Journ. Nurs., May, 1963, p. 85.

12. Jackson, G. D.: "How Blind Are Nurses to the Needs of the Visually Handicapped?" Nurs. Outlook, Sept., 1965, p. 34.

13. Jones, I.: "The Cataract Extraction Operation." Am. Journ. Nurs., Oct., 1960, p. 1433.

14. Miller, A.: "Helping Your Patient Who Dwells in Darkness." RN, Aug., 1962, p. 49.

15. Nader, A. F.: "Helping the Hard of Hearing." RN, Oct., 1961, p. 59.

16. Nordstrom, W.: "Adjusting to Cataract Glasses." Am. Journ. Nurs., July, 1966, p. 1578.

17. Ronnei, E. C.: "Hearing Aids." Am. Journ. Nurs., May, 1963, p. 90.

18. Rusk, H.: "Blindness — Some Facts about It." RN, Aug., 1962, p. 51.

19. Shafer, K. N., Sawyer, J. R., et al.: *Medical-Surgical Nursing*, 4th edition. St. Louis, Mo., C. V. Mosby Co., 1966.

20. Smith, D. W., and Gips, C. D.: *Care of the Adult Patient*, 2nd edition. Philadelphia, J. B. Lippincott Co., 1967.

21. Shepard, M. E.: *Nursing Care of Patients with Eye, Ear, Nose and Throat Disorders.* New York, The Macmillan Co., 1958.

SUGGESTED STUDENT READING

1. Bender, R. E.: "Communicating with Deaf Adults." Am. Journ. Nurs., April, 1966, p. 757.

2. Bosanko, L.: "Nursing Care of a Patient with a Cataract Extraction." Am. Journ. Nurs., Oct., 1960, p. 1435.

3. Carbary, L.: "When Your Patient Wears an Artificial Eye." Practical Nursing, July–Aug., 1962, p. 20.

4. Cooper, S.: "Giving Eye, Ear, and Nose Drops." RN, March, 1960, p. 69.

5. Covey, J. K., and Balanka, C.: "Myths and Facts about Eye Care." Today's Health, June, 1962, p. 49.

6. Miller, A.: "Helping Your Patient Who Dwells in Darkness." RN, Aug., 1962, p. 49.

7. Nader, A. F.: "Helping the Hard of Hearing." RN, Oct., 1961, p. 59.

8. Pamphlets from American Foundation for the Blind, 15 West 16th Street, N.W., Washington, D.C.

9. Rusk, H.: "Blindness — Some Facts about It." RN, Aug., 1962, p. 51.

OUTLINE FOR CHAPTER 19

Part I — Disorders of the Eyes

I. Introduction

A. Fundamentals of good eye care:
   1. Headache, burning, itching and redness of the eyes are symptoms of a visual defect.
   2. Adequate nutrition conserves but does not improve eyesight.
   3. Normal eyes do not require irrigations.
   4. Children do not outgrow crossed eyes.
   5. Every person over the age of 40 should have periodic eye examinations.
   6. Teaching eye safety to children in school could prevent many accidental injuries.
   7. Visual defects cannot always be corrected by eye glasses.

II. Diagnostic Tests and Examinations

A. Snellen chart — composed of increasingly smaller rows of type. Visual acuity expressed as a fraction comparing subject's distance (20 feet) with distance at which a person with normal vision can read the row. 20/20 is normal.

B. Near vision tested by a card with different sizes of types (Jaeger's Test Types).

C. Refraction — patient reads the Snellen chart through differently shaped lenses.

D. Intraocular pressure — tonometer measures amount of pressure being exerted by the aqueous humor within the chambers of the eye.

III. Common Visual Defects

A. Errors of refraction — light rays bent so that they do not focus properly on the retina.
   1. Myopia (nearsightedness) — light rays converge and focus in front of the retina. Individual has difficulty seeing distant objects.
   2. Hyperopia (farsightedness) — light rays focus behind the retina. Individual has difficulty seeing objects close at hand.
   3. Presbyopia is improper accomodation of the ciliary muscles and liga-

ments in switching between distant and near vision.

4. Astigmatism results from a warped lens or irregular curvature of the cornea.

IV. Injuries and Infections of the Eye

A. Foreign bodies—patient should be referred to physician if body is not easily removed.

B. Conjunctivitis is an inflammation of the mucous membrane lining the upper and lower lids and covering the front part of the eyeball.

1. Symptoms are redness, swelling of conjunctiva, watery secretion, burning and itching.
2. Treatment depends on organism causing infection. Antibiotic ointments, steroids and hot or cold moist compresses may help.

C. Sty (hordeolum) is an infection of a follicle of an eyelash.

1. Symptoms are redness, burning and itching of the eyelids. Pustule develops on the eyelid.
2. Warm, moist compresses usually cause rupture and draining of the pustule, or surgical incision may be made.

D. Cataract—an opacity of the lens of the eye.

1. Symptoms—blurring of vision.
2. Treatment—surgical removal of the affected lens and prescription of eyeglasses.
3. Nursing care
   a. Preoperative care—ophthalmic ointments and eye drops.
   b. Postoperative care—no stress on sutures by coughing, sneezing or suddenly turning head. Physical activity depending on orders of surgeon.
   c. Adjustment to cataract glasses which is frustrating and discouraging.

E. Glaucoma—a condition in which increased intraocular pressure produces varying degrees of visual impairment.

1. Cause is an obstruction to the outflow of aqueous humor in the anterior chamber of the eye.
2. Symptoms: in an acute attack the patient has severe headache or pain in affected eye, nausea and vomiting. Chronic glaucoma is characterized by vision that is blurred or hazy and then clears up after a while, trouble adjusting to dark, narrowing of vision, and seeing halos around objects and lights.
3. Treatment with myotics and drugs that decrease production of aqueous humor may help; otherwise removal of a section of the iris (iridectomy) may be necessary.

F. Detached retina—separation of the retina from the vascular wall of the eye.

1. Possible causes are sudden blow or penetrating injury, diabetic changes in the retina, myopia.
2. Symptoms: patient sees flashes of light and spots or moving particles and has cloudy vision or loss of central vision.
3. Treatment and nursing care—only treatment is surgical repair of tears or holes in retina, removing accumulated fluid and securing the retina in its normal position. Physical activity determined by directions of surgeon.

V. Nursing Care of the Patient Having Eye Surgery

A. Preoperative period: orient patient to his surroundings, explain procedures, watch for allergies or respiratory infection and cleanse intestinal tract. Ophthalmic drops or ointments exactly as ordered.

B. Postoperative period:

1. Position patient according to specific orders of surgeon, keep patient quiet and undisturbed and limit patient's activity.
2. Sudden pain in eye may indicate hemorrhage in operative area.
3. Instruct patient to avoid sudden, violent movements of the head.

VI. General Principles in the Care of the Blind

A. Emotional impact of blindness can be quite severe. Patient must be allowed to express his fears and to gradually adjust to his new way of life.

B. Special rules in helping blind person:

1. Do not shout.
2. Always speak as you enter his room and notify him when you are leaving.
3. Blind persons want to be treated as normal persons, not pitied.
4. Remember that whatever independence a blind person has acquired is

the result of hard work and determination.

Part II — Disorders of the Ears

I. Introduction

A. One with hearing difficulties tends to withdraw and live in a world of his own due to difficulty in communicating with others.

B. Loss of hearing can be due to a nerve defect (sensorineural) or to a barrier to the conduction of sound waves through the ear.

II. Special Diagnostic Tests and Examinations

A. Tuning fork tests:
    a. Weber test compares hearing acumen in each ear.
    b. Rinne test determines whether hearing loss is sensorineural or conductive.

B. Audiometry — audiometer measures sound perception.

III. Infections of the Ear

A. Otitis media, or tympanitis, is an inflammation of the middle ear; often a result of acute infection of the throat or sinuses.
    1. Symptoms are pain, fever and drainage from ear.
    2. Treatment includes rest, analgesics and antibiotics and possibly myringotomy (incision and drainage).

B. Mastoiditis is inflammation of the mastoid bone. Infection is usually streptococcal.
    1. Symptoms are earache with tenderness in the area of the mastoid bone, fever and congestion of ear drum.
    2. Treatment involves myringotomy and antibiotics and possibly mastoidectomy (surgical removal of infected mastoid cells).
    3. Nursing care of the patient having a mastoidectomy:
        a. Preoperative care — wash hair and shave area around ear. Become acquainted with children and make them feel secure after surgery.
        b. Postoperative care — prevent disturbance of drains or bandages, watch for bleeding, elevation of temperature or change in vital signs and give soft diet requiring little chewing.

IV. Disorders of the Inner Ear

A. Introduction. Inner ear is concerned with hearing and maintenance of equilibrium. Inaccessibility makes disorders difficult to treat.

B. Labyrinthitis — inflammation involving the labyrinths of the inner ear.
    1. Symptoms — loss of hearing in affected ear, dizziness, nausea, vomiting and nystagmus.
    2. Treatment — antibiotics, bed rest and drugs to control nausea. Possibly mastoidectomy for patients with chronic mastoiditis.

C. Meniere's syndrome — group of symptoms occurring as a result of increased fluid in labyrinthine spaces with swelling and congestion of mucous membranes of the cochlea.
    1. Symptoms — tinnitus, headache, poor coordination, loss of hearing and nausea and vomiting when head is moved.
    2. Treatment — bed rest, anti-emetics, restriction of fluid intake and sometimes surgical destruction of eighth nerve.

D. Otosclerosis — a fixation of the stapes due to destruction of normal bone and the laying down of sclerotic bone cells.
    1. Peculiar type of hearing loss in which patient's own voice seems much louder than others'.
    2. Treated surgically. Patient kept quiet after surgery and positioned so that operative ear is uppermost. Coughing, sneezing, or sudden movements of head to be avoided.

V. Nursing Care of the Patient Having Surgery of the Ear

A. Preoperative care: shave operative area, clean ear and pin hair back securely.

B. Postoperative care: patient is usually kept flat in bed with head kept still. Put side rails on bed.
    1. Watch for signs of injury to facial nerve.
    2. Avoid postoperative infection; it could spread to brain or meninges.
    3. Patient should avoid sneezing, coughing or blowing his nose.

VI. General Principles in the Care of the Deaf

A. Deafness is total loss of hearing. Many

people are "hard of hearing" but do have some sense of hearing.

B. Signs of hearing loss include listless or weary facial expression, inattention or inability to understand what is being said, voice or speech peculiarities, mispronunciation of words, continued failure in school and tendency to avoid others.

VII. The Nurse and the Deaf

A. Offer understanding and consideration; not pity.

B. Avoid shouting.

C. Face the person when you speak to him.

D. Keep questions to a minimum and phrase them so that more is required than yes or no answer.

E. Frequent visits to the patient while in the hospital will help him feel more secure and less isolated from others.

F. The hearing aid must be fitted properly and patient given adequate instruction in its use and care.

Part III — Disorders of the Throat

I. Pharyngitis (Inflammation of the Throat)

A. Symptoms — dryness, irritation in back of throat, slight fever and malaise.

B. Treatment — hot saline gargles and aspirin, and antibiotics or sulfonamides for severe infection.

II. Tonsillitis

A. An inflammation of the tonsils, usually streptococcal or staphylococcal.

B. Symptoms — sore throat, fever, chills, general malaise. Chronic infection can lead to enlargement of tonsils and adenoids.

C. Treatment — acute: hot saline gargles, bed rest and antibiotics. Chronic tonsillitis with enlargement of adenoids may require tonsillectomy and adenoidectomy.

III. Nursing Care of Patient Having Tonsillectomy and Adenoidectomy

A. Preoperative — temperature checked.

B. Postoperative — vital signs checked frequently. Patient kept on his side or abdomen as long as there is drainage from the throat. Diet restricted to soft, nonirritating foods until throat is healed.

IV. Cancer of the Larynx

A. Most easily cured of all malignancies.

B. Predisposing factors — smoking, chronic laryngitis and abuse of vocal cords.

C. Symptoms — hoarseness at first. Later, pain in throat, difficulty in swallowing, lump in throat, and pain in region of Adam's apple.

D. Treatment — partial or total laryngectomy.

   1. Patient who has had partial laryngectomy retains function of speech.

   2. Total laryngectomy patient has permanent opening in trachea and must learn new speech pattern.

Chapter 20

ACCIDENT AND EMERGENCY NURSING, DISASTER NURSING

PREVENTION OF ACCIDENTS

Home Safety. According to statistics compiled by the U.S. Department of Health, Education, and Welfare, home accidents cause more than one fourth of all accidental deaths. The principal victims of accidental deaths occurring in the home are children under 5 years of age and elderly persons over 65. Since persons in these age groups spend a large percentage of their time in the house it is imperative that safety hazards be removed from their environment if these accidental deaths are to be prevented.

Nurses, physicians, and other persons concerned with the safety and welfare of others must take an active part in the education of the public in regard to home accidents and the ways in which they can be eliminated. The two most dangerous rooms in the house are the kitchen and the bathroom. Falls account for almost one half of the accidental injuries sustained in the home. Figure 20-1 shows some of the most common hazards and how they can be avoided.

Highway Safety. Motor vehicle accidents are the leading cause of accidental death in the United States. The National Safety Council estimates that automobile accidents kill a person every 15 minutes and injure someone every 30 seconds. This means that every year there are over 38,000 Americans killed

and over one million disabled by some type of injury sustained in a traffic accident.

The two major causes of motor vehicle accidents are human failure and mechanical failure. Of these two, human failure is by far the greater danger. Improper driving, which causes almost 90 per cent of all accidents, may be due to drinking alcohol, taking drugs, lack of alertness and fatigue, excessive speed or emotional instability of the driver. Mechanical failure often is not detected as the cause of an accident; however, there has been much interest recently in the lack of built-in safety devices and inspection for safety hazards in new automobiles, and it is hoped that many instances of mechanical failure as the cause of accidents will soon be greatly reduced.

Water Safety. The advent of the 40-hour work week and extended vacations have provided more leisure time and more opportunity for Americans to enjoy water sports. With this increased participation in water-centered activities there has been a proportionate increase in accidental deaths and injuries in or on the water. Many of these accidents could have been prevented if the simple rules of water safety had been observed. These rules include using good judgment about the choice of swimming area, proper supervision of children and adults who are not strong swimmers, diving only in areas where

HOME SAFETY CHART

KITCHEN

For gas or coal stove, have vents or flues; keep windows open a crack

Never light stove with kerosene or gasoline

Turn off all flames after cooking

Repair any gas leakage

Use potholders, asbestos pads

Keep handles of pots and pans turned in

Keep knives, sharp instruments and poisons such as bleach out of children's reach

Wipe up spills on floor

Keep electric appliances in good working order

STORAGE AREAS

Always keep cellars, attics, garages neat

Throw out newspapers and oily rags at once: they can start fires

Clean and disinfect area where garbage is kept, and dispose of it frequently

Never place poisonous substances in drinking glasses, cold drink bottles or other containers that have been used for food or drink

Always label poisonous compounds; read labels of poisons you have purchased

LIVING ROOM

Be sure floors are not slippery

Replace frayed or torn carpets

Use rubber mats under rugs to prevent slipping

Cover electric sockets

Replace frayed electric cords

Keep electric cords off floor where people walk

Place heaters a safe distance from walls

Use screens around fireplace

Remove sharp edges from furniture

Check ashtrays for lit matches or cigarettes

FURNACE

Have it checked every year, especially for leaks in tank of oil-burning furnaces

Never light furnace with gasoline or kerosene

BATHROOM

Use rubber mat in tub

Keep soap in sturdy container

Store medicines out of children's reach

Keep all medicines capped and labeled

Throw out old medicines

Dispose of razor blades immediately after use

BEDROOMS

Do not smoke in bed

Use rubber mats under scatter rugs

STAIRWAYS

Cover with carpeting or rubber safety treads

Replace torn or frayed carpeting

Keep stairs cleared of toys and cleaning equipment

Install handrails, proper lighting

Use gates at top and bottom if there are young children

Figure 20-1.

the water is sufficiently deep and is free of rocks or other obstacles, and avoiding overexertion or swimming distances beyond one's ability. Above all one should know how to handle an emergency should it arise. Panic and unthinking actions frequently cause the loss of the life of the person in trouble as well as the would-be rescuer.

Rescue for a drowning person requires a cool head and deliberate action. First the rescuer should call for help. If possible, he should try to reach the victim without going in water over his head. It often is possible to reach him by extending an arm, towel, rope or pole, or any long and sturdy object that is handy. When the victim has grasped the object he can be pulled slowly to shore. If a boat is available, it should be used for rescue of the person who is beyond reach by other methods.

A swimming rescue is very difficult even for the most experienced swimmer, primarily because the victim is frightened and is abnormally strong in such a situation and is quite capable of drowning both himself and his rescuer. After the rescued person is brought out of the water he must be given artificial respiration if he is not breathing. If he is breathing he should be placed in a reclining position and covered with a blanket or coat. His head should be turned to one side so that if he vomits he will not aspirate the vomitus into his lungs. If the person is conscious, he may be given plain water, tea or coffee to drink. He should not be given any alcoholic beverages. The ordeal of nearly drowning can place an added burden on the heart and circulatory system. For this reason it is advisable to have the victim continue to lie down and rest even though he appears to be all right.

GENERAL PRINCIPLES
OF FIRST AID

1. Try to keep calm and think before acting.

2. Concentrate on what should be done first and the manner in which to proceed step by step. Move slowly and deliberately so that you can gain time to think things through and at the same time instill confidence in those you are trying to help.

3. Identify yourself as a nurse. This will serve to reassure the victim and onlookers.

4. Summon help or have someone call the local police department or physician or ambulance if necessary.

5. Make a careful but quick examination and evaluation of the extent of injuries sustained by the victim or victims. Obviously the more serious condition such as stoppage of breathing or severe bleeding must have top priority in the order of treatment. The following list of actions shows their order of importance:

    a. Maintain a patent airway.

    b. Stop bleeding.

    c. Prevent or treat shock.

    d. Protect wounds with a dressing if a sterile or clean bandage is available.

    e. Keep the victim in a reclining position. If he is found in another position and damage to the spine is a possibility do not attempt to force the person to lie straight.

    f. Keep the victim covered.

    g. Reassure the victim and make him as comfortable as possible.

    h. Observe the victim frequently and re-evaluate his condition at regular intervals until a physician or ambulance arrives.

ARTIFICIAL RESPIRATION

In any emergency situation in which there is respiratory failure, the first step to be taken is opening an airway so that proper exchange of oxygen and carbon dioxide can take place. Within 3 to 5 minutes after breathing has stopped the brain may suffer permanent damage from lack of oxygen and death will rapidly follow. Before you attempt to force air into the lungs, make sure that the air passages are open. Place the palm of your hand over the victim's mouth and feel for the movement of air. If none is apparent, check the nose and mouth for obstruction by mucus, water, or foreign objects. Loosen clothing that may constrict the neck. Begin artificial respiration by one of the methods listed below, being sure that the victim's chest is moving slightly with each breath. If you still do not see evidence of an air exchange, you should turn the victim on his side and give him several sharp blows between the shoulder blades. A child can be suspended by his ankles and then slapped sharply on the back in an attempt to dislodge any foreign body obstructing his air passages.

Mouth-to-Mouth Resuscitation. This method of artificial respiration is one of the oldest methods known and is now recommended by authorities as the most effective and practical technique for reinstating breathing. Other methods are used only when circumstances such as severe mouth injury prevent proper technique, or when for personal reasons a person cannot bring himself to place his mouth on the victim's mouth. The following list gives the steps of mouth-to-mouth resuscitation:

1. Clear the mouth and throat of mucus and foreign objects.
2. Place the victim on his back, elevate his shoulders and tilt his head back.
3. Insert your thumb between the patient's upper and lower teeth and grasp the lower jaw with the fingers,

Figure 20-2. Techniques for mouth-to-mouth and mouth-to-nose resuscitation. (From Gordon: Journal of the American Medical Association, May, 1958.)

pulling the jaw upward and forward so that the lower teeth are in front of the upper teeth. NOTE: The proper positioning of the lower jaw is extremely important and is necessary for proper exchange of air.

4. Close the patient's nose with the other hand. If the victim is a small child, the nose and mouth are both covered with the mouth of the resuscitator and the nose is not pinched closed.

5. Open your mouth wide and place it well over the victim's mouth.

6. Blow steadily into the victim's mouth until you see his chest rise.

7. Turn your head to the side and *watch* for movement of the chest. *Listen* for the escape of air from the lungs through the mouth.

8. The cycle of *blow, watch* and *listen* is repeated at the rate of about 12 times per minute for adults and 20 times per minute for infants and small children. Do not blow too hard or too rapidly or you may become dizzy.

9. If for some reason you do not wish to place your mouth directly on the victim's, put a clean cloth over his mouth. This will not greatly affect the flow of air into his lungs.

Chest Pressure—Arm Lift (Silvester) Method. This technique of artificial

CHEST PRESSURE-ARM LIFT (SILVESTER) METHOD

1. Place the victim in a face-up position and put something under his shoulders to raise them and to allow his head to drop backward.

2. Kneel at the victim's head, grasp his wrists, cross them, and press them over the lower chest. This should cause the air to flow out.

3. Immediately pull the arms outward and upward over his head and backward as far as possible. This should cause the air to rush in. Repeat the whole cycle about 12 times a minute, checking the mouth frequently for obstructions.

4. If a second rescuer is available, have him hold the victim 's head so that the jaw is jutting out. The helper should be alert to detect the presence of any stomach contents in the mouth and keep the mouth as clean as possible at all times.

Figure 20-3. (From *The Modern Medical Encyclopedia,* Western Publishing Company, Inc., New York.)

BACK PRESSURE-ARM LIFT (HOLGER-NIELSEN) METHOD

1. Place the victim face-down with one hand on the other as shown. Turn his head slightly to one side and make sure the chin is jutting out. Kneel at the victim's head. Place your hands on his back so the palms lie just below an imaginary line running between the armpits.

2. Rock forward until the arms are about vertical and allow the weight of the upper part of your body to exert steady, even pressure downward upon the hands.

3. Immediately draw his arms upward and toward you, applying enough lift to feel resistance and tension at his shoulders. Then lower the arms to the ground. Repeat the whole cycle 12 times a minute, checking the mouth frequently for obstruction.

4. If a second rescuer is available, have him hold the victim's head so that the jaw continues to jut out. The helper should be alert to detect any stomach contents in the mouth and keep the mouth as clean as possible at all times.

Figure 20-4. (From *The Modern Medical Encyclopedia*, Western Publishing Company, Inc., New York.)

respiration requires considerable physical strength on the part of the operator. It generally is less effective than the mouth-to-mouth method.

Back Pressure–Arm Lift (Holger-Nielsen) Method. This method also demands considerable strength and stamina to continue administering artificial respiration long enough to be effective. The description presented in Figure 20-4 is approved by the American Red Cross.

HEART-LUNG RESUSCITATION

This emergency measure is indicated when there has been cardiac arrest;

that is, when the heart has stopped beating and respirations have ceased. At present there is some controversy over the advisability of nurses' administering cardiac massage because of the serious complications that can develop. Since the practical nurse cannot be sure that she will never be called upon to administer heart-lung resuscitation, the basic steps of the emergency measure and some general information about it are presented here.

Symptoms of Cardiac Arrest. The symptoms of cardiac arrest must be recognized quickly and resuscitation begun immediately before anoxia produces permanent or fatal damage to the brain and nervous system. Within 20 to 30 seconds after loss of consciousness due to cardiac arrest there is cessation of breathing and circulatory failure. A pulse beat cannot be felt and no heart beat can be heard. The pupils become dilated and the patient has a deathlike appearance.

External Cardiac Massage. This involves external pressure over the heart region in an effort to stimulate the heart and cause it to resume its normal contraction and relaxation. As soon as cardiac arrest has been recognized initial treatment must be started. This consists of administering a sharp blow or two to the area over the heart. Oxygenation of the patient by artificial respiration using the mouth-to-mouth

method must also be administered immediately. After about five breaths have been blown into the patient's lungs a firm support should be placed under his chest. This support can be a board, food tray, or any flat, firm object. If the patient is already lying on the floor or firm ground, no additional support will be needed. If he is in bed and no firm support is available, he can be moved to the floor.

External cardiac massage essentially involves (1) depression of the lower third of the sternum to a depth of one and one-half to two inches, (2) holding the sternum down for one-half second, and (3) rapid release of pressure without completely removing the hand from the sternum. This depression-release cycle is repeated at a rate of 60

Figure 20-5. Technique of closed cardiac massage. Heavy circle in heart drawing shows area of application of force. Circles on supine figure show points of application of electrodes for defibrillation. (From Brainerd, Morgan, and Chattou: *Current Diagnosis and Treatment*, Lange Medical Publications, Los Altos, California.)

EMERGENCY MEASURES
Heart-Lung Resuscitation

Airway - **Open by tilting head back**

Breathe - **Inflate lungs rapidly 3-5 times**

mouth-to-mouth
mouth-to-nose

mouth-to-airway adjunct or bag and mask

IF CAROTID PULSE IS PRESENT

continue 12 lung inflations per minute

IF PULSE IS ABSENT

Pupils dilated and deathlike appearance

Circulate

press here

Depress Sternum 1½" to 2" once per second

CONTINUE RESUSCITATION until spontaneous pulse returns

ONE OPERATOR – alternate 2 quick inflations with 15 compressions

TWO OPERATORS – interpose one inflation after every fifth compression

Figure 20-6. Steps A, B, and C of heart-lung resuscitation emergency treatment. (Prepared by the Committee on Cardiopulmonary Resuscitation, American Heart Assocation.)

to 70 times per minute. It is recommended that the pressure be exerted by the heel of the left hand with the right hand over the left.

Ideally, there should be two persons performing heart-lung resuscitation; one to apply artificial respiration and the second to apply external cardiac massage. If two persons are not available, the cardiac massage must be interrupted every 25 to 30 seconds and

several breaths blown into the patient's lungs.

Heart-lung resuscitation most often fails for one of the following reasons: (1) the patient has not been oxygenated properly, (2) there has been ineffectual massage due to failure to place a firm support under the patient or inadequate pressure, or (3) the patient has had cardiac arrest for too long a period of time.

Contraindications and Complications.
External cardiac massage is contraindicated when the chest is surgically
opened or when the patient has suffered
a severe blunt injury to the chest wall.
Complications include fracture of the
ribs or sternum from too much pressure, rupture of the liver, diaphragm
or stomach, tearing of a large blood
vessel and development of emboli in
the bone marrow.

CONTROL OF BLEEDING

The only emergency conditions that
have priority over control of hemorrhage are cessation of breathing and a
sucking wound of the chest. Severe
bleeding can rapidly lead to irreversible shock resulting from reduced circulating blood volume and circulatory
collapse.

Application of Pressure. Bleeding
usually can be controlled by placing a
sterile or clean cloth over the wound
and applying firm, steady pressure with
the palm of your hand. Or, the area may
be wrapped snugly with a clean bandage
over several layers of cloth placed over
the wound. Do not wrap the area so
tightly as to constrict circulation completely. This would, in effect, be the
same as applying a tourniquet, a measure that is used only as a last resort
(see below). The flow of blood to the
wound can be decreased somewhat by
elevating the injured part and immobilizing it in some way.

If the bleeding is copious and impossible to stop with a pressure bandage,
the artery leading to the wounded area
should be compressed. The six principal
pressure points for control of arterial
bleeding are pictured in Figure 20-7.
These pressure points are extremely

Figure 20-7.   Location of the more commonly used digital pressure points. Shaded areas are those
within which hemorrhage may be controlled by pressure on the specific artery. *A*, Carotid artery; *B*,
temporal artery; *C*, external maxillary artery; *D*, subclavian artery; *E*, brachial artery; *F*, femoral artery.
(From Crawford: *Nursing Clinics of North America*, June, 1967.)

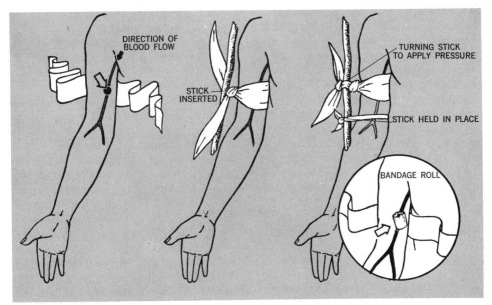

Figure 20-8. To apply a tourniquet for control of arterial bleeding of the arm: Wrap a gauze pad twice with a strip of cloth just below the armpit and tie with a half knot; tie a stick at the knot with a square knot. Slowly twist stick to tighten. Loosen tourniquet every ten minutes. (From *The Modern Medical Encyclopedia,* Western Publishing Company, Inc., New York.)

important because uncontrolled bleeding from an artery can be fatal in a very short time. Blood issuing from an artery will be bright red in color and will gush forth in spurts at regular intervals; blood from a severed vein leaks slowly and steadily and is dark red in color.

Use of Tourniquets. Application of a tourniquet to prevent hemorrhage is recommended *only as a last resort* when other methods have failed and hemorrhage threatens the life of the victim, or when an injured extremity has been amputated or severely crushed or mangled. The tourniquet has been used more often than it should have been, so if you are in doubt, do not apply one. The reason for this is obvious when we realize that a tourniquet can, by obstructing the flow of blood to a part, deprive its tissues of vital nutrients and permanently damage them, resulting in loss of the limb.

To apply a tourniquet, one needs several thicknesses of gauze or cloth to make a pad to be placed under the tourniquet, a wide strip of fabric long enough to go twice around the limb and a stick for tightening the tourniquet. Place the pad on the inside of the limb above the point of bleeding. Wrap the tourniquet around the limb over the pad, and then tie the loose end with a half knot (overhand knot). Insert the stick and tie again with a full knot. The tourniquet is then tightened by twisting the stick until bleeding stops (see Fig. 20-8). Once the tourniquet has been applied it should be released by a physician. Always leave the tourniquet uncovered so that it can be seen by others who may not be aware it has been applied. If this is not possible, write a note to the effect that a tourniquet has been applied, giving the location and the time of application of the tourniquet.

SHOCK

The term shock is extremely difficult, if not impossible, to define precisely. It has become something of a catch-all word that is used to cover a multitude of clinical situations and a variety of symptoms. These situations may vary from simple fainting to total circulatory collapse and death. In emergency nursing shock is usually *neurogenic* (caused by psychological factors such as pain, fright or trauma) or *hematogenic* (caused by decreased blood volume, as in severe bleeding, or loss of plasma, as in burns). Shock also may be caused by a "heart attack" which greatly reduces cardiac output and results in collapse of the peripheral vascular system.

Symptoms. The symptoms indicative of shock are the result of complex pathologic and psychological mechanisms. These involve inadequate blood volume, reduction of the cardiac output, loss of tone in and collapse of the blood vessels near the surface of the body, increased permeability of the capillaries with a shift of the body fluids from one compartment to another, and alterations in the chemical characteristics of the blood.

Not all of the signs and symptoms of shock need be present in every patient; they can occur in varying combinations and in different degrees of severity, depending on the cause of shock and the individual's response to it. The classic symptoms and signs of shock include cold, moist skin, especially of the extremities, pallor, especially of the lips and fingers, and rapid and weak pulse, decreased blood pressure, listlessness, thirst and oliguria.

Management of Shock. Whenever possible in an emergency situation, the nurse must do what she can to prevent shock or at least to lessen its severity. She can do this by acting quickly to control bleeding, relieving pain through proper splinting or positioning and treating the wound. There are several defense mechanisms of the body which are automatically called into action as soon as an injury occurs. By supporting these mechanisms through simple nursing measures, the nurse can reduce the

severity of shock and diminish its effects upon an accident victim.

Since most emergency cases are accompanied by some degree of psychogenic shock, it is extremely important to reassure and comfort the victim. This will help to keep him calm and reduce physical tension and activity so that his energies can be fully utilized by the natural defense mechanisms of the body. Maintaining normal body heat helps to ensure adequate circulation. To do this one must protect the patient from cold and dampness, but remember that applications of extreme heat to the surfaces of the body only serve to aggravate circulatory collapse and tend to increase loss of vital body fluids through perspiration. The "shock position" (with the head slightly lower than the feet) will improve circulation to the brain and heart. This position is contraindicated in head injuries.

As soon as the patient arrives at a hospital or clinic where equipment is available, other measures are taken to control shock. These may include administration of whole blood or plasma to restore the circulating blood volume, oxygen to relieve respiratory embarrassment, and narcotics for the control of pain.

BURNS

The two hazards to be guarded against in the emergency treatment of burns are infection and shock. All burns must be considered potentially dangerous because the skin is one of the body's first lines of defense against the invasion of pathogenic organisms. It also plays an important role in the maintenance of fluid balance and body temperature. The destruction of relatively large areas of skin can cause loss of vital body fluids and electrolytes, produce profound changes in the blood vessels and alter the chemical activities of the cells and tissues of the internal organs.

The severity of complications of a

burn will depend on the amount of body surface destroyed by the burn and the depth of the burn. The degrees of burn (first, second and third) and the means by which the extent of a burn are determined are discussed in Chapter 10 of this text.

Minor Burns. If the burned area is small and appears to be a first degree burn, the affected area should be immersed in cold water immediately. An alternative to this is applications of cold compresses, using ice cubes and a sterile gauze pad or clean cloth. By applying cold it is possible to reduce somewhat the pain of the burn. A minor burn should be covered with sterile petroleum jelly or a paste of baking soda and water and then loosely bandaged.

Major Burns. The burned area should be covered with a clean, dry dressing. This can be a sheet, towel or other freshly laundered piece of linen. It should be made of tightly woven cotton so that air is kept from the wound and the possibility of infection is reduced. The victim should be transported to a hospital as soon as possible.

No attempt should be made to remove clothing from a burned area. Never apply absorbent cotton, oily substances or ointments to a major burn. Blisters should not be disturbed because they serve as a protective covering over the wound.

If there is an unavoidable delay in getting the patient to a hospital and he is conscious and able to swallow, he should be given fluids to drink. The ideal is a solution of a half teaspoonful each of salt and baking soda in one quart of water. The patient is encouraged to drink small amounts of the solution at 10 to 15 minute intervals unless nausea develops and vomiting seems likely. Intravenous fluid therapy and more extensive medical treatment of major burns are discussed in Chapter 10 of this text.

Chemical Burns. Strong chemicals capable of burning the skin and mucous membranes will continue to destroy tissue unless they are diluted and removed immediately. For this reason one must act quickly to irrigate the area with large amounts of water until all traces of the chemical have been removed. Once this has been done the burned area is covered with a dressing and the patient is then transported to a hospital.

Chemical burns of the eye also require extensive irrigation followed by application of a clean dressing.

POISONING

The annual number of cases of poisoning in the United States is almost one half million. Of these, approximately two thousand are fatal, and a large majority are accidental. Prevention of accidental poisoning begins with a realization that there are literally hundreds of thousands of poisonous substances in our environment. Every home has a variety of poisons sitting on the shelves of the medicine cabinet, under the kitchen sink, or in the laundry room, utility room and garage. Children are the most frequent victims of poisoning, and medicines account for one half of all accidental poisonings of children under the age of five years. Aspirin has consistently been the cause of death in accidental poisoning in children of this age. Other poisons frequently ingested by children include bleaches, soaps and detergents, insecticides, and vitamin and iron preparations. Recently there has been an increase of poisoning in children who have ingested their mothers' birth control pills.

Prevention. As a member of the health team the practical nurse must do all she can to educate the public in the ways in which accidental poisoning can be prevented. She should remember the simple rules given below and use every opportunity to teach them to her friends and neighbors.

1. Destroy all medicines that are no longer being used. An overdose can be fatal, especially to a child. In some instances drugs undergo chemical changes with age and become toxic compounds.

2. Store poisons and inedible products separately from edible foods.

3. Do not transfer poisonous substances from their original container to an unmarked one. NEVER place a poison in a container (such as a soft drink bottle) that is normally used for edible solids or liquids.

4. Never tell a child that the medicine he is being given is candy. Tell him it is a drug to make him feel better and that it must be taken only as the doctor has directed.

5. Always read the labels of chemical products before using them.

Symptoms of Poisoning. The symptoms of poisoning vary according to the poison taken and the time that has elapsed since it first entered the body. Poisoning should be suspected if the victim becomes ill very suddenly and there is nearby an open container of a poison or a drug. In children one should be alert to the possibility of poisoning when there is a peculiar odor to the breath or when there is evidence that the child has eaten leaves or wild berries. Always remember that children are naturally very curious, and that a substance need not taste good for a child to place it in his mouth and swallow it.

Other symptoms of poisoning include pain or burning sensation in the mouth and throat, nausea, vomiting, disorientation, visual disturbances, loss of consciousness or a deep unnatural sleep.

General Principles of First Aid for Poisoning. All cases of poisoning demand immediate action. The longer the delay in treatment, the greater the chance of the poison being absorbed in the body and permanently damaging body tissues.

Always save the container and any of its contents that may help in identification of the poison. If the container cannot be found and the type of poison is not known, try to save a sample of vomitus for analysis and identification.

Swallowed Poisons. Generally, the first step is *dilution* of the poison, immediately followed by *removal* of the stomach contents. In the absence of a stomach pump, one must induce vomiting. A liquid such as water or milk will serve to dilute the poison. (Exceptions to this rule are listed below.) Vomiting is induced by placing a spoon or an index finger down the back of the throat to stimulate the gag reflex. An emetic such as 2 tablespoons of salt in a glass of warm water can be used. Be sure that during the vomiting episode the victim is positioned so that the vomitus will not be aspirated into the lungs and cause damage there.

Antidotes to specific poisons are often printed on the label. The specific antidote should be administered as soon as the stomach has been emptied of the poison. If the poison cannot be identified, a *universal antidote* can be given. This consists of one part strong tea, one part milk of magnesia, and two parts burnt crumbled toast. Using $\frac{1}{4}$ cup each of tea and milk of magnesia and $\frac{1}{2}$ cup of toast provides a sufficient amount.

When a patient has swallowed a *corrosive poison*, for example, a strong acid or alkali, vomiting is contraindicated because there is the danger of further irritating and damaging the upper intestinal tract. There is also the possibility of aspiration of the corrosive substance into the respiratory tract during vomiting. Antidotes for corrosive compounds are as follows: for *strong acids* use milk, water or milk of magnesia (1 to 2 cups for children, up to 1 quart for adults). For *strong alkalies* use milk, water, any fruit juice or vinegar (1 to 2 cups for children, up to 1 quart for patients five years or older).

Other cases in which *vomiting should not be induced* include when the victim is in a coma or unconscious, is having a convulsion, or has swallowed petroleum products, such as gasoline, kerosene, lighter fluid and some furniture polishes.

Inhaled Poisons. Transport the patient to fresh air immediately: do not let him walk. Loosen tight clothing. Apply artificial respiration as needed. Keep the patient warm and quiet. Do not give alcohol or any stimulant.

Barbiturate Poisoning. The barbiturate drugs are those most frequently used in suicide attempts. Approximately 50,000 cases of barbiturate poisoning are hospitalized every year in the United States. Symptoms include depression of respirations and reflexes, stupor or coma, dilated pupils and flushed face. The patient may be able to respond to questions, but his answers will be very slow. Without adequate treatment the patient succumbs to respiratory failure and cerebral edema. Pneumonia is a common sequela to barbiturate poisoning that has not proved fatal.

Emergency treatment must be instituted quickly if the patient's life is to be saved. The drug should be removed from the stomach by inducing vomiting or using a stomach pump. Artificial respiration is administered if breathing has ceased or is irregular and shallow. In the hospital, drugs that stimulate circulation are given and efforts are made to maintain a normal fluid and electrolyte balance. To counteract the depressing effect of barbiturates on the central nervous system, analeptic drugs (stimulants or restoratives) are given. Drugs of this type include picrotoxin, strychnine and bemegride. If the barbiturate is a long-acting type, an artificial kidney may be used to remove the drug from the blood stream.

There often is a delayed reaction to barbiturate poisoning, and the patient must be watched closely for several days after ingestion for signs of depression of the central nervous system.

Poisoning by Morphine, Bromides, and Other Sedatives. The patient who has taken or been given an overdose of a sedative drug will suffer from severe depression of the central nervous sytem, with resultant depression of respiration, involuntary reflexes and some voluntary actions. The symptoms are similar to those listed above for barbiturate poisoning. Emergency measures include administration of strong coffee or tea to provide a stimulant (caffeine) and attempts to keep the patient awake; he should not, however, be forced to walk, as this will only tire him and deplete his energies. If the patient is unconscious, it will be necessary to keep the air passages open, and artificial respiration should be administered if respiration has ceased.

Hospital treatment includes administration of oxygen, use of a respirator as needed, frequent suctioning, and administration of stimulants. A tracheostomy is sometimes required when depression is severe. The patient's vital signs must be noted at frequent intervals and any changes reported to the physician in charge. To facilitate drainage of bronchial secretions the patient is positioned so that the head is slightly lower than the feet. He must be turned frequently to prevent the development of pneumonia, which is always a hazard in cases of this type.

Poisoning by Carbon Monoxide and Other Lethal Gases. The inhalation of poisonous gases brings about an emergency situation in which death can occur in a matter of minutes. Carbon monoxide unites readily with hemoglobin, thereby replacing vital oxygen in the blood stream and rapidly producing a depletion of oxygen supply to body tissues. The first tissues to be affected are those of the nervous system, which cannot survive more than a few minutes once their supply of oxygen is gone. The patient first becomes drowsy, has a headache and experiences visual disturbances; he then sinks rapidly into a coma. The skin is a bright cherry red in color due to the presence of the carbon monoxide in the blood.

As soon as the victim of an inhaled

poison is found he must be carried to a source of fresh air, such as an open window or door, or outside and away from polluted air. The rescuer must be careful that he, too, is not overcome by inhaling the poisonous gas. Artificial respiration is begun immediately if the victim is not breathing. He should be kept warm and quiet and must not be allowed to walk about.

Hospital treatment includes administration of oxygen and supportive measures to prevent shock and maintain normal respiration. The patient must be observed carefully for signs of central nervous system damage and heart failure. Although he may appear to have recovered once oxygen has been administered, there can be residual effects of the poisoning that may be fatal.

Food Poisoning. This type of poisoning is produced by the toxins of bacteria present in contaminated food. The term "ptomaine poisoning," so frequently associated with food poisoning, is actually a misnomer. Ptomaines are substances formed by the decomposition or "spoilage" of protein foods. The digestive system is able to cope with these substances and they do not necessarily cause illness. Decomposing food is not of itself necessarily harmful, but since foods in the process of decomposition frequently harbor pathogenic organisms and serve as an excellent media for their growth, they should be avoided.

Prevention. Cleanliness, good personal hygiene, and proper preparation and handling of foods are essential to the prevention of food poisoning. Figure 20-9 presents the basic rules of prevention.

Symptoms and Treatment. Food poisoning should be suspected when more than one person in a group, family, or community is affected by an acute febrile gastrointestinal disturbance. The onset is sudden with nausea, vomiting, diarrhea and abdominal cramps. Emergency treatment generally consists of lavage or the induction of vomiting (if not already present) to remove the poisonous food from the stomach. Food is withheld, drugs are administered to control the diarrhea if it is present and sedation and parenteral fluids are administered. If diarrhea is not a symptom, a saline cathartic may be given to remove the bacteria from the lower intestinal tract.

Types. Food poisoning may be bacterial or chemical; however, the chemical types are not true food poisonings but a toxic condition caused by poisonous mushrooms, toxic berries, or foods that have not been cleansed of insecticides or other chemicals.

Botulism is the most dangerous type of food poisoning; about 65 percent of the cases are fatal. It is caused by *Clostridium botulinum*, which most often grows in foods that have not been properly canned at home. A neurotoxin produced by the organism affects muscular coordination and causes an inability to swallow, talk or breathe. Early recognition and emergency treatment are necessary to prevent death. The patient is given an antitoxin that neutralizes the neurotoxin. Supportive measures include use of a respirator to facilitate breathing and intravenous fluids to maintain normal fluid and electrolyte balance.

A strain of Staphylococcus known as *Staphylococcus aureus* frequently grows in creamed foods that have not been refrigerated adequately. Custards, cream pies, mayonnaise and processed foods of the type used for picnics are often the source of this type of food poisoning. The illness is rarely fatal and symptoms are usually limited to nausea, vomiting, diarrhea and abdominal cramps. The patient should be kept quiet and given sedation and parenteral fluids as necessary.

FRACTURES

A fracture is a break in the continuity of a bone. The types of fracture

CERTAIN BASIC RULES ARE IMPORTANT IN PREVENTING FOOD POISONING

PERSONAL HYGIENE

PERSONAL CLEANLINESS AND NEATNESS

NAILS CLEAN AND TRIMMED

HANDS WASHED BEFORE HANDLING FOOD

COVER COUGHS AND SNEEZES

HANDLING OF FOOD

SEPARATE TOWELS FOR WIPING DISHES AND DRYING HANDS

DO NOT PUT SPOON BACK IN MIXTURE AFTER TASTING

CUTS AND SCRATCHES COVERED WITH WATERPROOF BANDAGE

KEEP PETS AWAY FROM FOOD

HOME CANNING AND FREEZING

WASH FOOD PROPERLY BEFORE PRESERVING

BOIL REQUIRED LENGTH OF TIME TO REMOVE AIR FROM JARS

INSPECT BEFORE USING— THROW OUT ALL DEFECTIVE JARS

WRAP FOOD PROPERLY BEFORE FREEZING

STORAGE AND DISPOSAL OF FOOD

THROW OUT SPOILED FOOD IN REFRIGERATOR

KEEP MEAT, DAIRY PRODUCTS, MAYONNAISE, REFRIGERATED

FOOD KEPT OUT OF REFRIGERATOR SHOULD BE COVERED

SCRAPE AND RINSE DISHES AS SOON AS MEAL IS OVER. DISPOSE OF GARBAGE DAILY

Figure 20-9. Basic rules for prevention of food poisoning. (From *The Modern Medical Encyclopedia*, Western Publishing Company, Inc., New York.)

and their specific treatments are discussed in Chapter 11 of this text.

Symptoms of a fracture include pain and swelling in the area, deformity and limited motion. One should always treat a suspected fracture as a real one since proper first aid measures will be beneficial whether or not a true fracture is present.

Emergency treatment is aimed at immobilization of the affected part so that soft tissues in the areas adjacent to the bone will not be damaged further. The term "splint it as it lies" means exactly that. An inexperienced person should never attempt to straighten or set a broken bone. The injured part is immobilized in the position in which it is found at the time of injury and is supported firmly so that it will not be jarred when the victim is being moved to the hospital or doctor's office.

If the broken bone has pierced the skin and bleeding is severe, apply direct pressure over the wound (see Control of Bleeding, p. 454). Try to avoid introducing infectious agents into the wound and remember also the need for the prevention and treatment of shock.

HEAD INJURY

The victim of a blow to the head may suffer a skull fracture or concussion. In either case he should be kept quiet and no stimulants should be given. Since there can be a delayed reaction in injury to the brain, all head injuries should be considered serious and should have the attention of a physician. The symptoms, treatment and nursing care of head injuries are discussed in Chapter 18.

ELECTRIC SHOCK

When an electric current passes through the body, it can cause severe shock to the entire body, cessation of breathing, circulatory failure and serious burns.

Figure 20-10. To separate a victim from live electric wire without suffering similar shock, stand on rubber mat or dry board in rubber-soled shoes. Move wire with dry stick held with dry paper or dry gloves. Don't touch until sure wire contact is broken. (From *The Modern Medical Encyclopedia,* Western Publishing Company, Inc., New York.)

Emergency treatment involves artificial respiration if breathing has ceased, general measures to treat shock, and emergency treatment of a major burn when one is present. The proper procedure for separating a victim from a live conductor of electricity is described in Figure 20-10. Remember that water serves as a conductor of electricity and wet objects can transmit a fatal electric current to a person trying to rescue the victim of electric shock.

A person who is struck by lightning suffers from electric shock.

EMERGENCY CHILDBIRTH

It is often assumed that practical nurses should be able to assist a mother and infant in an emergency delivery outside the hospital environment. Such an assumption can be foolish if the nurse has not yet studied obstetrical nursing or has been allowed only to observe but never participate in the delivery of an infant in the hospital. The simple steps given here are presented only as emergency first aid measures to be undertaken when a physician or more experienced individual is not available.

1. Place the mother on her back in a comfortable position.

2. Keep the vaginal area as clean and free from contamination as possible.

3. Do not attempt to pull or push the infant through the birth canal.

4. Wipe the infant's nose and mouth with a clean cloth to remove mucus from his air passages.

5. Leave the infant between the mother's knees and cover him with a blanket or clean cloth.

6. The cord does not require attention unless a physician cannot be available within an hour. After that length of time the cord should be cut if the placenta (afterbirth) has been expelled. Tie the cord securely about two inches from the navel and again at about six inches. Cut the cord between the two places, using a knife or scissors that has been sterilized by boiling or soaking in a disinfectant.

7. Savé the placenta for the physician's inspection.

8. If there is no medical help available after the placenta is expelled, gently massage the fundus of the uterus to stimulate contraction and reduce bleeding. The fundus can be felt as a fairly large lump in the mother's abdomen just below her navel.

ANIMAL BITES

Family pets, especially dogs and cats, are the most common source of animal bites. When a wild animal such as a squirrel or fox attacks and bites a human being without provocation, one should always suspect rabies as the cause of the animal's unusual behavior. All animal and human bites should be treated as potentially dangerous because of the presence of pathogenic microorganisms in the mouth which can cause a serious infection.

Treatment. The wound should be washed immediately with soap and hot running water for 5 to 10 minutes. It is then covered with a clean bandage and a physician is consulted. If medical help is not readily available, it is best to make the wound bleed, probing it with a sharp, sterile instrument if necessary. Later the physician may decide to give tetanus toxin or toxoid to provide adequate immunity.

The possibility of rabies must always be considered in an animal bite. The animal must be confined and observed for signs of the disease. If he has been killed, his head should be sent to a laboratory for examination. If a diagnosis of rabies in the animal has been confirmed, or if there is no proof that the animal has been immunized against rabies, the victim is given passive immunization through a series of injections known as the Pasteur treatment. This treatment has serious complications and can be fatal, but since rabies itself is always fatal, the Pasteur treatment is recommended by most authorities.

SNAKE BITE

Although bites from poisonous snakes are rare in the United States, one should be able to differentiate between venomous and nonvenomous bites and should initiate treatment immediately when a snake bite does occur. The poisonous snakes in the United States are the pit vipers (copperheads, rattlesnakes and cottonmouths or water moccasins) and the coral snake, a brightly colored snake found in the southern regions of this country.

A venomous snake bite is distinguished by two fang marks, the immediate sensation of pain in the area and swelling and discoloration at the site of injection of venom. Nonpoisonous snake bites appear as small scratches or lacerations.

Treatment. Nonpoisonous snake bites are treated as simple wounds and require washing with soap and water and the application of a mild antiseptic. Venomous snake bites, which can be fatal, demand immediate and vigorous treatment. The formula TISA is used to designate the steps of treatment; i.e., *tourniquet, incision, suction* and *antivenin.* Since bodily activity increases circulation and subsequent distribution of the venom throughout the body, the victim must be kept quiet and given no stimulants.

TOURNIQUET.   The tourniquet (see page 455 for details) is applied between the fang marks and the trunk of the body. It should be moderately tight so as to impede venous flow but not to stop arterial flow of blood. It must be loosened every ten minutes for one full minute, and is left in place until a physician has administered antivenin or given further treatment.

INCISION.   A cut about ¼ inch deep and ¼ inch long is made directly over each fang mark.

SUCTION.   Removal of the venom from the site of injection can be done by applying a suction cup from a snake bite kit or with the mouth. The latter is quite safe if there are no open sores or cuts on the lips or mouth through which the venom can enter the blood stream.

ANTIVENIN.   This is an immunizing agent made of horse serum and as such is capable of causing a serious allergic reaction in hypersensitive individuals. For this reason the antivenin should be administered only by a physician under conditions in which the allergic reaction can be controlled.

INSECT BITES OR STINGS

Insect attacks, especially multiple stings from bees or wasps, can be quite serious or even fatal in small children or in persons who are highly allergic to the venom. If signs of anaphylactic shock—extreme swelling, respiratory difficulty or loss of consciousness—develop, the patient must receive medical treatment immediately. Serious al-

lergic reactions are discussed in Chapter 2.

Less serious stings of bees, wasps, yellow jackets, and hornets are treated by application of a paste of baking soda and water and cold compresses.

Bites from venomous spiders, scorpions and other poisonous insects are treated in the same manner as poisonous snake bites.

A tick, which can carry diseases such as Rocky Mountain spotted fever, is removed by placing a drop of turpentine or mineral oil on its body, and removing it with tweezers once its head has been withdrawn from the skin. If the tick is removed too quickly, his mouthpiece will be left in the skin and will serve as a source of irritation and infection. After the tick is removed, wash the area with soap and water and apply a mild disinfectant. If there is some question as to whether or not the tick may be carrying an infectious disease in a particular area of the country, a physician should be consulted.

INJURIES DUE TO EXTREME HEAT

Heatstroke. This rare condition, also called sunstroke is the result of a serious disturbance of the heat-regulating center in the brain. Normally the body will respond to higher environmental temperatures by increased perspiration and other internal mechanisms which keep the body temperature within normal limits. In heat stroke these mechanisms fail to function properly and the patient's temperature rises, the skin becomes dry and hot and there may be convulsions and collapse. Since the body temperature may go as high as 108 to 110° F. (42° C.) the patient is likely to die if his condition is not treated.

He should be placed in a shady, cool place and cooled immediately by sprinkling with water and fanning. As soon as possible, he should be immersed in cold water or have ice packs applied to lower his temperature. Care must be taken that his temperature is not lowered too quickly. The extremities are massaged so that adequate circulation is maintained.

The person with this disorder of the heat-regulating center may experience heatstroke any time he is exposed to extremely high temperature and he may need to adjust his life so that he can avoid repeated episodes of heatstroke.

Heat Exhaustion (Heat Prostration). This condition is caused by excessive sweating, which removes large quantities of salt and water from the body. The patient appears to be in shock with cool, damp skin, pallor, increased pulse and heart beat, dizziness or stupor. There also may be muscle cramps and poor coordination. Treatment is aimed at replacing the essential salts and fluids. He should be placed in a cool place and kept quiet. As much salt and water or tomato juice (one teaspoon of salt to a glass of liquid) as he can drink is administered. If he is unable to swallow the salt solution, replacement fluids are administered intravenously. Muscular cramps may be relieved by gently massaging the affected muscles.

Sunburn. Immediate treatment of a minor sunburn involves cool compresses using a solution of magnesium sulfate (Epsom salts) or sodium bicarbonate (baking soda) to relieve the discomfort. If chills, fever, swelling or gastrointestinal disturbances occur, the patient should receive medical attention.

INJURIES DUE TO EXTREME COLD

Prolonged exposure to cold can bring about a serious lowering of the body temperature *(hypothermia)* or a localized injury to tissues that is known as *frostbite.*

In hypothermia the victim has suffered from a generalized reaction to the cold. The emergency treatment is aimed at returning the body temperature to normal limits as soon as possible. It is now believed that gradual rewarming is not necessary and may be more harmful than rapid rewarming. The patient is placed in a warm bath and then wrapped in warm blankets. Do not apply hot water bottles or electric heating pads directly to the skin. The use of hypothermia in certain surgical procedures is discussed in Chapter 5.

Frostbite produces a constriction of blood vessels, damages the vessel walls and tissue cells and leads to the formation of blood clots (thrombosis). It occurs most often on the fingers, toes, cheeks and nose, where exposure is usually greatest and blood supply is most easily restricted by cold. Symptoms include numbness and pallor in the area, a prickling sensation and eventually edema as fluid escapes from damaged vessel walls.

The affected area should be warmed by immersion for about ten minutes in water heated to a temperature of between 90 and 100° F. Handle the part gently and *never* rub or massage the area. The practice of rubbing with ice or snow is dangerous and completely ineffectual. Rubbing the area can cause further damage to the tissues. Wrap the area in sterile or clean bandages, being sure to separate skin surfaces, as between the fingers. Give the patient hot coffee or tea to drink. Hospital treatment may include surgical debridement of dead tissue and skin grafting if the deeper tissues are destroyed by gangrene due to inadequate circulation.

THE HOSPITAL EMERGENCY ROOM

In recent years the hospital emergency room has become a combination doctor's office, outpatient clinic and facility for treatment of minor as well as major emergencies. Surveys show that there is an increasing number of patients going to emergency clinics with ailments that should be treated by a family doctor. There are various reasons for this trend but the most common factor seems to be the certainty of medical help in an emergency room regardless of the hour of day or night.

This additional burden of non-emergency cases somewhat changes the roles of the various members of the emergency room staff. Since the main purpose of nursing is to help meet the needs of those who require medical attention, the nurse is in no position to be critical of those who come to the emergency room seeking such help. She must be able to screen patients rapidly, use good judgment in discerning their individual needs and handle each case with tact and diplomacy. When a true emergency arises she must work quickly and effectively, remembering the basic principles and techniques she has learned in her classes. In some instances the nurse may be expected to go beyond the limits of the traditional functions of a nurse in order to save a life. Certainly then, the emergency room nurse must be a mature, thinking person, able to cope with a tremendous variety of situations.

The general procedures and policies in regard to keeping records, obtaining diagnostic x-rays and laboratory examinations and carrying out the final disposition of the patient will vary in each institution. The practical nurse must familiarize herself with these policies and procedures as soon as she is assigned to the emergency unit, and certainly *before* attempting to assist in the care of an emergency in which time is precious and a few minutes can mean the difference between life and death. In addition to this orientation to policies, the practical nurse must know the location of each item of emergency equipment and exactly what her duties will be in operating such equipment. She should become familiar with the drugs most commonly used in emergency situations and she must know where these drugs are stored, how they are administered, and by whom. She should learn her responsibilities in assisting

with various emergency procedures such as tracheostomy, thoracotomy, transfusions and suturing of wounds. And, above all else, she must maintain a calm, dignified attitude, deal with her distressed patients tactfully, and at the same time work quickly and efficiently.

Conduct of the staff in the emergency unit is one of the most important and perhaps least understood aspects of emergency care. The patient and his family may be experiencing one or more of a variety of emotions—anger, guilt, anxiety, fright or depression—and cannot be expected to be in complete control of their emotions. The personnel in an emergency unit are, in effect, "living in a fish bowl." Their every movement, facial expression and attitude become magnified and are under close scrutiny by individuals in a highly sensitive state of mind and mood. These distraught individuals need moral support and reassurance that everything possible is being done for the injured person in the quickest and most efficient way possible. Relatives and friends of injured persons sometimes spend what seems to them endless hours sitting in corridors and waiting rooms. So do the non-emergency cases who are waiting to see a doctor. They naturally become resentful and upset if they observe emergency clinic personnel indulging in social conversation, reading or drinking coffee together in apparent oblivion of the distress of those around them. These practices are, unfortunately, not uncommon, and each member of the staff should be aware of the need for professional conduct in the emergency room. The nurse must be careful of her choice of words and the tone of her voice when answering questions and she must always try to convey the impression that she is indeed interested in each patient as a person and sincerely concerned about his welfare.

DISASTER NURSING

Introduction. A disaster may be defined as any catastrophe in which

If help is available, what should be done for the apparent fracture?

If help is not available, what would you say to the victim with the fracture? How is moderate bleeding controlled?

2. While working in the Emergency Unit late one evening there is not much work to do and you hear one member of the staff complaining in a loud voice about "people who don't seem to know what the word emergency means." She is referring to several persons who have come in with non-emergency ills and are waiting to see a physician.

What impressions are being given by the complaining nurse's comments? What can you do to use your time productively while there is a lull in activity in the Emergency Room? Have you or has a member of your family ever been a patient in a serious emergency situation?

3. A friend of yours who is a Red Cross volunteer driver tells you about a course being offered by the Civil Defense Office and asks you to join her in taking the course.

Do you think you could gain anything by taking a course in civil defense planning? What do you know about disaster nursing plans in your community? What would you do if a hurricane hit your community one night while you were asleep?

REFERENCES

1. Beland, I. L.: *Clinical Nursing: Pathophysical and Psychosocial Approaches.* New York, The Macmillan Co., 1965.
2. Brunner, L. S., et al.: *Textbook of Medical-Surgical Nursing.* Philadelphia, J. B. Lippincott Co., 1964.
3. Cowan, L.: "Emergency." Am. Journ. Nurs., April, 1964, p. 123.
4. Elcherly, E. E.: "Living and Nursing in a Fallout Shelter." Am. Journ. Nurs., Nov., 1965, p. 123.
5. Kilpatrick, H. M.: "The Frightened Patient in the Emergency Room." Am. Journ. Nurs., May, 1966, p. 1031.
6. Magnussen, A.: "Who Does What in Defense, in Natural Disaster." Am. Journ. Nurs., March, 1965, p. 118.
7. Miller, R. R., and Johnson, S. R.: "Poison Control Now and in the Future." Am. Journ. Nurs., Sept., 1966, p. 1984.
8. *Modern Medical Encyclopedia.* New York, Golden Press, 1965.
9. Mushlin, H. R.: "Drugs and Food for the Disaster Shelter." Am. Journ. Nurs., Oct., 1964, p. 116.
10. Russel, F. E.: "Injuries by Venomous Animals." Am. Journ. Nurs., June, 1966, p. 1322.
11. Skellinger, W. C.: "Treatment of Poisoning in Children." Am. Journ. Nurs., Nov., 1965, p. 108.
12. Sullivan, C. M.: "Preparedness May Mean Survival." Am. Journ. Nurs., Nov., 1965, p. 121.
13. Weaver, O. J., and Robinson, R. C.: "Nursing Responsibilities in Community Disaster Nursing." *Nursing Clinics of North America,* vol. 2, no. 2, June, 1967.

SUGGESTED STUDENT READING

1. Journal of Practical Nursing: "The Emergency Room Nurse." March, 1966, p. 20.
2. U.S. Department of Health, Education, and Welfare, Public Health Service: "The Role of the Licensed Practical Nurse in National Disaster." 1967.

OUTLINE FOR CHAPTER 20

I. Prevention of Accidents

A. Home safety.
  1. More than one fourth of all accidental deaths occur in the home.
  2. Principal victims are children and the elderly.
  3. Education of the public will help prevent accidents.

B. Highway safety.
  1. Motor vehicle accidents are leading cause of death in this country.
  2. Two major causes of such accidents are human failure and mechanical failure.

C. Water safety.
  1. Observing the common-sense rules of water safety helps prevent accidents.
  2. Rescue methods vary. Attempt a swimming rescue only if you are experienced.
  3. Artificial respiration may be necessary.
  4. Have individual lie down and treat for shock.

II. General Principles of First Aid

A. Think before acting

B. Move slowly and deliberately and act with confidence.

C. Evaluate injuries and summon help.

D. Treat respiratory failure and hemorrhage first.

E. Prevent or treat shock.

F. Observe victim carefully and frequently for signs of change in his condition.

III. Artificial Respiration

A. Open an airway by clearing nose and mouth of obstructions and loosening tight clothing.

B. Mouth-to-mouth resuscitation is the best method. Elevate shoulders, tilt head back and pull lower jaw upward and forward. Repeat blow-watch-listen cycle 12 to 20 times per minute.

C. Two alternate methods are chest pressure-arm lift and back pressure arm-lift.

IV. Heart-Lung Resuscitation

A. Indicated in cardiac arrest.

B. Symptoms of cardiac arrest are loss of consciousness, absence of pulse and heart sounds and dilation of pupils.

C. External cardiac massage:
1. Depress lower third of sternum 1½ to 2 inches.
2. Release pressure.
3. Repeat cycle 60 to 70 times per minute.
4. Administer mouth-to-mouth resuscitation simultaneously. If only one operator is available, interrupt cardiac massage every 25 to 30 seconds and give artificial respiration for 3 to 5 breaths.

D. Failure of heart-lung resuscitation is usually due to inadequate oxygenation, ineffective massage or too long a period of cardiac arrest before initial treatment.

V. Control of Bleeding

A. Place clean or sterile dressing over wound and apply firm, steady pressure with hand or wrapping. Do not wrap wound so tightly as to constrict circulation to distal parts.

B. Elevate and immobilize the injured part.

C. If pressure to wound does not decrease blood loss from wound, apply pressure to pressure point above the artery serving the wounded area.

D. Use of tourniquet must be last resort, as when other methods fail and victim's life is in danger or when limb is amputated, severely mangled or crushed.
1. Tourniquet should be removed only by physician.
2. Do not cover tourniquet.

VI. Shock

A. Types are neurogenic and hematogenic.

B. Symptoms due to inadequate blood volume, loss of tone and then collapse of peripheral vessels and shift of body fluids. They are pallor, weak pulse, clammy skin and thirst.

C. Management of shock:
1. Reassure and comfort the patient.
2. Maintain body heat.
3. Place head lower than feet.
4. Restore circulating blood volume, relieve respiratory embarrassment and control pain.

VII. Burns

A. Two dangers are shock and infection.

B. Minor burns should be immersed in ice water or covered with cold compresses. Apply sterile petroleum jelly or a paste of baking soda and water and cover with loose bandage.

C. Major burns.
1. Cover with clean, dry dressing and transport victim to hospital or clinic.
2. Give him fluids to drink.
3. Never apply ointments or disturb blisters.

D. Chemical burns.
1. Flush with water.
2. Cover with a dressing and transport victim to hospital.

VIII. Poisoning

A. Education can help prevent accidental poisoning.

B. Symptoms — poisoning should be suspected if victim becomes suddenly ill and if there is a peculiar odor to the breath and an open container nearby. Save container or vomitus for identification.

C. Swallowed poisons.
1. Induce vomiting, except for corrosive poisons or petroleum products.
2. Give specific antidote if it is known or give universal antidote.

D. Inhaled poisons.

1. Transport victim to source of fresh air.
2. Give artificial respiration as necessary.
3. Keep victim warm and quiet; do not give alcohol or stimulants.

E. Barbiturate poisoning.
1. Most frequent in suicide attempts.
2. Induce vomiting.
3. Obtain medical help immediately or patient may die of respiratory failure.

F. Poisoning by Morphine and other sedatives which cause severe depression of the central nervous system.
1. Administer coffee or strong tea.
2. Give artificial respiration as needed.
3. Obtain medical help immediately.

G. Poisoning by carbon dioxide and other lethal gases.
1. Transport victim to source of fresh air.
2. Administer artificial respiration and oxygen.
3. Keep victim warm and avoid stimulation.

H. Food poisoning due to toxins produced by bacteria in contaminated foods.
1. Prevented by proper preparation, storage and handling of food.
2. Onset is acute with severe gastrointestinal disturbances.
3. Treatment—remove from intestinal tract and begin supportive measures.

IX. Head Injury

A. Keep patient quiet.
B. Have a doctor see victim.

X. Electric Shock

A. Give artificial respiration and treat burns as needed.
B. Use caution in separating victim from source of electric current.

XI. Emergency Childbirth

A. Avoid contamination as much as possible.
B. Do not pull infant through birth canal.
C. Cut cord if medical help is not available within an hour.
D. Save placenta for physician's inspection.
E. Massage the fundus after expulsion of the placenta.

XII. Animal Bites

A. Treat wound immediately.
B. Pasteur treatment may be necessary if examination of the animal reveals the possibility of rabies.

XIII. Snake Bite

A. Nonpoisonous snake bite is treated as minor wound.
B. Poisonous snake bite is treated by tourniquet, incision, suction and antivenin.

XIV. Insect Bites or Stings

A. Serious stings require immediate attention.
B. Apply paste of baking soda and water and cold compresses to less serious stings.
C. Apply a drop of turpentine or mineral oil to ticks and remove. Wash the area with soap and water and apply an antiseptic.

XV. Injuries Due to Extreme Heat

A. Heatstroke (sunstroke)—a disturbance in the heat-regulating mechanism in the brain allows patient's body temperature to become extremely high. Cool with cool water.
B. Heat exhaustion (heat prostration) is caused by excessive loss of salt and water through perspiration. Treated by replacement of these substances.
C. Sunburn—treat minor burn with solution of baking soda or Epsom salts and water. Major burns require medical attention as soon as possible.

XVI. Injuries Due to Extreme Cold

A. Hypothermia is a drastic lowering of body temperature. Patient is rewarmed by warm bath and blankets.
B. Frostbite is a local condition associated with constriction of blood vessels and damage to tissue and vessel walls.
1. Rewarm quickly by immersion in warm water.
2. Do not rub; handle very gently.

XVII. The Hospital Emergency Room

A. Increasing number of non-emergency cases being treated in the hospital emergency units.
B. Become familiar with procedures, policies and equipment of the institution.

XVIII. *Disaster Nursing*

A. A disaster involves loss of property, physical injuries, and interruption in activities of daily living on a large scale.

B. Agencies involved in planning disaster nursing are Office of Civil Defense, Red Cross, and other local voluntary organizations.

C. Nurse's responsibilities:
1. Know community disaster plans.
2. Provide leadership and nursing care.

D. Functions of the nurse:
1. Provide for emotional and physical comfort and safety of victims.
2. Work to increase effectiveness of local disaster planning agency.

GLOSSARY

Abduction — The withdrawal of a part away from the center of the body.

Absorption — The taking up of fluids or other substances.

Adduction — The act of drawing a part toward the center of the body.

Aerosols — Solutions of a drug or a bactericide that can be atomized into a fine mist.

Albumin — One of a group of simple proteins that yield only amino acids or their derivatives on hydrolysis.

Alkali — One of a group of compounds that form salts when united with acids and soaps when combined with fats. A base, or substance capable of neutralizing acids.

Alopecia — Loss of hair from a part of the body that normally is hairy.

Altruistic — Unselfishly thoughtful or working for the welfare of others.

Amino acids — A group of organic compounds that form the chief structure of proteins.

Anaerobic — Able to grow only in the presence of oxygen.

Analgesic — Relieving pain.

Aneurysm — A bulging outward of a portion of a blood vessel that has been damaged by disease or weakened by a congenital defect in the vessel wall.

Ankylosis — Abnormal fixation and immobility of a joint.

Antigen — A substance that stimulates the formation of a specific antibody and which reacts specifically with its antibody.

Anxiety — A feeling of extreme uncertainty and fear.

Aphasia — A defect in or the loss of the power of speech.

Apprehension — A mental state of fear in which danger or harm to oneself is anticipated.

Arteriography — X-ray filming of an artery following injection of a contrast medium.

Aspiration — The act of breathing or drawing in.

Asepsis — Absence of infectious material; freedom from infection.

Atelectasis — Incomplete expansion or collapse of the alveoli of a segment or entire lobe of the lung.

Atom — The smallest part of an element that can exist and still retain the chemical properties of the element.

Atrophy — A wasting away or reduction in size of a cell, organ or part of the body.

Audiology — The science concerned with the sense of hearing.

Autoclave — An apparatus used to apply steam under pressure for the purpose of sterilization.

473

Autoimmunity – The immune reaction of an organism to its own tissues.

Avitaminosis – A condition due to a lack of one or more vitamins in the diet.

Balanitis – Inflammation of the glans penis, usually associated with phymosis.

Benign – Not malignant; not having a tendency to recur; having a favorable outcome.

Bilirubin – A red bile pigment formed from the hemoglobin of red blood cells.

Biology – The science of physical life of living matter in all its forms and phenomena.

Blepharitis – Inflammation of the edges of the eyelids.

Bradycardia – Abnormal slowness of the heart beat and pulse.

Bronchioles – The smaller subdivisions of the bronchial tubes.

Bursa – A sac or sac-like structure filled with fluid that acts as a cushion and prevents friction between two moving parts.

Calorie – A unit of heat. In the study of metabolism a calorie is the amount of heat required to raise the temperature of 1 kg. of water 1° centigrade.

Cannula – A tube for insertion into the body. It usually encases a trocar that is used during insertion and then removed.

Capillary – Any one of the minute, hair-like vessels that connect the smaller arteries with the smaller veins.

Carrier – An individual who harbors in his body the specific organisms of a disease but does not have the symptoms and thus can spread the infection.

Catalyst – A substance that alters the speed of a reaction but does not form part of the final product.

Caustic – Burning or corrosive; capable of destroying living tissue.

Cauterize – Applying a caustic substance, hot iron or electric current as a means of killing tissue.

Cerebrospinal – Pertaining to the brain and spinal cord.

Cervix – Neck or neck-like part.

Coma – A state of unconsciousness in which the individual is unresponsive to even the most powerful stimuli.

Concussion – A severe jar or shock, or the condition that results from such an injury.

Conduction – The transmission or transfer of sound waves, nerve impulses or electrical charges.

Contour – The outline or configuration of the body or one of its parts.

Contracture – A condition in which there is fixed resistance to the stretching of a muscle. It results from fibrosis of the tissues surrounding a joint or from disorders of the muscle fibers.

Curettage – Scraping the walls of a cavity such as the uterus.

Cyst – A sac or sac-like structure, usually abnormal and containing liquid or semi-solid matter and often caused by blockage of a passage.

Cytology – Study of cells.

Cytotoxic – An agent poisonous to cells.

Debilitated – Weak; lacking strength.

Debridement – The removal of all dead tissue and foreign matter in or near a wound.

Defibrillator – An apparatus used to counteract convulsive twitching of the heart muscle by application of electric impulses to the heart.

Dehydration — Removal of water from the body or a tissue; or, the condition resulting from excessive loss of water.

Delusion — A false belief that cannot be changed by reason, argument or persuasion.

Dermatology — The branch of medicine concerned with diagnosis and treatment of skin disorders.

Deviation — A turning away from the center or from the normal course.

Diaphragm — 1. The dome-shaped muscle separating the thoracic and abdominal cavities and aiding in the function of respiration. 2. Thin partition.

Diastole — The period of dilation of the heart when the ventricles fill with blood.

Diathermy — The generation of heat produced by the resistance of body tissues to the passage of high frequency electric impulses.

Diffusion — The process of passing through or spreading widely through a tissue or structure.

Dilatation — The condition of being stretched beyond normal dimensions.

Disability — A condition in which one is deprived of power or crippled.

Disinfectant — An agent that destroys pathogenic organisms.

Distention — The state of being enlarged.

Duct — A tube, pipe or channel for conveying liquid, air or other matter.

Dysphagia — Difficulty in swallowing.

Dyspnea — Difficult or labored breathing.

Dysuria — Painful or difficult urination.

Ectopic — Located away from the normal position.

Electrolyte — A compound which, when in solution, will conduct an electrical current by means of its ions.

Element — Any one of the basic parts or constituents of a thing. In chemistry, a simple substance that cannot be broken down by ordinary chemical means.

Embolism — The obstruction of a blood vessel by a clot, plug of fat, or other substances brought there by the blood.

Empathy — Entering through imagination into the feelings or motives of another.

Enzyme — A complex protein produced in living cells and able to act as a catalyst in chemical change, particularly in the changing of a substrate for which the enzyme is specific.

Epiphysis — The end of a long bone, usually wider than the shaft and resembling a knob. It is either made up of cartilage or separated from the shaft by a disc of cartilage.

Equilibrium — A state of balance.

Erythema — Redness of the skin produced by congestion of the capillaries.

Eschar — A hard crust or scab produced by a burn or corrosive agent.

Euphoria — An exaggerated feeling of well-being or bodily comfort.

Exacerbation — Increase in severity of a symptom or disease.

Excreted — Thrown off as waste matter in a normal discharge.

Exfoliate — To fall off in scales or layers.

Expiration — The act of exhaling air from the lungs.

Extension — A stretching out or prolonging in time, space or direction.

Exudate — Material that has escaped from blood vessels and been deposited in or on tissues, usually as a result of inflammation.

Facade — A front or outward part of anything.

Facies — The appearance of or expression on a face.

Febrile — Pertaining to fever.

Fibrin — A whitish, insoluble protein that forms the essential protein of a blood clot.

Filtration — The passage of a liquid through a straining device.

Fissure — A cleft or groove.

Fistula — An abnormal passage.

Flaccid — Weak or limp.

Flatus — Gas in the intestinal tract.

Flexion — The bending of a limb or other part.

Fulguration — Destruction of tissues by the application of electric sparks that are controlled by a movable electrode.

Fundus — The base or part of a hollow organ that is farthest removed from its mouth.

Geriatrics — The branch of medicine concerned with problems peculiar to old age and aging.

Gerontology — The scientific study of all the problems of aging.

Gingivitis — Inflammation of the gums.

Globulin — Any one of a class of proteins. Gamma globulins are plasma proteins that react with specific harmful agents such as bacteria, viruses or toxins that invade the body.

Glycosuria — The presence of abnormal amounts of glucose in the urine.

Gynecology — That branch of medicine concerned with the diagnosis and treatment of disorders of the female genital tract.

Hematinic — An agent that increases the hemoglobin level and the number of red blood cells.

Hematoma — A tumor containing blood that has escaped from an injured vessel.

Hematuria — Blood in the urine.

Hemiplegia — Paralysis of one side of the body.

Hemolysis — Destruction of red blood cells with the liberation of hemoglobin.

Hemoptysis — The spitting of blood or blood-stained sputum.

Hepatic — Pertaining to the liver.

Hormone — A chemical substance, formed in certain parts of the body, that has a specific effect on the activity of a certain "target" organ.

Hydrocele — A collection of fluid, especially in the scrotal sac.

Hydrolysis — The splitting of a compound into fragments by the addition of water.

Hypercalcemia — Excessive amount of calcium in the blood.

Hyperpnea — Abnormal increase in the rate and depth of respiration.

Hypersensitive — Having an abnormally increased sensitivity, especially in regard to a reaction to certain substances which are innocuous to a normal person.

Hypothalamus — That portion of the brain that forms the floor and part of the lateral wall of the third ventricle. It exerts control over visceral activities, water balance, body temperature and sleep.

Idiopathic — Without a known cause, self-originating.

Idiosyncrasy – 1. A feeling, liking or aversion peculiar to a single person or group. 2. An abnormal sensitivity to some drug, protein or other agent that is peculiar to an individual.

Immunity – Security against a particular disease or poison.

Impaction – The condition of being firmly lodged or wedged.

Incoherent – Confused, disconnected.

Inspiration – The act of drawing air into the lungs.

Intercostal – Situated between the ribs.

Interdependent – Mutually dependent.

Interstitial – Pertaining to or situated in the interstices or interspaces of a tissue.

Intracranial – Within the skull.

Intraocular – Within the eye.

Intussusception – A telescoping of one part of the intestine into the lumen of an immediately adjacent segment.

Isotopic – Any of two or more forms of a chemical element having the same chemical properties and the same atomic number, but different weights or radioactive behavior.

Lacrimal – Pertaining to the tears.

Leiomyoma – A benign tumor arising from smooth muscle.

Lipoid – Resembling fat.

Lumen – The space within a tubular organ such as a blood vessel.

Lymphatic – Pertaining to or containing lymph.

Malignant – Tending to become progressively worse and to have a fatal outcome.

Mediastinum – 1. Septum or partition. 2. A partition formed by the two pleurae between the lungs, including the enclosed space in which are all the viscera of the thorax except the lungs.

Menarche – The beginning of menstruation.

Menopause – Cessation of menstruation.

Meninges – The three membranes that cover the brain and spinal cord: the dura mater, pia mater and arachnoid.

Necrotic – Pertaining to the death of tissue.

Neoplasm – Any new or abnormal growth, such as tumor.

Nevus – A mole or birthmark.

Nodular – Pertaining to a swelling or protuberance.

Occiput – The back of the head.

Occlusion – The state of being closed or shut off.

Occult – Concealed from observation.

Ocular – Pertaining to the eye.

Oxidation – The act of combining or causing to combine with oxygen.

Palliative – Providing relief, but not a cure.

Palsy — Paralysis.

Paracentesis — Surgical puncture of a cavity for the aspiration of fluid.

Pathogenic — Producing disease.

Pectoral — Pertaining to the chest or breast.

Pedicle — A base or stem-like part.

Penetration — The act or power of going into or through.

Perineum — The area between the anus and the genital organs.

Phagocyte — Any cell that ingests microorganisms or other cells and foreign particles.

Phimosis — Restriction of the foreskin so that it cannot be drawn back from over the glans penis.

Placebo — A pill or injection given to a person as medicine but actually containing no active ingredients.

Platelet — A circular disc that is one of the blood elements and concerned with coagulation of blood.

Poultice — A soft, hot, moist mass of mustard, herbs or other medicines applied to the body for therapy.

Prophylaxis — Prevention of disease; preventive treatments.

Radiopaque — Not transparent to x-rays or other radioactive substances.

Reaction — The response of a part to stimulation.

Reflex — An involuntary action in direct response to stimulation of a nerve.

Remission — An abatement or lessening of the symptoms of a disease; also, the period during which such an abatement occurs.

Residue — That which remains after the removal of other substances.

Resistance — The act of withstanding or opposing.

Resorption — The act of absorbing again.

Sclerosis — A hardening, especially hardening of a part from inflammation.

Secrete — To separate or elaborate cell products.

Sinus — 1. A cavity or hollow space. 2. An abnormal channel or opening allowing for the escape of pus.

Spermatozoon — The male germ cell produced by the testes.

Spore — A single cell which becomes free and is capable of reproduction. It can flourish without oxygen and can develop resistance to pasteurization.

Stasis — A stoppage of the flow of blood or other body fluids in any part.

Stoma — Any minute pore, orifice or opening on a free surface.

Supine — Lying with the face upward.

Susceptible — Readily affected or acted upon.

Synthesis — The artificial building up of a chemical compound by uniting its elements.

Systemic — Pertaining to or affecting the body as a whole.

Systole — The period of contraction of the heart, especially contraction of the ventricles.

Tachycardia — Excessively rapid action of the heart.

Therapeutic — Pertaining to the art of healing; curative.

Thoracentesis — Surgical puncture of the chest wall with drainage of fluid.

Thromboplastin — A factor essential to the production of thrombin and proper coagulation of blood.

Tinnitus — A noise or ringing in the ears.
Toxic — Poisonous.
Transmitted — Transferred; carried across.
Trauma — A wound or injury.
Tremor — An involuntary trembling or quivering.
Trocar — A sharp-pointed instrument used with a cannula for piercing a part of the body.

Vascular — Pertaining to or full of vessels.
Virulent — Exceedingly pathogenic, noxious or harmful.
Vital — Necessary to or pertaining to life.
Volvulus — A knotting or twisting of the bowel producing intestinal obstruction.

INDEX

Italic numbers indicate pages on which illustrations appear. The letter "t" immediately following a page number indicates tabular information.